Ocular Differential Diagnosis

Seventh Edition

Ocular Differential Diagnosis

Seventh Edition

Frederick Hampton Roy, M.D., F.A.C.S.

Department of Ophthalmology
University of Arkansas Medical Center
Little Rock, Arkansas
Baptist Medical Center
St. Vincent Infirmary
Arkansas Children's Hospital
Little Rock Surgery Center
Little Rock, Arkansas

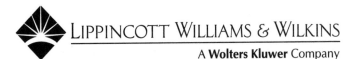

LIPPINCOTT WILLIAMS & WILKINS
A **Wolters Kluwer** Company
Philadelphia · Baltimore · New York · London
Buenos Aires · Hong Kong · Sydney · Tokyo

Acquisitions Editor: Jonathan Pine
Developmental Editor: Selina M. Bush
Production Editor: Thomas Boyce
Manufacturing Manager: Timothy Reynolds
Cover Designer: Christine Jenny
Compositor: Maryland Composition
Printer: Victor Graphics

© **2002 by LIPPINCOTT WILLIAMS & WILKINS**
530 Walnut Street
Philadelphia, PA 19106 USA
LWW.com

Previous editions: 1972, 1977, 1982, 1987, 1992, 1997
Printed in the USA

Library of Congress Cataloging-in-Publication Data

ISBN 0-7817-3607-2

Care has been taken to confirm the accuracy of the information presented and to describe generally accepted practices. However, the author and publisher are not responsible for errors or omissions or for any consequences from application of the information in this book and make no warranty, expressed or implied, with respect to the currency, completeness, or accuracy of the contents of the publication. Application of this information in a particular situation remains the professional responsibility of the practitioner.

The author and publisher have exerted every effort to ensure that drug selection and dosage set forth in this text are in accordance with current recommendations and practice at the time of publication. However, in view of ongoing research, changes in government regulations, and the constant flow of information relating to drug therapy and drug reactions, the reader is urged to check the package insert for each drug for any change in indications and dosage and for added warnings and precautions. This is particularly important when the recommended agent is a new or infrequently employed drug.

Some drugs and medical devices presented in this publication have Food and Drug Administration (FDA) clearance for limited use in restricted research settings. It is the responsibility of the health care provider to ascertain the FDA status of each drug or device planned for use in their clinical practice.

10 9 8 7 6 5 4 3 2 1

To Mary Michelle
To my children:
Nichols, Robert, Kimberly, Frederick, Jr., Charles, and Helena
To Dr. Arlington Krause,
molder and questioner in my early formative academic life
To Dr. Philip Lewis and Dr. Roger Hiatt
for guidance and direction

Contents

Preface

The first edition of *Ocular Differential Diagnosis* was published in 1972, and various editions have been translated in Spanish, Turkish, Chinese, Portuguese, and Italian. All previous editions have been my work. Dr. Gonzolo Murillo of La Paz, Bolivia, helped in edition four and five with the diagnostic decision tables. In edition six, section editors helped to standardize the language and made helpful suggestions. I feel this is the best edition of *Ocular Differential Diagnosis* thus far. This text would not have been possible without the superb efforts of Renee Tindall, Dr. Fernando Murillo, Angie Brown, and Dr. Kae Chatman.

The *Ocular Differential Diagnosis* book provides comprehensive lists of causes for symptoms or findings. Frequently more information is needed and hopefully *Ocular Syndromes and Systemic Diseases* will furnish additional information to make a better diagnosis. I hope the ophthalmologist and optometrist using this book will bring any errors in this edition to my attention.

Frederick Hampton Roy, M.D.
Little Rock, Arkansas

How to Use This Book

This book can be used easily and quickly by following the directions presented below.

1. If the sign or symptom relates to a particular region of the eye, turn to the table of contents preceding this page to find the number of the page on which listings of the signs and symptoms pertaining to the specific region begins. This latter page (or those immediately following) will refer the user to that (or those) on which the various causes of the condition are listed. For example, let us assume that the patient has pigmentation of the cornea. The table of contents on page vii shows that the cornea section begins on page 241. Turning to page 241 the user finds references to page 248 on which the causes of corneal pigmentation are listed according to type. In the subject index, this topic is listed as Cornea, pigmentation of, 248.

2. If the symptom, such as binocular diplopia or night blindness, does not relate to a particular region of the eye, look for it either in the subject index at the back of the book or under General Signs and Symptoms beginning on page 619.

   Various features of a disease may be crosschecked. For instance, a "pulsating exophthalmos with orbital bruit and conjunctival edema" may be sought under orbit, page 3, where the user of the book is referred to exophthalmos, page 4, and orbital bruit, page 31, and under conjunctiva, page 183, where the user is referred to conjunctival edema, page 202. The terms "exophthalmos," "orbital bruit" (under orbit, bruit of) and "conjunctival edema" (under conjunctiva, edema of) may also be found in the subject index. Terms such as "secondary glaucoma" are indexed under the noun, e.g., glaucoma, secondary.

3. Following some of the differential diagnosis lists are diagnostic decision tables. These tables list the history, physical signs, and laboratory tests that differentiate each possible diagnosis. These can be identified in the subject index because they are followed by a *t*.

Ocular Differential Diagnosis

Seventh Edition

PART I

Regional Signs and Symptoms

1

Orbit

CONTENTS

PSEUDOPROPTOSIS (APPEARANCE OF EXOPHTHALMOS)

*1. Asymmetry of bony orbits
 2. Congenital cystic eyeball
*3. Contralateral enophthalmos (see p. 15)
 4. Facial asymmetry as progressive facial hemiatrophy (Parry–Romberg syndrome)
 5. Harlequin orbit (shallow orbit with arched superior and lateral wall) as with hypophosphatasia
 6. Hypoplastic supraorbital ridges as in trisomy (Edward syndrome)
 7. Retraction of upper lid as with thyroid disease
 8. Slight blepharoptosis as with Horner syndrome of contralateral eye
 9. Shallow orbit as in Crouzon disease (craniofacial dysostosis)
10. Unilateral congenital glaucoma
11. Unilateral high-axial myopia
12. Unilateral secondary glaucoma resulting from ocular trauma during childhood

Newell FW. *Ophthalmology: principles and concepts*, 7th ed. St. Louis: CV Mosby, 1992.
Rootman J. *Diseases of the orbit*. Philadelphia: JB Lippincott, 1988.

EXOPHTHALMOS

1. Drugs, including the following:

adrenal cortex injection	hydrocortisone	paramethasone
aldosterone	iodide and iodine solution	poliovirus vaccine
beclomethasone	and compounds	prednisolone
betamethasone	levothyroxine	prednisone
carbimazole	liothyronine	propranolol
cocaine	liotrix	propylthiouracil
cortisone	lithium carbonate	radioactive iodides
desoxycorticosterone	medrysone succinylcholine	thyroglobulin
dexamethasone	meprednisone	thyroid
dextrothyroxine	methimazole	triamcinolone
fludrocortisone	methylprednisolone	vitamin A
flu-prednisolone	methylthiouracil	
fluorometholone	oral contraceptives	

2. Inflammation
    A. Acute—orbital cellulitis
    B. Acute suppurative—mucormycosis (diabetic or debility)
    C. Allergic fungal sinusitis
    D. Benign lymphoepithelial lesion (Mikulicz disease)
   *E. Chronic (nongranulomatous—pseudotumor)
    F. Chronic (granulomatous—tuberculosis, sarcoid (Schaumann syndrome), syphilis (lues), parasites, aspergillosis)
    G. Relapsing polychondritis
3. Injuries
    A. Foreign body
    B. Orbital hemorrhage
    C. Orbital roof fracture
    D. Secondary carotid cavernous sinus fistula
    E. Thermal burns

4. Systemic disease
    A. Acute intracranial hypertension
    B. Amyloidosis (Lubarsch–Pick syndrome)
    C. Chloroma
    D. Cretinism (hypothyroidism)
    E. Hydrocephalus and ventriculoperitoneal syndrome
    F. Hypervitaminosis A
    G. Hypophosphatasia (phosphoethanolaminuria)
  *H. Thyroid disorder
    I. Myasthenia gravis (Erb–Goldflam syndrome)
    J. Obesity
5. Tumors
    A. Cartilaginous tumors
        (1) Cartilaginous hamartoma
        (2) Chondroma
        (3) Chondrosarcoma
        (4) Mesenchymal chondrosarcoma
    B. Cystic lesions
        (1) Colobomatous cyst
        (2) Dermoid cyst
        (3) Hematocele
        (4) Hydatid cyst
        (5) Meningocele and meningoencephalocele
        (6) Mucocele
        (7) Optic nerve sheath cyst
        (8) Simple epithelial cyst
        (9) Teratoma
    C. Fibrocytic tumors
        (1) Fibroma
        (2) Fibrosarcoma
        (3) Fibrous histiocytoma
        (4) Juvenile fibromatosis
        (5) Nodular fasciitis
    D. Histiocytic lesions
        (1) Others
            a. Juvenile xanthogranuloma (JXG, nevoxanthoendothelioma)
            b. Sinus histiocytosis with massive lymphadenopathy
        (2) Systemic histiocytoses (histiocytosis X) (Hand–Schüller–Christian disease)
    E. Inflammatory pseudotumor of orbit
        (1) Ectopic cerebellar tissue in orbit
        (2) Local, such as fungus or foreign body
        (3) Systemic such as sarcoidosis syndrome (Schaumann syndrome) or collagen disease
        (4) Unknown cause
    F. Lacrimal gland (fossa) lesions
        (1) Epithelial tumors
            a. Adenoid cystic carcinoma
            b. Mucoepidermoid carcinoma

* = most important

      c. Pleomorphic adenocarcinoma (malignant mixed tumor)
      d. Pleomorphic adenoma (benign mixed tumor)
    (2) Nonepithelial lesions
      a. Infectious
      b. Inflammatory
      c. Lymphoid and leukemia
      d. Systemic (sarcoid)

G. Lipocytic and myxoid tumors
    (1) Lipoma
    (2) Liposarcoma
    (3) Myxoid liposarcoma
    (4) Myxoma

H. Lymphoid tumors and leukemias (excluding lacrimal gland lesions)
    (1) Benign reactive lymphoid hyperplasia
    (2) Burkitt lymphoma
    (3) Lymphoblastic leukemia
    (4) Myelogenous leukemia (granulocytic sarcoma)
    (5) Non-Hodgkin lymphoma

I. Metastatic tumors of the orbit
    (1) Malignant melanoma of skin
    (2) Neuroblastoma (child)
    (3) Other sites such as Ewing sarcoma
    (4) Primary in breast (adult female)
    (5) Primary in lung (adult male)
    (6) Primary in prostate (adult male)

J. Nonepithelial lesions
    (1) Benign reactive lymphoid hyperplasia
    (2) Inflammatory pseudotumors (dacryoadenitis)
    (3) Lymphoma
    (4) Plasmacytoma

K. Optic nerve and meningeal tumors
    (1) Juvenile pilocytic astrocytoma (optic nerve glioma)
    (2) Meningioma
      a. Primary optic nerve sheath
      b. Secondary
    (3) Malignant optic nerve glioma

L. Osseous and fibroosseous tumors
    (1) Aneurysmal bone cyst
    (2) Benign osteoblastoma
    (3) Brown tumor of hyperparathyroidism
    (4) Fibrous dysplasia (Albright syndrome)
    (5) Giant cell granuloma
    (6) Giant cell tumor (osteoclastoma)
    (7) Infantile cortical hyperostosis
    (8) Ossifying fibroma
    (9) Osteoma
    (10) Osteosarcoma

M. Peripheral nerve tumors
    (1) Alveolar soft-part sarcoma

(2) Amputation neuroma
(3) Granular cell myoblastoma
(4) Neurilemoma
   a. Benign
   b. Malignant
(5) Neurofibroma
   a. Plexiform
   b. Solitary
(6) Paraganglioma (chemodectoma)
N. Primary melanocytic tumors
   (1) Blue nevus
   (2) Melanocytic hamartoma
   (3) Melanotic progonoma (retinal tumor)
   (4) Primary orbital melanoma
O. Rhabdomyoma and rhabdomyosarcoma
   (1) Rhabdomyoma
   (2) Rhabdomyosarcoma
P. Secondary orbital tumors from adjacent structures
   (1) Conjunctival origin
      a. Melanoma
      b. Mucoepidermoid carcinoma
      c. Squamous cell carcinoma
   (2) Eyelid origin
      a. Basal cell carcinoma
      b. Melanoma
      c. Sebaceous carcinoma
      d. Squamous cell carcinoma
   (3) Intracranial origin
      a. Astrocytoma
      b. Meningioma
   (4) Intraocular origin
      a. Medulloepithelioma
      b. Neurilemoma
      c. Retinoblastoma
      d. Uveal melanoma
   (5) Nasopharyngeal origin
      a. Angiofibroma
      b. Carcinoma
      c. Melanoma
   (6) Paranasal sinus origin
      a. Ethmoid sinus carcinoma
      b. Inverting papilloma
      c. Maxillary sinus carcinoma
      d. Rhabdomyosarcoma
Q. Vasculogenic lesions
   (1) Capillary hemangioma
   (2) Cavernous hemangioma
   (3) Hemangiopericytoma
   (4) Hemangiosarcoma

(5) Kaposi sarcoma

(6) Lymphangioma

(7) Varices

(8) Vascular leiomyoma

(9) Vascular leiomyosarcoma

6. Vascular disorders

   A. Allergic vasculitis

   B. Angioedema (Quincke disease)

   C. Arteriovenous aneurysm or varices

   D. Arteriovenous fistula (varicose aneurysm)

   E. Collagen disease—lupus erythematosus (Kaposi–Libman–Sacks syndrome), periarteritis nodosa (Kussmaul disease), or dermatomucomyositis (Wagner–Unverricht syndrome)

   F. Cranial arteritis

   G. Thrombophlebitis

   H. Scurvy causing bilateral orbital hemorrhage

Archer KF, et al. Orbital nonchromaffin paraganglioma. *Ophthalmology* 1989;96:1659–1666.

Carter K, et al. Ophthalmic manifestations of allergic fungal sinusitis. *Am J Ophthalmol* 1999;127:189–195.

Fraunfelder FT, Fraunfelder FW. *Drug-induced ocular side effects.* Woburn, MA: Butterworth-Heinemann, 2001.

Luxenberg MN. Chloroma. *Arch Ophthalmol* 1991;109:734–736.

Lyon DB, et al. Epithelioid hemangioendothelioma of the orbital bones. *Ophthalmology* 1993;99:1773–1778.

Newman NJ, et al. Ectopic brain in the orbit. *Ophthalmology* 1986;93:268–272.

Shields JA, et al. Classification and incidence of space-occupying lesions of the orbit. *Arch Ophthalmol* 1984;102:1606–1611.

Sloan B, et al. Scurvy causing bilateral orbital hemorrhage. *Arch Ophthalmol* 1999;117:842.

SYNDROMES AND DISEASES ASSOCIATED WITH EXOPHTHALMOS

1. Actinomycosis
2. Albright syndrome (fibrous dysplasia)
3. Amyloidosis (Lubarsch–Pick syndrome)
4. Apert syndrome (sphenoacrocraniosyndactyly)
5. Arteriovenous fistula (varicose aneurysm)
6. Aspergillosis
7. Bacillus cereus
8. Bloch–Sulzberger disease (incontinentia pigment I)
9. Bonnet–Dechaume–Blanc syndrome (neuroretinoangiomatosis syndrome)
10. Bourneville syndrome (tuberous sclerosis)
11. Caffey syndrome (infantile cortical hyperostosis)
12. Carotid artery–cavernous sinus fistula
13. Clostridium perfringens
14. Coenurosis
15. Craniostenosis
16. Cretinism (hypothyroidism)
17. Crouzon disease (craniofacial dysostosis)
18. Cryptococcosis
19. Cushing syndrome (adrenocortical syndrome)

20. Dejean sign (orbital floor fracture)
21. de Lange syndrome (congenital muscular hypertrophy-cerebral syndrome)
22. Dermatomucomyositis (polymyositis dermatomyositis)
23. Dermoid
24. Diencephalic epilepsy syndrome (autonomic epilepsy syndrome)
25. Dirofilariasis
26. Dracontiasis (Guinea worm infection)
27. Engelmann syndrome (diaphyseal dysplasia)
28. Ewing sarcoma
29. Feer disease (infantile acrodynia)
30. Fibrosarcoma
31. Fibrous dysplasia (Albright syndrome)
32. Foix syndrome (cavernous sinus thrombosis)
33. Gardner syndrome
34. Grönblad–Strandberg syndrome (pseudoxanthoma elasticum)
35. Hallermann–Streiff–François syndrome (oculomandibulofacial dyscephaly)
36. Hand–Schüller–Christian disease (histiocytosis X)
37. Heerfordt syndrome (uveoparotid fever)
38. Hemangiomas
39. Herpes zoster
40. Hodgkin disease
41. Hollenhorst syndrome (chorioretinal infarction syndrome)
42. Horner syndrome (cervical sympathetic paralysis syndrome)
43. Hunter syndrome (MPS [mucopolysaccharidosis] II)
44. Hurler (MPS I-H) syndrome
45. Hutchinson disease (adrenal cortex neuroblastoma with orbital metastasis)
46. Hydatid cyst
47. Hydrocephalus chondrodystrophicus congenita (extreme hydrocephalus syndrome)
48. Hypertension
49. Hyperthyroidism (Basedow syndrome)
50. Hypervitaminosis A
51. Hypophosphatasia (phosphoethanolaminuria)
52. Jansen disease (metaphyseal dysostosis)
53. JXG (nevoxanthoendothelioma)
54. Kleeblattschädel syndrome (cloverleaf skull)
55. Leiomyoma
56. Leopard syndrome (multiple lentigines syndrome)
57. Leprechaunism
58. Leukemia
59. Linear nevus sebaceous of Jadassohn
60. Lupus erythematosus (Kaposi–Libman–Sacks syndrome)
61. Lymphoid hyperplasia
62. Lymphangioma
63. Lymphosarcoma
64. Melnick–Needles syndrome (osteodysplasty)
65. Meningioma
66. Mikulicz syndrome (dacryosialoadenopathy)
67. Möbius disease (congenital paralysis of sixth and seventh nerves)

68. Mucocele
69. Mucormycosis
70. Multiple myeloma
71. Mumps
72. Myasthenia gravis (Erb–Goldflam syndrome)
73. Neurilemoma
74. Noonan syndrome (male Turner syndrome)
75. Osteopetrosis (Albers–Schönberg syndrome)
76. Paget syndrome (osteitis deformans)
77. Periarteritis nodosa (Kussmaul syndrome)
78. Periocular and ocular metastatic tumors
79. Pfeiffer syndrome
80. Pierre–Robin syndrome (micrognathia-glossoptosis syndrome)
81. Progeria (Hutchinson–Gilford syndrome)
82. Pyknodysostosis
83. Quincke disease (angioedema)
84. Relapsing polychondritis
85. Retinoblastoma
86. Rhabdomyosarcoma
87. Rochon–Duvigneaud syndrome (superior orbital fissure syndrome)
88. Rollet syndrome (orbital apex–sphenoidal syndrome)
89. Sarcoidosis syndrome (Schaumann syndrome)
90. Scaphocephaly syndrome
91. Scheie syndrome (MPS I-S)
92. Scurvy (avitaminosis C)
93. Sebaceous gland carcinoma
94. Seckel syndrome (bird-headed dwarf syndrome)
95. Sézary syndrome (mycosis fungoides syndrome)
96. Shy–Gonatas syndrome (orthostatic hypotension syndrome)
97. Siegrist sign (pigmented choroidal vessels)
98. Silverman syndrome (battered baby syndrome)
99. Sphenocavernous syndrome
100. Streptococcus
101. Sturge–Weber syndrome (encephalofacial angiomatosis)
102. Syphilis (lues)
103. Thermal burns
104. Trichinellosis
105. Trisomy syndrome (Edward syndrome)
106. Tuberculosis
107. Turner syndrome (gonadal dysgenesis)
108. von Hippel–Lindau syndrome (retinocerebral angiomatosis)
109. von Recklinghausen disease (neurofibromatosis)
110. Wegener syndrome (Wegener granulomatosis)

Goodman RM, Gorlin RJ. *The face in genetic disorders.* St. Louis: CV Mosby, 1970.

Miller NR, et al. Lytic Paget disease as a cause of orbital cholesterol granuloma. *Arch Ophthalmol* 1999;117: 1084–1085.

Roy FH. *Ocular syndromes and systemic diseases*, 3rd ed. Philadelphia: Lippincott Williams & Wilkins, 2002.

SPECIFIC EXOPHTHALMOS

1. Age
   A. Newborn—most common
      - *(1) Orbital sepsis
      - (2) Orbital neoplasm including congenital malignant teratoid neoplasm
   B. Neonatal—osteomyelitis of the maxilla
   C. Early childhood (up to 1 year of age—most common)
      - *(1) Dermoid
      - *(2) Hemangioma
      - (3) Dermolipoma
      - (4) Histiocytosis X including Hand–Schüller–Christian disease
      - *(5) Orbital extension of retinoblastoma
   D. One to five years—most common
      - *(1) Dermoid
      - (2) Metastatic neuroblastoma
      - (3) Rhabdomyosarcoma
      - (4) Epithelial cyst, such as sebaceous cyst and epithelial inclusion cyst
      - (5) Glioma of optic nerve
      - (6) Sphenoid wing meningioma
      - *(7) Orbital extension of retinoblastoma
      - (8) Fibrous dysplasia (Albright syndrome)
      - (9) Metastatic embryonal sarcoma
      - *(10) Hemangioma
   E. Five to ten years—most common
      - (1) Pseudotumor
      - (2) Orbital extension of retinoblastoma
      - (3) Malignant lymphomas and leukemias
      - *(4) Dermoid
      - *(5) Hemangioma
      - (6) Meningioma
      - (7) Fibrous dysplasia (Albright syndrome)
      - (8) Rhabdomyosarcoma
      - (9) Orbital hematoma
      - (10) Glioma of optic nerve
   F. Ten to thirty years—most common
      - *(1) Pseudotumor
      - (2) Mucocele
      - (3) Meningioma
      - *(4) Endocrine ophthalmopathy (thyroid-related ophthalmopathy)
      - (5) Lacrimal gland tumor
      - (6) Malignant lymphomas and leukemias
      - (7) Dermoid
      - (8) Hemangioma
      - (9) Peripheral nerve tumors
      - (10) Undifferentiated sarcomas
      - (11) Osteoma
      - (12) Fibrous dysplasia (Albright syndrome)
      - (13) Rhabdomyosarcoma

* = most important

       (14) Glioma of optic nerve
- G. Thirty to fifty years—most common
    - *(1) Pseudotumor
    - (2) Mucocele
    - (3) Malignant lymphomas and leukemias
    - *(4) Hemangioma
    - *(5) Endocrine ophthalmopathy (thyroid-related ophthalmopathy)
    - (6) Lacrimal gland tumors
    - (7) Rhinogenic carcinoma
    - (8) Malignant melanoma
    - (9) Osteosarcoma
    - (10) Fibrosarcoma
    - (11) Metastatic carcinoma
    - (12) Meningioma
    - (13) Dermoid
- H. Fifty to seventy years—most common
    - *(1) Pseudotumor
    - *(2) Mucocele
    - *(3) Malignant lymphomas and leukemias
    - (4) Dermoid
    - (5) Carcinoma of palpebral or epibulbar origin
    - *(6) Meningioma
    - *(7) Endocrine ophthalmopathy (thyroid-related ophthalmopathy)
    - (8) Lacrimal gland tumor
    - (9) Osteosarcoma
    - (10) Fibrosarcoma
    - (11) Undifferentiated sarcoma
    - (12) Metastatic carcinoma
    - (13) Osteoma
    - (14) Fibrous dysplasia (Albright syndrome)
    - (15) Neurofibroma
    - (16) Hemangioma
- I. More than seventy years—most common
    - (1) Melanoma
    - (2) Pseudotumor
    - *(3) Lymphoma
    - *(4) Metastatic tumor
    - (5) Basal cell carcinoma
    - (6) Mucocele
2. Unilateral exophthalmos—most common
    - A. Anatomical conditions
        - (1) Unilateral myopia of high degree
        - (2) Defects in the vault of the orbit: meningocele, encephalocele, hydroencephalocele
        - (3) Exophthalmos associated with arterial hypertension
        - (4) Recurrent exophthalmos from retrobulbar hemorrhage, lymphangioma
        - (5) Intermittent exophthalmos associated with venous anomalies within the cranium
        - (6) Disease of the pituitary gland; meningiomas involving sphenoid ridge

*(7) Unilateral exophthalmos associated with endocrine or thyroid-related ophthalmopathy

B. Traumatic conditions
    (1) Contralateral floor fracture with enophthalmos
    (2) Fracture of the orbit with retrobulbar hemorrhage
    (3) Laceration and rupture of the tissues of the orbit and the extraocular muscles
    (4) Intracranial trauma sustained at birth; aneurysm in orbit
    (5) Pulsating exophthalmos from carotid–cavernous aneurysm
    (6) Spontaneous retrobulbar hemorrhage as seen in whooping cough
    (7) Chronic subdural hematoma bulging into orbit
    (8) Posterior exophthalmos (orbital apex lesion)
        a. Pseudotumor
        b. Malignant tumor
        c. Benign tumor
        d. Vascular disease
        e. Infection

C. Inflammatory conditions
    (1) Retrobulbar abscess and cellulitis
    (2) Thrombophlebitis of the orbital veins
    (3) Cavernous sinus thrombosis
    (4) Erysipelas (St. Anthony fire)
    (5) Tenonitis
    (6) Periostitis (syphilitic or tuberculous)
    (7) Orbital mucocele, pyocele; cholesteatoma
    (8) Orbital exostosis
    (9) Paget disease with hyperostosis
   (10) Actinomycosis, trichinosis, mycotic pseudotumor
   (11) Herpes (HSV-1) with acute retinal necrosis

D. Disease of blood, lymph, and hematopoietic system
    (1) Rickets (avitaminosis D)
    (2) Scurvy (avitaminosis C)
    (3) Hemophilia (factor VIII deficiency)
    (4) Lymphosarcoma
    (5) Chloroma
    (6) Hodgkin disease

E. Space-taking lesions
    (1) Vascular anomalies
        a. Congenital orbital varix (young patient with systemic abnormalities)
        b. Cavernous hemangioma (middle age)
        c. Capillary hemangioma (young children) Kasabach–Merrit syndrome
        d. Lymphangiomas
    (2) Orbital tumors: pseudotumors, orbital cysts, meningocele, lymphangioma, orbital meningioma, lacrimal gland tumor, sarcoma, metastatic carcinoma, metastatic adrenal tumors, osteomas arising in the accessory nasal sinuses, tumors of the nasopharynx (benign and malignant)
    (3) Intracranial tumor with orbital extension including chordoma and meningioma

F. Unilateral exophthalmos in children
    (1) Inflammation

* = most important

(2) Vascular disorders

(3) Neoplasms

(4) Metabolic diseases

(5) Developmental anomalies

(6) Others

*(7) Orbital cellulitis

3. Bilateral exophthalmos—most common

  *A. Thyroid or endocrine ophthalmopathy

  B. Orbital myositis (owing to causes other than thyroid dysfunction)

  C. Cavernous sinus thrombosis (Foix syndrome)

  D. Metastatic neuroblastoma

  E. Hand–Schüller–Christian disease (histiocytosis X)

  F. Crouzon disease (craniofacial dysostosis)

  G. Paget disease (osteitis deformans)

4. Type proptosis—most common

  A. Straightforward—glioma of optic nerve, intraconal cavernous hemangioma

  B. Down and temporal—mucocele of frontal sinus

  C. Down and nasal—lacrimal gland lesion

  D. Downward—tumor of roof of orbit

  E. Upward—tumor of floor of orbit

5. Transient exophthalmos

  *A. Orbital varices

  B. Orbital varices with intracranial extension

  C. Arteriovenous malformations

  D. Cavernous hemangioma

  E. Intraorbital arteriovenous malformation

6. Pulsating exophthalmos—most common

  *A. Carotid-cavernous fistula

  B. von Recklinghausen disease associated with bony defect of skull

  C. Large frontal mucocele

  D. Meningoencephalocele

  E. Blow-in fracture of roof of orbit

  F. Neurofibromatosis

  G. Fistula

  H. Malignancies

  I. Mucoceles

  J. Orbital varix

  K. Dermoid cysts

  L. Aneurysm

7. Recurrent exophthalmos

  A. Recurrent orbital inflammation (pseudotumor) or hemorrhage

  B. Orbital cysts that rupture

  C. Lymphangioma (children)

  D. Syndrome of intermittent exophthalmos-congenital venous malformations of the orbit: venous angioma and orbital varix

  E. Temporal lobe tumor with orbital extension

  F. Neurofibromatosis

  G. Vascular neoplasm

8. Intermittent exophthalmos
   A. Orbital varices
   B. Recurrent hemorrhage
   C. Vascular neoplasm
   D. Lymphangioma
9. Exophthalmos associated with conjunctival chemosis, restricted movement of eyes because of pain—pseudotumor
10. Exophthalmos in an acutely ill patient—cavernous sinus thrombosis
11. Exophthalmos associated with engorged conjunctival episcleral vessels
    A. Nonpulsating—cerebral arteriovenous angioma, ophthalmic vein thrombosis, or cavernous sinus thrombosis
    B. Pulsating exophthalmos—carotid-cavernous sinus fistula
12. Exophthalmos associated with a palpable mass in region of the lacrimal gland
    A. Primary inflammatory exophthalmos
    B. Neoplasm
    C. Sarcoidosis syndrome (Schaumann syndrome)
    D. Hodgkin disease
13. Exophthalmos in patient with uncontrolled diabetes, usually with acidosis, who develops unilateral lid edema, ptosis, internal and external ophthalmoplegia, proptosis, and severe vision loss—orbital mucormycosis
14. Exophthalmos in an infant with ecchymosis of the eyelids
    A. Metastatic neuroblastoma
    B. Orbital leukemia infiltration
15. Bilateral exophthalmos from bilateral orbital pseudotumor
    A. Eosinophilic granuloma
    B. Retroperitoneal fibrosis
    C. Myasthenia gravis (Erb–Goldflam syndrome)

Henderson JW. *Orbital tumors*. New York: Thieme-Stratton, 1980.

Jones IS, Jakobiec FA. *Diseases of the orbit*. Philadelphia: Harper & Row, 1979.

Katz SE, et al. Combined venous lymphatic malformations of the orbit (so-called lymphangiomas). *Ophthalmology* 1998;105:176–184.

Klapper SR, et al. Orbital involvement in allergic fungal sinusitis. *Ophthalmology* 1997;104:2094–2100.

Krohel GB, et al. *Orbital disease: a practical approach*. Stewart WB, Chavis RM, eds. New York: Grune & Stratton, 1981.

Moin M, et al. Spontaneous hemorrhage in an intraorbital arteriovenous malformation. *Ophthalmology* 2000;107: 2215–2219.

Nicholson DH, Green WR, eds. *Pediatric ocular tumors*. New York: Masson, 1981.

Steinkuller PG, Font RL. Congenital malignant teratoid neoplasm of the eye and orbit. *Ophthalmology* 1997;104: 38–42.

Tornerup NR, et al. HV-1 induced acute retinal necrosis syndrome presenting with severe inflammatory orbitopathy proptosis and optic nerve involvement. *Ophthalmology* 2000;107:397–401.

Wright JE, et al. Orbital venous anomalies. *Ophthalmology* 1997;104:905–913.

ENOPHTHALMOS

1. Senility (common)
2. Wasting diseases—loss of orbital fat
*3. Injury—blowout fracture of floor of orbit (most common)
4. Orbital varices—transient exophthalmos with fat atrophy

* = most important

Exophthalmos (up to 1 year)

	Dermoid	Hemangioma	Histiocytosis X on Hand-Schüler- Christian Disease	Retinoblastoma (Orbital Extension)
History				
1. Bilateral				S
2. Congenital	S	U		S
3. Familial				U
4. More in females		U		
5. More in males			U	
6. Present at birth		S		
Physical Findings				
1. Astigmatism	S	S		
2. Bluish lid/conjunctiva		U		U
3. Bullous keratopathy			S	
4. Cataract			S	
5. Corneal opacity				S
6. Glaucoma		R		U
7. Hypopyon	U			S
8. Keratitis	S	S		
9. Lid ecchymosis	S			R
10. Microphthalmos	S			
11. Papilledema			S	R
12. Phthisis bulbi				S
13. Ptosis	S	S		
14. Retinal detachment			S	
15. Retinal hemorrhage			U	
16. Uveitis			U	
17. Vitreous hemorrhage				S
Laboratory Data				
1. Biopsy	U	U	S	U
2. Computed tomographic scan				
A. Calcific densities	U			U
B. Tumor	S	U	S	S
3. Orbital roentigenogram				
A. Cystic defects	U			
B. Diffusely enlarged orbit		U		
C. Enlarged optic canal				U
D. Expansion of orbital margin	U	U		
E. Fossa formation of orbit	U			
F. Orbital bone destruction			U	U
G. Orbital mass				U
4. Thrombocytopenia		U		
5. Ultrasonography				
A. Cystic tumor	U			
B. Orbital mass		U		

R = rarely; S = sometimes; and U = usually.

Exophthalmos (1—5 years)

	Dermoid*	Metastatic Neuroblastoma	Rhabdomyosarcoma	Sebaceous Carcinoma	Glioma of Optic Nerve	Sphenoid Wing Meningioma	Retinoblastoma (Orbital Extension)*	Fibrous Dysplasia	Metastatic Embryomal Sarcoma	Hemangioma*
History										
1. Bilateral		U			S	S	S			
2. Congenital		S					S			U
3. Familial			U				U			
4. More in females				U	U	S				U
5. More in males			U						S	
6. Painful			S				S			
7. Painless						U	S	U		
Physical Findings										
1. Anosmia						S		S		
2. Associated with neurofibromatosis					S	S		S		
3. Astigmatism	S									S
4. Bluish lid/conjunctiva								U		U
5. Corneal opacity								S		
6. Choroidal folds			S		S					
7. Edema lids/conjunctiva	S		S					S		
8. Extraocular muscle paralysis	S		S	S	S					
9. Glaucoma		R	S		S			U		S
10. Hearing defects, nasal obstruction, and epiphora			S					S		
11. Heterochromia of iris		S								
12. Horner syndrome		S								
13. Hypermetropia					S	S				
14. Hypopyon	U							S		
15. Keratitis	S		S	S					S	S
16. Lid ecchymosis	S	U	S					R	U	
17. Located in superior nasal quadrant			U							
18. Located in superior temporal quadrant		U								
19. Marcus Gunn pupil sign						S	U			
20. Microphthalmos	S									
21. Nystagmus						S				
22. Optic nerve atrophy		S				S	S	U		
23. Optic neuritis		S								
24. Papilledema		S		S			U	R	S	
25. Palsy of third cranial nerve						U				
26. Palsy of sixth and seventh cranial nerves		S								
27. Phthisis bulbi								S		
28. Ptosis	S	S	U							S
29. Retinal hemorrhage		U								
30. Strabismus		S	S	S	S	S	S			
31. Vitreous hemorrhage								S	U	

Exophthalmos (1–5 years) (Continued)	Dermoid*	Metastatic Neuroblastoma	Rhabdosarcoma	Sebaceous Carcinoma	Glioma of Optic Nerve	Sphenoid Wing Meningioma	Retinoblastoma (Orbital Extension)*	Fibrous Dysplasia	Metastatic Embryonal Sarcoma	Hemangioma*
Laboratory Data										
1. Biopsy	S	U	S	U	R	U	U	S	U	S
2. Computed tomographic scan										
A. Enlargement optic nerve/sheath					U					
B. Orbital mass	U	S			U			S	S	U
C. Tumor between optic nerve and lateral rectus										U
D. Tumor with bony erosion			U							
3. In urine										
A. Catecholamines		U								
B. Vanillylmandelic acid		U								
4. Orbital roentgenogram										
A. Calcific densities	S		U			U				
B. Cystic defect	S									
C. Diffusely enlarged orbit					U		U	U		U
D. Enlargement of superior orbital fissure								U		
E. Expansion of optic canal					U		U			
F. Expansion of orbital margin	U					U				U
G. Fossa formation of orbit	U									
H. Hyperostosis						U	U			
I. Narrowing of superior orbital fissure								U		
J. Orbital mass that involves sphenoid bone								U		
K. Osteolysis	U									
5. Ultrasonography										
A. Cystic tumor	U							U		U
B. Orbital mass		S	U					S	U	S
C. Enlarged optic nerve shadow					U	U				

* R = rarely; S = sometimes; and U = usually.

Exophthalmos (5–10 years)

	Pseudotumor	Retinoblastoma*	Leukemia and Lymphomas	Dermoid*	Hemangioma*	Meningioma	Fibrous Dysplasia	Rhabdomyosarcoma	Orbital Hematoma	Glioma of Optic Nerve
History										
1. Bilateral	S	S	S				S			S
2. Familial		U								
3. Following blunt trauma								S	U	
4. More in females					U	U				U
5. More in males			U					U		
6. Painful	U					S		S	S	
7. Painless		U	U	U	U	U	U	U		S
8. Rapid onset	S								U	S
Physical Findings										
1. Anosmia							S			
2. Associated with neurofibromatosis						S	S			S
3. Astigmatism				S	S					
4. Bluish lid/conjunctiva		U			U				S	
5. Central retinal artery thrombosis	S									
6. Corneal opacity		S								
7. Choroidal folds						S		S		S
8. Edema of lids/conjunctiva	U	S		S		S		S	S	
9. Epibulbar lesions			U							
10. Extraocular muscle paralysis: Limitation/Restriction	S		S	S		S		S		S
11. Glaucoma	S	U	U		S			S		S
12. Globe displacement (down)	S									
13. Hypermetropia	S					S	U			S
14. Hypopyon		S	S							
15. Involvement of trigeminal nerve	U									
16. Intraorbital bleeding			S							
17. Keratitis				S	S	S	S	S		
18. Lid ecchymosis	S	R	R	S				S	S	
19. Located in superior nasal quadrant									U	
20. Marcus Gunn pupil sign						S				S
21. Microphthalmos				S						
22. Nystagmus										S
23. Ophthalmoplegia	S									
24. Optic nerve atrophy	S		S			U	U			S
25. Optic neuritis	S		S							
26. Optociliary venous shunts on disc						S				S
27. Orbital myositis	S									
28. Papilledema	S	R	S			S	S	S		S
29. Phthisis bulbi		S	S							
30. Ptosis	S			S	S	R	S	U	S	
31. Retinal detachment		S								
32. Soft retinal exudate			U							
33. Strabismus		S				S	S			S
34. Uveitis		S	U							
35. Vitreous hemorrhage		S							S	

* = most important

Exophthalmos (5–10 years) (Continued)

	Pseudotumor	Retinoblastoma*	Leukemia and Lymphomas	Dermoid*	Hemangioma*	Meningioma	Fibrous Dysplasia	Rhabdomyosarcoma	Orbital Hematoma	Glioma of Optic Nerve
Laboratory Data										
1. Biopsy	U	S	U	U	U	S	S	S	S	R
2. Computed tomographic scan										
A. Calcific densities		U		U				U		
B. Diffuse radiodensity blends with normal structure	U									
C. Enlargement optic nerve/sheath						U				U
D. Extraocular muscle enlargement	U							S		
E. Orbital mass		S	S	U	U		S	S	S	
F. Tumor with bony erosion							S	U		
3. Orbital roentgenogram										
A. Calcific densities		U		U				U		
B. Diffusely enlarged orbit		S			S			R		
C. Enlarged optic canal							S			S
D. Expansion of orbital margin				U						
E. Fossa formation of orbit				U						
F. Hyperostosis		S				S	S			S
G. Hyperostosis sphenoid bone						S	U			
H. Narrowing of superior orbital fissure							U			
I. Osteolysis			S	S						
J. Periosteal reaction										
4. Thrombocytopenia						S				
5. Ultrasonography										
A. Cystic tumor				U	U					
B. Enlarged optic nerve						U				U
C. Orbital mass			S	U	S	S		U	U	
D. Uniform dense diffuse mass	U		U				U			

R = rarely; S = sometimes; and U = usually.

Exophthalmos (10–30 years)

	Pseudotumor*	Mucocele	Meningioma	Thyroid Ophthalmopathy*	Lacrimal Gland Tumor	Malignant Lymphomas and Leukemias	Dermoid	Hemangioma	Peripheral Nerve Tumors	Undifferentiated Sarcomas	Osteoma	Fibrous Dysplasia	Rhabdomyosarcoma	Glioma of Optic Nerve
History														
1. Bilateral	S			S		S								R
2. Common in females			U	S				U						S
3. Common in males						U			U		S		U	
4. Familial													U	
5. Painful	U		S		S								S	
6. Painless		U	U					U	U	U	U	U	U	R
7. Slow onset									U					
Physical Findings														
1. Anosmia			S									S		
2. Associated with neurofibromatosis									U			S		S
3. Astigmatism					R		S	S						
4. Bluish lids/conjunctiva								U						
5. Central retinal artery occlusion	S													
6. Corneal opacity												R		
7. Choroidal folds		S	S					S					R	S
8. Edema lids/conjunctiva	U		S	S			R					S	S	
9. Epibulbar lesion							U		S					
10. Extraocular muscle restriction	S	S	S	U	R	S	S	S	R				S	
11. Glaucoma	S			S		S		R				R	S	R
12. Globe displacement (down)	S	S		U			S		R		S	S		
13. Hemangioma of conjunctiva, iris, or disc								U						
14. Hyperopia	S		U					S						
15. Hypopyon							S							
16. Infrequent blinking				U										
17. Intraorbital bleeding								S	R	S				
18. Involvement of trigeminal nerve	U				S									
19. Keratitis			S	U			S	S	S					
20. Lacrimation	S	S		S	S									
21. Lid ecchymosis	S						R	S					S	
22. Lid lag				U										
23. Lid retraction				U										
24. Marcus Gunn pupil sign			S											S
25. Microphthalmos							S							
26. Nystagmus														S
27. Neurocutaneous melanosis									U					
28. Optic nerve atrophy	S	R	U				S		S		S	S	S	S
29. Optic neuritis	S						S							
30. Optociliary venous shunts on disc			S											
31. Orbital myositis	S				S									
32. Panophthalmitis														

* = most important

Exophthalmos (10—30 years) (Continued)

Physical Findings	Pseudotumor*	Mucocele	Meningioma	Thyroid Ophthalmopathy*	Lacrimal Gland Tumor	Malignant Lymphomas and Leukemias	Dermoid	Hemangioma	Peripheral Nerve Tumors	Undifferentiated Sarcomas	Osteoma	Fibrous Dysplasia	Rhabdomyosarcoma	Glioma of Optic Nerve
33. Papilledema	S	R	S	R		S		S			S	S	S	
34. Poor fixation on lateral gaze	S			U										
35. Ptosis			S	S			S	S					S	
36. Retinal detachment						S					S			
37. Soft retinal exudate						U								
38. Strabismus	S		S	S										S
39. Tremor of closed lids				U										
40. Uveitis	R					U								

R = rarely; S = sometimes; and U = usually.

Exophthalmos (30–50 years)

	Pseudotumor*	Mucocele	Malignant Lymphomas and Leukemias	Hemangioma	Thyroid Ophthalmopathy*	Lacrimal Gland Tumor	Rhinogenic Carcinoma	Malignant Melanoma	Osteosarcoma	Fibrosarcoma	Metastatic Carcinoma	Meningioma	Dermoid
History													
1. Bilateral	S		S		S						S		
2. Chinese extraction							U						
3. Common in females				S	S							U	
4. Common in males			U				U						
5. Familial					S				S	S	S		
6. More in whites				S				U					
7. Painful	U				S	S				U	S		
Physical Findings													
1. Astigmatism					S	S					S		S
2. Bluish lids/conjunctiva				U									
3. Central retinal artery occlusion	S												
4. Choroidal folds		S			S						S	S	

Exophthalmos (30–50 years) (Continued)

Physical Findings

Physical Findings	Pseudotumor*	Mucocele	Malignant Lymphomas and Leukemias	Hemangioma	Thyroid Ophthalmopathy*	Lacrimal Gland Tumor	Rhinogenic Carcinoma	Malignant Melanoma	Osteosarcoma	Fibrosarcoma	Metastatic Carcinoma	Meningioma	Dermoid
5. Choroidal nevus								S					
6. Conjunctivitis	S				S								
7. Cranial nerve palsies							S				R		
8. Degenerative changes in retinal pigment epithelium								S			S		
9. Edema of lids/conjunctiva	S				S					S	S	S	R
10. Epibulbar subconjunctival lesion			S								R		
11. Fibrosarcoma of lids, lacrimal sac, or sclera										U			
12. Glaucoma	S		S	S				R	S		R		
13. Globe displacement (down)	S	S	R	R	S	U				S	S		R
14. Hemangioma of conjunctiva, iris, or disc				S									
15. Horner syndrome							S						
16. Hypermetropia	S											U	
17. Hypopyon			S										U
18. Increased pigmentation of lids			S	S				S					
19. Infrequent blinking					U								
20. Intraorbital bleeding			S							R	R		
21. Involvement of trigeminal nerve	U						S		S				
22. Keratitis					S	U			S			R	R
23. Lacrimation	S				S	S							S
24. Lid ecchymosis	S		R										
25. Lid lag					U								
26. Marcus Gunn pupil sign					S							S	
27. Microphthalmos													S
28. Nasolacrimal obstruction								U		S	S	R	
29. Orbital myositis	S				S				S	S			
30. Ophthalmoplegia	S	R			S	R	U		S	S	S		
31. Optic nerve atrophy	R	R	S	R	S				S	S		U	
32. Optic neuritis	S		S								R		
33. Optociliary venous shunts on the disc												S	
34. Panophthalmitis									S		S		
35. Papilledema	S		S	R						S		U	
36. Phthisis bulbi			S										
37. Pigmented or amelanotic choroidal mass								U					
38. Poor fixation on lateral gaze			S		U								

R = rarely; S = sometimes; and U = usually.

* = most important

Exophthalmos (50–70 years)

	Pseudotumor*	Mucocele	Malignant Lymphomas and Leukemias	Dermoid	Carcinoma of Palpebral and Epibulbar Origin	Meningioma	Thyroid Ophthalmopathy	Lacrimal Gland Tumor	Osteosarcoma	Fibrosarcoma	Undifferentiated Sarcoma	Metastatic Carcinoma	Osteoma	Fibrous Dysplasia	Neurofibroma	Hemangioma
History																
1. Bilateral	S		S				S					S				
2. Common in females						U	S									U
3. Common in males			U										S			
4. Familial							S									
5. Painful	S		S		S	R	S	U				S	S		S	
Physical Findings																
1. Associated with neurofibromatosis														S	U	
2. Bluish lids/conjunctiva																U
3. Central retinal artery occlusion	S		R									R				
4. Chalazions					S											
5. Choroidal folds		S				S						S			S	S
6. Chronic blepharitis					S											
7. Conjunctivitis	S				S											
8. Disc pallor	R					S										
9. Ectropion					S										S	
10. Edema of lids/conjunctiva	S		S			S	S	S						S	S	
11. Entropion					S										S	
12. Epibulbar subconjunctival vessels			U		U											
13. Extraocular muscle paralysis	S	R	S				S				S				S	
14. Fibrosarcoma of lids, lacrimal sac, and sclera											U					
15. Glaucoma	S		U					S				R			S	S
16. Globe displacement (down and temporal)	S	S										S	S		S	
17. Globe displacement (down and nasal)								U				S			S	
18. Hemangioma of conjunctiva, iris, or disc																S
19. Hypermetropia	S					U										S
20. Hypopyon			S		S							S				
21. Involvment of trigeminal nerve	U						S	S							S	
22. Increased pigmentation of lids							S									
23. Intraorbital bleeding			S						S			S				
24. Infrequent blinking							U									
25. Keratitis				S	S	S	U		U	S		S		S	S	S
26. Lacrimation	S						S	S								
27. Lid ecchymosis	S		R	S	S										S	
28. Lid lag							U									
29. Lid notching					S											
30. Lid retraction					S		U									
31. Loss of vision	S	S				U	S		S		S	S		U	S	
32. Madarosis				U												
33. Marcus Gunn pupil sign						S	S									
34. Microphthalmos			S													
35. Nasolacrimal obstruction								S				R			S	

Exophthalmos (50–70 years) (Continued)

	Pseudotumor*	Mucocele	Malignant Lymphomas and Leukemias	Dermoid	Carcinoma of Palpebral and Epibulbar Origin	Meningioma	Thyroid Ophthalmopathy	Lacrimal Gland Tumor	Osteosarcoma	Fibrosarcoma	Undifferentiated Sarcoma	Metastatic Carcinoma	Osteoma	Fibrous Dysplasia	Neurofibroma	Hemangioma
Physical Findings																
36. Nodular or nodular ulcerative lid lesion					U											
37. Nystagmus														S		
38. Ophthalmoplegia	S						S	R	S							
39. Optic nerve atrophy	S	R	S			U			S		S		S	U	S	
40. Optic neuritis	S		S									R				
41. Optociliary venous shunts on the disc						S										
42. Orbital myositis	S							S	S							
43. Panophthalmitis						S						S				
44. Papilledema	S	R	S						S				S	S	S	
45. Phthisis bulbi			S													
46. Poor fixation on lateral gaze	S						U									
47. Ptosis			S			S	S								S	S
48. Retinal detachment	R		S									S				
49. Soft retinal exudates			U									S				
50. Tremor of closed lids							U									
51. Uveitis	S		U						S			S			S	
52. Vitreous hemorrhage												S				U
Laboratory Data																
1. Biopsy	U	U	U	U	U	S		U	S	S	S	U	U	S	U	U
2. Computed tomographic scan																
A. Calcific densities		S			S				S		R					
B. Diffuse radiodensity blends with normal structure	U															
C. Enlargement optic nerve sheath						U										
D. Extraocular muscle enlargement	U						U					S				
E. Orbital mass		U	U	U	U			U	U	U	U		U	S	U	U
F. Tumor between optic nerve and lateral rectus																U
G. Tumor superior lateral orbit		R						U				S				
3. In blood																
A. 32 Phosphorus uptake elevated												U				
B. T3–T4 level increased, thyrotropin-releasing hormone test positive							S									
4. Orbital roentgenogram																
A. Calcific densities		S		S									U	S		
B. Cystic defects			S													
C. Diffusely enlarged orbit	S													S		
D. Expansion of optic canal						U									U	
E. Expansion of orbital margins						S		U							U	U
F. Fossa formation of orbit			S					S								
G. Frontal sinus bone dense/destruction		U												S		

* = most important

Exophthalmos (50—70 years) (Continued)

	Pseudotumor*	Mucocele	Malignant Lymphomas and Leukemias	Dermoid	Carcinoma of Palpebral and Epibulbar Origin	Meningioma	Thyroid Ophthalmopathy	Lacrimal Gland Tumor	Osteosarcoma	Fibrosarcoma	Undifferentiated Sarcoma	Metastatic Carcinoma	Osteoma	Fibrous Dysplasia	Neurofibroma	Hemangioma
Laboratory Data																
H. Hyperostosis						S							U			
I. Narrowing of superior orbital fissure						U		U					U	U		
J. Orbital mass											S	S			S	
K. Osteolysis			U	S	U	S										
L. Periosteal reaction	S															
5. Ultrasonography																
A. Cystic tumor		U		U												U
B. Enlarged extraocular muscle	S															
C. Orbital mass			U						U	U	U	U	U			
D. Uniform diffuse dense mass	U		U		U							U				

R = rarely; S = sometimes; and U = usually.

Exophthalmos (more than 70 years)

	Malignant Melanoma	Pseudotumor	Malignant Lymphoma and Leukemia*	Metastatic Carcinoma*	Basal Cell Carcinoma	Mucocele
History						
1. Bilateral		S		S		
2. Common in females				S		S
3. Common in males		S		S		
4. More in whites	U			U		
5. Ocular pain		U	S	S	S	
Physical Findings						
1. Central retinal artery occlusion				S	R	
2. Choroidal folds				S	S	
3. Choroidal nevus	S					
4. Degenerative changes in retinal pigment epithelium	S					
5. Ectropion					S	S
6. Edema of lids/conjunctiva		S	U	S		
7. Entropion					S	S

Exophthalmos (more than 70 years) (Continued)

	Malignant Melanoma	Pseudotumor	Malignant Lymphoma and Leukemia*	Metastatic Carcinoma*	Basal Cell Carcinoma	Mucocele
Physical Findings						
8. Extraocular muscle limatation	S	S	S	S		S
9. Glaucoma	S	S		S		
10. Globe displacement (down and temporally)		S				S
11. Hypermetropia	U	S				
12. Increased lid pigmentation	S					
13. Intraorbital bleeding				S		
14. Involvement of trigeminal nerve		U		S		S
15. Lacrimation					S	U
16. Lid ecchymosis		S		S	S	
17. Nodular/ulcerative lid lesion					U	
18. Optic nerve atrophy	S	R		S		S
19. Optic neuritis		S				
20. Orbital myositis		S		S		
21. Papilledema	S	S	S	S		S
22. Pigmented or amelanotic choroidal mass	S					
23. Retinal detachment	S	S				
24. Retinal hemorrhages			S	S		
25. Uveitis		S	U	S		
26. Vitreous hemorrhage	U					
Laboratory Data						
1. Biopsy	U	U	U	U	U	U
2. Computed tomographic scan						
A. Diffuse radiodensity blends with normal structures		S				
B. Extraocular muscle enlargement		U		U		U
C. Orbital mass	U			U		U
3. Orbital roentgenogram						
A. Calcific densities						U
B. Diffusely enlarged orbit	U	U	U	U	U	
C. Enlargement of superior orbital fissure				U		
D. Erosion of optic canal	U					U
E. Frontal sinus bone dense/destruction						U
F. Osteolysis	U			U	U	
G. Periosteal reaction		U				
4. Ultrasonography						
A. Orbital mass			S	U	S	
B. Uniform dense diffuse mass			U		U	

R = rarely; S = sometimes; and U = usually.

Pulsating exophthalmos (most common)

	Carotid-cavernous Aneurysm	Von-Recklinghausen Disease with Bony Defect of Skull	Large Frontal Mucocele	Meningoencephalocele	Blow-out Fracture of Orbital Root
History					
1. Activated at puberty, pregnancy, and menopause		S			
2. Congenital				U	
3. Diplopia			U		U
4. Hereditary		U			
5. Ocular pain	S				U
6. Slow progression	U				
7. Trauma					U
8. Unilateral	U	R	U		S
Physical Findings					
1. Cataracts		S			
2. Displacement of the globe		U	U	U	U
3. Elephantiasis of lids		U			
4. Hamartoma of retina		S			
5. Hydrophthalmos		S			
6. Hypertelorism				U	
7. Intraorbital hemorrhage					U
8. Lacrimation, excessive			U		
9. Lid ecchymosis/edema					U
10. Loss of facial sensation	U				
11. Mass fluctuant to palpation in the orbid				U	
12. Nodular swelling of corneal nerves		U			
13. Ophthalmoplegia	U				U
14. Optic atrophy		S			S
15. Optic nerve edema	S				
16. Orbital edema					U
17. Orbital emphysema					U
18. Ptosis		U			S
Laboratory Data					
1. Carotid angiography	U			S	
2. Cerebral arteriography	U				
3. Computed tomographic orbit scan	U	U	U	U	U
4. Pneumoencephalography	U			S	
5. Roentgenogram, orbit	U	U	U	U	U
6. Ultrasonography (ocular)				U	
7. Venography	S				

R = rarely; S = sometimes; and U = usually.

Recurrent exophthalmos

	Recurrent Ocular Inflammation or Hemorrhage	Orbital Cysts That Rupture	Lymphangioma	Syndrome of Intermittent Exophthalmos—Congenital Malformation of Orbit, Venous Angioma, Orbital Varix	Temporal Lobe Tumor with Orbital Extension	Neurofibromatosis	Vascular Neoplasms
History							
1. Alterations in visual field					U		
2. Apparently healthy individuals	U				U		
3. Associated with upper respiratory infection		S					
4. Congenital				S			
5. Diplopia	S		S	S			S
6. Hematologic history	U		R				
7. Hereditary						U	
8. More in males	S	S					U
9. Most in children					U		
10. Traumatic history		U	S				R
11. Unilateral	U	S	U		R		
12. Visual hallucinations					U		
Physical Findings							
1. Blood cysts of orbit	S	U	U				
2. Bluish color lids/conjunctiva							U
3. Conjunctival ecchymosis	U		R				
4. Ectropion uvea						U	
5. Glaucoma				S		S	S
6. Hemangioma conjunctiva/disc							U
7. Keratitis						S	S
8. Lid ecchymosis	U		R				
9. Narrowing of the palpebral fissure					U		
10. Neurofibroma of eyelids						U	
11. Nystagmus						S	S
12. Optic nerve atrophy			S	S	S	S	S
13. Prominent corneal nerves						S	
14. Ptosis			R		R	U	S
15. Pupil dilated					U		
16. Retrobulbar hemorrhage	S	R		R	R		S
17. Venous malformation in lids, fornix, and canthal areas				U			
18. Vitreous hemorrhage							S
Laboratory Data							
1. Carotid angiography					U		R
2. Complete blood count	U						
3. Computed tomographic scan	U	U	U		U	S	U
4. Histopathology			S	U	U	U	S
5. Ultrasonography	U	U	U		S	U	U
6. Venous angiography				U			
7. Roentgenogram (orbit and skull)		R		U	S	S	S

R = rarely; S = sometimes; and U = usually.

5. Chronic or severe liver or gallbladder disease (usually in right eye owing to increased tone of orbicularis muscle and extraocular muscles)
6. Iatrogenic
    A. Orbital decompression
    B. Sinus surgery
7. Superior sulcus deformity
    A. Traumatic bony loss
    B. Atrophy of the orbital tissues
    C. Levator detachment with ptosis
    D. Migration of muscle cone implant
    E. Herniated orbital fat secondary to an orbital fracture
8. Associated syndromes
    A. Arthrogryposis (amyoplasia congenital)
    B. Babinski–Nageotte syndrome (medullary tegmental paralysis)
    C. Cestan–Chenais syndrome (lesion in the lateral portion of medulla oblongata)
    D. Cockayne syndrome (dwarfism with retinal atrophy and deafness)
    E. Craniocervical syndrome (whiplash injury)
    F. Cretinism (hypothyroidism)
    G. Cryptophthalmia syndrome
    H. Dejean syndrome (orbital floor syndrome)
    I. Dejerine–Klumpke syndrome (thalamic hyperesthetic anesthesia)
    J. Duane retraction syndrome
    K. Freeman–Sheldon syndrome (craniocarpotarsal dysplasia)
    L. General fibrosis syndrome
    M. Greig syndrome (ocular hypertelorism syndrome)
    N. Hemifacial microsomia syndrome (François–Haustrate syndrome)
    O. Horner syndrome (cervical sympathetic paralysis syndrome)
    P. Klippel–Trenaunay–Weber syndrome (angioosteohypertrophy syndrome)
    Q. Krause syndrome (encephaloophthalmic syndrome)
    R. Maple syrup urine disease (branched chain ketoaciduria)
    S. Morquio syndrome (MPS IV)
    T. Naffziger syndrome (scalenus anticus syndrome)
    U. Pancoast syndrome (superior pulmonary sulcus syndrome)
    V. Parry–Romberg syndrome (progressive facial hemiatrophy)
    W. Passow syndrome (Bremer status dysraphicus)
    X. Raeder syndrome (paratrigeminal paralysis)
    Y. Retroparotid space syndrome
    Z. Silent sinus syndrome
    AA. Vernet syndrome (jugular foramen syndrome)
    BB. von Herrenschwand syndrome (sympathetic heterochromia)
    CC. Wallenberg syndrome (dorsolateral medullary syndrome)
9. Apparent enophthalmos with horizontal conjugate gaze
10. Metastatic adenocarcinoma of orbit (cicatricial)
11. Neurofibromatosis: pulsating enophthalmos
12. Typhoid fever (abdominal typhus)

Albert DM, Jakobiec FA. *Principles and practice of ophthalmology*. Philadelphia: WB Saunders, 1994:1881–2095.

Cline RA, Rootman J. Enophthalmos: a clinical review. *Ophthalmology* 1984;91:229–237.

Roy FH. *Ocular syndromes and systemic diseases*, 3rd ed. Philadelphia: Lippincott Williams & Wilkins, 2002.

Stasior OG, Roen JL. Traumatic enophthalmos. *Ophthalmology* 1982;89:1267.

INTRAORBITAL CALCIFICATIONS

1. Calcification of more irregular configuration and texture
    A. Cysticercosis
    B. Orbital hematoma
    C. Plexiform neurofibroma
    D. Toxoplasmosis
    E. Tuberculosis
2. Calcification of orbital vessels
    A. Atheromatous plaque
    B. Monkeberg sclerosis
    C. Secondary to metabolic-endocrine disturbances such as hyperparathyroidism or hypervitaminosis
    D. Band-shaped keratopathy
3. Chronic inflammatory and parasitic disease of the orbit
4. Hemangiopericytoma
5. Intraocular calcifications following
    A. Congenital deformity
    B. Malignant lacrimal gland tumor
    C. Recurrent iritis and keratitis
    D. Retinal detachment
    E. Trauma (perforating, nonperforating, or surgical)
6. Intraocular sarcoma
7. Mucocele
8. Myositis ossificans
9. Orbital phleboliths: helical form in veins—smooth, round, or oval
10. Organized hematomas of the orbit
*11. Retinoblastoma
12. Retrolental fibroplasia
13. Sites of intraocular calcification
    A. Cyclitic membrane
    B. Lens
    C. Peripapillary choroid
    D. Posterior pole to ora serrata in region of choroid and pigment epithelium
    E. Retina
    F. Vitreous

Albert DM, Jakobiec FA. *Principles and practice of ophthalmology*. Philadelphia: WB Saunders, 1994:1881–2095.

Basta LL, et al. Focal choroidal calcification. *Ann Ophthalmol* 1981;13:447–450.

Garrity JA, Kennerdell JS. Orbital calcification associated with hemangiopericytoma. *Am J Ophthalmol* 1986;102:126.

Zizmor J, Lombardi G. *Atlas of orbital radiology*. Birmingham: Aesculapius, 1973.

ORBITAL BRUIT (NOISE HEARD OVER ORBIT WITH STETHOSCOPE)

1. Bilateral
    A. Hyperthyroidism
    B. Severe anemias
2. Unilateral
    *A. Abnormal communication in the cavernous sinus (i.e., bilateral carotid-cavernous sinus)

* = most important

Orbital bruit (noise heard over orbit with stethoscope)

	Hyperthyroidism	Severe Anemias	Arteriovenous Aneurysm	Stenosis of Carotid Artery	Aneurysmal Angiomas of Orbit or Fundus	Abnormal Communication in Cavernous Sinus	Intermittent or Pulsating Exophthalmos
History							
1. Amaurosis fugax							
2. Bilateral					U		
3. Congenital	U	S					S
4. Diplopia						S	S
5. Familial	S						
6. Middle age	U						
7. Older patients	U					U	
8. Traumatic						U	S
Physical Findings							
1. Arteriovenous malformations of retina						U	S
2. Central or branch retinal artery occlusion					U		
3. Chemosis of conjunctiva	S					U	S
4. Conjunctival vessels dilated						U	S
5. Cotton-wool spots		U			U		
6. Enlargement periorbital veins of lids, forehead, temple						S	U
7. Exposure keratopathy	S						
8. Hollenhorst plaques					U		
9. Increased intraocular pressure						U	S
10. Increased lid pigmentation	U						
11. Infrequent blinking	U						
12. Lid edema	S						
13. Lid lag	U						
14. Neurofibromas in lids, conjunctiva, and cornea							S
15. Nodules in iris							S
16. Ophthalmoplegia	S						
17. Restriction of extraocular myaels	U						
18. Papilledema		U					
19. Retinal hemorrhage		S	U	S			
20. Retraction of upper lid	U						
21. Tremor of closed lids	U						
Laboratory Data							
1. Carotid arteriography							
2. Cerebral angiography				S			
3. Computed tomographic scan					U	U	
4. Orbital ultrasonogram	U						
5. Orbital venography	U						
6. Orbital roentgenogram							U
7. Platelet levels and hemoglobin low counts		U					S
8. T3–T4	U						

R = rarely; S = sometimes; and U = usually.

B. Aneurysmal angioma of orbit or fundus such as in Wyburn–Mason syndrome (Bonnet–Dechaume–Blanc syndrome)

C. Arteriovenous aneurysm (arteriovenous fistula)

D. Intermittent or pulsating exophthalmos

E. Stenosis of carotid artery including thrombosis, sclerosis, or external pressure such as that due to an outer-ridge sphenoidmeningioma

Albert DM, Jakobiec FA. *Principles and practice of ophthalmology.* Philadelphia: WB Saunders, 1994:1881–2095.

Grobb WE, et al. Facial hamartomas in children: neurofibroma, lymphangioma, and hemangiomia. *Plast Reconstr Surg* 1980;66:509.

Kushner FH. Carotid-cavernous fistula as a complication of carotid endarterectomy. *Ann Ophthalmol* 1981;13:979.

Lloyd GA. Vascular anomalies in the orbit: C T and angiographic diagnosis. *Orbit* 1982;1:45.

ORBITAL EMPHYSEMA (AIR FOUND IN ORBITAL TISSUES AND ADNEXA USUALLY DEMONSTRABLE BY PALPATION)

*1. Due to fracture of ethmoid sinuses or orbital floor

2. Following forceful blowing of nose

3. Injury from compressed air

4. Orbital cellulitis and abscess with gas formation by infecting organism

5. Osteomyelitis and infected sinus with fistulous communication with gas formation by infecting organism

6. Resulting from use of high-speed dental drill and air-water spray during oral operation

7. Subconjunctival emphysema seen with mechanical ventilation

Buckley MJ, et al. Orbital emphysema causing vision loss after a dental extraction. *J Am Dent Assoc* 1990;120: 421–422.

Hunts JH, et al. Orbital emphysema: staging and acute management. *Ophthalmology* 1994;101:960–966.

Zimmer-Galler IE, Bartley GB. Orbital emphysema: case reports and review of the literature. *Mayo Clin Proc* 1994; 69:115–121.

ORBITAL PAIN

1. Acute dacryoadenitis

2. Amputation neuroma of the orbit

3. Associated syndromes

    A. Cavernous sinus thrombosis syndrome

    B. Charlin syndrome (nasal nerves syndrome)

    C. Erysipelas

    D. Ophthalmoplegic migraine syndrome

    E. Raeder syndrome (paratrigeminal paralysis)

    F. Tolosa–Hunt syndrome (painful ophthalmoplegia).

4. Break-bone fever (dengue fever)

5. Clostridium perfringens

6. Eye strain from uncorrected errors of refraction

7. Myositis

    A. Collagen diseases

    B. Infectious myositis

    C. Trichinosis

8. Orbital cellulitis or abscess

9. Orbital periostitis because of injury, tuberculosis, syphilis, extension of sinus disease, or other conditions

* = most important

*10. Pseudotumor or tumor of the orbit—pain infrequently present
11. Retrobulbar neuritis
12. Trauma
13. Tumors of cerebellopontine angle, frequent lesion of seventh nerve

Albert DM, Jakobiec FA. *Principles and practice of ophthalmology*. Philadelphia: WB Saunders, 1994:1881–2095.

Bullen CL, Younge BR. Chronic orbital myositis. *Ophthalmology* 1982;89:1749.

Lanzino G, et al. Orbital pain and unruptured carotid-posterior communicating artery aneurysms: the role of sensory fibers of the third cranial nerve. *Acta Neurochir (Wien)* 1993;120:7–11.

Roy FH. *Ocular syndromes and systemic diseases*, 3rd ed. Philadelphia: Lippincott Williams & Wilkins, 2002.

SHALLOW ORBITS OR DIMINISHED ORBITAL VOLUME (ILLUSION OF PROPTOSIS OR GLAUCOMA)

1. Aminopterin-induced syndrome
2. Apert syndrome (acrocephalosyndactyly)
3. Carpenter syndrome
4. Cerebrohepatorenal syndrome (Smith–Lemli–Opitz syndrome)
5. Craniostenosis
6. Crouzon disease (craniofacial dysostosis)
7. Diseases of nasal passages and sinuses
    A. Dentigerous cysts
    B. Fibrous dysplasia (Albright syndrome)
    C. Hypoplasia of maxilla associated with chronic maxillary sinusitis
    D. Rhinoscleroma
8. Dubowitz syndrome
9. Early enucleation of eye
*10. Familial hypoplasia of orbital margin
11. Frontometaphyseal dysplasia (FMD)
12. Hyperostosis (hypertrophy of orbital bones)
13. Hypophosphatasia–harlequin orbit (shallow orbit with arched superior and lateral wall)
14. Kleeblattschädel syndrome
15. Lateral displacement of medial orbital wall by hypertrophic polypoid nasal sinus disease
16. Marshall–Smith syndrome
17. Oculoauriculovertebral dysplasia (Goldenhar syndrome)
18. Osteogenesis imperfecta (van der Hoeve syndrome)
19. Radiation injury of bone
20. Robert syndrome (pseudothalidomide syndrome)
21. Saethre–Chotzen syndrome
22. Secondary to fracture
23. Stanesco dysostosis syndrome
24. Trisomy 13-(trisomy D) (Patau syndrome)
25. Trisomy (Edward syndrome)
26. Zellweger syndrome
27. 6q- D syndrome
28. 9p- syndrome

Cursiefen C, et al. Adenoma of the nonpigmented ciliary epithelium mimicking a malignant melanoma of the iris. *Arch Ophthalmol* 1999;117:113–118.

Roy FH. *Ocular syndromes and systemic diseases*, 3rd ed. Philadelphia: Lippincott Williams & Wilkins, 2002.

Smith DW. *Recognizable patterns of human malformation*, 4th ed. Philadelphia: WB Saunders, 1988.

PSEUDOHYPERTELORISM (ILLUSION OF INCREASED DISTANCE BETWEEN BONY ORBITS AND INCREASED INTERPUPILLARY DISTANCE)

1. Blepharophimosis
*2. Epicanthal skin folds
3. Exotropia
*4. Flat nasal bridge of nose
5. Increased distance between the inner canthi (telecanthus)
6. Widely spaced eyebrows

DeMyer W. The median cleft face syndrome. *Neurology* 1967;17:961.

HYPERTELORISM (INCREASED DISTANCE BETWEEN BONY ORBITS AND INCREASED INTERPUPILLARY DISTANCE)

1. Aarskog syndrome (faciodigitogenital syndrome)
2. Acrocollosal syndrome
3. Acrodysostosis syndrome
4. Albers–Schönberg disease (osteopetrosis)
5. Aminopterin-induced syndrome
*6. Apert syndrome (acrodysplasia)
*7. Association of hypertelorism, microtia, and facial clefting
*8. Baraitser–Winter syndrome
9. BBB syndrome (hypertelorism–hypospadias syndrome)
10. Blatt syndrome (cranioorbitoocular dysraphia)
11. Blepharonosofacial syndrome
12. Camptomelic dysplasia syndrome
13. Carpenter syndrome (acrocephalopolysyndactyly II)
14. Cat's-eye syndrome (Schachenmann syndrome)
15. Cerebral gigantism (Sotos syndrome)
16. Cerebrohepatorenal syndrome (Zellweger)
17. Cherubism
18. Chromosome partial long-arm deletion syndrome (de Grouchy syndrome)
19. Chromosome partial short-arm deletion syndrome [monosomy partial (short-arm) syndrome]
20. Chromosome short-arm deletion
21. Chondrodystrophia calcificans congenita (Conradi syndrome)
22. Cleft lip and palate sequence
23. Clefting, ectropion, and conical teeth syndrome
24. Cleidocranial dysostosis syndrome
25. Coffin–Lowry syndrome
26. Congenital hemihypertrophy
27. Craniocarpotarsal syndrome (Freeman–Sheldon syndrome)
28. Craniocleidodysostosis syndrome (Marie–Sainton syndrome)
29. Craniosynostosis–radial aplasia (Baller–Gerold syndrome)
30. Cretinism (hypothyroidism)
31. Cri-du-chat syndrome (Cry of the cat syndrome)
32. Crouzon disease (craniofacial dysostosis)
33. Cryptophthalmos syndrome
34. Curtius syndrome (ectodermal dysplasia with ocular malformations)
35. Diamond–Blackfan syndrome

* = most important

36. DiGeorge sequence
37. Down syndrome (mongolism)
38. Dubowitz syndrome (dwarfism–eczema–peculiar facies)
39. Duplication 14Q syndrome
40. Ehlers–Danlos syndrome (fibrodysplasia elastica generalisata)
41. Engelmann syndrome (diaphyseal dysplasia)
42. 18P syndrome
43. Faciooculoacousticorenal syndrome
44. Familial characteristic
45. Familial metaphyseal dysplasia (Pyle disease)
46. Fetal alcohol syndrome
47. Fetal aminopterin effects
48. Fetal hydantoin effects
49. Fish odor syndrome
50. 4Q syndrome
51. Frontonasal dysplasia syndrome (median cleft face syndrome)
52. Frontal encephaloceles
53. Gorlin syndrome (orodigitofacial dysostosis)
54. Greig syndrome (hypertelorism)
55. Haney–Falls syndrome (congenital keratoconus posticus circumscriptus)
56. Holt–Oram syndrome
57. Hurler syndrome (MPS I-H)
58. Hydrocephalus
59. Hypomelanosis of Ito syndrome (systematized achromic nevus)
60. Ichthyosis (collodion baby)
61. Infantile gigantism
62. Infantile hypercalcemia with supravalvular aortic stenosis (Williams–Beuren syndrome)
63. Iris dysplasia–hypertelorism–psychomotor retardation syndrome
64. Jacobs syndrome (triple X syndrome)
65. KBG syndrome (initials of family studied)
66. Kleeblattschädel syndrome (extreme hydrocephalus syndrome)
67. Klein syndrome
68. Klinefelter XXY syndrome (gynecomastia–aspermatogenesis syndrome)
69. Klippel–Feil syndrome (synostosis cervical vertebrae)
70. Larsen syndrome
71. Leprechaunism
72. Lissencephalia (Miller–Dieker syndrome)
73. Little syndrome (nail–patella syndrome)
74. Mandibulofacial dysostosis (Franceschetti syndrome)
75. Maple syrup urine disease (branched-chain ketoaciduria)
76. Marfan syndrome (arachnodactyly–dystrophia–mesodermalis congenita)
77. Marshall–Smith syndrome
78. Meckel–Gruber syndrome
79. Melnick–Needles syndrome (osteodysplasty)
80. Metaphyseal dysostosis (Jansen disease)
81. McFarland syndrome
82. Morquio–Ullrich syndrome (MPS IV)
83. Multiple basal cell nevi (Gorlin–Goltz syndrome)

84. Multiple lentigines syndrome (Leopard syndrome)
85. Myelomeningocele–Chiari malformations
86. Noonan syndrome (male Turner syndrome)
87. Oculodentodigital syndrome
88. Oculomandibulofacial dyscephaly (Hallermann–Streiff syndrome)
89. Optic nerve hypoplasia
90. Orofaciodigital (OFD) type I and type II (Mohr syndrome)
91. Osteogenesis imperfecta (van der Hoeves syndrome)
92. Otopalatodigital syndrome (OPD syndrome)
93. Pallister–Killian syndrome
94. Pena-shokeir type I syndrome
95. Pfeiffer syndrome
96. Potter syndrome (renofacial syndrome)
97. Ring B chromosome
98. Ring chromosome
99. Rieger syndrome (dysgenesis mesostromalis)
100. Robert syndrome (pseudothalidomide syndrome)
101. Robinow syndrome (fetal face syndrome)
102. Saethre–Chotzen syndrome (acrocephalosyndactyly type III)
103. Sjögren–Larson syndrome (oligophrenia-ichthyosis-spastic diplegia syndrome)
104. Sprengel syndrome
105. Traumatic nasoorbital fracture
106. Triploidy syndrome
107. Trisomy syndrome
108. Trisomy 6 q syndrome
109. Trisomy 9q syndrome
110. Trisomy 13- (Patau syndrome)
111. Trisomy 17p syndrome
112. Trisomy syndrome
113. Turner–Bonnevie–Ullrich–Nielsen syndrome
114. Turner syndrome (gonadal dysgenesis)
115. Waardenburg syndrome (embryonic fixation syndrome)
116. Weaver syndrome
117. Williams syndrome
118. XXXX syndrome
119. XXXXX syndrome
120. XXXXY syndrome
121. 4p- syndrome (Wolf syndrome)
122. 4p- D syndrome
123. 6p- D syndrome
124. 9p- syndrome
125. 10q- syndrome
126. 13q- syndrome
127. 18q- syndrome

Pallotta R. Iris coloboma ptosis, hypertelorism, and mental retardation: a new syndrome possibly localized on chromosome 2. *J Med Genet* 1991;28:342–344.

Roy FH. *Ocular syndromes and systemic diseases*, 3rd ed. Philadelphia: Lippincott Williams & Wilkins, 2002.

Seaver LH, Cassidy SB. New syndrome: mother and son with hypertelorism, downslanting palpebral fissures, malar hypoplasia, and apparently low-set ears associated with joint and scrotal anomalies. *Am J Med Genet* 1991;41: 405–409.

HYPOTELORISM (DECREASED DISTANCE BETWEEN BONY ORBITS AND DECREASED INTERPUPILLARY DISTANCE)

1. Arrhinencephaly (holoprosencephaly)
2. Cebocephalia
3. Cockayne syndrome (dwarfism with retinal atrophy and deafness)
4. Coffin–Siris syndrome
5. Ethmocephalus
*6. Familial
7. François diencephalic syndrome (Hallerman–Streiff syndrome)
8. Goldenhar syndrome (oculoauriculovertebral dysplasia)
9. Maternal phenylketonuria fetal effects
10. Meckel–Gruber syndrome
11. Median cleft lip (frontonasal dysplasia syndrome)
12. Median philtrum-premaxilla anlage
13. Ocular–dental–digital dysplasia (Meyer–Schivickerath and Weyers syndrome)
14. Ring syndrome
15. Trigonocephaly (C syndrome, Opitz trigonocephaly syndrome)
16. Trisomy 13- (Patau syndrome, trisomy D syndrome)
17. Trisomy 20p syndrome
18. Trisomy (Down syndrome, mongolism)
19. Turner syndrome (gonadal dysgenesis)
20. Williams syndrome
21. Wolf syndrome (monosomy partial syndrome)
22. 5p- D syndrome
23. 18p- syndrome

Evans DG. Dominantly inherited microcephaly, hypotelorism and normal intelligence. *Clin Genet* 1991;39:178–180.

Judisch GF, et al. Orbital hypotelorism. *Arch Ophthalmol* 1984;102:995–997.

Richieri-Costa A, et al. Mental retardation, microbrachycephaly, hypotelorism, palpebral ptosis, thin/long face, cleft lip, and lumbosacral/pelvic anomalies. *Am J Med Genet* 1992;43:565–568.

Roy FH. *Ocular syndromes and systemic diseases*, 3rd ed. Philadelphia: Lippincott Williams & Wilkins, 2002.

DEEP-SET EYES

1. Cockayne syndrome (dwarfism with retinal atrophy and deafness)
2. Craniocarpotarsal syndrome (Freeman–Sheldon syndrome)
3. Familial
4. Marfan syndrome (dolichostenomelia–arachnodactylyhyperchon–droplasia–dystrophia mesodermalis congenita)
5. Mesodermal dysmorphodystrophy (Weill–Marchesani syndrome)
6. Oculocerebrorenal syndrome (Lowe syndrome)
7. Pyknodysostosis
8. Syndrome of blepharophimosis with myopathy

Aita JA. *Congenital facial anomalies with neurologic defects*. Springfield, IL: Charles C Thomas, 1969.

PROMINENT SUPRAORBITAL RIDGES

1. Apert syndrome (acrocephalosyndactylism syndrome)

2. Basal cell nevus syndrome (Gorlin–Goltz syndrome)
3. Cleidocranial dysostosis (Marie–Sainton syndrome)
4. Congenital lipodystrophy
5. Congenital syphilis (congenital lues)
6. Ectodermal dysplasia (Curtius syndrome)
*7. Frontometaphyseal dysplasia
8. Hurler syndrome (MPS I-H)
9. Marfan syndrome (arachnodactyly-dystrophia mesodermalis congenita)
10. Otopalatodigital syndrome (Taybi syndrome)
11. Pyle metaphyseal dysplasia syndrome

Albert DM, Jakobiec FA. *Principles and practice of ophthalmology*. Philadelphia: WB Saunders, 1994:1881–2095.

Roy FH. *Ocular syndromes and systemic diseases*, 3rd ed. Philadelphia: Lippincott Williams & Wilkins, 2002.

OSTEOLYSIS OF BONY ORBIT

1. Autoimmune diseases, such as Wegener granulomatosis
2. Congenital
3. Hyperparathyroidism
4. Injury, such as blowout fracture of orbital floor
5. Meningocele and encephalocele of orbit
6. Metastasis from remote primary neoplasms
7. Primary orbital disease
    A. Infectious, including tuberculosis and syphilis
    B. Neoplastic, including neurofibroma and lacrimal gland tumor
    C. Cystic, including dermoid and epidermoid cyst
8. Reticuloendotheliosis as histiocytosis X (Hand–Schüller–Christian disease)
9. Secondary extension of infectious or neoplastic disease from adjacent sinuses, brain, skin, bone, nasopharynx, and esophagus
10. Sinus disease including mucoceles

Albert DM, Jakobiec FA. *Principles and practice of ophthalmology*. Philadelphia: WB Saunders, 1994:1881–2095.

Margo CE, et al. Psammomatoid ossifying fibroma. *Arch Ophthalmol* 1986;107:1347–1351.

Oh KT, et al. Adenocarcinoma of the esophagus presenting as orbital cellulitis. *Arch Ophthalmol* 2000;118:986–988.

FOSSA FORMATION OF ORBIT (LOCAL EXPANSION OF BONY ORBITAL WALL CAUSED BY PERSISTENT PRESSURE; BONY CORTEX IS INTACT)

1. Encapsulated benign lacrimal gland tumor
2. Encapsulated malignant lacrimal gland tumor
3. Orbital dermoid

Albert DM, Jakobiec FA. *Principles and practice of ophthalmology*. Philadelphia: WB Saunders, 1994:1881–2095.

Jacobs L, et al. *Computerized tomography of the orbit and sella turcica*. New York: Raven Press, 1980.

Zizmor J. Orbital radiology in unilateral exophthalmos. In: Turtz AI. *Proceedings of the Centennial Symposium: Manhattan Eye, Ear, and Throat Hospital, Vol I*. St. Louis: CV Mosby, 1969.

SUBPERIOSTEAL ORBITAL HEMORRHAGE

1. Generalized diseases with bleeding diatheses
2. Paranasal sinusitis

* = most important

3. Sudden elevation of cranial venous pressure
4. Trauma

Atalla ML, et al. Nontraumatic subperiosteal orbital hemorrhage. *Ophthalmology* 2001;108:183–189.

Hunt KE, Ross JJ. Orbital hemorrhage in the nonoperated eye as a complication of general endotracheal anesthesia. *Arch Ophthalmol* 1998;116L:105–106.

ORBITAL HEMORRHAGE

1. Idiopathic
2. Other
    A. General endotracheal anesthesia
    B. Late migration of orbital implant
3. Preexisting vascular tumors
    A. Cholesterol granuloma
    B. Cystic lymphangiomas
    C. Hemorrhagic varix
4. Surgery
    A. Retrobulbar injection
    B. Rhinoplasty
    C. Subtentorial infusion anesthesia
5. Systemic
    A. Heparin
    B. Thrombolytic
6. Trauma

Chorich LJ, et al. Hemorrhagic ocular complications associated with the use of systemic thrombolytic agents. *Ophthalmology* 1998;105:428–431.

Polito E, et al. Diagnosis and treatment of orbital hemorrhagic lesions. *Ann Opthalmol* 1994;26:85–93.

EXPANSION OF ORBITAL MARGINS (USUALLY ASSOCIATED WITH BENIGN TUMORS OF THE ORBIT)

1. Dermoid
2. Hemangioma
3. Lacrimal gland tumors
4. Meningioma
5. Neurofibroma

Albert DM, Jakobiec FA. *Principles and practice of ophthalmology.* Philadelphia: WB Saunders, 1994:1881–2095.

Coleman DJ, et al. *Ultrasonography of the eye and orbit.* Philadelphia: Lea & Febiger, 1977.

Katz BJ, Nerad JA. Ophthalmic manifestations of fibrous dysplasia. *Ophthalmology* 1998;105:2207–2215.

Zizmor J. Orbital radiology in unilateral exophthalmos. In: Turtz AI, ed. *Proceedings of the Centennial Symposium: Manhattan Eye, Ear, and Throat Hospital, Vol I.* St. Louis: CV Mosby, 1969.

HYPERTROPHY OF ORBITAL BONES (HYPEROSTOSIS OR SCLEROSIS OR BOTH)

1. Acromegaly
2. Anemias of childhood (severe: Cooley, sickle cell, spherocytosis, iron deficiency)
3. Cerebral atrophy (childhood)
4. Craniostenosis

5. Engelmann disease (hereditary diaphyseal dysplasia)
6. Hyperostosis frontalis interna
7. Idiopathic
8. Infantile cortical hyperostosis (Caffey disease)
9. Microcephaly
10. Myotonia atrophica (myotonic dystrophy, Curschmann–Steinert syndrome)
11. Osteopetrosis (Albers–Schönberg disease)
12. Paget disease (osteitis deformans)
13. Tumors of orbit, including osteoma, fibrous dysplasia (Albright syndrome), meningioma, metastatic neuroblastoma, mixed tumors of lacrimal gland, transitional cell carcinomas of the nasopharynx

Albert DM, Jakobiec FA. *Principles and practice of ophthalmology.* Philadelphia: WB Saunders, 1994:1881–2095.

Jacobs L, et al. *Computerized tomography of the orbit and sella turcica.* New York: Raven Press, 1980.

Teplick JG, Hoskin ME. *Roentgenologic diagnosis*, 3rd ed. Philadelphia: WB Saunders, 1976.

EXPANSION OF OPTIC CANAL

1. Increased intracranial pressure
2. Inflammatory lesions
    A. Chiasmatic arachnoiditis
    B. Nonspecific granuloma
    C. Sarcoid granuloma
    D. Tuberculoma
3. Tumors
    A. Meningioma
    B. Metastatic sarcoma to choroid
    C. Neurofibromatosis (von Recklinghausen syndrome)
    D. Optic nerve glioma
    E. Retinoblastoma
4. Vascular lesions
    A. Arteriovenous malformation
    B. Ophthalmic artery aneurysm

Levin LA, Rubin PD. Advances in orbital imaging. *Int Ophthalmol Clin* 1992;32:1–25.

Potter GD, Trakel SL. Optic canal. In: Newton TH, Potts DG, eds. *Radiology of the skull and brain*, Vol 1, Book 2. St. Louis: CV Mosby, 1971.

Zizmor J. Orbital radiology in unilateral exophthalmos. In: Turtz AI, ed. *Proceedings of the Centennial Symposium: Manhattan Eye, Ear, and Throat Hospital, Vol I.* St. Louis: CV Mosby, 1969.

SMALL OPTIC CANALS

1. Developmental abnormalities
    A. Anophthalmos or microphthalmos
    B. Enucleation
    C. Craniosynostosis (CSO)
2. Dysostoses
    A. Osteopetrosis (Albers–Schönberg syndrome)
    B. Fibrous dysplasia (Albright syndrome)
    C. Pyle disease (craniometaphyseal dysplasia syndrome)
    D. Paget disease (osteitis deformans)

3. Inflammatory lesions—osteitis
4. Tumor—meningioma

Albert DM, Jakobiec FA. *Principles and practice of ophthalmology*. Philadelphia: WB Saunders, 1994:1881–2095.

Potter GD, Trokel SL. Optic canal. In: Newton TH, Potts DG, eds. *Radiology of the skull and brain*, Vol 1, Book 2. St. Louis: CV Mosby, 1971.

EROSION OF OPTIC CANAL

1. Lateral wall
   A. Pituitary tumor
   B. Aneurysm of internal carotid artery
   C. Craniopharyngioma
   D. Tumor of orbital apex
2. Medial wall
   A. Carcinoma of sphenoid sinus
   B. Mucocele of sphenoid sinus
   C. Granuloma of sphenoid sinus
3. Roof
   A. Tumor of anterior cranial fossa
   B. Surgical unroofing
4. Decrease in length
   A. Tumor of orbital apex
5. Complete destruction
   A. Malignant tumor
   B. Eosinophilic granuloma

Albert DM, Jakobiec FA. *Principles and practice of ophthalmology*. Philadelphia: WB Saunders, 1994:1881–2095.

Potter GD, Trakel SL. Optic canal. In: Newton TH, Potts DG, eds. *Radiology of the skull and brain*, Vol 1, Book 2. St. Louis: CV Mosby, 1971.

Zizmor J. Orbital radiology in unilateral exophthalmos. In: Turtz AI, ed. *Proceedings of the Centennial Symposium: Manhattan Eye, Ear, and Throat Hospital, Vol I*. St. Louis: CV Mosby, 1969.

ENLARGEMENT OF SUPERIOR ORBITAL FISSURE

1. Carotid cavernous fistula
2. Chronic increased intracranial pressure
3. Extension of infraorbital mass into fissure
4. Intracavernous carotid aneurysm
5. Intracranial chordoma
6. Masses within middle fossa
7. Metastatic carcinoma to sphenoid wings
8. Nasopharyngeal carcinoma—rare
9. Neurofibromatosis including optic nerve glioma
10. Orbital dysplasia
11. Orbital varix
12. Pituitary neoplasm—changes in sella and clinoid process
13. Posterior orbital encephalocele
14. Sarcomas, neurilemoma, or other orbital malignancies

Albert DM, Jakobiec FA. *Principles and practice of ophthalmology*. Philadelphia: WB Saunders, 1994:1881–2095.

Grimson BS, Perry DD. Enlargement of the optic disk in childhood optic nerve tumors. *Am J Ophthalmol* 1984; 97:627–631.

Shields JA, et al. Orbital neurilemoma with extension through the superior orbital fissure. *Arch Ophthalmol* 1986; 104:871–873.

NARROWING OF SUPERIOR ORBITAL FISSURE

1. Chronic hemolytic anemias of childhood
2. Fibrous dysplasia (Albright syndrome)
3. Meningioma
4. Osteitis
5. Osteoblastoma
6. Osteoma
7. Osteopetrosis (Albers–Schönberg syndrome)
8. Paget disease (osteitis deformans)

Albert DM, Jakobiec FA. *Principles and practice of ophthalmology.* Philadelphia: WB Saunders, 1994:1881–2095.

Jacobs L, et al. *Computerized tomography of the orbit and sella turcica.* New York: Raven Press, 1980.

Kieffer SA. Superior orbital fissure. In: Newton TH, Potts DG, eds. *Radiology of the skull and brain*, Vol 1, Book 2. St. Louis: CV Mosby, 1971.

SMALL ORBIT

1. Anophthalmos
2. Enucleation
3. Microphthalmos
4. Mucocele

Kieffer SA. Orbit. In: Newton TH, Potts DG, eds. *Radiology of the skull and brain*, Vol 1, Book 2. St. Louis: CV Mosby, 1971.

Sarnat BG. Eye and orbital size in the young and adult. *Ophthalmologica* 1982;185:74–89.

LARGE ORBIT

1. Congenital
   A. Dysplasia
   B. Glaucoma
   C. Serous cysts
2. Pseudotumor
3. Tumors within the muscle cone
   A. Hemangiomas
   B. Neurofibroma
   C. Optic glioma
   D. Orbital varix
   E. Retinoblastoma

Albert DM, Jakobiec FA. *Principles and practice of ophthalmology.* Philadelphia: WB Saunders, 1994:1881–2095.

Kieffer SA. Orbit. In: Newton TH, Potts DG, eds. *Radiology of the skull and brain*, Vol 1, Book 2. St. Louis: CV Mosby, 1971.

HEMATIC ORBITAL CYSTS (BLOOD CYST OF ORBIT)

1. Blood dyscrasia
2. Cavernous hemangioma

3. Childbirth
4. Lymphangioma
5. Orbital blunt trauma
6. Spontaneous hemorrhage
7. Vascular disease

Albert DM, Jakobiec FA. *Principles and practice of ophthalmology*. Philadelphia: WB Saunders, 1994:1881–2095.

Jacobson DM, et al. Maternal orbital hematoma associated with labor. *Am J Ophthalmol* 1988;105:547–553.

Shapiro A, et al. A clinicopathologic study of hematic cysts of the orbit. *Am J Ophthalmol* 1986;102:237–241.

2

Lids

CONTENTS

MONGOLOID PALPEBRAL FISSURE (TEMPORAL CANTHUS HIGHER THAN NASAL CANTHUS)

1. Esotropia syndrome
2. Exotropia syndrome
3. Amniogenic band syndrome (Streeter dysplasia)
4. Anhidrotic ectodermal dysplasia
5. Cebocephalia (fetalis hypoplastica)
6. Chondrodystrophia (Conradi syndrome)
7. Chromosome short-arm deletion
8. Congenital spherocytic anemia
9. Crouzon syndrome (hereditary craniofacial dysostosis)
10. Duplication 14Q syndrome
11. Femoral-facial syndrome
12. Fetal hydantoin syndrome
13. Hereditary ectodermal dysplasia syndrome (Siemen syndrome)
14. Jacobs syndrome (triple X syndrome)
15. Jarcho–Levin syndrome
16. Klinefelter XXY syndrome (gynecomastia–aspermatogenesis syndrome)
17. Laurence–Moon–Biedl syndrome (retinitis pigmentosa–polydactyl–adiposogenital syndrome)
18. Meckel syndrome (dysencephalia–splanchnocystic syndrome)
19. Miller–Dieker syndrome
*20. Mongoloid (trisomy or Down syndrome)
*21. Asian persons
22. Peters trisomy 5p (Peters anomaly)
23. Otopalataodigital syndrome
24. Pfeiffer syndrome
25. Pleonosteosis syndrome (Leri syndrome, carpal tunnel syndrome)
26. Prader–Willi syndrome
27. Rhizomelic chondrodysplasia punctata syndrome
28. Trisomy mosaic and 9p- syndromes
29. Trisomy syndrome
30. Trisomy 6Q syndrome
31. Trisomy 9Q syndrome
32. Trisomy and 18q syndrome

* = most important

33. Trisomy 20p syndrome
34. XXXXX syndrome
35. XXXXY syndrome
36. 4p- syndrome
37. 5p- syndrome

Isenberg SJ. *The eye in infancy*. Chicago: Year Book Medical, 1989.

Roy FH. *Ocular syndromes and systemic diseases*, 3rd ed. Philadelphia: Lippincott Williams & Wilkins, 2002.

ANTIMONGOLOID PALPEBRAL FISSURE (DOWNWARD DISPLACEMENT OF TEMPORAL CANTHUS)

1. Aarskog syndrome (faciodigitogenital syndrome)
2. Acrocephalosyndactylia (Apert syndrome)
3. Esotropia and exotropia
4. Bird-headed dwarf syndrome (Seckel syndrome)
5. Baraitser–Winter syndrome
6. Cardiofaciocutaneous syndrome
7. Cerebral gigantism (Sotos syndrome)
8. Cleft palate
9. Chromosome short-arm deletion
10. Cloverleaf cranium
11. Coffin–Lowry syndrome
12. Cohen syndrome
13. Congenital facial hemiatrophy (Möbius syndrome)
14. Craniocarpotarsal dysplasia (Freeman–Sheldon syndrome; whistling face syndrome)
15. Craniofacial dysostosis (Crouzon syndrome)
16. Cri-du-chat syndrome (Cry of the cat syndrome)
17. De Lange syndrome (congenital muscular hypertrophy–cerebral syndrome)
18. Di George syndrome
19. Epidermal nevus syndrome (ichthyosis hystrix)
20. Lethal multiple pterygium syndrome (LMPS)
21. Linear nevus sebaceous of Jadassohn (Jadassohn-type anetoderma)
22. Mandibulofacial dysostosis (Franceschetti syndrome and Treacher–Collins syndrome)
23. Marchesani syndrome (dystrophia mesodermalis congenita hyperplastica)
24. Maxillofacial dysostosis
25. Nager syndrome
26. Noonan syndrome (male Turner syndrome)
27. Obesity–cerebral–ocular–skeletal anomalies syndrome
28. Oculoauriculovertebral dysplasia (Goldenhar syndrome)
29. Oculomandibulofacial dyscephaly (Hallermann–Streiff syndrome)
30. Organoid nevus syndrome
31. Otopalatodigital syndrome (OPD)
32. Pyknodysostosis
33. Partial trisomy of long arm of chromosome 630. Pseudo-Ullrich–Turner syndrome
34. Ring D chromosome
35. Rubinstein–Taybi syndrome (broad thumbs syndrome)
36. Ruvalcaba syndrome
37. Saethre–Chotzen syndrome
38. 3-P syndrome

*39. Trauma
40. Trisomy 9p syndrome
41. Trisomy syndrome
42. Trisomy 17p syndrome
43. Trisomy 20P syndrome
44. Trisomy syndrome (E syndrome)
45. Turner syndrome (gonadal dysgenesis)
46. Wolf syndrome (chromosome partial deletion syndrome)
47. 4q- syndrome
48. 21q syndrome
49. 9p syndrome

Isenberg SJ. *The eye in infancy*. Chicago: Year Book Medical, 1989.

Roy FH. *Ocular syndromes and systemic diseases*, 3rd ed. Philadelphia: Lippincott Williams & Wilkins, 2002.

PSEUDOPTOSIS

Pseudoptosis includes conditions that simulate ptosis, but lid droop is not the result of levator malfunction, and ptosis is usually corrected when the causative factors are cleared up or removed.

1. Due to globe displacement
    A. Anophthalmia including poorly fitting prosthesis
    *B. Enophthalmos such as that resulting from blowout fracture of the floor of the orbit or atrophy of orbital fat
    *C. Microphthalmia
    *D. Phthisis bulbi
    E. Hypotony and inward collapse of eye
    F. Cornea plana
    G. Hypotropia of that eye or hypertropia of the other eye
2. Due to mechanical displacement of the lid
    A. Inflammation
        (1) Trachoma—thick, heavy lid
        *(2) Chalazion or hordeolum
        (3) Elephantiasis
        (4) Chronic conjunctivitis–conjunctival thickening
        (5) Traumatic or infectious edema involving the lid
        *(6) Blepharitis
        (7) Corneal foreign body
        (8) Contact lens
        (9) Sinusitis, cellulitis
    B. Tumors, especially fibromas, lipomas, or hemangiomas
    C. Scar tissue due to burns, physical trauma, and lacerations that can bind the lid down
    D. Tumors of lacrimal gland—S-shaped lid
*3. Dermatochalasis (ptosis adiposa, baggy lids, "puffs"—senile atrophy of the lid skin)
4. Blepharochalasis—a rare condition occurring in young persons, characterized by recurrent bouts of inflammatory lid edema with subsequent stretching of the skin
5. The oriental lid—the palpebral fissure is narrower than normal and the upper lid rarely has a furrow; hence, the fold usually hangs down to or over the lid margin.

6. Dissociated vertical deviation (DVD)
7. Duane syndrome (retraction syndrome)
8. Blepharospasm—eyebrow lower than normal, hemifacial spasm
9. Contralateral widening of the lid fissure as pseudoproptosis (see p. 4), exophthalmos, or lid retraction (see p. 62)
10. Vertical strabismus

Beard C. *Ptosis*. St. Louis: CV Mosby, 1969.

Beyer CK, et al. Naso-orbital fractures, complications, and treatment. *Ophthalmology* 1982;89:456.

Crawford JS. Ptosis: is it correctable and how? *Ann Ophthalmol* 1971;3:452–456.

Huber A. *Eye symptoms in brain tumors*, 2nd ed. St. Louis: CV Mosby, 1971.

BLEPHAROPTOSIS (PTOSIS, DROOPY UPPER LID; WEAK LEVATOR PALPEBRAE SUPERIORIS MUSCLE)

1. Congenital ptosis
    *A. Simple (most congenital ptosis)—may be the result of autosomal dominant inheritance
    B. Complicated ptosis
        (1) Ptosis with ophthalmoplegia (most congenital ptosis)—the most commonly involved muscle is the superior rectus
        (2) Ptosis with other lid deformities such as epicanthus, blepharophimosis, microphthalmia, and lid coloboma—may be hereditary
        (3) Synkinetic (paradoxical) ptosis-aberrant nervous connections from the other extrinsic muscles of the eye and jaw to the levator muscle
            a. Marcus Gunn phenomenon (jaw-winking reflex)—motor root of the fifth cranial nerve to the muscle of mastication also is misdirected through the third nerve to the levator muscle.
            b. Phenomenon of Marin Amat (reverse jaw-winking reflex)
            c. Misdirected third nerve syndrome—bizarre eyelid movements that may accompany various eye movements; the ptotic eyelid may rise as the medial rectus, the inferior rectus, or the superior rectus muscle contracts.
        (4) Horner syndrome
    C. Involutional ptosis
    D. Mechanical
        (1) Periorbital tumor
        (2) Neuroma, neurofibroma
        (3) Cicatricial skin changes
2. Acquired ptosis
    A. Traumatic ptosis
        (1) Eyelid laceration
        (2) Postsurgical ptosis
            a. Anterior transposition of inferior oblique muscle
            b. Enucleation
            c. Orbital operation
            d. Cataract operation
            e. Radial keratotomy

* = most important

      (3) Foreign bodies lying in the roof of the orbit

      (4) Fracture of orbital roof, also following contusion with resulting hematoma but without fracture

      (5) Air-blast injury

      (6) Botulinum toxin treatment of strabismus and blepharospasm

      (7) Prolonged hard contact lens wear

      (8) Infratemporal fossa foreign body

B. Neurogenic ptosis

      (1) Peripheral involvement of the third nerve

      (2) Basilar, cortical, and nuclear lesions

      (3) Cerebral hemorrhages, tumors, or abscesses

      (4) Multiple neuritis, nerve syphilis, or multiple sclerosis

      (5) Horner syndrome—lower lid higher than other lower lid

      (6) Familial dysautonomia (Riley–Day syndrome)

      (7) Misdirected third nerve syndrome—following third nerve palsy the fibers do not regrow into their respective muscles.

      (8) Aseptic meningitis, transient

      (9) Pituitary tumor

C. Myogenic ptosis

      (1) Primary muscular atrophy (late familial ptosis); ptosis is usually the only symptom.

      (2) Dystrophia myotonia, in which there is dystrophia not only of the extraocular muscles but also of the face, neck, and extremities

      (3) Myasthenia gravis, nonfamilial acquired ptosis

      (4) The congenital fibrosis syndrome characterized by bilateral ptosis and gradual fibrosis of all the extraocular muscles

      (5) Oculopharyngeal muscular dystrophy characterized by dysphagia and progressive bilateral ptosis

      (6) Progressive familial myopathic ptosis and involvement of one, some, or all extraocular (and no other) muscles of one or both eyes

      (7) Late spontaneous unilateral ptosis

      (8) Amyloid degeneration with involvement of the levator muscle

    *(9) Senility—loss of general muscle tone and atrophy of orbital fat

    (10) Ptosis and normal pregnancy

    (11) Hyperthyroidism and ptosis—following active stages

    (12) Drugs, including the following:

adenine arabinoside	butalbital	desoxycorticosterone
adrenal cortex injection	butallylonal	dexamethasone
alcohol	butethal	dextrothyroxine
aldosterone	carbon dioxide	digitalis
allobarbital	carbromal	dimethyl tubocurarine
amobarbital	chloral hydrate	diphtheria and tetanus
amodiaquine	chloroquine	toxoids and pertussis
aprobarbital	cocaine(?)	(DPT)
aurothioglucose	cortisone	disulfiram(?)
aurothioglycanide	cyclobarbital	fludrocortisone
barbital	cyclopentyl allylbarbituric	fluorometholone
betamethasone	acid	flu-prednisolone
butabarbital	cyclopentobarbital	F3T

* = most important

gold Au-198
gold sodium thiomalate
heptabarbital
hexethal
hexobarbital
hydrocortisone
hydroxychloroquine
idoxuridine
isocarboxazid
isosorbide dinitrate(?)
loxapine
measles virus vaccine (live)
medrysone
mephenesin
mephobarbital
metharbital
methitural
methohexital

methyl alcohol
methylpentynol
methylprednisolone
metocurine iodide
nalidixic acid(?)
nialamide
opium
oral contraceptives
paramethasone
pentobarbital
phencyclidine
phenelzine
phenobarbital
phenoxybenzamine
prednisolone
prednisone
primidone
probarbital

secobarbital
succinylcholine
sulthiame
talbutal
tetraethylammonium
thiamylal
thiopental
tolazoline
tranylcypromine
triamcinolone
trichloroethylene
trifluorothymidine
tubocurarine
vidarabine
vinbarbital
vinblastine
vincristine

(13) Corticosteroid ptosis—prolonged use of topical corticosteroid therapy
(14) Mascara ptosis—due to subconjunctival deposits of mascara
(15) Ptosis associated with chronic conjunctivitis and uveitis
(16) Use of botulinum toxin
   D. Protective ptosis following injury to the eye
   E. Mechanical ptosis
      (1) Tumor
         a. Benign tumor—such as neurofibroma or hemangioma
         b. Malignant tumor—such as basal cell carcinoma, squamous cell carcinoma, malignant melanoma, or rhabdomyosarcoma
         c. Metastatic lesion—such as from breast or lung
         d. Sinus extension—such as mucocele of frontal sinus
      (2) Blepharochalasis—hereditary with recurrent attacks of severe edema and residual damage to the tissues
      (3) Cicatricial ptosis—such as that secondary to cicatricial conjunctivitis (see p. 49–50) or surgical trauma to the superior fornix
      (4) Contact lens migration
      (5) Palpebral form of vernal conjunctivitis
      (6) Intracranial extension—such as chordoma

Bodker FS, et al. Acquired blepharoptosis secondary to essential blepharospasm. *Ophthalmic Surgery* 1993;24: 546–550.

Fraunfelder FT, Fraunfelder FW. *Drug-induced ocular side effects.* Woburn, MA: Butterworth-Heinemann, 2001.

Frueh BR. The mechanistic classification of ptosis. *Ophthalmology* 1980;87:1019.

Grant CA, et al. An infratemporal fossa foreign body presents as an infraorbital mass. *Arch Ophthalmol* 2000;118: 993–995.

Hertle RW, et al. Congenital unilateral fibrosis, blepharoptosis, and enophthalmos syndrome. *Ophthalmology* 1992; 99:347–355.

Kushner BJ. The effect of anterior transposition of the inferior oblique muscle on the palpebral fissure. *Arch Ophthalmol* 12000;18:1542–1544.

Roy FH. *Ocular syndromes and systemic diseases*, 3rd ed. Philadelphia: Lippincott Williams & Wilkins, 2002.

Vaughn GL, et al. Variable diplopia and blepharoptosis after orbital floor fracture repair. *Am J Ophthalmol* 1994; 117:407–409.

SYNDROMES AND DISEASES ASSOCIATED WITH PTOSIS

1. Aarskog syndrome (faciogenital dysplasia)—x-linked
2. Acquired immunodeficiency syndrome
3. Addison disease (idiopathic hypoparathyroidism)
4. Alacrima congenital with distichiasis, conjunctivitis, keratitis—autosomal dominant
5. Albers–Schönberg syndrome (marble bone disease)
6. Albright syndrome (osteitis fibrosa disseminata)
7. Amyloidosis (Lubarsch–Pick syndrome)
8. Apert syndrome (acrocephalosyndactylia syndrome)
9. Arteriovenous fistula
10. Axenfeld–Schurenberg syndrome (cyclic oculomotor paralysis)
11. Babinski–Nageotte syndrome (medullary tegmental paralysis)
12. Basal cell carcinoma
13. Bassen–Kornzweig syndrome (abetalipoproteinemia)
14. Bell palsy (idiopathic facial paralysis)
15. Bing–Neel syndrome (Bing disease)
16. Blepharophimosis syndrome
17. Bonnet–Dechaume-Blanc syndrome (neuroretinoangiomatosis)
18. Bonnevie–Ullrich syndrome (pterygolymphangiectasia)
19. Botulism
20. Brown syndrome (superior oblique tendon sheath syndrome)
21. Carpenter syndrome (acrocephalopolysyndactyly II)
22. Cavernous sinus syndrome (Foix syndrome)
23. Cerebral palsy
24. Cestan–Chenais syndrome (Cestan syndrome)
25. Chromosome long-arm deletion syndrome
26. Chromosome partial deletion (long-arm) syndrome (de Grouchy syndrome)
27. Chromosome short-arm deletion syndrome
28. Congenital fibrosis syndrome (all extraocular muscles)
29. Congenital fibrosis of the inferior rectus with ptosis—autosomal dominant
*30. Congenital ptosis
    A. Simple failure of peripheral differentiation of muscles—dominant
    B. Ptosis with blepharophimosis—dominant
    C. Ptosis due to ophthalmoplegia—autosomal dominant
31. Craniocarpotarsal dysplasia (Freeman–Sheldon syndrome)
32. Craniocervical syndrome (whiplash injury)
33. Cretinism (juvenile hypothyroidism)
34. Creutzfeldt–Jakob syndrome (spastic pseudosclerosis)
35. Cri-du-chat syndrome (Cry of the cat syndrome)
36. Crouzon syndrome (craniofacial dysostosis)
37. Cushing syndrome (2) (cerebellopontine angle syndrome)
38. Dandy–Walker syndrome (atresia of foramen Magendie)
39. Dawson disease (subacute sclerosing panencephalitis)
40. Dejerine–Klumpke syndrome (lower radicular syndrome)
41. de Lange syndrome (congenital muscular hypertrophy—cerebral syndrome)
42. Devic syndrome (ophthalmoencephalomyelopathy)
43. Diphtheria
44. Dubowitz syndrome (dwarfism–eczema–peculiar facies)

45. Duck-bill lips, low-set ears—autosomal dominant
46. Eaton–Lambert syndrome (myasthenic syndrome)
47. Eclampsia and preeclampsia
48. Ehlers–Danlos syndrome (fibrodysplasia elastic generalisata)
49. Engelmann syndrome (osteopathia hyperostotica scleroticans multiplex infantalis)
50. Epidermal nevus syndrome (ichthyosis hystrix)
51. Erb–Goldflam syndrome (myasthenia gravis)
52. Erysipelas (St. Anthony fire)
53. Fabry syndrome
54. Faciorenal acromesometic syndrome
55. Fisher syndrome (ophthalmoplegia–ataxia–areflexia syndrome)
56. Fetal alcohol syndrome
57. Fetal trimethadione
58. Foramen lacerum syndrome (aneurysm of internal carotid artery syndrome)
59. Freeman–Sheldon syndrome
60. Garcin syndrome (half-base syndrome)
61. Gerlier disease (paralytic vertigo)
62. Gillum–Anderson syndrome (dominant blepharoptosis, high myopia)
63. Guillain–Barré syndrome (acute infectious neuritis)
64. Hairy elbow syndrome
65. Hemangiomas
66. Herpes zoster
67. Hodgkin disease
68. Horner syndrome (cervical sympathetic paralysis)
69. Hunter syndrome [mucopolysaccharidosis (MPS) II]
70. Hurler disease (MPS I)
71. Hyperammonemia
72. Hyperparathyroidism
73. Hyperthyroidism (Basedow syndrome)
74. Hypocalcemia
*75. Hypoparathyroidism
76. Hysteria
77. Infectious mononucleosis
78. Influenza
79. Jugular foramen syndrome (Vernet syndrome)
80. Kearns–Sarne syndrome
81. Kiloh–Nevin syndrome (muscular dystrophy of external ocular muscles)
82. Kohn–Romano syndrome (blepharoptosis, blepharophimosis, epicanthus inversus, telecanthus)
83. Komoto syndrome (congenital eyelid tetrad)
84. Krause syndrome (congenital encephaloophthalmic dysplasia)
85. Kugelberg–Welander syndrome (progressive proximal muscle atrophy)
86. Kussmaul disease (necrotizing angiitis)
87. Laurence–Moon–Bardet–Biedl syndrome (retinitis pigmentosa–polydactyly–adiposo-genital syndrome)
88. Leigh disease (subacute necrotizing encephalomyelopathy)
89. Little syndrome (nail–patella syndrome)
90. Lymphangioma
91. Lymphedema

* = most important

92. Malaria
93. Malignant hyperthermia syndrome
94. Maple-syrup urine disease (branched-chain ketoaciduria)
95. Marcus Gunn syndrome (jaw-winking syndrome)
96. Marin Amat syndrome (inverted Marcus Gunn syndrome)
97. MERRF syndrome
98. Micro syndrome
99. Misdirected third nerve syndrome
100. Möbius syndrome (congenital paralysis of the sixth and seventh nerves)
101. Morquio syndrome (keratosulfaturia)
102. Mucormycosis
103. Multiple sclerosis (disseminated sclerosis)
104. Myopathy, centronuclear with external ophthalmoplegia—autosomal dominant
105. Myotonic dystrophy syndrome (Curschmann–Steinert syndrome)
106. Myotubular myopathy—autosomal recessive or x-linked
107. Naffziger syndrome (scalenus anticus syndrome)
108. Neurilemoma
109. Neuroblastoma
110. Neurofibromatosis
111. Nonne–Milroy–Meige disease (congenital trophedema)
112. Noonan syndrome (male Turner syndrome)
113. Oculopharyngeal muscular dystrophy
114. Ophthalmoplegic migraine syndrome
115. Ophthalmoplegic—retinal degeneration (Kearns–Sayre syndrome)
116. Orodigital–facial syndrome (Papillon–Léage and Psaume syndrome)
117. Pachydermoperiostosis (Touraine–Solente–Gole syndrome)
118. Pancoast syndrome (superior pulmonary sulcus syndrome)
119. Parinaud syndrome (paralysis of vertical movements)
120. Parkinson syndrome (paralysis agitans)
121. Parry–Romberg syndrome (progressive facial hemiatrophy)
122. Periocular and ocular metastatic tumors
123. Pierre–Robin syndrome (micrognathia–glossoptosis syndrome)
124. Poliomyelitis
125. Progressive intracranial arterial occlusion syndrome
126. Purpura and ptosis—combined inheritance with male-to-male transmission
127. Raeder syndrome (paratrigeminal paralysis)
128. Retraction syndrome (Duane syndrome)—autosomal dominant
129. Retroparotid space syndrome
130. Riley–Day syndrome (congenital familial dysautonomia)
131. Ring D chromosome
132. Rollet syndrome (orbital apex–sphenoidal syndrome)
133. Rubinstein–Taybi syndrome (broad thumbs syndrome)
134. Scleroderma (progressive systemic sclerosis)
135. Scurvy (vitamin C deficiency)
136. Shy–Gonatas syndrome (similar to Hunter and Refsum syndrome)
137. Smith–Lemli–Opitz syndrome (cerebrohepatorenal syndrome)
138. Smith syndrome (facioskeletogenital dysplasia)
139. Sparganosis
140. Spider bites

Ptosis

	Congenital Ptosis	Traumatic Ptosis	Neurogenic Ptosis as Horner Syndrome	Myogenic Ptosis as Myasthenia Gravis	Drugs as Steroid Ptosis	Mechanical Ptosis as Neurofibroma	Cicatricial Ptosis as Following Conjunctivitis
History							
1. Bilateral	S			U	S		U
2. Birth injury		U					
3. Familial	S			S		S	
4. Trauma/surgery		U					
5. More in females				U			S
6. Photophobia							U
7. Prolonged use of topical corticosteroids					U		
8. Transient diplopia				U		S	
9. Visual loss		S					
10. Weakness/fatigability	S	S		U		S	
Physical Findings							
1. Accomodative insufficiency				R			
2. Amblyopia	S						
3. Astigmatism	S					S	S
4. Blepharophimosis-ptosis syndrome	S						
5. Conjunctival discharge							U
6. Disc hypoplasia	R						
7. Enophthalmos	S		U				
8. Epiphora							U
9. Extraocular muscle fibrosis	S						
10. Heterochromia of iris			S				
11. Involved lid higher in downgaze	U						
12. Lagophthalmos	S						
13. Levator disinsertion		U				S	S
14. Lid crease absent	U	S	U				
15. Lid crease present		U			U	U	U
16. Lid lag in downgaze	U	S					
17. Lower lid somewhat elevated			U				
18. Miotic pupil			U				
19. Moderate/marked ptosis with fair/poor levator function	S						
20. Myopia	S						
21. Nystagmus	S				S		
22. Orbicularis oculi weakness				U			
23. Paradoxical lid retraction				U			
24. Ptosis decreases downgaze	U						
25. Ptosis increases upgaze	U					U	U
26. Ptosis same in upgaze and downgaze		U					
27. Slight ptosis with good levator function	U			U		U	U
28. S-shaped lid margin						U	

Ptosis (Continued)	Congenital Ptosis	Traumatic Ptosis	Neurogenic Ptosis as Horner Syndrome	Myogenic Ptosis as Myasthenia Gravis	Drugs as Steroid Ptosis	Mechanical Ptosis as Neurofibroma	Cicatricial Ptosis as Following Conjunctivitis
Physical Findings							
29. Strabismus	S						
30. Transient hyperemic, anhidrotic, warm ipsilateral face			U				
31. Transient increased accommodation			S				
32. Upper salcus deeper uninvolved side		U					
Laboratory Data							
1. Hydroxyamphetamine or cocaine 4% drops pharmacologic test			U				
2. Positive tensilon test				U			

R = rarely; S = sometimes; and U = usually.

141. Strabismus and ectopic pupils—autosomal dominant
142. Subclavian steal syndrome
143. Syphilis (acquired lues)
144. Syringomyelia (Passow syndrome)
145. Temporal arteritis syndrome (Hutchinson–Horton–Magath–Brown syndrome)
146. Thirteen Q syndrome (microcephaly, high nasal bridge, thumb hypoplasia)
147. Tolosa–Hunt syndrome (painful ophthalmoplegia)
148. 3p syndrome
149. Trachoma
150. Treft syndrome (optic atrophy and hearing loss)
151. Triploidy (chromosomes instead of 46)
152. Trisomy (E syndrome)
153. Tuberculosis
154. Tunbridge–Paley disease (juvenile diabetes, optic atrophy and hearing loss)
155. Turner syndrome (gonadal dysgenesis)
156. van Bogaert–Hozay syndrome
157. Vertebral fusion, posterior lumbosacral with ptosis—autosomal dominant
158. von Herrenschwand syndrome (sympathetic heterochromia)
159. von Recklinghausen syndrome (neurofibromatosis)
160. Waardenburg syndrome (embryonic fixation syndrome)
161. Wallenberg syndrome (dorsolateral medullary syndrome)
162. Weber syndrome (cerebellar peduncle syndrome)
163. Wernicke syndrome (hemorrhagic polioencephalitis superior syndrome)

Larned DC, et al. The association of congenital ptosis and congenital heart disease. *Ophthalmology* 1986;93:492–494.

McKusick VA. *Mendelian inheritance in man*, 12th ed. Baltimore: Johns Hopkins University Press, 1998.

Roy FH. *Ocular syndromes and systemic diseases*, 3rd ed. Philadelphia: Lippincott Williams & Wilkins, 2002.

SPECIFIC BLEPHAROPTOSIS

1. Unilateral ptosis with dilated pupil—tumor or abscess of temporal lobe and third nerve palsy
2. Unilateral ptosis with miosis—midbrain lesion near the posterior commissure and Horner syndrome
3. Ptosis with disturbance of integrated ocular movement—lesion near superior colliculus
4. Bilateral ptosis with small immobile pupils and loss of upward rotation of eyeballs—lesion near posterior commissure
5. Ptosis with loss of voluntary elevation but normal involuntary elevation of the lid when the eye looks up—supranuclear lesion
6. Ptosis in repose and normal elevation with active motion—hereditary cerebellar ataxia of Pierre-Marie
7. Ptosis onset in adolescent—familial chronic external ophthalmoplegia
8. Ptosis may be early and only sign of nuclear paralysis in:
    A. Botulism
    B. Multiple sclerosis (disseminated sclerosis)
    C. Hemorrhagic superior poliomyelitis of Wernicke
    D. Tabes
    E. Vasospasm of ophthalmoplegic migraine
9. Ptosis with cranial nerve dysfunction suggests a basal lesion, such as the following:
    A. Aneurysm

    B. Epidemic paralyzed vertigo (Gerlier disease)
    *C. Herpes zoster
    D. Meningitis
    E. Polyneuritis of cranial nerves
    *F. Trauma
10. Transient ptosis
    A. Acute exanthema
    B. Acute infection such as erysipelas
    *C. Botulinum toxin injection
    D. Eclampsia
    E. Exogenous poisons such as those due to alcohol, lead, carbon monoxide, arsenic, snake venom
    F. Hematoma
    G. Influenza
    H. Scurvy (vitamin C deficiency)
11. Ptosis with orbicularis weakness—muscle disease
12. S-shaped ptosis
    A. Chronic chalazion
    B. Cyst on lateral border of tarsus
    C. Dermoid
    D. Floppy eyelid syndrome
    E. Lacrimal gland enlargement or prolapse
    F. Lateral levator palpebrae superioris muscle dehiscence
    G. Neurofibromatosis
    H. Trachoma
    I. Drugs, including the following:

acebutolol
acetophenazine
alseroxylon
atenolol
auronofin
beclomethasone
botulinum A toxin
bupivacaine butaperazine
carphenazine
carteolol
chloroprocaine
chlorpromazine
cisplatin
combination products of
  estrogens and
  progestogens
contraceptives
dapiprazole hydrochloride
deserpidine
diacetylmorphine
diethazine
estradiol
ethopropazine

etidocaine
fluvoxamine
gold sodium thiosulfate
guanethidine
labetalol
levodopa
levothyroxine
liothyronine
liotrix
loxapine
medroxyprogesterone
meperidine
mepivacaine
meprednisone
mesoridazine
methdilazine
methotrimeprazine
methoxyflurane
metoprolol
nadolol
perphenazine
phenytoin
pindolol
piperacetazine

practolol
procaine
prochlorperazine
promazine
promethazine
propiomazine
propoxycaine
propranolol
rauwolfia serpentina
rescinnamine
reserpine
syrosingopine
thiethylperazine
thiopropazate
thioproperazine
thioridazine
thyroglobulin
tobramycin
trifluridine
trifluromazine
trimeprazine
trimethadione
trimethaphan

* = most important

Dunn WJ, et al. Botulinum toxin for the treatment of dysthyroid ocular myopathy. *Ophthalmology* 1986;93: 4770–4775.

Gerner EW, Hughes SM. Floppy eyelid with hyperglycinemia. *Am J Ophthalmol* 1984;98:614–615.

Haessler FH. *Eye signs in general disease.* Springfield, IL: Charles C Thomas, 1960.

HORNER SYNDROME

Horner syndrome comprises paralysis of sympathetic nerve supply with lid ptosis, miosis, apparent enophthalmos, frequently dilatation of the vessels with absence of sweating (anhidrosis) on homolateral side; the pupil demonstrates a decreased sensitivity to cocaine and hypersensitivity to adrenalin and may have heterochromia with congenital Horner syndrome.

1. Region of first neuron—lesions of hypothalamus and diencephalic region also suggest diabetes insipidus, disturbed temperature regulation, adiposogenital syndrome, and autonomic epidemic epilepsy of Penfield.
    A. Arnold–Chiari malformation
    B. Basal meningitis, such as in syphilis
    C. Base-of-skull tumors (e.g., melanoma)
    D. Multiple sclerosis
    E. Pituitary tumor
    F. Tumor of the third ventricle
    G. Midbrain, such as in syphilis
    H. Pons, such as in intrapontine hemorrhage
    I. Medulla, such as in Wallenberg syndrome (lateral medullary syndrome)—thrombosis of posterior inferior cerebellar artery
    J. Cervical region
        (1) Syringomyelia
        (2) Tumor
        (3) Injury as traumatic dislocation of cervical vertebrae or dissection of the vertebral artery
        (4) Syphilis (acquired lues)
        (5) Poliomyelitis
        (6) Meningitis
        (7) Amyotrophic lateral sclerosis
        (8) Related to scleroderma and facial hemiatrophy
        (9) Vascular malformation such as agenesis of internal carotid artery
2. Region of second neuron
    A. Spinal birth injury—Klumpke paralysis with injured lower brachial plexus
    B. Cervical rib
    C. Charcot–Tobias syndrome
    D. Thoracic lesions
        (1) Pancoast tumor—in apex of lung, such as carcinoma or tuberculosis
        (2) Aneurysm of aorta, subclavian, or carotid artery
        (3) Central venous catheterization
        (4) Mediastinal tumors
        (5) Lymphadenopathy of Hodgkin disease, leukemia, lymphosarcoma, or tuberculosis
        (6) Stellate ganglion block
        (7) Tube thoracostomy

   E. Neck
- *(1) Enlarged lymph gland, tumors, aneurysm, and thyroid gland
- (2) Carcinoma of esophagus
- (3) Retropharyngeal tumors
- (4) Neuroma of sympathetic chain
- (5) Intraoral trauma with damage to internal carotid plexus
- (6) Thin intervertebral foramina of spinal cord, such as in pachymeningitis, hypertrophic spinal arthritis, ruptured intervertebral disc, and meningeal tumors
- (7) Traction of sternocleidomastoid muscle, such as from positioning on operating table
- (8) Complications of tonsillectomy
- (9) Mandibular tooth abscess
- *(10) Lesions of middle ear, such as in acute purulent otitis media and petromastoid operation
- (11) Carotid artery dissection
- (12) Internal carotid artery occlusion

3. Region of third neuron
   A. Aneurysm of internal carotid and its branches
   B. Paratrigeminal syndrome (Raeder syndrome)
   C. Cavernous sinus syndrome (Foix syndrome)
   D. Tumors of cysts of orbit
   E. Drugs can affect any region and include the following:

acetophenazine	levodopa	promethazine
alseroxylon	lidocaine	propiomazine
bupivacaine	mepivacaine	propoxycaine
butaperazine	mesoridazine	rauwolfia serpentina
carphenazine	methdilazine	rescinnamine
chloroprocaine	methotrimeprazine	reserpine
chlorpromazine	oral contraceptives	syrosingopine
deserpidine	perazine	thiethylperazine
diacetylmorphine	pericyazine	thiopropazate
diethazine	perphenazine	thioproperazine
ethopropazine	piperacetazine	thioridazine
etidocaine	prilocaine	trifluoperazine
fluphenazine	procaine	triflupromazine
guanethidine	prochlorperazine	trimeprazine
influenza virus vaccine	promazine	

   F. Cluster headaches (migrainous neuralgia)
   G. Herpes zoster
   H. Migraine
   I. Fetal varicella syndrome

Fraunfelder FT, Fraunfelder FW. *Drug-induced ocular side effects.* Woburn, MA: Butterworth-Heinemann, 2001.

Roy FH. *Ocular syndromes and systemic diseases*, 3rd ed. Philadelphia: Lippincott Williams & Wilkins, 2002.

Ryan FH, et al. Congenital Horner's syndrome resulting from agenesis of the internal carotid artery. *Ophthalmology* 2000;107:185–188.

Smith EF, et al. Herpes zoster ophthalmicus as a cause of Horner syndrome. *J Clin Neuro-Ophthalmol* 1993;13: 250–253.

* = most important

Horner syndrome

	Region of First Neuron as Pituitary Tumor	Region of Second Neuron as Pancoast Tumor	Region of Third Neuron as Cluster Headaches
History			
1. Begins during second to third decades			U
2. Cervical trauma/surgery		U	
3. Common during fourth to seventh decades	U		
4. Common–bronchogenic carcinoma		S	
5. Common in males		U	U
6. Common—meningioma and internal carotid aneurysm			U
7. Common—single intracranial neoplasm (adenoma)	U		
8. Family			U
9. Head trauma			S
10. Visual loss in one or both eyes	S		
Physical Findings			
1. Anhidrosis homolateral side	U	U	S
2. Apparent enophthalmos	U	U	S
3. Bitemporal hemianopia	U		
4. Extraocular muscle palsies	U		
5. Failure of pupil dilation with hydroxyamphetamine 1%	U		S
6. Heterochromia of iris			U
7. Increased accommodation	R	R	
8. Ipsilateral lacrimation	U	U	
9. Miosis			U
10. Narrowing of palpebral fissure	U	U	U
11. Ocular hypotony		U	
12. Optic disc pallor	U	U	S
13. Papilledema	S		
14. Proptosis	R		
15. Ptosis	S		
16. Pupil dilates little with cocaine 4%	U	U	U
17. Recurrent ocular pain	U	U	U
18. Third nerve palsy			U
19. Transient dilated vessels conjunctiva/face			U
20. Trigeminal anesthesia	U	U	U
Laboratory Data			
1. Carotid arteriography			U
2. Computed tomographic scan of head	U	U	U
3. Cervical planigrams		U	
4. Pituitary panel—serum prolactin, growth hormone, adrenocorticotropic hormone, follicle-stimulating hormone, luteinizing hormone, thyroid-stimulating hormone	S		
5. Pneumoencephalography	S		S
6. Visual field test	U		
7. Roentgenogram of chest		U	
8. Roentgenogram of skull	U		S

R = rarely; S = sometimes; and U = usually

PTOSIS OF LOWER LID (UNCOMMON DROOPING OF LOWER LID SO THAT LID MARGIN IS ADJACENT TO GLOBE BUT BELOW LIMBUS)

1. Blepharophimosis syndrome
*2. Cicatricial with mechanical displacement by scar, tumor, or skin disease; may be associated with ectropion
*3. Paralytic due to lower lid lagophthalmos
4. Pseudoptosis such as in exophthalmos and higher degrees of myopia
5. Idiopathic

Fox SA. Idiopathic blepharoptosis of lower eyelid. *Am J Ophthalmol* 1972;74:330–331.

Leatherbarron B, Collin JR. Eyelid surgery in facial palsy. *Eye* 1991;5:585–590.

LAGOPHTHALMOS (INABILITY TO CLOSE EYELIDS VOLUNTARILY)

*1. Physiologic—many people sleep with their eyes open, especially Asian people
2. Orbital—extreme proptosis
3. Mechanical—scarring of the lids or retractor muscles
4. Paralytic
    A. Seventh nerve palsy (see p. 66)
    B. Leprosy
    C. Lesions of cerebral cortex and its projections, including bilateral frontal lesions
5. Psychological
    A. Failure to comprehend the command
    *B. Unwillingness to comply with the command

Harvey JT, Anderson RL. Lid lag and lagophthalmos. *Ophthalmol Surg* 1981;12:338.

Lessell S. Supranuclear paralysis of voluntary lid closure. *Arch Ophthalmol* 1972;88:241–244.

PSEUDO–LID RETRACTION

*1. Exophthalmos
2. Unilateral high axial myopia
3. Unilateral congenital glaucoma
4. Congenital cystic eyeball
5. Abnormalities of orbit
    A. Asymmetry
    B. Shallow such as in Crouzon disease (dysostosis craniofacialis)
    C. Harlequin—shallow orbit with arched superior and lateral wall, such as in hypophosphatasia
6. Ptosis of other eyelid

Fox SA. The palpebral fissure. *Am J Ophthalmol* 1966;62:73–78.

Walsh FB, Hoyt WF. *Clinical neuro-ophthalmology*, 4th ed. Baltimore: Williams & Wilkins, 1985.

LID RETRACTION

Lid retraction is defined normally as more than 85% of vertical palpebral fissures and 10 mm or less with the eyelids just concealing the corneoscleral limbus at the 12 and 6 o'clock meridians.

1. Lid retraction with upward movement of eye

    A. Congestive dysthyroid disease

    B. Deficiency in upward gaze—following rectus operation or weakness of superior rectus

    C. Excessive stimulation of levator muscles in Bell phenomenon with seventh nerve palsy

    D. Levator muscles receive excessive stimuli from nerve fiber of superior rectus

    E. Pretectal or periaqueductal lesion in midbrain

2. Lid retraction with downward movement of eye

    A. Aberrant regeneration of third nerve of inferior rectus to levator (pseudo-Graefe phenomenon)—elevation of lid in downward gaze

    B. Brown syndrome (superior oblique tendon sheath syndrome)

    C. Extrapyramidal syndrome of postencephalic parkinsonism and progressive supranuclear palsy

    D. Failure of levator to relax on downward movement of eye

        (1) Secondary neuromuscular

      *(2) Mechanical, such as from a scar

    E. Noncongestive type of dysthyroid exophthalmos (Graefe sign)—lid lag in downward gaze

3. Lid retraction with horizontal gaze

    A. Duane syndrome (retraction syndrome)

    B. Underaction of lateral rectus muscle and spillover to levator causing widening

4. Lid retraction because of supranuclear lesions—usually bilateral when due to lesion in or about posterior commissure (Collier sign, tucked lids, posterior fossa stare)

    A. Bulbar poliomyelitis

    B. Chorea (Huntington hereditary chorea)

    C. Closed head injury associated with defective adduction of eyes, coarse nystagmus, nuclear palsy, pyramidal signs

    D. Coma due to disease of ventral midbrain and pons

    E. Craniostenosis

    F. Epidemic encephalitis

    G. Hydrocephalic infants

    H. Hydrophobia

    I. Hysteria

    J. Malingering

    K. Meningitis

    L. Multiple sclerosis (disseminated sclerosis)

    M. Parinaud syndrome (divergence paralysis)

    N. Parkinson disease (paralysis agitans)

    O. Russell syndrome

    P. Sylvian aqueduct syndrome (Koerber–Solus–Elschnig syndrome)

    Q. Syphilis (tabes)

    R. Tumors of the midbrain; meningiomas of sphenoid wing; sellar, parasellar, and suprasellar tumors; and frontal or temporal lobe tumors

    S. von Economo syndrome (encephalitis lethargica)

5. Lid retraction because of neuromuscular disease—commonly asymmetric or unilateral

    A. Drugs

        (1) Phenylephrine and other sympathomimetics

        (2) Prostigmin and Tensilon, especially with myasthenic levator involvement

* = most important

(3) Succinylcholine, subparalytic doses

(4) Thyroid extract

B. Fuch phenomenon—healing of injured third nerve, previously ptotic lid has involuntarily spastic raising with movements of eyes

C. Infant lid retraction—transient because of maternal hyperthyroidism

D. Irritation of cervical sympathetic nerve (Horner syndrome)

*E. Mechanical suspension of lid such as that due to scar, tumor, surgical attachment to frontalis muscle, or shortening of levator muscle or following glaucoma filtering procedures

F. Peripheral seventh nerve paresis with loss of orbicularis oculi muscle tone

6. Lid retraction with myopathic disease

A. Associated with hepatic cirrhosis

B. Thyroid myopathy (Graves disease, Basedow syndrome)

(1) Dalrymple sign—widening of palpebral fissure

(2) Stellwag sign—retraction of upper lid associated with infrequent or incomplete blinking

7. Lid retraction following operations on vertical muscles, such as recession of superior rectus muscle or simultaneous recession and restriction of the levator by common fascial check ligament between the two muscles

8. Paradoxical lid retraction because of paradoxical levator innervation

A. Defective ocular abduction with abducens palsy

B. Lid retraction associated with ptosis of the opposite eyelid (levator denervation supersensitivity)

C. Misdirection of third nerve axons (following acquired or congenital lesions)—occurs on attempt to adduct, elevate, or depress eye

D. Movement of lower jaw

(1) Contraction of external pterygoid muscle by opening mouth (Marcus Gunn)

(2) Contraction of internal pterygoid muscle by closing the mouth

9. Physiologic

A. Act of surprise

B. Slow onset of blindness, such as that secondary to glaucoma and optic atrophy

C. Time of attention

Collins JR, et al. Congenital eyelid retraction. *Br J Ophthalmol* 1990;74:542–544.

Dixon R. The surgical management of thyroid-related upper eyelid retraction. *Ophthalmology* 1982;89:52.

Roy FH. *Ocular syndromes and systemic diseases*, 3rd ed. Philadelphia: Lippincott Williams & Wilkins, 2002.

Walsh FB, Hoyt WF. *Clinical neuro-ophthalmology*, 4th ed. Baltimore: Williams & Wilkins, 1985.

LID LAG

Lig lag is defined as occurring when the patient looks down and the eyelids lag behind briefly.

1. Congenital—usually in association with congenital ptosis
2. Hepatic failure
3. Iatrogenic—following ptosis surgery
4. Mechanical—scars of the upper lid
5. Myopathic disease

*A. Graefe sign—thyroid myopathy—the upper lid pauses and then follows the eye downward (Basedow syndrome)

* = most important

B. Myotonic dystrophia

C. Periodic myotonic lid lag—familial (hyperkalemic) myotonic periodic paralysis

6. Neuromuscular disease

A. Excessive intake of thyroid extract

B. Physiologic lagophthalmos—short upper tarsus in some Asian and some white persons with incomplete descent of the lid during sleep

7. Supranuclear origin—extrapyramidal syndromes have defective inhibition of lids in downward gaze

A. Congenital supranuclear lid lag

B. Guillain–Barré syndrome

C. Postencephalitic parkinsonism, Parkinson syndrome (shaking palsy)

D. Progressive supranuclear palsy

Kirkali P, Kansu T. Lid lag in hyperkalemic periodic paralysis. *Ann Ophthal* 1991;23:422–423.

Roy FH. *Ocular syndromes and systemic diseases*, 3rd ed. Philadelphia: Lippincott Williams & Wilkins, 2002.

Tan E, et al. Lid lag and the Guillain-Barré syndrome. *J Clin Neuro-Ophthal* 1990;10:121–123.

BLEPHAROSPASM (SPASMODIC EYELID CLOSURE)

Most common and important: Psychogenic onset commonly in children and young adults

1. Addison disease (adrenal cortical insufficiency)
2. Associated with syphilis, tetanus, and tetany
3. Basal ganglion dysfunction—onset usually after middle age; including Parkinson disease (shaking palsy)
4. Cerebral palsy
5. Cogan syndrome (nonsyphilitic interstitial keratitis) with vestibuloauditory symptoms
6. Drugs, including the following:

acetophenazine
amitriptyline
amodiaquine
amoxapine(?)
amphetamine
antazoline
brompheniramine
butaperazine
carbinoxamine
carphenazine
chloroquine
chlorpheniramine
chlorpromazine
clemastine
clomipramine
desipramine
dexbrompheniramine
dexchlorpheniramine
dextroamphetamine
dextrothyroxine
diethazine
dimercaprol

dimethindene
diphenhydramine
diphenylpyraline
doxepin
doxylamine
dronabinol
droperidol
emetine
ethopropazine
fluphenazine
haloperidol
hashish
hydroxychloroquine
imipramine
levodopa
levothyroxine
liothyronine
liotrix
lorazepam
marihuana
mesoridazine
methamphetamine

methdilazine
methotrimeprazine
nortriptyline
pentylenetetrazol
perazine
pericyazine
perphenazine
pheniramine
phenmetrazine
phenylephrine
piperacetazine
prochlorperazine
promazine
promethazine
propiomazine
protriptyline
pyrilamine
selegiline
tetrahydrocannabinol
thiethylperazine
thiopropazate
thioproperazine

thioridazine	trifluperidol	tripelennamine
thyroglobulin	triflupromazine	triprolidine
thyroid	trimeprazine	vidarabine
trifluoperazine	trimipramine	vinblastine

   7. Electrical injury
   8. Encephalitis
   9. Epidemic keratoconjunctivitis
10. Hallervorden–Spatz
11. Hereditary reflex blepharospasm
12. Idiopathic (essential)
13. Leprosy (Hansen disease)
14. Meige syndrome
15. Obsessive–compulsive disorder
*16. Pain or light sensitivity following injury or inflammation or foreign bodies of lids, conjunctiva, cornea, or iris
17. Photosensitivity and sunburn
18. Poison ivy dermatitis
19. Postencephalitic blepharospasm
20. Psychogenic obsessive–compulsive disorder—onset commonly in children and young adults
21. Psychologic reflex blepharospasm—seen in premature infants with tactile stimulation of lids
22. Sparganosis
23. Systemic scleroderma (progressive systemic sclerosis)
24. Thomsen syndrome (congenital myotonia syndrome)
25. Tourette syndrome (coprolalia, generalized tic)

Defazio G, et al. Genetic contribution to idiopathic adult-onset blepharospasm and cranial-cervical dystonia. *Eur Neurol* 1993;33:345–350.

Fraunfelder FT, Fraunfelder FW. *Drug-induced ocular side effects.* Woburn, MA: Butterworth-Heinemann, 2001.

Larumbe R, et al. Reflex blepharospasm associated with bilateral basal ganglia lesion. *Movement Disorders* 1993; 8:198–200.

Patel BC, Anderson RL. Blepharospasm. *Ophthalmic Practice* 1993;11:293–302.

Roy FH. *Ocular syndromes and systemic diseases*, 3rd ed. Philadelphia: Lippincott Williams & Wilkins, 2002.

FACIAL PALSY

Facial palsy is defined as paralysis of facial muscles supplied by the seventh nerve; orbicularis oculi paralysis may result in epiphora and ectropion.

1. Congenital
2. Birth injury with nerve crushed at exit of stylomastoid foramen
3. Myogenic paralysis
    A. Myotonic atrophia
    B. Facioscapulohumeral type of muscular dystrophy
    C. Myasthenia gravis (Erb–Goldflam syndrome)
    D. Hypokalemia, periodic
    E. Curare poisoning
    F. Botulism
    G. Congenital facial diplegia (Möbius syndrome)

H. Infants, from maternal ingestion of thalidomide

I. Kugelberg–Welander syndrome

4. Neurologic paralysis

    A. Supranuclear paralysis—upper face, including orbicularis relatively unaffected with affected lower face

        (1) Voluntary movement—pyramidal fibers involved, such as in Weber syndrome, with contralateral hemiplegia of face and limbs and ipsilateral oculomotor paralysis

        (2) Weakness or abolition of the emotional movements of the face with retention of full voluntary activity, such as with lesion of anterior part of frontal lobe or near optic thalamus

    B. Peripheral paralysis—involvement of upper and lower face

        (1) Pontine lesion—associated structures involved include sixth nerve, conjugate ocular deviation to the same side, ipsilateral paralysis of jaw muscles, and pyramidal tract in paralysis of limb of opposite side

            a. Acute nuclear lesions, such as with anterior poliomyelitis, Landry paralysis, or degenerative conditions

            b. Foville syndrome—ipsilateral sixth nerve with loss of conjugate deviation to same side and hemiplegia of the opposite limbs

            c. Millard–Gubler syndrome—ipsilateral sixth nerve paralysis and hemiplegia of the opposite limbs

            d. Parotid gland surgery

            e. Progressive muscular atrophy

            f. Syringobulbia

            g. Tumors

            h. Vascular lesions

        (2) Posterior fossa—associated with nerve deafness, loss of taste on anterior two thirds of tongue, and occasionally diminution of tears

            a. Acoustic neuroma

            b. CHARGE (coloboma, heart disease, atresia choanae, retarded growth and retarded development or central nervous system anomalies, genital hypoplasia, and ear anomalies or deafness) syndrome association

            c. Facial neuritis due to polyneuritis cranialis, beriberi, encephalitis, diabetes, or intrathecal anesthesia

            d. Fracture of the skull

            e. Meningitis, including syphilitic and tuberculous

            f. Preauricular cyst associated with congenital cholesteatoma

            g. Tumors of facial nerve

        (3) Petrous temporal bone—associated with decreased lacrimation and salivary secretion, loss of taste on anterior two thirds of tongue, and intensified sensation of loud noises

            *a. Arteriosclerosis

            *b. Bell palsy—inflammation of facial nerve of unknown cause

            c. Cephalic tetanus

            d. Diabetes mellitus (Willis disease)

            e. Fractures

            f. Herpes zoster, spread from geniculate ganglion

            g. Hypertension

* = most important

    h. Nerve leprosy (Hansen disease)
  *i. Otitis media
    j. Secondary syphilis
  (4) Facial lesions at or beyond the stylomastoid foramen
    a. Fracture of the ramus of the mandible
    b. Melkersson–Rosenthal syndrome (Melkersson idiopathic fibroedema)
    c. Neoplasia or inflammatory swelling of parotid, such as in uveoparotid fever (Heerfordt disease) and Mikulicz disease
    d. Supporting lymph nodes behind the angle of the jaw

Eggenberger ER. Facial palsy in Lyme disease. *N Engl J Med* 1993;328:1571.

Lacombe D. Facial palsy and cranial nerve abnormalities in CHARGE association. *Am J Med Genet* 1993;15: 351–353.

Roy FH. *Ocular syndromes and systemic diseases*, 3rd ed. Philadelphia: Lippincott Williams & Wilkins, 2002.

INFREQUENT BLINKING

 *1. Contact lens use
  2. Encephalitis, acute
  3. Encephalitis or mild postencephalitic states
 *4. Ethanol intake
  5. Infants in first few months of life
  6. Parkinson syndrome, including mycostatic paresis of parkinsonism
  7. Psychotic states
  8. Progressive supranuclear palsy
  9. Thyrotoxicosis including exophthalmic ophthalmoplegia (Stellwag sign)

Roy FH. *Ocular syndromes and systemic diseases*, 3rd ed. Philadelphia: Lippincott Williams & Wilkins, 2002.

Walsh FB, Hoyt WF. *Clinical neuro-ophthalmology*, 4th ed. Baltimore: Williams & Wilkins, 1985.

FREQUENT BLINKING

 *1. Reflex—strong lights, sudden approach of objects toward eyes, loud noises, and touching the cornea; reflex blinking common in albinos and light intolerance
  2. Spontaneous—mental state and environment
    A. Children with habit spasm and facial tic
    B. Blepharospasm
   *C. Older persons with inadequate lacrimation and local irritation of the eyes
  3. Disorders of central nervous system disease, such as parkinsonism or various forms of pseudobulbar palsy
  4. Drugs, including the following:

acetylcholine	carbachol	etidocaine
allobarbital	carbamazepine	heptabarbital
ambenonium	chloroprocaine	hexethal
amobarbital	chloroquine	hexobarbital
amodiaquine	clofibrate	hydroxychloroquine
aprobarbital	cyclobarbital	isoflurophate
barbital bupivacaine	cyclopentobarbital	levodopa
butabarbital	demecarium	lidocaine
butalbital	dibucaine	mephobarbital
butallylonal	echothiophate	mepivacaine
butethal	edrophonium	methacholine

metharbital	pilocarpine	secobarbital
methitural	piperocaine	talbutal
methohexital	prilocaine	tetracaine
methylphenidate	primidone	thiamylal
neostigmine	probarbital	thiopental
pentobarbital	procaine	vinbarbital
phenobarbital	propoxycaine	
physostigmine	pyridostigmine	

Fraunfelder FT, Fraunfelder FW. *Drug-induced ocular side effects.* Woburn, MA: Butterworth-Heinemann, 2001.

Moses RA. *Adler's physiology of the eye*, 8th ed. St. Louis: CV Mosby, 1986.

Walsh FB, Hoyt WF. *Clinical neuro-ophthalmology*, 4th ed. Baltimore: Williams & Wilkins, 1985.

LID EDEMA (PUFFINESS OR BAGGINESS OF LIDS)

*1. Noninflammatory or minimally inflammatory swelling
    A. Acosta syndrome (Mountain climbers syndrome)
    B. Allergic gastroenteropathy with protein loss
    C. Arteriovenous fistula
    D. Cardiac and renal disease
        (1) Nephrosis and acute glomerulonephritis—early morning edema
        (2) Starvation and cachexia
    E. Dermatochalasis
    F. Elephantiasis
        (1) Chronic eczema or infection (erysipelas)
        (2) Hemolymphangioma
        (3) Leprosy (Hansen disease)
        (4) Lues (syphilis)
        (5) Melkersson–Rosenthal syndrome (Melkersson idiopathic fibroedema)
        (6) Nonne–Milroy–Meige disease (idiopathic hereditary lymphedema)
        (7) von Recklinghausen disease (neurofibromatosis)
        (8) Traumatic disruption of the lymph drainage system
        (9) Tuberculosis
    G. Endocrine exophthalmos (hyperthyroidism)
    H. Foix syndrome (cavernous sinus syndrome)
    I. Granulomatous ileocolitis
    J. Hutchinson syndrome (adrenal cortex neuroblastoma with orbital metastasis)
    K. Infectious generalized diseases
        (1) Diphtheria
        (2) Infectious mononucleosis
        (3) Malaria
        (4) Meningococcal meningitis
        (5) Pertussis (whooping cough)
        (6) Rheumatic fever
        (7) Scarlet fever
        (8) Trypanosomiasis
        (9) Tuberculosis
        (10) Yellow fever
    L. Melkersson-Rosenthal syndrome
    M. Nasal nerve syndrome (Charlin syndrome)

* = most important

N. Parasitic infestations
  (1) Anthrax
  (2) Ascariasis
  (3) Chlamydia
  (4) Dermatophytosis
  (5) Myiasis
  (6) Onchocerciasis syndrome (river blindness)
  (7) Tapeworms
  (8) Toxocariasis
  (9) Trichinosis
O. Protrusion of fat through orbital fascia
P. Retinoblastoma
Q. Stasis, including premenstrual edema
R. Superior vena cava syndrome
S. Systemic scleroderma (progressive systemic scleroderma)
*T. Tumors and pseudotumors
  (1) Benign and malignant ectodermal and mesodermal tumors
  (2) Brill–Symmers disease (lymphosarcoma)
  (3) Hemangiomas
  (4) Hodgkin disease
  (5) Leukemic deposit
  (6) Liposarcoma
  (7) Meningiomas of sphenoid ridge with impediment of venous circulation of ophthalmic veins or cavernous sinus
  (8) Neurofibromatosis
  (9) Pseudotumors
     a. Amyloid degeneration
     b. Eosinophilic or basophilic granulomas
U. Trauma
  (1) Basilar skull fractures
  (2) Injury
  *(3) Surgery
V. Angioneurotic edema caused by drugs, including the following:

acenocoumarol
acetaminophen
acetanilid
acetophenazine
acetyldigitoxin
acyclovir
adrenal cortex injection
albuterol
alcohol
aldosterone
allobarbital
alprazolam
aluminum nicotinate
aminosalicylate(?)
aminosalicylic acid(?)
amiodarone

amitriptyline
amobarbital
amoxapine
amoxicillin
ampicillin
anisindione
antazoline
antimony lithium thiomalate
antimony potassium tartrate
antimony sodium tartrate
antimony sodium
   thioglycolate
antipyrine
aprobarbital
aspirin
atropine

auranofin
aurothioglucose
aurothioglycanide
azatadine
bacitracin
barbital
belladonna
bendroflumethiazide
benzalkonium
benzathine penicillin G
benzphetamine
benzthiazide
betamethasone
betaxolol
bleomycin
botulinum A toxin

* = most important

brimonidine tartrate
brompheniramine
bupivacaine
busulfan
butabarbital
butalbital
butallylonal
butaperazine
butethal
cactinomycin
capreomycin
captopril
carbamazepine
carbenicillin
carbimazole
carbinoxamine
carisoprodol
carphenazine
cefaclor
cefadroxil
cefamandole
cefazolin
cefonicid
cefoperazone
ceforanide
cefotaxime
cefotetan
cefoxitin
cefsulodin
ceftazidime
ceftizoxime
ceftriaxone
cefuroxime
cephalexin
cephaloglycin
cephaloridine
cephalothin
cephapirin
cephradine
chloral hydrate
chlorambucil
chloramphenicol
chlordiazepoxide
chloroform
chloroprocaine
chlorothiazide
chlorpheniramine
chlorphentermine
chlorpropamide

chlorprothixene
chlortetracycline
chlorthalidone
chrysarobin
ciprofloxacin
cisplatin
clindamycin
clofibrate
clomipramine
clonazepam
clonidine
clorazepate
cloxacillin
cobalt
codeine
colloidal silver combination
    products
cortisone
cyclobarbital
cyclopentobarbital
cyclophosphamide
cyclosporine
cyclothiazide
cyproheptadine
cytarabine
dacarbazine
dactinomycin
danazol
dantrolene
dapiprazole hydrochloride
dapsone
daunorubicin
deferoxamine
demecarium
demeclocycline
desipramine
deslanoside
desoxycorticosterone
dexamethasone
dexbrompheniramine
dexchlorpheniramine
dextrothyroxine
dextran
DHT
diacetylmorphine
diatrizoate meglumine and
    sodium
diazepam
dichlorphenamide

dicloxacillin
dicumarol
diethazine
diethylcarbamazine
diethylpropion
digitalis
digitoxin
digoxin
diltiazem
dimethindene
dimethyl sulfoxide
diphenadione
diphenhydramine
diphenylpyraline
diphtheria and tetanus
    toxoids (adsorbed)
diphtheria and tetanus
    toxoids and pertussis
    vaccine (adsorbed)
disulfiram
doxepin
doxorubicin
doxycycline
doxylamine
droperidol
echothiophate
emetine
enalapril
ergonovine
ergotamine
erythromycin
ether
ethionamide
ethopropazine
ethosuximide
ethotoin
ethyl biscoumacetate
etidocaine
etretinate
F3T
fenfluramine
flecainide
floxuridine
fludrocortisone
fluorescein
fluorometholone
fluorouracil
fluphenazine
fluprednisone

flurazepam
gitalin
glyburide
gold Au 198
gold sodium thiomalate
gold sodium thiosulfate
griseofulvin
guanethidine
homatropine
hydralazine
halazepam
haloperidol
heparin
heptabarbital
hetacillin
hexethal
hexobarbital
hydrabamine penicillin V
hydrocortisone
ibuprofen
IDU (idoxuridine)
imipramine
indomethacin
insulin
iodide and iodine solution
  and compounds
iodipamide
  meglumine
iothalamate
  meglumine
iron dextran
isoniazid
isopropyl unoprostone
isosorbide
isotretinoin
ketoprofen
lanatoside C
latanoprost
leuprolide acetate
levodopa
levothyroxine
lidocaine
liothyronine
liotrix
lincomycin
lithium carbonate
loxapine
lorazepam
mannitol

maprotiline
measles and rubella virus
  vaccine (live)
measles, mumps, and rubella
  virus vaccine (live)
measles virus vaccine (live)
mecamylamine
medroxyprogesterone
medrysone
mefenamic acid mepivacaine
melphalan
mephenytoin
mephobarbital
meprednisone
meprobamate
mercuric oxide
methyldopa
mesoridazine
methacycline
metharbital
methdilazine
methicillin
methitural
methohexital
methotrimeprazine
methsuximide
methyl scopolamine
methysergide
methylene blue
methylergonovine
methylprednisolone
metoclopramide
metrizamide
metronidazole
mexiletine
mianserin
midazolam
minocycline
mitomycin
moxalactam
mumps virus vaccine (live)
nafcillin
nalidixic acid
naltrexone
naproxen
niacin
niacinamide
nicotinic acid
nicotinyl alcohol

nifedipine
nitrazepam
nitrofurantoin
nitromersol of estrogens and
  progestogens
olapatadine hydrochloride
oxprenolol
oral contraceptives
ouabain
oxacillin
oxyphenbutazone
oxytetracycline
paramethadione
paramethasone
penicillin
pentazocine
pentobarbital
perazine
pericyazine
perphenazine
phenacetin
phenobarbital
phenoxymethyl penicillin
phensuximide
phenylbutazone
phenylmercuric acetate
phenylmercuric nitrate
pimozide
piperacetazine
piperazine
piroxicam
poliovirus vaccine
polymyxin B prazosin
potassium penicillin G
potassium penicillin V
potassium phenethicillin
potassium phenoxymethyl
prazepam
prednisolone
prednisone
primidone
probarbital procaine
  penicillin G
procaine
prochlorperazine
promazine
promethazine
propiomazine
propofol
propoxycaine

protriptyline
quinacrine
quinidine
quinine
rabies immune globulin
rabies vaccine
radioactive iodides
ranitidine
rifampin
rubella and mumps virus
   vaccine (live)
rubella virus vaccine (live)
scopolamine
secobarbital
silver nitrate
silver protein
smallpox vaccine
sodium antimony gluconate
sodium iothalamate acid
   isoflurophate
sodium salicylate

streptomycin
succinylcholine
sulindac
suramin
talbutal
temazepam
tetanus immune globulin
tetanus toxoid
tetracycline
tetraethylammonium
thiabendazole
thiamylal
thiethylperazine
thimerosal
thyroglobulin
tolazamide
tolbutamide
tretinoin
trichloroethylene
trifluridine
trimethaphan

thiopental
thiopropazate
thioproperazine
thioridazine
thiotepa
thiothixene
tocainide
triamcinolone
triazolam
trifluoperazine
trifluperidol
triflupromazine
trimeprazine
trimethadione
trimethidium
trimipramine
vidarabine
vancomycin
verapamil
vinbarbital
vinblastine

2. Inflammatory edema
    A. Acute hemorrhagic conjunctivitis
    B. Allergic eczema (contact dermatitis)
        (1) Anesthetics
      *(2) Atropine (topical)
        (3) Eczematous keratoconjunctivitis
        (4) Iodine
        (5) Mercury
        (6) Neurodermatitis
        (7) Penicillin
        (8) Photodermatitis
        (9) Quincke edema
      (10) Tuberculosis (scrofula)
    C. Anthrax
    D. Bee sting of the cornea
    E. Dacryoadenitis
        (1) Acute dacryoadenitis
        (2) Chronic dacryoadenitis
    F. Epidemic keratoconjunctivitis
    G. Erysipelas
    H. Herpes simplex
    I. Hollenhorst syndrome (chorioretinal infarction syndrome)
    J. Hordeolum, chalazion
    K. Lymphogranuloma venereum
    L. Mycoses
    M. Ophthalmic zoster

* = most important

N. Other causes of lid edema
   (1) Conjunctival inflammations
      a. Diphtheria
      b. Newcastle disease (fowlpox)
      c. Ophthalmia neonatorum
      d. Parinaud syndrome (conjunctiva-adenitis syndrome)
   (2) Keratitis
   (3) Orbital inflammation
   (4) Periostitis
   (5) Scleritis (see p. 237–239)
      a. Posterior scleritis
      b. Scleromalacia perforans
   (6) Thermal, chemical, mechanical, or radiation injury
      a. Hypothermal injury
      b. Polychlorinated biphenyl (PCB)
O. Scalded skin syndrome (Ritter disease)
P. Serum sickness—systemic reaction to foreign serum, serum products, vaccines, penicillin, and sulfa drugs
Q. Silverman syndrome (battered-baby syndrome)
R. Spider bites
S. Urticaria due to drugs, including the following:

acenocoumarin	aurothioglycanide	cefadroxil
acetaminophen	azatadine	cefamandole
acetanilid	bacitracin	cefazolin
acetazolamide	barbital	cefonicid
acyclovir	Bacille Calmette-Guérin	cefoperazone
albuterol	(BCG) vaccine	ceforanide
allobarbital	bendroflumethiazide	cefotaxime
allopurinol	benzathine penicillin G	cefotetan
alprazolam	benzphetamine	cefoxitin
aluminum nicotinate	benzthiazide	cefsulodin
amiodarone	betamethasone	ceftazidime
amitriptyline	betaxolol	ceftizoxime
amobarbital	bleomycin	ceftriaxone
amoxapine	brompheniramine	cefuroxime
amoxicillin	bupivacaine	cephalexin
ampicillin	busulfan	cephaloglycin
anisindione	butabarbital	cephaloridine
antazoline	butalbital	cephalothin
antimony lithium thiomalate	butallylonal	cephapirin
antimony potassium tartrate	cactinomycin	cephradine
antimony sodium tartrate	capreomycin	chlorambucil
antimony sodium	captopril	chloramphenicol
thioglycollate	carbamazepine	chlordiazepoxide
antipyrine	carbenicillin	chloroprocaine
aprobarbital	carbimazole	chlorothiazide
aspirin	carbinoxamine	chlorpheniramine
auranofin	carisoprodol	chlorphentermine
aurothioglucose	cefaclor	chlorporthixene

chlortetracycline
chlorthalidone
cimetidine
cisplatin
clemastine
clindamycin
clofibrate
clomiphene
clomipramine
clonazepam
clonidine
clorazepate
cloxacillin
cobalt
codeine
cyclobarbital
cyclopentobarbital
cyclophosphamide
cyclosporine
cyclothiazide
cyproheptadine
cytarabine
dacarbazine
dactinomycin
danazol
dantrolene
dapsone
daunorubicin
deferoxamine
demeclocycline
desipramine
dexamethasone
dexbrompheniramine
dexchlorpheniramine
dextran
diacetylmorphine
diatrizoate meglumine and
    sodium
diazepam
dichlorphenamide
dicloxacillin
dicumarol
diethylcarbamazine
diethylpropion
digitalis
diltiazem
dimethindene
dimethyl imidazole
    carboxamide (DIC)

dimethyl sulfoxide (DMSO)
diphenadione
diphenhydramine
diphenylpyraline
diphtheria and tetanus
    toxoids (adsorbed)
diphtheria and tetanus
    toxoids and pertussis
    (DPT) vaccine (adsorbed)
diphtheria toxoids (adsorbed)
disulfiram
DPT vaccine
doxepin
doxorubicin
doxycycline
doxylamine
emetine
enalapril
erythromycin
ethionamide
ethotoin
ethoxzolamide
ethyl biscoumacetate
etidocaine
etretinate
fenfluramine
fenoprofen
flecainide
fluorescein
fluorouracil
flurazepam
flurbiprofen
framycetin
furosemide
gentamicin
glutethimide
gold Au 198
gold sodium thiomalate
gold sodium thiosulfate
griseofulvin
halazepam
heparin
heptabarbital
hetacillin
hexethal
hexobarbital
hydrabamine penicillin V
hydralazine
hydrochlorothiazide

hydrocortisone
hydroflumethiazide
hydromorphone
ibuprofen
imipramine
indapamide
indomethacin
influenza virus vaccine
insulin
interferon
iodide and iodine solutions
    and compounds
iodipamide meglumine
iophendylate
iothalamate meglumine and
    sodium
iothalamic acid
iron dextran
isoniazid
isosorbide
isotretinoin
ketoprofen
labetalol
levallorphan
levobunolol
lidocaine
lincomycin
lorazepam
loxapine
mannitol
maprotiline
measles and rubella virus
    vaccine (live)
measles, mumps, and rubella
    virus vaccine (live)
measles virus vaccine (live)
melphalan
meperidine
mephenytoin
mephobarbital
mepivacaine
meprobamate
mercuric oxide
methacycline
methadone
methaqualone
metharbital
methazolamide

methicillin
methimazole
methitural
methocarbamol
methohexital
methotrexate
methyclothiazide
methyldopa
methylphenidate
methylprednisolone
methylthiouracil
methyprylon
metoclopramide
metocurine iodide
metolazone
metoprolol
metrizamide
metronidazole
mianserin
midazolam
minocycline
mitomycin
morphine
moxalactam
mumps virus vaccine (live)
nafcillin
nalidixic acid
nalorphine
naloxone
naltrexone
naproxen
neomycin
neostigmine
niacin
niacinamide
nicotinyl alcohol
nifedipine
nitrazepam
nitrofurantoin
nitromersol
nortriptyline
opium
oral contraceptives
oxacillin
oxazepam
oxymorphone
oxyphenbutazone
oxytetracycline
penicillamine

pentazocine
pentobarbital
phenacetin
phendimetrazine
phenindione
pheniramine
phenobarbital
phenprocoumon
phentermine
phenylbutazone
phenylmercuric acetate
phenylmercuric nitrate
piperazine
piroxicam
poliovirus vaccine
polythiazide
potassium penicillin G
potassium penicillin V
potassium phenethicillin
practolol
prazepam
prazosin
prilocaine
primidone
probarbital
procaine
procaine penicillin G
procarbazine
propoxycaine
propranolol
propylthiouracil
protriptyline
pyrilamine
quinacrine
quinethazone
quinidine
quinine
rabies immune globulin
rabies vaccine
radioactive iodides
ranitidine
rifampin
rubella and mumps virus
    vaccine (live)
rubella virus vaccine (live)
secobarbital
smallpox vaccine
sodium antimonylgluconate
sodium salicylate

stibocaptate
stibogluconate
stibophen
streptomycin
succinylcholine
sulfacetamide
sulfachlorpyridazine
sulfacytine
sulfadiazine
sulfadimethoxine
sulfamerazine
sulfameter
sulfamethazine
sulfamethizole
sulfamethoxazole
sulfamethoxypyridazine
sulfanilamide
sulfaphenazole
sulfapyridine
sulfasalazine
sulfathiazole
sulfisoxazole
sulindac
suramin
talbutal
temazepam
tetanus immune globulin
tetanus toxoid
tetracycline
thiabendazole
thiamylal
thimerosal
thiopental
thiotepa
thiothixene
timolol
triamcinolone
triazolam
trichlormethiazide
trimethaphan
trimipramine
tripelennamine
triprolidine
tubocurarine
vancomycin
verapamil
vinbarbital
warfarin

T. Wegener syndrome (Wegener granulomatosis)

U. Vaccination

    (1) Ocular vaccina

    (2) Postvaccinial ocular syndrome

    (3) Variola

Cockerham KP, et al. Melkersson-Rosenthal syndrome. *Arch Ophthalmol* 2000;118:227–230.

Fraunfelder FT, Fraunfelder FW. *Drug-induced ocular side effects*. Woburn, MA: Butterworth-Heinemann, 2001.

Newell F. *Ophthalmology, principles and concepts*, 7th ed. St. Louis: CV Mosby, 1991.

Roy FH. *Ocular syndromes and systemic diseases*, 3rd ed. Philadelphia: Lippincott Williams & Wilkins, 2002.

Yeatts RP, White WL. Granulomatous blepharitis as a sign of Melkersson-Rosenthal syndrome. *Ophthalmology* 1997;104:1185–1190.

BLEEDING OF THE EYELID

1. Drugs, including the following:

acetazolamide
acetohexamide
allopurinol
alprazolam
amantadine
amitriptyline
aspirin
auranofin
aurothioglucose
aurothioglycanide
BCG vaccine
bendroflumethiazide
benzthiazide
betamethasone
betaxolol
carbamazepine
chlordiazepoxide
chlorothiazide
chlorpropamide
chlorthalidone
cimetidine
clofibrate
clonazepam
clorazepate
cyclothiazide
cytarabine
danazol
dapsone
desipramine
dexamethasone
diazepam
dichlorphenamide
diltiazem

emetine
ethoxzolamide
flurazepam
furosemide
glutethimide
glyburide
gold Au 198
gold sodium thiomalate
gold sodium thiosulfate
halazepam
hydrochlorothiazide
hydrocortisone
hydroflumethiazide
ibuprofen
imipramine
indapamide
indomethacin
influenza virus vaccine
interferon
ketoprofen
levobunolol
lorazepam
measles and rubella virus
  vaccine (live)
measles, mumps, and rubella
  virus vaccine (live)
measles virus vaccine (live)
methaqualone
methazolamide
methyclothiazide
methylprednisolone
methyprylon
metolazone

metoprolol
midazolam
mumps virus vaccine (live)
naproxen
nifedipine
nitrazepam
nortriptyline
oxazepam
oxprenolol
phenytoin
piperazine
piroxicam
polythiazide
prazepam
procarbazine
propranolol
protriptyline
quinethazone
quinine
rifampin
rubella and mumps virus
  vaccine (live)
rubella virus vaccine (live)
smallpox vaccine
sodium salicylate
sulfacetamide
sulfachlorpyridazine
sulfacytine
sulfadiazine
sulfadimethoxine
sulfamerazine
sulfameter
sulfamethazine

sulfamethizole	sulfathiazole	tolbutamide
sulfamethoxazole	sulfisoxazole	triamcinolone
sulfamethoxypyridazine	temazepam	triazolam
sulfanilamide	tetanus immune globulin	trichlormethiazide
sulfaphenazole	tetanus toxoid	verapamil
sulfapyridine	timolol	
sulfasalazine	tolazamide	

   2. Hutchinson syndrome (adrenal cortex neuroblastoma with orbital metastasis)

*3. Trauma

Fraunfelder FT, Fraunfelder FW. *Drug-induced ocular side effects*. Woburn, MA: Butterworth-Heinemann, 2001.

ECTROPION (LID MARGIN TURNED OUTWARD FROM THE EYEBALL)

1. Congenital ectropion
   - A. With distichiasis
   - B. With tight septum; microblepharon
   - C. With partial coloboma
   - D. With mandibulofacial dysostosis (Franceschetti syndrome)
   - E. With megaloblepharon (euryblepharon)
   - F. With microphthalmos or buphthalmos
   - G. Cerebrooculofacioskeletal syndrome
   - H. Down syndrome (mongolism)
   - I. Hartnup syndrome (niacin deficiency)
   - J. Lowe syndrome (oculocerebrorenal syndrome)
   - K. Miller syndrome
   - L. Milroy disease (oromandibular dystonia)
   - M. Robinow syndrome
   - N. Sjögren–Larrson syndrome
2. Acquired ectropion
   - A. Spastic ectropion
     - *(1) Acute spastic ectropion
     - (2) Blepharophimosis syndrome
     - *(3) Chronic spastic ectropion becoming cicatricial ectropion
     - (4) Hypothermal injury
     - (5) Myasthenia gravis—afternoon onset (Erb–Goldflam syndrome)
     - (6) Siemen syndrome (hereditary ectodermal dysplasia syndrome)
   - B. Atonic ectropion
     - (1) Anophthalmic socket
     - (1) Bell palsy (Idiopathic facial paralysis)
     - (2) Guillain–Barré syndrome (acute infectious neuritis)
     - (3) Paralytic ectropion—lagophthalmos, such as in seventh nerve palsy
     - *(4) Senile ectropion—tissue relaxation
   - C. Cicatricial ectropion
     - (1) Amendola syndrome
     - (2) Blastomycosis
     - (3) Collodion baby syndrome (congenital ichthyosis)
     - (4) Chronic dermatitis
     - (5) Cutaneous T-cell

    (6) Etretinate therapy

    (7) Excessive skin excision

    (8) Facial burns and scarring

    (9) Hydroa vacciniforme

    (10) Kabuki makeup syndrome

    (11) Leprosy (Hansen disease)

    (12) Orbital fracture repair

    (13) Palmoplantar keratodermia

    (14) Postblepharoplasty ectropion

    (15) Psoriasis (psoriasis vulgaris)

    (16) Radiation

    (17) Sézary syndrome (malignant cutaneous reticulosis syndrome)

    (18) Systemic fluorouracil

    (19) Thermal burns

    (20) Trauma

    (21) Transformation from chronic spastic ectropion

    (22) Zinsser–Engman–Cole syndrome (dyskeratosis congenita with pigmentation)

  D. Allergic ectropion-anaphylactic, contact, and microbial (usually temporary)

    (1) Danbolt–Closs syndrome (acrodermatitis enteropathica)

    (2) Elschnig syndrome

  E. Mechanical

    (1) Kaposi disease (multiple idiopathic hemorrhagic sarcoma)

    (2) Leiomyoma

    (3) Lumps (chalazion, cysts, neurofibroma)

Hurwitz BS. Cicatricial ectropion: a complication of systemic fluorouracil. *Arch Ophthal* 1993;111:1608–1609.

Isenberg SJ. *The eye in infancy.* Chicago: Year Book Medical, 1989.

Roy FH. *Ocular syndromes and systemic diseases*, 3rd ed. Philadelphia: Lippincott Williams & Wilkins, 2002.

Stratakis CA, et al. A variant of the cerebro-oculo-facio-skeletal syndrome with congenital ectropion and a case of lamellar ichthyosis in the same family. *Clin Genet* 1994;45:162–163.

ENTROPION (INVERSION OF LID MARGIN)

1. Congenital, including congenital epiblepharon—inferior oblique insufficiency; ectrodactyly, ectodermal dysplasia, cleft lip-palate syndrome, including with and without lower eyelid retractor insertion

  A. Inferior oblique insufficiency syndrome

  B. Dental–ocular–cutaneous syndrome

  C. Siemen syndrome (anhidrotic ectodermal dysplasia)

2. Acquired

  *A. Spastic entropion—acute, affecting lower lid, precipitated by acute inflammation or prolonged patching

  B. Mechanical entropion

    (1) Anophthalmos

    (2) Enophthalmos

    (3) Microphthalmos

    (4) Lymphedema

  *C. Senile entropion—relative enophthalmos secondary to fat atrophy

  D. Cicatricial entropion—physical and chemical burns of conjunctiva and cicatrizing diseases, including trachoma and leprosy

* = most important

    (1) Chronic cicatricial conjunctivitis
    (2) Leprosy (Hansen disease)
    (3) Radiation
    (4) Thermal burns
    (5) Trachoma
    (6) Following cryosurgery of the eyelid
    (7) Amendola syndrome
    (8) Variola

Bartley GB, et al. Congenital entropion with intact lower eyelid retractor insertion. *Am J Ophthalmol* 1991;112: 437–441.

Roy FH. *Ocular syndromes and systemic diseases*, 3rd ed. Philadelphia: Lippincott Williams & Wilkins, 2002.

Westfall CT, et al. Operative complications of the transconjunctival inferior fornix approach. *Ophthalmology* 1991; 98:1525–1528.

EPICANTHUS (FOLD OF SKIN OVER INNER CANTHUS OF EYE)

1. Types
   - A. Epicanthus inversus—fold arises in the lower lid and extends upward to a point slightly above the inner canthus; it is accompanied by long medial canthal tendons, blepharophimosis, and ptosis—autosomal dominant
   - *B. Epicanthus palpebralis (common type)—epicanthal fold arises from the upper lid above the tarsal region and extends to the lower margin of the orbit
   - C. Epicanthus supraciliaris (unusual type)—epicanthal fold arises near brow and runs toward tear sac
   - *D. Epicanthus tarsalis (Mongolian eye)—epicanthal fold arises from the tarsal (lid) fold and loses itself in the skin close to the inner canthus—autosomal dominant
2. Associated conditions
   - A. Aminopterin-induced syndrome
   - B. Basal cell nevus syndrome (Gorlin syndrome)
   - C. Bassen-Kornzweig syndrome (familial hypolipoproteinemia)
   - D. Bilateral renal agenesis
   - E. Blepharophimosis, ptosis, epicanthus inversus syndrome
   - F. Bonnevie-Ullrich syndrome (pterygolymphangiectasia)
   - G. Carpenter syndrome (acrocephalopolysyndactyly II)
   - H. Cat-eye syndrome (partial G-trisomy syndrome)
   - I. Cerebrofacioarticular syndrome of van Maldergen
   - J. Cerebrohepatorenal syndrome (Smith–Lemli–Opitz syndrome)
   - K. Chondrodystrophia (Conradi syndrome)
   - L. Chromosome long-arm deletion syndrome
   - M. Chromosome deletion (deletion 18)
   - N. Chromosome partial short-arm deletion syndrome (Wolf syndrome)
   - O. Chromosome short-arm deletion syndrome
   - P. Chromosome 13q partial deletion syndrome
   - Q. Congenital facial paralysis (Möbius syndrome)
   - R. Craniocarpotarsal syndrome (whistling face syndrome)
   - S. Craniosynostosis-radial aplasia (Baller–Gerold syndrome)
   - T. Cri-du-chat syndrome (Cry of the cat syndrome)
   - U. Dubowitz syndrome
   - V. Down syndrome (trisomy 21, mongolism)

* = most important

W. Drummond syndrome (idiopathic hypercalcemia, blue diaper syndrome)
X. Ehlers–Danlos syndrome (fibrodysplasia elastica generalisata)
Y. 18q syndrome
Z. Familial blepharophimosis
AA. Fetal alcohol syndrome
BB. Freeman–Sheldon syndrome (whistling face syndrome)
CC. 4Q syndrome
DD. Gansslen syndrome (hematologic-metabolic bone disorder)
EE. Greig syndrome (ocular hypertelorism syndrome)
FF. Hurler syndrome (dysostosis multiplex)
GG. Infantile hypercalcemia
HH. Jacobs syndrome (triple X syndrome)
II. Klinefelter XXY syndrome (gynecomastia-aspermatogenesis syndrome)
JJ. Kohn–Romano syndrome (ptosis, blepharophimosis, epicanthus inversus, and telecanthus)
KK. Komoto syndrome (congenital eyelid tetrad)
LL. Laurence–Moon–Bardet–Biedl syndrome (retinitis pigmentosa-polydactyly-adiposogenital)
MM. Leopard syndrome (multiple lentigines syndrome)
NN. Leroy syndrome (mucopolysaccharide excretion)
OO. Little syndrome (nail patella syndrome)
PP. Michel syndrome
QQ. Mohr–Claussen syndrome (similar to orodigitofacial syndrome)
RR. Noonan syndrome (Turner syndrome in males)
SS. Oculocerebrorenal syndrome (Lowe syndrome)
TT. Oculodentodigital dysplasia (microphthalmos syndrome)
UU. Potter syndrome (renofacial syndrome)
VV. Ring chromosome syndrome
WW. Ring chromosome syndrome
XX. Ring chromosome (microcephaly, hypertelorism, epicanthus)
YY. Ring chromosome in the D group (13–15)
ZZ. Robinow–Silverman–Smith syndrome
AAA. Rubinstein–Taybi syndrome (broad thumbs syndrome)
BBB. Schonenberg syndrome (dwarf-cardiopathy syndrome)
CCC. Smith syndrome (facioskeletogenital dysplasia)
DDD. TAR (thrombocytopenia absent radius) syndrome
EEE. Thalassemia
FFF. Trisomy syndrome (Edward syndrome)
GGG. Turner syndrome (gonadal dysgenesis)
HHH. Waardenburg syndrome (embryonic fixation syndrome)
III. X-linked mental retardation syndrome
JJJ. XXXXX syndrome

McKusick VA. *Mendelian inheritance in man*, 12th ed. Baltimore: Johns Hopkins University Press, 1998.

Roy FH. *Ocular syndromes and systemic diseases*, 3rd ed. Philadelphia: Lippincott Williams & Wilkins, 2002.

HYPOPIGMENTATION (DEPIGMENTATION OF EYELIDS)

1. Drugs, including the following:

adrenal cortex injection
alcohol
aldosterone beclomethasone
amodiaquine
arsenic
betamethasone
carbimazole
chloramphenicol
chloroquine
corticosteroids
cortisone
desoxycortiscosterone

dexamethasone
fludrocortisone
fluorometholone
fluprenisolone
gentamicin(?)
hydrocortisone
hydroquinone
hydroxychloroquine
isoflurophate
medrysone
meprednisone
mercaptoethylamine

methimazole
methotrexate
methylprednisolone
methylthiouracil
neostigmine
paramethasone
physostigmine
prednisolone
prednisone
propylthiouracil
thiotepa
triamcinolone

2. Genetic factors
   A. Albinism
   B. Chediak–Higashi syndrome (anomalous leukocytic inclusions with constitutional stigmata)
   C. Cross–McKusick–Breen syndrome
   D. Fanconi syndrome (amino diabetes)
   E. Hermansky–Pudlak syndrome (oculocutaneous albinism and hemorrhagic diathesis)
   F. Histidinemia
   G. Homocystinuria
   H. Incontinentia pigmenti achromians (hypomelanosis of Ito syndrome)
   I. Menkes syndrome (kinky hair syndrome)
   J. Nevus depigmentosus
   K. Phenylketonuria (Folling syndrome)
   L. Tuberous sclerosis (Bourneville syndrome)
   M. Vitiligo
   N. Vogt–Koyanagi–Harada syndrome (uveitis-vitiligo-alopecia-poliosis syndrome)
   O. Waardenburg syndrome (embryonic fixation syndrome)
   P. Woolf syndrome (chromosome partial deletion syndrome)
   Q. Ziprkowski–Margolis syndrome
3. Following cryosurgery of the eyelid
4. Burns (thermal, ultraviolet, ionizing, radiation)
5. Trauma
6. Kwashiorkor—malnutrition in children
7. Chronic protein deficiency or loss and malabsorption of vitamin B_{12}
8. Endocrine factors
   A. Hypopituitarism (Simmond syndrome)
   B. Addison disease (adrenal cortical insufficiency)
   C. Hyperthyroidism (Graves disease)
9. Inflammation and infection
   A. Discoid lupus erythematosus
   B. Eczematous dermatitis
   C. Leprosy (Hansen disease)
   D. Onchocerciasis syndrome (river blindness)
   E. Pinta

F. Pityriasis alba
G. Postinflammatory hypomelanoses
H. Post-kala-azar
I. Psoriasis
J. Sarcoidosis syndrome (Schaumann syndrome)
K. Syphilis (acquired lues)
L. Tinea versicolor
M. Vagabond leukoderma
N. Vitiligo
O. Yaws

10. Scleroderma (progressive systemic sclerosis)

Fraunfelder FT, Fraunfelder FW. *Drug-induced ocular side effects*. Woburn, MA: Butterworth-Heinemann, 2001.

Roy FH. *Ocular syndromes and systemic diseases*, 3rd ed. Philadelphia: Lippincott Williams & Wilkins, 2002.

HYPERPIGMENTATION (DISCOLORATION OF LIDS)

1. Deposits of the eyelids as caused by drugs, including:
2. Hyperpigmentation as caused by drugs, including the following:

acetophenazine
acid bismuth sodium tartrate
Alcian blue
actinomycin C
aluminum nicotinate
aminopterin
amiodarone
amodiaquine
amphotericin B
antipyrine
aurothioglucose
aurothioglycanide
bismuth oxychloride
bismuth sodium tartrate
bismuth sodium
   thioglycollate
bismuth sodium
   triglycollamate
bismuth subcarbonate
bismuth subsalicylate
   chloroquine
bleomycin
busulfan
butaperazine
calcitriol
carphenazine
chlorpromazine
chlortetracycline
chrysarobin

clofazimine
colloidal silver
cyclophosphamide
cytarabine
dactinomycin
demeclocycline
diethazine
doxycycline
dromostanolone
enalapril
epinephrine
ergocalciferol
ethopropazine
ferrocholinate
ferrous fumarate
ferrous gluconate
ferrous succinate
ferrous sulfate
floxuridine
fluorescein
fluorouracil
fluoxymesterone
fluphenazine
gold Au 198
gold sodium thiomalate
gold sodium thiosulfate
hydroxychloroquine
iron dextran
iron sorbitex

ketoprofen
mercaptopurine
mercuric oxide
mesoridazine
methacycline
methdilazine
methotrexate
methotrimeprazine
methylene blue
mild silver protein
minocycline
minoxidil
niacinamide
nicotinic acid
nicotinyl alcohol
nitromersol
oxytetracycline
penicillamine
perazine
pericyazine
perphenazine
phenylmercuric acetate
phenylmercuric nitrate
piperacetazine
pipobroman
polysaccharide-iron complex
practolol
procarbazine
prochlorperazine

promazine	sulfamethizole	thioproperazine
promethazine	sulfisoxazole	thioridazine
propiomazine	testolactone	trifluoperazine
quinacrine	testosterone	triflupromazine
rifampin	tetracycline	trimeprazine
rose bengal	thiethylperazine	uracil mustard
silver nitrate	thimerosal	vitamin A
silver protein	thimerosal thiopropazate	vitamin D_2
sulfacetamide	thioguanine	vitamin D_3

3. Periorbital hyperpigmentation—dark circles around the eye
    *A. Allergic rhinitis
    *B. Familial (autosomal dominant)
    C. Medium and dark complexioned white persons
4. Brown hyperpigmentation
    A. Genetic factors
        (1) Acanthosis nigricans
        (2) Albright syndrome (fibrous dysplasia)
        (3) Cafe-au-lait and freckle-like macules in neurofibromatosis
        (4) Dyskeratosis congenita
        (5) Fanconi syndrome (amino diabetes)
        (6) Freckles
        (7) Lentigines
        (8) Melanocytic nevus
        (9) Neurocutaneous melanosis
        (10) Seborrheic keratosis
        (11) Xeroderma pigmentosum
    B. Metabolic factors
        (1) Gaucher syndrome (cerebroside lipidosis)
        (2) Hemochromatosis
        (3) Niemann–Pick disease (essential lipoid histiocytosis)
        (4) Porphyria (cutanea tarda)
        (5) Wilson disease (hepatolenticular degeneration)
    C. Endocrine factors
        (1) adrenocorticotropic hormone (ACTH) therapy
        (2) Addison disease (adrenal cortical insufficiency)
        (3) Estrogen therapy
        (4) Melanoma
        (5) Pituitary tumors
        (6) Pregnancy
    D. Nutritional factors
        (1) Kwashiorkor (hypoproteinemia syndrome)
        (2) Pellagra (avitaminosis B_2)
        (3) Sprue
        (4) Vitamin B_{12} deficiency (Addison pernicious anemia)
    E. Chemical and pharmacologic agents
        (1) Arsenic
        (2) Berlock dermatosis
        (3) Bleomycin

       (4) Busulfan
       (5) Nitrogen mustard, topical
       (6) Photochemical agents
  F. Physical agents
       (1) Ionizing radiation
       (2) Thermal radiation
     *(3) Trauma
       (4) Ultraviolet light
  G. Inflammation and infection
       (1) Atopic dermatitis
       (2) Lichen planus
       (3) Lichen simplex chronicus
       (4) Lupus erythematosus discoid (Kaposi–Libman–Sacks syndrome)
       (5) Psoriasis
       (6) Tinea versicolor
  H. Neoplasms
       (1) Acanthosis nigricans
       (2) Malignant melanoma
       (3) Mastocytosis
  I. Miscellaneous factors
       (1) Autosomal recessive ectodermal dysplasia
       (2) Catatonic schizophrenia
       (3) Chronic hepatic insufficiency
       (4) Cronkhite-Canada syndrome
       (5) Encephalitis
       (6) Erythema dyschromicum perstans
       (7) Liver spots
       (8) Systemic scleroderma (progressive systemic sclerosis)
       (9) Whipple syndrome (intestinal lipodystrophy)
5. Blue, gray or slate hyperpigmentation
  A. Genetic factors
       (1) Blue melanocytic nevus
       (2) Dermal melanocytosis (Mongolian spot)
       (3) Franceschetti–Jadassohn syndrome (reticular pigmented dermatosis)
       (4) Incontinentia pigmenti (Bloch–Sulzberger syndrome)
       (5) Oculodermal melanocytosis
  B. Metabolic factors
       (1) Amyloidosis, cutaneous macular (Lubarsch–Pick syndrome)
       (2) Hemochromatosis
  C. Nutritional factors
       (1) Chronic nutritional insufficiency
  D. Inflammation and infection
       (1) Erythema dyschromicum perstans
       (2) Pinta
       (3) Riehl melanosis
  E. Chemical and pharmacologic agents
       (1) Chlorpromazine
       (2) Gold
       (3) Phenothiazine

* = most important

(4) Sulfonamides

(5) Tetracycline

F. Neoplasms

    (1) Slate-gray dermal pigmentation with metastatic melanoma and melano-genemia

G. Other

    (1) Blue dye

    (2) Cyanosis

Fraunfelder FT, Fraunfelder FW. *Drug-induced ocular side effects.* Woburn, MA: Butterworth-Heinemann, 2001.

Haddock N, Wilkin JK. Periorbital hyperpigmentation. *JAMA* 1981;246:835.

Pau H. *Differential diagnosis of eye diseases*, 2nd ed. New York: Thieme Medical, 1988.

Schwartz MP. Blue Christmas. *JAMA* 1987;257:3229–3230.

TUMORS OF EYELIDS

1. Molluscum contagiosum—small, greasy-appearing elevation that is usually umbilicated or any other granuloma

2. Neoplasm

    A. Basal cell epithelioma—common; may be a red, circumscribed, lobulated growth involving the lid margin or may have an umbilicated center (rodent ulcer)

    B. Squamous cell or Zeis cell epithelioma—hard pearly appearing lesion, usually without increased vascularity

    C. Meibomian-gland carcinoma—resembles a chalazion

    D. Metastatic tumors of the lid—respiratory tract, breast, skin (melanoma), gastrointestinal tract, or kidney

    E. Keratoacanthoma—benign, hemispherical, elevated tumor with a central keratin-filled crater; develops within several months

    F. Hemangioma—rubor of vascular tumor, usually having a smooth surface with tufts of vessels near the surface

    G. Benign mixed tumor of the lacrimal (palpebral) gland

    H. Trichilemmoma

    I. Lymphangioma

    J. Juvenile xanthogranuloma

3. Metaplasia or hyperplasia

    A. Trichoepithelioma

    B. Syringoma

   *C. Sebaceous adenoma

   *D. Papilloma-smooth, rounded, or pedunculated elevation

   *E. Nevus—usually pigmented, raised, and smooth surfaced; however, may be papillomatous or contain hair

    F. Benign calcifying epithelioma

    G. Inverted follicular keratosis

    H. Blue nevus—blue–black and velvet-like in appearance

    I. Freckles

    J. Lentigo simplex

    K. Solar lentigo

    L. Melasma

Tumors of eyelids	Molluscum Contagiosum*	Neoplasm as Basal Cell*	Metaplasia/Hyperplasia as Trichoepithelioma	Cyst as Sebacemon*	Lipoid Proteinosis	Pseudotumor of Lids
History						
1. Foreign body history						U
2. Hereditary			S		U	
3. Malignancy previously		U				
4. More frequent lower lid		U				
5. Viral etiology	U					
Physical Findings						
1. A rise in hair-bearing skin		U				
2. Bead-like excrescences with loss of cilia at lid margins					U	
3. Chalazion		U				
4. Chronic blepharitis		U			U	
5. Conjunctivitis	U					
6. Cystic nodules filled with sebaceous/serious material				U		
7. Ectropion		S				
8. Encysted contact lens						U
9. Entropion		S				
10. Flesh-colored, rounded papules—some pigmented			U			
11. Foreign body sensation						U
12. Keratitis	U					
13. Lid notching		U				
14. Lid retraction		U				
15. Madarosis		U			U	
16. Nodular hyperemic lid lesion						U
17. Nodular/nodular ulcerative lid lesion		U				
18. Small umbilicated tumor	U					
19. Yellow-white nodule				U	U	
Laboratory Data						
Histopathology						
Epithelial cyst walls have serous/sebaceous material				U		
Granuloma	U					
Granulomatous infiltrates with micro-organisms						U
Large, nuclear forms, including multinucleated cells and monstrous cellular forms				U		
Lower lipid content					U	
Narrow strand of basaloid cells like adenoid basal cell carcinomas, keratinizing cysts with pilar differentiation			U			
Tumor cells in nests, cords, sheets; peripheral cells may palisade		U		S		

R = rarely; S = sometimes; and U = usually.

* = most important

4. Cyst
   *A. Sebaceous
   B. Sudoriferous
   C. Traumatic
   D. Congenital inclusion
5. Lipoid proteinosis—wax-like, pearly nodules
6. Pseudotumor of lid-encysted contact lens
7. Amyloidosis (Lubarsch–Pick syndrome)

Boynton JR, Markowitch W. Porocarcinoma of eyelid. *Ophthalmology* 1997;104:1626–1628.

Cook BE, Bartley GB. Epidemiologic characteristics and clinical course of patients with malignant eyelid tumors in an incidence cohort in Olmsted County, Minnesota. *Ophthalmology* 1999;106:746–750.

Kerten RC, et al. Accuracy of clinical diagnosis of cutaneous eyelid lesions. *Ophthalmology* 1997;104:479–484.

Pau H. *Differential diagnosis of eye diseases*, 2nd ed. New York: Thieme Medical, 1988.

XANTHELASMA (SMOOTH YELLOW DEPOSITS IN THE EYELID, ESPECIALLY THE SUPERIOR NASAL AND INFERIOR NASAL AREAS)

1. Xanthelasma with hyperlipemia (primary or secondary)
   *A. Type II—familial hyper-B-lipoproteinemia (familial hypercholesterolemia)
   *B. Type III—familial hyper-B- and hyper-pre-B-lipoproteinemia (familial hyperlipemia with hypercholesterolemia)
   C. Other types are infrequent, including type I, familial fat-induced hyperlipoproteinemia (hyperchylomicronemia); type IV, familial hyper-pre-B-lipoproteinemia (carbohydrate-induced hyperlipemia); type V, familial hyperchylomicronemia with hyper-pre-B-lipoproteinemia (mixed hyperlipemia), lichen sclerosis et atrophicus.
2. Xanthelasma without hyperlipemia
   A. Generalized
   B. Histiocytosis X (eosinophilic granuloma, Hand–Schüller–Christian disease, and Letterer-Siwe disease)
   C. Local (no systemic disease)
   D. Reticulohistiocytoma cutis
   E. Xanthoma disseminatum

Depot MJ, et al. Bilateral and extensive xanthelasma palpebrarum in a young man. *Ophthalmology* 1984;91:522–527.

Roy FH. *Ocular syndromes and systemic diseases*, 3rd ed. Philadelphia: Lippincott Williams & Wilkins, 2002.

CHRONIC BLEPHARITIS (INFLAMMATION OF LIDS)

*1. Seborrheic—lid margin covered with small, white or gray scales
   A. Associated with seborrheic dermatitis of the scalp
   B. Aggravated by chemical fumes, smoke, and smog
   C. May be associated with uncorrected refractive errors (especially hyperopia)
   D. May be due to *Pityrosporon ovale*
   E. *Aspergillus fumigatus* may be its cause
   F. Associated with systemic diseases
      (1) Acne rosacea
      (2) *Acinetobacter* Iwoffi
      (3) Acrodermatitis chronica atrophicans
      (4) Aspergillosis

(5) Candidiasis
(6) Cretinism (hypothyroidism)
(7) Demodicosis
(8) Dermatophytosis
(9) Diphtheria
(10) Erysipelas
(11) Herpes simplex
(12) Hypocalcemia
(13) Hypoparathyroidism
(14) Listerellosis
(15) Malaria
(16) Moraxella lacunata
(17) Pellagra (avitaminosis B$_2$)
*(18) Seborrheic dermatitis
(19) Sporotrichosis
(20) Staphylococcus
(21) Streptococcus
(22) Syphilis (acquired lues)
(23) Scleroderma (systemic scleroderma)
(24) Tuberculosis
(25) Vaccinia
(26) Xeroderma pigmentosum

G. Associated with syndromes
(1) Danbolt–Closs syndrome (acrodermatitis enteropathica)
(2) Down syndrome (mongolism)
(3) Goldscheider syndrome (epidermolysis bullosa)
(4) Hand–Schüller–Christian syndrome (lipoid granuloma syndrome)
(5) Lyell syndrome (toxic epidermal necrolysis)
(6) Myotonic dystrophy syndrome (Curschmann–Steinert syndrome)
(7) Parkinson syndrome (paralysis agitans)
(8) Sézary syndrome (mycosis fungoides syndrome)
(9) Siemens syndrome (hereditary ectodermal dysplasia syndrome)
(10) Syndrome of Beal (acute follicular conjunctivitis)
(11) Wernicke syndrome
(12) Thiamine deficiency
(13) Wiskott–Aldrich syndrome
(14) Zinsser–Engman–Cole syndrome (dyskeratosis congenita with pigmentation)

H. Drugs, including the following:

acyclovir
benzalkonium
F3T idoxuridine
isosorbide
mannitol
meperidine
mercuric oxide
nitromersol
phenylmercuric acetate
phenylmercuric nitrate
thimerosal
trifluridine
vidarabine

2. Ulcerative—suppurative inflammation of the follicles of the lashes and the associated glands of Zeis and Moll
   A. *Staphylococcus aureus* or *S. albus* may be responsible
   B. Due to mixed infection of a staphylococcus and *P. ovale*
   C. Associated with vaccinia

* = most important

D. Due to *Blastomyces dermatitidis*

E. Herpes simplex—vesicles at lash line, then ulceration

*3. Angular—inflammation of the angles of the lids, usually associated with an angular conjunctivitis

    A. *Candida albicans*

    B. *Moraxella lacunata*

    C. Stannus cerebellar syndrome (riboflavin deficiency)

    D. *Staphylococcus aureus*

4. Exfoliative dermatitis owing to drugs, including the following:

acetohexamide
acetophenazine
acid bismuth sodium tartrate
adiphenine
allobarbital
allopurinol
ambutonium
aminosalicylate(?)
aminosalicylic acid
amithiozone
amobarbital
amodiaquine
amoxicillin
ampicillin
anisindione
anisotropine
antipyrine
aprobarbital
atropine methylnitrate
auranofin
aurothioglucose
aurothioglycanide
barbital
bismuth carbonate
bismuth oxychloride
bismuth salicylate
bismuth sodium tartrate
bismuth sodium
  thioglycollate
bismuth sodium
  triglycollamate
bismuth subcarbonate
bismuth subsalicylate
bupivacaine
busulfan
butabarbital
butalbital
butallylonal
butaperazine

butethal
captopril
carbamazepine
carbenicillin
carbimazole
carisoprodol
carphenazine
cefaclor
cefadroxil
cefamandole
cefazolin
cefonicid
cefoperazone
ceforanide
cefotaxime
cefotetan
cefoxitin
cefsulodin
ceftazidime
ceftizoxime
ceftriaxone
cefuroxime
cephalexin
cephaloglycin
cephaloridine
cephalothin
cephapirin
cephradine
chlorambucil
chloroprocaine
chloroquine
chlorpromazine
chlorpropamide
chlorprothixene
cimetidine
ciprofloxacin
clidinium
clindamycin
cloxacillin

codeine
cyclobarbital
cyclopentobarbital
cyclophosphamide
dapsone
dicloxacillin
dicyclomine
diethazine
diltiazem
diphemanil
diphenadione
diphenylhydantoin
droperidol
enalapril
erythrityl tetranitrate
erythromycin
ethionamide
ethopropazine
ethosuximide
ethotoin
etidocaine
fenoprofen
flecainide
fluphenazine
furosemide
glutethimide
glyburide
glycopyrrolate
gold Au 198
gold sodium thiomalate
gold sodium thiosulfate
griseofulvin
haloperidol
heptabarbital
hetacillin
hexethal
hexobarbital
hexocyclium

* = most important

hydroxychloroquine
indomethacin
iodide and iodine solutions
   and compounds
isoniazid
isopropamide
isosorbide dinitrate
ketoprofen
lidocaine
lincomycin
mannitol hexanitrate
mechlorethamine
melphalan
mepenzolate
mephenytoin
mephobarbital
mepivacaine
meprobamate
mesoridazine
methantheline
metharbital
methdilazine
methicillin
methimazole
methitural
methixene
methohexital
methotrimeprazine
methsuximide
methylatropine nitrate
methylphenidate
methylthiouracil
methyprylon
moxalactam
nafcillin
naltrexone
naproxen(?)
nitroglycerin
oxacillin
oxyphenbutazone
oxyphencyclimine

oxyphenonium
paramethadione
pentaerythritol tetranitrate
pentobarbital
perazine
pericyazine
perphenazine
phenindione
phenobarbital
phensuximide
phenylbutazone
phenytoin
pimozide
pipenzolate
piperacetazine
piperidolate
piroxicam
poldine
practolol
prilocaine
primidone
probarbital
procaine
procarbazine
prochlorperazine
promazine
promethazine
propantheline
propiomazine
propoxycaine
propoxyphene
propranolol
propylthiouracil
quinacrine
quinidine
radioactive iodides
rifampin
secobarbital
streptomycin
sulfacetamide
sulfachlorpyridazine
sulfacytine

sulfadiazine
sulfadimethoxine
sulfamerazine
sulfameter
sulfamethazine
sulfamethizole
sulfamethoxazole
sulfamethoxypyridazine
sulfanilamide
sulfaphenazole
sulfapyridine
sulfasalazine
sulfathiazole
sulfisoxazole
sulindac
talbutal
thiabendazole
thiamylal
thiethylperazine
thiopental
thiopropazate
thioproperazine
thioridazine
thiothixene
tolazamide
tolbutamide
trichloroethylene
tridihexethyl
triethylenemelamine
trifluoperazine
trifluperidol
triflupromazine
trimeprazine
trimethadione
trolnitrate
uracil mustard
vancomycin
vinbarbital
vitamin A

5. Other types
    A. Due to mites (*Demodex folliculorum*)
    B. Due to pubic lice (*Phthirus pubis*)

6. Erythema due to drugs, including the following:

acebutolol
acetaminophen
acetanilid
acetazolamide
acyclovir
adrenal cortex injection
aldosterone
albuterol
allopurinol
alprazolam
amitriptyline
amoxapine
antazoline
atenolol
auranofin
aurothioglucose
aurothioglycanide
azatadine
BCG vaccine
Bis-chloroethyl-nitroso-urea
   (BCNU)
beclomethasone
benzalkonium
benzathine penicillin G
benzphetamine
betamethasone
betaxolol
bleomycin
bromide
brompheniramine
busulfan
cactinomycin
captopril
carbinoxamine
carmustine
chloroethyl-cyclohexyl-
   nitrosourea (CCNU)
cefaclor
cefadroxil
cefamandole
cefazolin
cefonicid
cefoperazone
ceforanide
cefotaxime
cefotetan

cefoxitin
cefsulodin
ceftazidime
ceftizoxime
ceftriaxone
cefuroxime
cephalexin
cephaloglycin
cephaloridine
cephalothin
cephapirin
cephradine
chlorambucil
chlordiazepoxide
chlorpheniramine
chlorphentermine
chlorphentermine
chlortetracycline
cimetidine
ciprofloxacin
dapiprazole hydrochloride
desoxycorticosterone
cisplatin
clemastine
clofibrate
clomipramine
clonazepam
clorazepate
cortisone
cyclophosphamide
cyclosporin
cyproheptadine
cytarabine
dacarbazine
dactinomycin
danazol
daunorubicin
deferoxamine
demeclocycline
desipramine
dexamethasone
dexbrompheniramine
dexchlorpheniramine
dextran
diacetylmorphine
diatrizoate

diazepam
diazoxide
DIC
DMSO
DPT vaccine
dichlorphenamide
diethylcarbamazine
diethylpropion
diltiazem
dimethindene
dimethyl sulfoxide
diphenhydramine
diphenylpyraline
diphtheria and tetanus
   toxoids (adsorbed)
diphtheria and tetanus
   toxoids and pertussis
   vaccine (adsorbed)
diphtheria toxoid (adsorbed)
disopyramide
disulfiram
doxepin
doxorubicin
doxycycline
doxylamine
enalapril
ergonovine
ergotamine
ethionamide
ethoxzolamide
etretinate
fenfluramine
fenoprofen
flecainide
floxuridine
fluorometholone
fluorouracil
flurazepam
flurbiprofen
framycetin
gold Au 198
gold sodium thiomalate
gold sodium thiosulfate
halazepam
hexachlorophene
hydrabamine penicillin V

hydralazine
hydrocortisone
hydroxyurea
ibuprofen
imipramine
influenza virus vaccine
insulin
iodipamide meglumine
iothalamate meglumine and
    sodium
iothalamic acid
iron dextran
isotretinoin
ketoprofen
labetalol
levallorphan
levobunolol
lomustine
lorazepam
maprotiline
measles and rubella virus
    vaccine (live)
measles virus vaccine (live)
measles, mumps, and rubella
    virus vaccine (live)
mechlorethamine
medrysone
mefenamic acid
meglumine and sodium
melphalan
meperidine
meprednisone
mercuric oxide
methacycline
methazolamide
methocarbamol
methotrexate
methoxsalen
methylergonovine
methylprednisolone
methysergide

metocurine iodide
metoprolol
metronidazole
mexiletine
mianserin
midazolam
minocycline
minoxidil
mitomycin
mitotane
moxalactam
mumps virus vaccine (live)
nadolol
nalorphine
naloxone
naltrexone
naproxen
neomycin
neostigmine
nifedipine
nitrazepam
nitromersol
nortriptyline
oxazepam
oxprenolol
oxytetracycline
paramethasone
pentazocine
phenacetin
phendimetrazine
pheniramine
phentermine
phenylephrine
phenylmercuric acetate
phenylmercuric nitrate
pindolol
piroxicam
poliovirus vaccine
potassium penicillin G
potassium penicillin V
potassium phenethicillin
practolol

prazepam
prazosin
prednisolone
prednisone
procaine penicillin G
procarbazine
propranolol
protriptyline
pyrilamine
rabies immune globulin
rabies vaccine
ranitidine
rifampin
rubella and mumps virus
    vaccine (live)
semustine
smallpox vaccine
spironolactone
streptomycin
streptozocin
succinylcholine
sulindac
temazepam
tetanus immune globulin
tetanus toxoid
tetracycline
thimerosal
thiotepa
timolol
tocainide
trazodone
triazolam
triethylenemelamine
trimipramine
trioxsalen
tripelennamine
triprolidine
tubocurarine
uracil mustard
verapamil

Fraunfelder FT, Fraunfelder FW. *Drug-induced ocular side effects.* Woburn, MA: Butterworth-Heinemann, 2001.

McCulley JP, et al. Classification of chronic blepharitis. *Ophthalmology* 1982;89:1173.

Roy FH. *Ocular syndromes and systemic diseases*, 3rd ed. Philadelphia: Lippincott Williams & Wilkins, 2002.

Yeatts RP, White WL. Granulomatous blepharitis as a sign of Melkersson-Rosenthal syndrome. *Ophthalmology* 1997;104:1185–1190.

ACUTE BLEPHARITIS (INFLAMMATION OF LIDS WITH RAPID ONSET)

1. Usual allergy to drugs, including the following:

acenocoumarin
acetaminophen
acetanilid
acetazolamide
acetohexamide
acetophenazine
acetyldigitoxin
actinomycin C
acyclovir
adenine arabinoside
adiphenine
allobarbital
allopurinol
alprazolam
aluminum nicotinate
ambutonium(?)
aminopterin
aminosalicylate(?)
aminosalicylic acid(?)
amithiozone
amobarbital
amodiaquine
amoxicillin
amphotericin B
ampicillin
amyl nitrite
anisindione
anisotropine
antazoline
antipyrine
aprobarbital
aspirin
atropine
atropine methylnitrate
auranofin
aurothioglucose
aurothioglycanide
bacitracin
barbital belladonna
bendroflumethiazide
benoxinate
benzalkonium
benzathine penicillin G
benzphetamine
benzthiazide

betamethasone
betaxolol
bishydroxycoumarin
bleomycin
bromide
bupivacaine
busulfan
butabarbital
butacaine
butalbital
butallylonal
butaperazine
butethal
cactinomycin
carbachol
carbamazepine
carbenicillin
carbimazole
carisoprodol
carmustine
carphenazine
cefaclor
cefadroxil
cefamandole
cefazolin
cefonicid
cefoperazone
ceforanide
cefotaxime
cefotetan
cefoxitin
cefsulodin
ceftazidime
ceftizoxime
ceftriaxone
cefuroxime
cephalexin
cephaloglycin
cephaloridine
cephalothin
cephapirin
cephradine
chloral hydrate
chlorambucil
chloramphenicol

chlordiazepoxide
chloroprocaine
chloroquine
chlorothiazide
chlorphentermine
chlorpromazine
chlorpropamide
chlorprothixene
chlortetracycline
chlorthalidone
chrysarobin
clidinium
clindamycin
clomiphene
clonazepam
clorazepate
cloxacillin
cobalt
cocaine
colistin
colloidal silver
cortisone
cyclobarbital
cyclopentobarbital
cyclopentolate
cyclophosphamide
cycloserine
cyclothiazide
cytarabine
dacarbazine
dactinomycin
daunorubicin
deferoxamine
demecarium
deslanoside
dexamethasone
diatrizoate meglumine and
   sodium
diazepam
diazoxide
dibucaine
dichlorphenamide
dicloxacillin
dicumarol
dicyclomine

diethazine
diethylcarbamazine
diethylpropion
digitalis
digitoxin
digoxin
dimercaprol
dimethyl sulfoxide
diphemanil
diphenadione
diphenylhydantoin
diphtheria and tetanus
   toxoids (adsorbed)
diphtheria and tetanus
   toxoids and pertussis
   vaccine (adsorbed)
diphtheria toxoid adsorbed
dipivefrin
disulfiram
doxorubicin
dromostanolone
droperidol
dyclonine
echothiophate
edrophonium emetine
ephedrine
epinephrine
ergonovine
ergotamine
erythromycin
ethionamide
ethopropazine
ethosuximide
ethotoin
ethoxzolamide
ethyl biscoumacetate
etidocaine
F3T
fenfluramine
fluorescein
fluorometholone
fluorouracil
fluoxymesterone
fluphenazine
flurazepam
framycetin
furosemide
gentamicin

gitalin
glutethimide
glyburide
glycopyrrolate
gold Au 198
gold sodium thiomalate
gold sodium thiosulfate
griseofulvin
halazepam
haloperidol
heparin
heptabarbital
hetacillin
hexethal
hexobarbital
hexocyclium
homatropine
hyaluronidase
hydrabamine penicillin V
hydralazine
hydrochlorothiazide
hydrocortisone
hydroflumethiazide
hydromorphone
hydroxyamphetamine
hydroxychloroquine
idoxuridine
indapamide
influenza virus vaccine
insulin
iodide and iodine solutions
   and compounds
iodipamide meglumine
iothalamate meglumine and
   sodium
iothalamic acid
isoflurophate
isoniazid
isopropamide
kanamycin
lanatoside C
levallorphan
levobunolol
levodopa
lidocaine
lincomycin
lomustine
lorazepam

measles and rubella virus
   vaccine (live)
measles, mumps, and rubella
   virus vaccine (live)
measles virus vaccine (live)
mechlorethamine
medrysone
melphalan
mepenzolate
meperidine
mephenytoin
mephobarbital
mepivacaine
meprobamate
mercuric oxide
mesoridazine
methacholine
methantheline
metharbital
methazolamide
methdilazine
methicillin
methimazole
methitural
methixene
methohexital
methotrexate
methotrimeprazine
methsuximide
methyclothiazide
methylatropine nitrate
methyldopa
methylergonovine
methylprednisolone
methylthiouracil
methyprylone
methysergide
metolazone
metrizamide
midazolam
mild silver protein
mitomycin
morphine
moxalactam
mumps virus vaccine (live)
nafcillin
nalorphine
naloxone

naltrexone
naphazoline
naproxen
neomycin
neostigmine
niacinamide
nicotinic acid
nicotinyl alcohol
nitrazepam
nitrofurantoin
nitromersol
nystatin
opium
oral contraceptives
ouabain
oxacillin
oxprenolol
oxymorphone
oxyphenbutazone
oxyphencyclimine
oxyphenonium
paramethadione
pentobarbital
perazine
pericyazine
perphenazine
phenacaine
phenacetin
phendimetrazine
phenindione
phenobarbital
phenprocoumon
phensuximide
phentermine
phenylbutazone
phenylephrine
phenylmercuric acetate
phenylmercuric nitrate
phenytoin
physostigmine
pilocarpine
pipenzolate
piperacetazine
piperazine
piperidolate
piperocaine
pipobroman

poldine
polymyxin B
polythiazide
potassium penicillin G
potassium penicillin V
potassium phenethicillin
potassium phenoxymethyl
  penicillin
prazepam
prednisolone
prilocaine
primidone
probarbital
procaine
procaine penicillin G
prochlorperazine
promazine
promethazine
propantheline
proparacaine
propiomazine
propoxycaine
propranolol
propylthiouracil
quinethazone
quinidine
quinine
rabies immune globulin
rabies vaccine
radioactive iodides
scopolamine
secobarbital
semustine
silver nitrate
silver protein
sodium salicylate
streptomycin
streptozocin
succinylcholine
sulfacetamide
sulfachlorpyridazine
sulfadiazine
sulfadimethoxine
sulfamerazine
sulfameter
sulfamethazine
sulfamethizole
sulfamethoxazole

sulfamethoxypyridazine
sulfanilamide
sulfaphenazole
sulfapyridine
sulfasalazine
sulfathiazole
sulfisoxazole
talbutal
temazepam
testolactone
testosterone
tetanus immune globulin
tetanus toxoid
tetracaine
tetracycline
tetrahydrozoline
thiabendazole
thiamylal
thiethylperazine
thimerosal
thiopental
thiopropazate
thioproperazine
thioridazine
thiotepa
thiothixene
timolol
tolazamide
tolbutamide
trazodone
triazolam
trichlormethiazide
tridihexethyl
triethylenemelamine
trifluoperazine
trifluorothymidine
trifluperidol
triflupromazine
trifluridine
trimeprazine
trimethadione
tropicamide
uracil mustard
vancomycin
vidarabine
vinbarbital
warfarin

*2. Infections, such as bacterial, fungal, and viral

Fraunfelder FT, Fraunfelder FW. *Drug-induced ocular side effects.* Woburn, MA: Butterworth-Heinemann, 2001.

Tasman W, Jaeger E, eds. *Duane's clinical ophthalmology.* Philadelphia: JB Lippincott, 1990.

THICKENED EYELIDS

1. Trachoma
2. Multiple chalazia
*3. Chronic conjunctivitis
*4. Blepharitis—lid margins thickened
5. Tarsitis—rare, such as in syphilis or tuberculosis
6. Trisomy (E syndrome)
7. Congenital hypothyroidism
8. Pheochromocytoma, medullary thyroid carcinoma, and neurofibromatosis

Baum JL, Adler ME. Pheochromocytoma, medullary thyroid carcinoma, and multiple mucosal neuroma. *Arch Ophthalmol* 1972;87:574–584.

Gellis SS, Feingold M. *Atlas of mental retardation.* Washington, DC: US Government Printing Office, 1968.

BLEPHAROPHIMOSIS (SHORT PALPEBRAL FISSURE)

1. Blepharochalasis
2. Blepharofacioskeletal syndrome
3. Blepharophimosis-amenorrhea syndrome (blepharophimosis, ptosis, epicanthus inversus syndrome)
4. Carpenter syndrome (acrocephalopolysyndactyly II)
5. Clefting syndrome with anterior chamber and lid anomalies
6. Craniocarpotarsal syndrome (Freeman–Sheldon syndrome; whistling face syndrome)
7. Down syndrome (trisomy 21, mongolism)
8. Dubowitz syndrome
9. 18P syndrome
10. Kaufman oculocerebrofacial syndrome
11. Klein–Waardenburg syndrome
12. Komoto syndrome (congenital eyelid tetrad)
13. Marden–Walker syndrome
14. Meyer-Schwickerath and Weyers syndrome
15. Michel syndrome
*16. Microphthalmos
17. Mohr syndrome (orofaciodigital syndrome II)
18. Mohr syndrome
19. Oculopalatoskeletal syndrome
20. Ohdo blepharophimosis syndrome
21. Pena–Shokeir type II syndrome
22. Progeria (Hutchinson–Gilford syndrome)
23. Rieger syndrome (dysgenesis mesostromalis)
24. Ring chromosome in the D group (13–15) (ring D syndrome)
25. Schonenberg syndrome (dwarf cardiopathy syndrome)
26. Schwartz-Jampel syndrome (osteochondromuscular dystrophy)
27. Simosa syndrome

* = most important

28. Syndrome of blepharophimosis with myopathy
*29. Traumatic
30. Trisomy (E syndrome) (Edward syndrome)
31. Waardenburg syndrome (embryonic fixation syndrome)
32. Young–Simpson syndrome
33. X-linked mental retardation syndrome
34. 3p- syndrome
35. 10q- syndrome

Bonthron DT, et al. Parental consanguinity in the blepharophimosis, heart defect, hypothyroidism, mental retardation syndrome (Young-Simpson syndrome). *J Med Genet* 1993;30:255–256.

Melnyk AR. Blepharophimosis, ptosis, and mental retardation: further delineation of Ohdo syndrome. *Clin Dysmorphol* 1994;3:121–124.

Roy FH. *Ocular syndromes and systemic diseases*, 3rd ed. Philadelphia: Lippincott Williams & Wilkins, 2002.

Suri M, et al. Blepharophimosis, telecanthus, microstomia, and unusual ear anomaly Simosa syndrome in an infant. *Am J Med Genet* 1994;51:222–223.

EURYBLEPHARON

Euryblepharon is defined as a horizontally elongated palpebral aperture (normal, 30 mm) and may be associated with ectropion and present in other family members.

1. Excessive tension of skin
2. Defective separation of the lids
3. Excessive pull of the platysma
*4. Localized displacement of the lateral canthi
5. Hypoplasia of tarsus

Feldman E, et al. Euryblepharon: a case report with photographs documenting the condition from infancy to adulthood. *J Pediatr Ophthalmol Strabismus* 1980;17:307–309.

Gupta AK, et al. Euryblepharon. *J Pediatr Ophthalmol* 1972;9:173–174.

McCord CD, et al. Congenital euryblepharon. *Ann Ophthalmol* 1979;11:1217–1224.

LID COLOBOMA

1. Amniogenic band syndrome (amniotic bands–Streeter anomaly)
2. Epidermal nevus syndrome
3. Facial clefting syndrome (Tessier syndromes)
4. Fraser syndrome
5. Frontonasal dysplasia syndrome
6. Goldenhar syndrome (oculoauriculovertebral dysplasia)
7. Miller syndrome
8. Nager syndrome
9. Nevus sebaceous of Jadassohn (linear sebaceous nevus syndrome)
10. Palpebral coloboma-lipoma syndrome
*11. Traumatic
12. Treacher Collins–Franceschetti syndrome (mandibulofacial dysostosis)

Braude LL, et al. Ocular abnormalities in the amniogenic band syndrome. *Br J Ophthalmol* 1981;65:299–303.

Burch JV, et al. Ichthyosis hystrix (epidermal nevus syndrome) and Coats' disease. *Am J Opthalmol* 1980;89:25–30.

Isenberg SJ. *The eye of infancy*. Chicago: Year Book Medical, 1989.

Roy FH. *Ocular syndromes and systemic diseases*, 3rd ed. Philadelphia: Lippincott Williams & Wilkins, 2002.

NECROSIS OF EYELIDS

1. Drugs, including the following:

acenocoumarol	diphenadione	phenprocoumon
amphotericin B	ethyl biscoumacetate	tobramycin
anisindione	nafcillin	warfarin
dicumarol	phenindione	

*2. Mechanical, electrical, or thermal trauma
3. Periorbital cellulitis-periorbital necrotizing cellulitis
4. Secondary to infection

Fraunfelder FT, Fraunfelder FW. *Drug-induced ocular side effects.* Woburn, MA: Butterworth-Heinemann, 2001.

Scott PM, Bloome MA. Lid necrosis secondary to streptococcal periorbital cellulitis. *Ann Ophthalmol* 1981;13:461.

POLIOSIS (WHITENING OF HAIR, EYEBROWS, AND EYELASHES)

1. Albino
2. Alopecia areata
*3. Aging
4. Drugs, including the following:

amodiaquine	dexamethasone	medrysone
betamethasone	epinephrine	prednisolone
chloroquine	fluorometholone	thiotepa
cortisone	hydrocortisone	
cyclosporin A	hydroxychloroquine	

5. Leprosy (Hansen disease)
6. Radiation therapy
7. Rubinstein–Taybi syndrome
8. Severe dermatitis
9. Stress
*10. Unknown etiology
11. Vitiligo
12. Vogt–Koyanagi–Harada syndrome (uveitis–vitiligo–alopecia–poliosis syndrome)
13. Waardenburg syndrome (embryonic fixation syndrome)
14. Werner syndrome (progeria of adults)

Fraunfelder FT, Fraunfelder FW. *Drug-induced ocular side effects.* Woburn, MA: Butterworth-Heinemann, 2001.

Rosner F. Can hair turn white overnight? *JAMA* 1981;246:2324.

Roy FH. *Ocular syndromes and systemic diseases,* 3rd ed. Philadelphia: Lippincott Williams & Wilkins, 2002.

Walsh FB, Hoyt WF. *Clinical neuro-ophthalmology,* 4th ed. Baltimore: Williams & Wilkins, 1985.

TRICHOMEGALY (LONG LASHES)

1. Associated with cataract and hereditary spherocytosis
2. Congenital with pigmentary retinal degeneration, dwarfism, and mental retardation
3. Cyclosporine induced
4. De Lange syndrome (congenital muscular hypertrophy—cerebral syndrome)
5. Ectodermal dysplasia (Curtius syndrome)
6. Human immunodeficiency virus (HIV)

* = most important

   7. Hypertrichosis (hirsutism)
   8. Isolated adrenal malfunction and ovarian atrophy
   9. Noonan syndrome (male Turner syndrome)
 *10. Normal
  11. Oliver–McFarlane syndrome
  12. Rubinstein–Taybi syndrome (broad thumbs syndrome)
  13. Schwartz syndrome

Chang TS, et al. Congenital trichomegaly, pigmentary degeneration of the retina and growth retardation Oliver-McFarlane syndrome year follow-up of the first reported case. *Can J Ophthal* 1993;28:191–193.

Isenberg SJ. *The eye in infancy*. Chicago: Year Book Medical, 1989.

McKusick VA. *Mendelian inheritance in man*, 12th ed. Baltimore: Johns Hopkins University Press, 1998.

Roy FH. *Ocular syndromes and systemic diseases*, 3rd ed. Philadelphia: Lippincott Williams & Wilkins, 2002.

MADAROSIS (LOSS OF EYELASHES)

  1. Chronic skin diseases, including psoriasis, neurodermatitis, exfoliative dermatitis, ichthyosis, alopecia areata, acne, lichen planus, epidermolysis bullosa, lupus erythematosus, acanthosis nigricans, dermatophytosis, hereditary ectodermal dysplasia syndrome and acrodermatitis
  2. Congenital atrichia
  3. Cryptophthalmos
  4. Cutaneous T cell lymphoma
  5. Demodicosis
  6. Drugs, including the following:

acebutolol(?)
acenocoumarin(?)
acetazolamide(?)
acetohexamide(?)
acid bismuth sodium tartrate
actinomycin C(?)
alcohol(?)
allopurinol(?)
aluminum nicotinate
amantadine(?)
aminopterin(?)
aminosalicylate(?)
aminosalicylic acid(?)
amiodarone(?)
amithiozone(?)
amitriptyline(?)
amodiaquine(?)
amoxapine(?)
amphetamine(?)
anisindione(?)
aspirin(?)
atenolol(?)
auranofin(?)
aurothioglucose(?)
aurothioglycanide(?)

azathioprine(?)
benzphetamine(?)
betaxolol
bishydroxycoumarin(?)
bismuth oxychloride(?)
bismuth sodium tartrate(?)
bismuth sodium
    thioglycollate(?)
bismuth sodium
    triglycollamate(?)
bismuth subcarbonate(?)
bismuth subsalicylate(?)
bleomycin(?)
broxyquinoline(?)
busulfan(?)
cactinomycin
captopril(?)
carbamazepine(?)
carbimazole(?)
carmustine
CCNU
chlorambucil(?)
chloroquine(?)
chlorphentermine(?)
chlorpropamide(?)

cimetidine(?)
cisplatin
clofibrate(?)
clomiphene(?)
clonazepam(?)
colchicine(?)
cyclophosphamide(?)
cytarabine(?)
dacarbazine
dactinomycin(?)
danazol(?)
daunorubicin
desipramine(?)
dextroamphetamine(?)
dextrothyroxine(?)
diacetylmorphine(?)
DIC
dichlorphenamide(?)
dicumarol(?)
diethylcarbamazine
diethylpropion(?)
diltiazem(?)
diphenadione(?)
divalproex sodium(?)
doxepin(?)

doxorubicin
dromostanolone(?)
droperidol(?)
enalapril(?)
epinephrine
ergonovine(?)
ergotamine(?)
ethionamide(?)
ethotoin(?)
ethoxzolamide(?)
ethyl biscoumacetate(?)
etretinate(?)
fenfluramine(?)
fenoprofen(?)
flecainide(?)
floxuridine(?)
fluorouracil(?)
fluoxymesterone(?)
gentamicin
glyburide
glycopyrrolate(?)
gold au 198
gold sodium thiomalate(?)
gold sodium thiosulfate(?)
guanethidine(?)
haloperidol(?)
HCNU
heparin(?)
hydroxychloroquine(?)
hydroxyurea(?)
ibuprofen(?)
imipramine(?)
indomethacin(?)
interferon(?)
iodochlorhydroxyquin(?)
iodoquinol(?)
isotretinoin(?)
ketoprofen(?)
labetalol(?)
levobunolol
levodopa(?)
lithium carbonate(?)
lomustine
maprotiline(?)

mechlorethamine(?)
melphalan(?)
mephenytoin(?)
methamphetamine(?)
methazolamide(?)
methimazole(?)
methotrexate(?)
methylergonovine(?)
methylthiouracil(?)
methysergide(?)
metoprolol(?)
mexiletine(?)
mianserin(?)
minocycline(?)
minoxidil(?)
mitomycin
mitotane(?)
morphine(?)
nadolol(?)
naltrexone(?)
naproxen(?)
niacin(?)
niacinamide(?)
nicotinyl alcohol(?)
nifedipine(?)
nitrofurantoin(?)
nortriptyline(?)
opium(?)
oral contraceptives(?)
oxprenolol(?)
paramethadione(?)
penicillamine(?)
phendimetrazine(?)
phenindione(?)
phenmetrazine(?)
phenprocoumon(?)
phentermine(?)
pindolol(?)
pipobroman(?)
prazosin(?)
piroxicam
procarbazine(?)
propranolol(?)
propylthiouracil(?)
protriptyline(?)

pyridostigmine(?)
ranitidine
semustine
sodium salicylate(?)
streptomycin(?)
streptozocin
sulfacetamide(?)
sulfachlorpyridazine(?)
sulfacytine(?)
sulfadiazine(?)
sulfadimethoxine(?)
sulfamerazine(?)
sulfameter(?)
sulfamethazine(?)
sulfamethizole(?)
sulfamethoxazole
sulfamethoxypyridazine(?)
sulfanilamide(?)
sulfaphenazole(?)
sulfapyridine(?)
sulfasalazine(?)
sulfathiazole(?)
sulfisoxazole
sulindac(?)
tamoxifen(?)
testolactone(?)
testosterone(?)
tetracycline(?)
thiotepa
timolol maleate
tocainide(?)
tolazamide(?)
tolbutamide(?)
triethylenemelamine(?)
trifluperidol(?)
trimethadione(?)
uracil mustard(?)
valproate sodium(?)
valproic acid(?)
verapamil(?)
vinblastine(?)
vincristine(?)
vitamin A
warfarin(?)

7. Ehlers–Danlos syndrome, unspecified type
*8. Endocrine disease, including hypothyroidism, hyperthyroidism, pituitary insufficiency,
   hypoparathyroidism, and pituitary necrosis syndrome (Simmonds–Sheehan syndrome)
9. Following eyelid tattooing

* = most important

Madarosis (loss of eyelashes)

	Drugs as Thiotepa	Vogt-Koyanagi Harada Disease	Endocrine Diseases (e.g., Hypothyroidism)	Inflammation and Infection (e.g., Blepharitis)	Radiation	Severe Systemic Diseases (e.g., Tuberculosis)	Chronic Skin Diseases (e.g., Psoriasis)
History							
1. Common in females							U
2. Common in whites							U
3. Congenital			S				
4. Hereditary							U
5. Japanese and Italian extraction		U					
6. Onset, 10 to 35 years							U
7. Seborrheic disease				U			
8. Thiotepa eyedrop usage	U						
9. Thyroidectomy/hypophysectomy			S				
10. Young adults		U					
Physical Findings							
1. Blepharitis				U	U	S	
2. Cataract		S	S		S		
3. Chalazion				S			S
4. Choroiditis		U					
5. Chronic dacryoadenitis and dacryocystitis						S	
6. Conjunctivitis, exudative				U			
7. Conjunctivitis, mucopurulent				U		S	
8. Conjunctival phlyctenules				S		U	
9. Corneal ulcer				S	S	S	
10. Decreased tear secretion			S	U	U		
11. Ectropion						S	S
12. Entropion						S	
13. Epiphora	U						
14. Excised pterygium	U						
15. Exophthalmos			R				
16. Exudative retinitis with periphlebitis						S	
17. Glaucoma		S				S	
18. Gray-white appearance of sclera			U				
19. Hypopyon						S	
20. Keratitis				S	S	S	
21. Lid abscess				S			
22. Lid carcinoma					S		
23. Lid collarettes/granuloma						S	S
24. Lid concretions				U			
25. Lid scaling						S	U
26. Lid thickening						S	
27. Loss of eyebrow hairs		U					
28. Lupus tuberculosis lids						S	
29. Meibomianitis				S		S	
30. Optic nerve atrophy						S	

Madarosis (loss of eyelashes) (Continued)

	Drugs as Thiotepa	Vogt-Koyanagi Harada Disease	Endocrine Diseases (e.g., Hypothyroidism)	Inflammation and Infection (e.g., Blepharitis)	Radiation	Severe Systemic Diseases (e.g., Tuberculosis)	Chronic Skin Diseases (e.g., Psoriasis)
Physical Findings							
31. Optic neuritis						S	
32. Panophthalmitis						S	
33. Pannus				S	S	S	S
34. Plaque-like lesions in lids/conjunctiva/cornea							U
35. Pruritus				S			
36. Retinal detachment		S					
37. Retinal hemorrhage		R					
38. Scleritis						S	
39. Sebaceous cyst lid				S			
40. Subconjunctival nodules (tuberculomas)						S	
41. Symblepharon					S		
42. Trichiasis						S	S
43. Tylosis ciliaris						S	
44. Uveitis		U			S	S	
45. Vitreous opacity		S					
46. White lashes (poliosis)		S			S	S	
Laboratory Data							
1. Fluorescein angiography		U				S	
2. Cerebrospinal fluid abnormal		U					
3. Red blood count, white blood count, hemoglobin, hematocrit	U						
4. Radioactive iodine uptake test			U				
5. T3 and T4 serum test			U				
6. Purified protein derivative and ELISA test						U	
7. Chest roentgenogram						U	

R = rarely; S = sometimes; and U = usually.

10. Generalized hypotrichosis
11. HIV (human immunodeficiency virus)
12. Hypocalcemia
13. Hypothermal injury
*14. Idiopathic
15. Inflammation and infection of the lids, including seborrheic blepharitis, squamous blepharitis, herpes zoster, sebaceous gland carcinoma, vaccinia, mycotic infection, furuncles, and erysipelas
16. Intoxication with arsenic, bismuth, thallium, gold, quinine and vitamin A
17. Isolated madarosis
18. Keratosis decalvans
19. Keratosis follicularis
20. Keratosis spinulosa
21. Lid colobomas
22. Leprosy
23. Lipoid proteinosis (Urbach–Wiethe syndrome)
24. Polymorphous light eruption
25. Pseudoprogeria syndrome
26. Radiation
27. Severe debilitating systemic diseases, including tuberculosis, syphilis, sickle cell anemia, cholera, and Hansen disease (leprosy)
28. Trauma
29. Vogt–Koyanagi–Harada disease (uveitis–vitiligo–alopecia–poliosis syndrome)

Dana MR, et al. Ocular manifestations of leprosy in a noninstitutionalized community in the United States. *Arch Ophthalmol* 1994;112:626–629.

Fraunfelder FT, Fraunfelder FW. *Drug-induced ocular side effects.* Woburn, MA: Butterworth-Heinemann, 2001.

Isenberg SJ. *The eye in infancy.* Chicago: Year Book Medical, 1989.

Roy FH. *Ocular syndromes and systemic diseases,* 3rd ed. Philadelphia: Lippincott Williams & Wilkins, 2002.

DISTICHIASIS (ACCESSORY ROW OF LASHES GROWING FROM OPENINGS OF MEIBOMIAN GLAND)

1. Acquired
    A. Chemical
    B. Immunologic
    C. Physical
*2. Congenital
    A. Anodontia–hypotrichosis syndrome
    B. Distichiasis, lymphedema syndrome
    C. Ectropion and distichiasis
    D. Idiopathic eyelid edema
    E. Pierre Robin syndrome
    F. Tristichiasis
3. Hereditary—autosomal dominant

Fraunfelder FT, Roy FH. *Current ocular therapy,* 5th ed. Philadelphia: WB Saunders, 2000.

Isenberg SJ. *The eye in infancy.* Chicago: Year Book Medical, 1989.

Kolin T, et al. Hereditary lymphedema and distichiasis. *Arch Ophthalmol* 1991;109:980–982.

Temple IK, Collin JR. Distichiasis-lymphoedema syndrome: a family report. *Clin Dysmorphol* 1994;3:139–142.

COARSE EYEBROWS

1. Congenital hypothyroidism (cretinism)
2. CPD syndrome (chorioretinopathy and pituitary dysfunction)
3. Hunter syndrome [mucopolysaccharidosis (MPS II)]
4. Hurler syndrome (MPS I)
*5. Normal variation
6. Rubinstein–Taybi syndrome (broad thumbs syndrome)
7. Sanfilippo syndrome (MPS III)

Roy FH. *Ocular syndromes and systemic diseases*, 3rd ed. Philadelphia: Lippincott Williams & Wilkins, 2002.

SYNOPHRYS (CONFLUENT EYEBROWS EXTENDING TO MIDLINE)

1. Basal cell nevus syndrome (Gorlin syndrome)
2. Cornelia De Lange syndrome (congenital muscular hypertrophy–cerebral syndrome)
3. Deletion 3p syndrome
4. Duplication 3q syndrome
5. Frontometaphyseal dysplasia
6. Hirschhorn–Cooper syndrome (chromosome partial deletion syndrome)
7. Labard syndrome
*8. Normal variation
9. Partial trisomy chromosome 15
10. Smith–Lemli–Opitz syndrome (cerebrohepatorenal syndrome)
11. Thirteen trisomy syndrome (Patau syndrome)
12. Waardenburg syndrome (interoculoiridodermatoauditive dysplasia)

Roy FH. *Ocular syndromes and systemic diseases*, 3rd ed. Philadelphia: Lippincott Williams & Wilkins, 2002.
Smith DW. *Recognizable patterns of human malformation*. Philadelphia: WB Saunders, 1970.

HERTOGH SIGN (LACK OF OUTER THIRD OF EYEBROWS)

1. Autonomic nervous system dysfunction
2. Diphtheria
*3. Endocrinopathies
4. Hypogonadism
5. Hypothyroidism
6. Neurodermatitis
7. Scleroderma (systemic scleroderma)

Pau H. *Differential diagnoses of eye diseases*, 2nd ed. New York: Thieme Medical, 1988.
Roy FH. *Ocular syndromes and systemic diseases*, 3rd ed. Philadelphia: Lippincott Williams & Wilkins, 2002.

LID MYOKYMIA (SPONTANEOUS FASCICULAR EYELID TREMOR WITHOUT MUSCULAR ATROPHY OR WEAKNESS)

*1. Not associated with organic disease
    A. Fatigue
    B. Lack of sleep
    C. Bright light dazzle

* = most important

D. Irritative corneal or conjunctival lesions
E. Debility or anemia
F. Excessive alcohol or smoking
G. Overwork
2. Followed by spastic paretic facial contracture—in dorsal pons in adult and children
3. Multiple sclerosis (disseminated sclerosis)
4. Trigeminal neuralgia
5. Myasthenia gravis (pseudoparalytic syndrome)
6. Familial occurrence
7. Autosomal dominant familial dystonia

Fraunfelder FT, Roy FH. *Current ocular therapy*, 5th ed. Philadelphia: WB Saunders, 2000.

PRESEPTAL CELLULITIS OF EYELID

 1. Eczema
*2. Hordeolum
 3. Neonatal conjunctivitis
 4. Otitis media
 5. Sinusitis
 6. *S. aureus*
 7. Toxic shock syndrome
 8. Trauma
 9. Upper respiratory tract
10. Varicella

Brower MF, et al. Preseptal cellulitis complicated by toxic shock syndrome. *Arch Ophthalmol* 1987;105:1631–1632.

Weiss A, et al. Bacterial periorbital and orbital cellulitis in childhood. *Ophthalmology* 1983;90:195– 203.

TELECANTHUS (DISPROPORTIONATE INCREASE IN DISTANCE BETWEEN MEDIAL CANTHI; MEASUREMENTS IN INFANTS ARE 18 TO 22 MM)

*1. Primary
 2. Secondary—may occur secondarily to an increased distance between the bony orbits (see hypertelorism)
     A. Aarskog syndrome
     B. Blepharonasofacial syndrome
     C. Blepharophimosis syndrome
     D. Camptomelic dysplasia
     E. Carpenter syndrome
     F. Cerebrofacioarticular syndrome of van Maldegem
     G. Coffin–Lowry syndrome
     H. de Lange syndrome
     I. Deletion 5g syndrome
     J. Dubowitz syndrome
     K. Facial–renal acromesomelic syndrome
     L. Faciooculoacousticorenal syndrome
     M. Fetal alcohol syndrome
     N. Fetal hydantoin syndrome
     O. Frontonasal dysplasia

   P. Lambotte syndrome
   Q. KBG syndrome (initials of family studied)
   R. Michel syndrome
   S. Nasopalpebral lipoma–coloboma syndrome
   T. Oculodentodigital syndrome
   U. Orofaciodigital (OFD) type I and type II (Mohr syndrome)
   V. Prader–Willi syndrome
   W. Rieger syndrome
   X. Simosa syndrome
   Y. Tetra-X syndrome
   Z. Trisomy syndrome
  AA. Toriello–Carey syndrome
  BB. Trauma
  CC. Waardenburg syndrome
  DD. Williams syndrome
  EE. 5p- syndrome (Cri-du-chat)
  FF. 10q- syndrome
  GG. Fetal hydantoin syndrome

Isenberg SJ. *The eye in infancy*. Chicago: Year Book Medical, 1989.

Suri M, et al. Blepharophimosis, telecanthus, microstomia, and unusual ear anomaly (Simosa syndrome) in an infant. *Am J Med Genet* 1994;51:222–223.

Tasman W, Jaeger E, eds. *Duane's clinical ophthalmology*. Philadelphia: JB Lippincott, 1990.

ANKYLOBLEPHARON (PARTIAL OR COMPLETE FUSION OF UPPER TO LOWER EYELIDS)

 *1. Ablepharon, macrostomia syndrome
  2. Ankyloblepharon ectodermal dysplasia, cleft lip and palate
  3. Curly hair, ankyloblepharon, nail dysplasia syndrome (CHANDS)
  4. Cryptophthalmos (complete fusion of lids)
  5. Diphtheritic conjunctivitis
  6. Ectodermal syndrome
  7. Edward syndrome
  8. Fraser syndrome
  9. Gastrointestinal anomalies
 10. Hay–Wells ectodermal pterygium syndrome
 11. Popliteal pterygium syndrome
 12. Smallpox
 13. Trachoma
 14. Trisomy 18
 15. Ulcerative blepharitis

Isenberg SJ. *The eye in infancy*. Chicago: Year Book Medical, 1989.

Roy FH. *Ophthalmic surgery: approaches by the masters*. Philadelphia: Lea & Febiger, 1995.

FLARING OF NASAL PART OF EYEBROW

  1. Blepharonasofacial syndrome
  2. Partial trisomy 10q syndrome

* = most important

*3. Waardenburg syndrome
4. Williams syndrome

Isenberg SJ. *The eye in infancy*. Chicago: Year Book Medical, 1989.

HIGH ARCHED BROW

1. Kabuki makeup syndrome
2. Shprintzen–Goldberg syndrome

Isenberg SJ. *The eye in infancy*. Chicago: Year Book Medical, 1989.

ABSENT BROW HAIR

1. Cryptophthalmos
2. Duplication 14q syndrome
3. Pallister-Killian syndrome
4. Pseudoprogeria syndrome

Isenberg SJ. *The eye in infancy*. Chicago: Year Book Medical, 1989.

TRICHIASIS (INWARD TURNING LASHES)

*1. Inflammation/infection
    A. Chronic blepharitis
    B. Herpes simplex or zoster
    C. Trachoma
2. Lid Tumors
    A. Basal cell carcinoma
    B. Capillary hemangioma
    C. Conjunctiva amyloidosis
3. Medications
    A. Epinephrine
    B. Idoxuridine
    C. Phospholine iodide
    D. Pilocarpine
    E. Practolol
    F. Trifluridine
    G. Vidarabine
4. Systemic/Immunologic Disorders
    A. Erythema multiforme
    B. Ocular cicatricial pemphigoid
    C. Stevens–Johnson syndrome
    D. Toxic epidermal necrolysis
    E. Vernal kertoconjunctivitis
5. Trauma
    A. Chemical injury (lye)
    B. Mechanical injury or repair of injury
        (1) Lower lid transconjunctival approach for floor fracture repair or blepharo-
            plasty

* = most important

    (2) After enucleation

    (3) After ectropion repair

    (4) Thermal burns to face/lids

C. Surgery

Byrnes GA. Congenital distichiasis. *Arch Ophthalmol* 1991;109:1752–1753.

Foster CS. Cicatricial pemphigoid. *Trans Am Ophthalmol Soc* 1986;84:527–663.

Roy FH. *Ophthalmic surgery: approaches by the masters.* Philadelphia: Lea & Febiger, 1995.

Udell IJ. Trifluridine-associated conjunctival cicatrization. *Am J Ophthalmol* 1976;82:117–121.

3

Lacrimal System

CONTENTS

DACRYOADENITIS (INFLAMMATION OF LACRIMAL GLAND)

1. Acute dacryoadenitis—rare catarrhal inflammation of the lacrimal gland that usually accompanies systemic disease
   A. In children—*mumps, measles, influenza, scarlet fever, erysipelas, typhoid fever
   B. In adults—gonorrhea, endogenous conjunctivitis and uveitis, infectious mononucleosis, typhoid fever, Crohn disease
   C. Secondary to inflammation from lids or conjunctiva, to include *Klebsiella pneumoniae*, coliform organisms, *Staphylococcus, *Streptococcus, Aedes aegypti, *Diplococcus pneumoniae*, and *Neisseria gonorrhea*
2. Chronic dacryoadenitis—proliferative inflammation of the lacrimal gland, usually because of specific granulomatous disease
   A. Boeck sarcoid (Schaumann syndrome)
   B. Heerfordt disease—chronic bilateral parotitis and uveitis, often associated with paresis of the cranial nerves, usually the seventh nerve, and other general symptoms
      *(1) Sarcoidosis syndrome (Schaumann syndrome)
      (2) Tuberculosis

C. Mikulicz syndrome—dacryoadenitis and parotitis manifested by chronic bilateral swelling of the lacrimal and salivary glands
   (1) Bang disease (brucellosis)
   (2) Hodgkin disease
   (3) Leukemia
   (4) Lymphoma
   (5) Lymphosarcoma (Brill–Symmers disease)
   (6) Reticuloendothelial disease
   (7) Mumps
  *(8) Sarcoidosis syndrome (Schaumann syndrome)
   (9) Syphilis
  (10) Tuberculosis
  (11) Waldenstrom macroglobulinemia
D. Miliary tuberculosis
E. Pseudotumor
F. Syphilis (gumma)
3. Painless enlargement of lacrimal gland
  A. Leukemia
  B. Mumps
4. Painful enlargement of lacrimal gland
  A. Autoimmunologically mediated syndrome
  B. Lymphomatous disease (25%)
  C. Chronic enlargement arising from sarcoid or orbital pseudotumor (25%)
  D. Lacrimal gland neoplasm (50%)
    (1) Benign
      a. Adenoma
      b. Mixed tumor
    (2) Malignant
      a. Carcinoma unrelated to mixed tumor
      b. Adenocarcinoma (adenoid cystic carcinoma)
      c. Mucoepidermoid carcinoma
      d. Squamous cell carcinoma
      e. Mixed tumor

Divine RD, et al. Metastatic carcinoid unresponsive radiation therapy presenting as a lacrimal fossa mass. *Ophthalmology* 1982;89:516.

Newell FW. *Ophthalmology, principles and concepts*, 7th ed. St. Louis: CV Mosby, 1992.

Rhem MN, et al. Epstein-Barr virus dacryoadenitis. *Am J Ophthalmol* 2000;129:372–375.

Roy FH. *Ocular syndrome and systemic diseases*, 3rd ed. Philadelphia: Lippincott Williams & Wilkins, 2002.

Shields CL, et al. Clinicopathologic review of cases of lacrimal gland lesions. *Ophthalmology* 1989;96:431–435.

BLOODY TEARS

1. Conjunctiva
  A. Application of a drug such as silver nitrate
  B. Cachectic conjunctivitis
  C. Focal dermal hypoplasia syndrome (Goltz syndrome)
  D. Fibroma
  *E. Giant papillary conjunctivitis secondary to contact lens wear or prosthesis wear

* = most important

Acute dacryoadenitis (inflammation of lacrimal gland)

	Children (e.g., Mumps)	Adult (e.g., Typhoid Fever)	Inflammation of Lids/Conjunctiva (e.g., Staphylococcus)
History			
1. Affects all ages			U
2. Contagious disease	U	U	
3. Virus infection	U		
Physical Findings			
1. Central retinal artery emboli		S	
2. Central scotoma		S	
3. Congenital punctal occlusion	R		
4. Conjunctivitis	U	U	U
5. Corneal ulcer	S	S	S
6. Cortical blindness	R		
7. Dacryocystitis		S	S
8. Ectropion			S
9. Endophthalmitis		S	S
10. Entropion			S
11. Exophthalmos	R		
12. Granuloma in lids			S
13. Hordeolum			S
14. Hypopyon		S	S
15. Keratitis	U		S
16. Lid abscess/cellulitis			S
17. Madarosis			S
18. Microphthalmos	R		
19. Optic atrophy	R		
20. Optic neuritis	S	S	
21. Panophthalmitis		S	S
22. Orbital vein thrombosis		S	
23. Paralysis of extraocular muscles	S	S	
24. Phlyctenules in conjunctiva			S
25. Ptosis			S
26. Retinal detachment		S	
27. Scleritis	S		
28. Tenonitis	U	U	
29. Uveitis	U	S	R
30. Dacryoadenitis	S	U	S
31. Vitreous hemorrhages	R	S	
Laboratory Data			
1. Stain and culture			
Gram-negative bacillus		U	
Gram-positive cocci			U

R = rarely; S = sometimes; and U = usually.

Mikulicz syndrome—chronic dacryoadenitis and parotitis

	Tuberculosis	Leukemia	Lymphosarcoma	Hodgkin Disease	Sarcoidosis	Lymphoma
History						
1. Children, young adults, and middle age		U	S	U		
2. Greater in blacks					U	
3. Greater in females					S	
4. Greater in males		S	U			
5. Infants, small children						
6. Malignant lymphoma association				U		
7. Occurs 20 to 40 years					U	
Physical Findings						
1. Blepharitis	U	U				
2. Cataract				U		
3. Central serous retinopathy		S				
4. Chronic dacryocystitis	U					
5. Cranial nerve paralysis (usually facial)					S	
6. Exophthalmos			U			U
7. Extraocular muscle paralysis					S	
8. Firm, elastic, orbital mass	S	U				U
9. Follicular, hypertropic granulomatous, papillary or purulent conjunctivitis	U				S	
10. Granulomatous uveitis, posterior synechiae	U	U			U	U
11. Hemorrhage in conjunctiva, choroid, sclera, orbital tissue, retina, and/or optic disc		U				
12. Hypopyon	U					
13. Keratitis				U		
14. Keratoconjunctivitis sicca					S	
15. Painless lid swelling			U		S	
16. Papilledema		S			S	S
17. Peripheral retinal neovascularization		S				
18. Perivascular retinal white lines		S				
19. Posterior synechiae	U				U	
20. Retinal detachment		S				
21. Soft retinal exudates		U				
22. Subconjunctival nodules	U				U	
23. Lids: nodules (milia), ptosis					S	S
24. Optic-nerve; optic atrophy	S				S	S
Laboratory Data						
1. Angiotensin-converting enzyme test					U	
2. Aqueous cytology		U				
3. Biopsy of gland	U	U	U	U	U	U
4. Blood count		U	U	U		
5. Bone marrow		U				S
6. Chest roentgenogram	U		S	S		
7. Gallium scan test					U	
8. Kveim test					U	
9. Orbit/skull roentgenogram						U
10. Peripheral blood smear		U				
11. Tuberculin skin test	U					
12. HIV	U					

R = rarely; S = sometimes; and U = usually.

Bloody tears

	Systemic Disease as Hemophilia	Local Trauma	Lid Disease as Pubic Lice/Nits on Lashes	Conjunctival Tumor as Granuloma	Subconjunctival Hemorrhage	Corneal Vascular Lesion
History						
1. Associated with systemic and local diseases						S
2. Hereditary	S					
3. Inflammation				U		
4. Skin disease			U			
5. Spontaneous appearance					U	
6. Trauma history	S	U			U	S
7. Aspirin intake					U	
Physical Findings						
1. Associated with sarcoid				U		
2. Conjunctival hemorrhage	S	S			U	U
3. Conjunctival keratinization		S		S		
4. Conjunctival necrosis		S				
5. Conjunctival nodules		S		S		
6. Corneal edema						S
7. Corneal opacity						S
8. Chemosis of conjunctiva		U		S	S	S
9. Epithelial inclusion cysts		S		S		
10. Exophthalmos	S	S				
11. Faulty closure of conjunctival surgical incisions				U		
12. Follicular conjunctivitis			U			
13. Glaucoma	S					
14. Infestation of lids (adult lice/nits on hair shifts)			U			
15. Leukoma of cornea						S
16. Lid hemorrhage	S	S	S			
17. Lid laceration		U			S	
18. Lid scaling			S			
19. Loss of vision	S	S				S
20. Low intraocular pressure		S			S	R
21. Madarosis			S			
22. Marginal keratitis			S	S		
23. Penetration/perforation of sclera		U			U	
24. Perforation/laceration of bulbar conjunctiva		U			U	
25. Pseudomembranous conjunctivitis		S		R		
26. Retained foreign bodies						
27. Retinal hemorrhages posttrauma	U	S				
28. Retinitis proliferans	S	R				
29. Retrobulbar hemorrhages	S	S				
30. Secondary to retinal/strabismus surgery				U	S	
31. Small rust-colored specks of excreta on the skin of the lids			U			
32. Superficial/deep corneal vessels						S
33. Vessels into old corneal lesion						S
34. Vitreous hemorrhage	S	U				
Laboratory Data						
1. Pulse transmission time and factor 8 assay	U					
2. Microscopic exam lid lice/nits			U			

R = rarely; S = sometimes; and U = usually.

    F. Gross disturbance of autonomic nervous system

    G. Hemangioma

    H. Hereditary hemorrhagic telangiectasis

    I. Inflammatory granuloma

    J. Malignant melanoma

    K. Metastatic carcinoid tumor

  *L. Severe conjunctivitis with marked hyperemia

 *M. Subconjunctival hemorrhage following sudden venous congestion of head from stooping, coughing, choking, Valsalva trauma, hemophilia or advanced athrombia

    N. Vicarious menstruation with ectopic tissue

2. Corneal vascular lesion or pannus

3. Lid

    A. Pubic lice and nits on the lashes

    B. Trauma

4. Other

    A. Familial telangiectasis

    B. Hemophilia

    C. Hysteria

    D. Jaundice

    E. Osler–Weber–Render

    F. Pathologic process of lacrimal gland

    G. Severe anemia

    H. Severe epistaxis with regurgitation through the lacrimal passages

Dutt S, et al. Acute dacryoadenitis and Crohn's disease: findings and management. *Ophthalmic Plastic & Reconstructive Surg* 1992;8:295–299.

Gritz DC, Rao NA. Metastatic carcinoid tumor diagnosis from a caruncular mass. *Am J Ophthalmol* 1991;112: 468–469.

Hornblass A, et al. The management of epithelial tumors of the lacrimal sac. *Ophthalmology* 1982;7:476.

Krohel GB, et al. Bloody tears associated with familial telangiectasis. *Arch Ophthalmol* 1987;105:1489–1490.

EXCESSIVE TEARS

1. Hypersecretion of tears—may be due to basic secretors (mucin, lacrimal, including secretion from glands of Kraus and Wolfring and oil, including secretion from Zeis, Moll, and Meibomian palpebral glands) or reflex secretors (main lacrimal glands and accessory palpebral glands)

    A. Primary (disturbance of lacrimal gland)

    B. Central or psychic

        (1) Central nervous system lues

        (2) Corticomeningeal lesions

        (3) Emotional states

        (4) Hysteria

        (5) Physical pain

        (6) Voluntary lacrimation, such as when acting

    C. Neurogenic

        (1) Ametropia, tropia, phoria, and eyestrain or fatigue

        (2) Caloric, lacrimal, and reflex tearing—bilateral lacrimation when syringing the ear with warm or cold water and during Tensilon testing

                                                                 * = most important

(3) Crocodile or alligator tears—unilateral profuse tearing when eating
   a. Congenital, often associated with ipsilateral paresis of lateral rectus muscle
   b. Acquired with onset in early stage of facial palsy (Bell palsy) or sequela with parasympathetic fibers to the otic ganglion growing back into superficial petrosal nerve
   c. Duane retraction syndrome
(4) Bell palsy (idiopathic facial paralysis)
(5) Marin–Amat syndrome (inverted Marcus Gunn Jaw-wink phenomenon)
(6) Melkersson–Rosenthal syndrome (Melkersson idiopathic fibro edema)
   d. Section of the greater superficial petrosal nerve
(7) Drugs, including the following:

acebutolol	doxorubicin	nalorphine
acetophenazine	edrophonium	naloxone
acetylcholine	epinephrine	neostigmine
adrenal cortex injection	ether	nifedipine
aldosterone	ethopropazine	nitrazepam
Apresoline	etretinate	opium
alcohol	floxuridine	oxazepam
alseroxylon	fludrocortisone	paramethasone
ambenonium	fluorometholone	pentazocine
antazoline	fluorouracil	perazine
atenolol	fluphenazine	pericyazine
beclomethasone	fluprednisolone	perphenazine
betamethasone	flurazepam	phenylephrine
bethanechol	glycerin	pindolol
bishydroxycoumarin	halazepam	piperacetazine
bleomycin	heparin	piperazine
butaperazine	hydralazine	piroxicam
carbachol	hydrocortisone	practolol
carphenazine	hydroxyamphetamine	prazepam
chloral hydrate	indomethacin(?)	prochlorperazine
chlordiazepoxide	isotretinoin	promazine
chlorpromazine	ketamine	promethazine
ciprofloxacin	labetalol	propiomazine
clonazepam	levallorphan	propoxyphene
clorazepate	lithium carbonate	propranolol
codeine	lorazepam	pyridostigmine quinidine
dactinomycin	meprednisone	pyridostigmine
dantrolene	mesoridazine	pyrilamine
desoxycorticosterone	methacholine	quinidine
dexamethasone	methaqualone	rauwolfia serpentina
dextran	methdilazine	rescinnamine
diazepam	methotrimeprazine	reserpine
diazoxide	methylprednisolone	rifampin
dicumarol	metoprolol	syrosingopine
diethazine	midazolam	temazepam
diethylcarbamazine	mitomycin	thiethylperazine
diltiazem	morphine	thiopropazate
disodium pamidronate	nadolol naltrexone	

thioproperazine   trifluoperazine   verapamil
thioridazine   triflupromazine   vinblastine
triazolam   trimeprazine   warfarin
trichloroethylene   tripelennamine

(8) Exposure to wind, cold, or bright light; photosensitivity and sunburn
(9) Glaucoma
(10) Horner syndrome (see p. 59) (cervical sympathetic paralysis syndrome)
(11) Inflammation or infection of the conjunctiva, uvea, cornea, orbit, lids, sinuses, teeth, or ears
    a. Acute hemorrhagic conjunctivitis
    b. Avitaminosis B (pellagra, niacin deficiency)
    c. Conjunctivochalasis
    d. Elschnig syndrome (I) (meibomian conjunctivitis)
    e. Epidemic keratoconjunctivitis
    f. Feer syndrome (acrodynia)
    g. Hanhart syndrome (recessive keratosis palmoplantaris)
    h. Keratodermia palmaris et plantaris
    i. Reiter syndrome (polyarthritis enteric)
    j. Stannus cerebellar syndrome (riboflavin deficiency)
    k. Thelaziasis
(12) Lesions affecting the lids
    a. Acrodermatitis chronic atrophicans
    b. Blepharoptosis
    c. Congenital distichiasis
    *d. Ectropion
    *e. Entropion
    f. Epiblepharon
    g. Eyelid retraction
    *h. Facial paralysis
    i. Lid imbrication syndrome
    j. Papilloma
    k. Punctal apposition
    l. Trachoma
    *m. Trichiasis
(13) Morquio–Brailsford syndrome (MPS IV)
(14) Myasthenia gravis—afternoon ectropion (Erb–Goldflam syndrome)
(15) Ophthalmorhinostomatohygrosis syndrome
(16) Parkinson disease–facial akinesia
(17) Reflex, such as vomiting or laughing
(18) Sjögren syndrome (secretoinhibitor syndrome)
(19) Stimulation of some cortical areas—thalamus, hypothalamus, cervical sympathetic ganglia, or the lacrimal nucleus
    a. Diencephalic epilepsy syndrome (Penfield syndrome)
    b. Encephalitis
    (1) acute
    (2) hemorrhagica superior
    (3) lethargy
    (4) periaxialis diffusa

* = most important

        c. Engelmann syndrome (diaphyseal dysplasia)

        d. Giant-cell arteritis (temporal arteritis)

        e. Hypothalamic tumors

        f. Meningitis

        g. Page syndrome (hypertensive diencephalic syndrome)

        h. Pseudobulbar palsy from Parkinson syndrome (shaking palsy)

        i. Sluder syndrome (lower facial neuralgia syndrome)

        j. Tic douloureux (trigeminal neuralgia syndrome)

        k. Various senile dementias

    (20) Gradenigo syndrome (temporal syndrome)

    (21) Raeder syndrome (paratrigeminal paralysis, cluster headache)

    (22) Retroparotid space syndrome (Villaret syndrome)

    (23) Rhabdomyosarcoma

    (24) Rothmund syndrome (telangiectasia–pigmentation–cataract syndrome)

    (25) Thermal burns

  D. Symptomatic

    (1) Bee sting of cornea

    (2) Tabes

    (3) Thyrotoxicosis (Basedow syndrome)

2. Inadequacy of lacrimal drainage system

  A. Congenital anomalies of lacrimal apparatus

    (1) Absence or atresia including ectrodactyly-ectodermal dysplasia-clefting syndrome

    (2) Amniotocele

  *(3) Fistulas of lacrimal sac and nasolacrimal duct

    (4) Lateral displacement of medial canthi with lateral displacement of puncta and lengthening of canaliculi as in Waardenburg syndrome (interoculoiridodermatoauditive dysplasia)

    (5) Obstruction of nasolacrimal drainage system, including Walker–Clodius syndrome (lobster claw deformity with nasolacrimal obstruction)

  *(6) Unformed puncta (punctal atresia)

  B. Complications from diseases such as pemphigus, Stevens–Johnson syndrome (dermatostomatitis), and lupus.

 *C. Dacryocystitis

 *D. Distended canaliculi with obstruction, such as from *Actinomyces israelii (Streptothrix foersteri)*, papilloma, or dacryolith

  E. Because of drugs, including the following:

acyclovir	isoflurophate
adenine arabinoside	neostigmine
colloidal silver	physostigmine
demecarium	quinacrine
DEP	silver nitrate
echothiophate	silver protein
epinephrine	thiotepa
F3T	trifluorothymide
floxuridine	trifluorothymidine (including Fuchs–Lyell
fluorouracil	syndrome) (allergic reaction due to drugs
idoxuridine	causing nasolacrimal obstruction)
IDU	

*F. Eversion of inferior lacrimal punctum, including involutional ectropion (horizontal lid laxity and retractors disinsertion)

G. Eversion of inferior lacrimal punctum secondary to ichthyosis or scleroderma

H. Goltz syndrome (focal dermal hypoplasia syndrome)

I. Inadequacy of physiologic lacrimal pump

J. Traumatic lesions of lacrimal drainage system

K. Tumor obstruction, including polyps, papillary hypertrophy, and neurofibromas

    (1) Botulinum toxin usage

    (2) Dyskeratosis congenita (Zinsser–Engman–Cole syndrome)

    (3) Gravity inversion

    (4) Irritation from dust and gases

    (5) Inflammation or destruction of turbinates

    (6) Inhalation cocaine abuse

    (7) Leprosy (Hansen disease)

    (8) Leukemia

    (9) Plasmoma

    (10) Rhinosporidiosis

    (11) Scleroma

    (12) Tuberculosis

    (13) Tumors

L. Primary neoplasms

    (1) Fibroma

    (2) Hemangiopericytoma

    (3) Melanoma

    (4) Papilloma

    (5) Squamous cell carcinoma

M. Secondary involvement by neoplasms

    (1) Basal cell carcinoma

    (2) Lethal midline granuloma

    (3) Leukemia

    (4) Lymphoma

    (5) Maxillary sinus tumors

    (6) Neurofibroma

    (7) Wegener granulomatosis

N. Nasal disease

    (1) Sinusitis

    (2) Hypertrophic rhinitis

    (3) Pseudoepiphora, such as wound fistula following intraocular operation with leak of aqueous

Baron EM, et al. Rhabdomyosarcoma manifesting as acquired nasolacrimal duct obstruction. *Am J Ophthal* 1993; 115:239–242.

Friberg TR, Weinreb RN. Ocular manifestations of gravity inversion. *JAMA* 1985;253:1755–1758.

Fraunfelder FT, Fraunfelder FW. *Drug-induced ocular side effects.* Woburn, MA: Butterworth-Heinemann, 2001.

Glatt HJ. Epiphora caused by blepharoptosis. *Am J Ophthalmol* 1991;111:649–650.

Roy FH. *Ocular syndromes and systemic diseases*, 3rd ed. Philadelphia: Lippincott Williams & Wilkins, 2002.

Wojno TH. Allergic lacrimal obstruction. *Am J Ophthalmol* 1988;106:48–52.

* = most important

Excessive tears

	Psychic as Hysteria	Neurogenic as Glaucoma	Hyperthyroidism	Congenital Lesion Drainage as Unformed Puncta	Dacryocystitis	Traumatic Lesion as Cut Canaliculi	Obstruction by Actinomyces Israeli	Drugs as Idoxuridine	Eversion—Lower Punctum as Ectropion
History									
1. Anxiety state	U								
2. Bilateral	U	U	U	S				U	S
3. Common 30 to 50 years			U						
4. Common in females			U		U				
5. Common in males						U			S
6. Common in rural midwest United States							U		
7. Common in whites					U				
8. Congenital		S		U					S
9. Dyschromatopsia	S								
10. Exaggeration of symptoms without physical cause	U								
11. Familial		U				S			
12. Night blindness	S								
13. Onset at 2 weeks					U				
14. Topical idoxuridine during 2 weeks								U	
15. Trauma						U			S
Physical Findings									
1. Accommodative spasm	S								
2. Amaurosis fugax	S								
3. Angioneurotic lid edema	S								
4. Anisocoria	S	S							
5. Optic neuritis	S								
6. Avulsion of medial canthal tendon						U			
7. Canaliculitis				S	S		U		
8. Cataract		S							
9. Central serous retinopathy	S								
10. Closed anterior chamber angle		U							
11. Conjunctivitis					S		U		U
12. Conjunctivitis, self-induced	S								
13. Contact dermatitis	S								
14. Corneal abscess			S						
15. Corneal edema		U							
16. Corneal filaments								U	
17. Corneal hypesthesia	S	U							
18. Corneal superficial neovascularization								S.	
19. Corneal ulcer					S		S	S	
20. Creamy pus from punctum often with sulfur granules							U		
21. Cyst of lacrimal gland						S			
22. Lid/lacrimal sac tenderness					U		U		S
23. Turbid tear					U	S	U		S
24. Dye clearance delay				U	U	U	U	S	U
25. Lid imbrication									S
26. Dacryocystitis				U	U	U	R		
27. Disc hemorrhage		S							
28. Ectropion of puncta							U		

Excessive tears (Continued)

	Psychic as Hysteria	Neurogenic as Glaucoma	Hyperthyroidism	Congenital Lesion Drainage as Unformed Puncta	Dacryocystitis	Traumatic Lesion as Cut Canaliculi	Obstruction by Actinomyces Israeli	Drugs as Idoxuridine	Eversion—Lower Punctum as Ectropion
Physical Findings									
29. Edema/hyperemia/pain of surrounding lacrimal sac					U				
30. Exposure keratopathy			S						
31. Extraocular muscles involvement			U						
32. Fine punctate keratopathy								U	
33. Fistula of lacrimal sac/gland						U			
34. Folds in Descemet membrane		U							
35. Follicular conjunctivitis								S	
36. Glaucomatous disc cupping		S							
37. Herpetic keratitis	S								
38. Hypopyon							U		
39. Increased intraocular pressure	S	U	S						
40. Lacrimal gland enlargement			S						
41. Lid abscess							S		
42. Lid cicatrization inner canthus						U			S
43. Lid lag			U						
44. Lid retraction			U						
45. Mild dilated and fixed pupil		S							
46. Mucopurulent material from the sac at pressure					U				
47. Nystagmus	S								
48. Optic nerve atrophy		U	S						
49. Orbital cellulitis						S			
50. Panophthalmitis					S				
51. Papilledema			S						
52. Peripheral anterior synechiae		U							
53. Pouting of the punctum							U		
54. Proptosis (axial)			U						
55. Ptosis	S							S	
56. Stenosis of lacrimal punctum							U	S	
57. Strabismus	S								
58. Traumatic corneal epithelial erosions	U								
59. Uveitis							S		
60. Visual field defects		U	S						

R = rarely; S = sometimes; and U = usually.

DRUGS FOUND IN TEARS

Drugs, including the following:

alcian blue	fluorouracil	sodium salicylate
amodiaquine	hydroxychloroquine	trypan blue
aspirin	methotrexate	vitamin A
chloroquine	minocycline	
fluorescein	rose bengal	

Fraunfelder FT, Fraunfelder FW. *Drug-induced ocular side effects.* Woburn, MA: Butterworth-Heinemann, 2001.

Tabbara KF, Cooper H. Minocycline levels in tears of patients with active trachoma. *Arch Ophthalmol* 1989;107: 93–95.

DRY EYE (PAUCITY OR ABSENCE OF TEARS)

1. Xerosis—local tissue changes
    A. Cicatricial degeneration of conjunctiva and mucous tissues
        (1) General—diphtheria
        (2) Upper lid—trachoma
        (3) Lower lid
            a. Avitaminosis A
            b. Chemical irritation (especially due to alkali)
            c. Dermatitis herpetiformis (Duhring–Brocq disease)
            d. Epidermolysis bullosa (Weber–Cockayne syndrome)
            e. Erythema multiforme (Stevens–Johnson syndrome)
            f. Ocular pemphigoid
            g. Plummer–Vinson syndrome (sideropenic dysphagia syndrome)
            h. Radium burns
            i. Reiter syndrome (conjunctivourethrosynovial syndrome)
            j. Sjögren syndrome (secretoinhibitor syndrome)
            k. Uyemura syndrome (fundus albipunctatus with hemeralopia and xerosis)
    B. Exposure keratitis
        (1) Anterior lamella shortage secondary to trauma or facial burn
        *(2) Deficient lid closure as part of facial palsy
        *(3) Ectropion (see p. 81)
        (4) Eyelid retraction-Graves ophthalmopathy (incomplete blink)
        (5) Exophthalmos
        (6) Following botulism
        *(7) Infrequent blinking, such as with progressive supranuclear palsy
        (8) Lack of blinking as during coma
        (9) Levator spasm
        (10) Melkersson–Rosenthal syndrome (Melkersson idiopathic fibroedema)
        (11) Methylmalonic aciduria
        (12) Ocular proptosis
        (13) Rapid evaporation in hot, dry areas
        (14) Stiff, immobile, retracted lids, such as those occurring secondary to tuberculoid leprosy (Hansen disease)
2. Keratoconjunctivitis sicca—primary tear diminution of main and accessory lacrimal glands
    A. Congenital
        (1) Congenital absence of lacrimal gland as in Bonnevie–Ullrich syndrome

* = most important

(2) Neurogenic
(3) Associated with generalized disturbance
   a. Anhidrotic type of ectodermal dysplasia
   b. Familial dysautonomia (Riley–Day syndrome)
   c. Cri-du-chat syndrome (Cry of the cat syndrome)
   d. Cystic fibrosis syndrome (fibrocystic disease of pancreas)
B. Neurogenic hyposecretion
   (1) Central—aplasia of lacrimal nucleus or lesion of seventh nerve between nucleus and geniculate ganglion
      a. Pontine lesions
      b. Basal fractures
      c. Otitis media
   (2) Peripheral—greater superficial petrosal nerve, sphenopalatine ganglion, or lacrimal branch
      a. Skull fractures
      b. Associated with neoplasms
      c. Neurologic lesion of fifth nerve (neuroparalytic keratitis)
   (3) Herpes zoster of the geniculate ganglion (Ramsey–Hunt syndrome)
   (4) Parasympathetic blocking drugs, such as atropine and scopolamine, may decrease an already barely adequate secretion.
   (5) Botulism
   (6) Deep anesthesia
   (7) Debilitating disease, such as typhus and cholera, and high temperature
   (8) Allergy
C. Systemic disease
   (1) Allgrove syndrome
   (2) Acquired immunodeficiency syndrome (AIDS)
   (3) Amyotrophic lateral sclerosis
   (4) Danbolt–Closs syndrome (acrodermatitis enteropathica)
   (5) Disseminated lupus erythematosus (Kaposi–Libman–Sacks syndrome)
   (6) Drugs, including the following:

acebutolol
acetophenazine
albuterol
aluminum nicotinate(?)
amitriptyline
antazoline
astemizole
atenolol
atropine
azatadine
belladonna
bendroflumethiazide
benzalkonium
benzthiazide
brimonidine
brompheniramine
busulfan

butaperazine
carbinoxamine
carphenazine
chlorisondamine
chlorothiazide
chlorpheniramine
chlorpromazine
chlorthalidone
cimetidine(?)
clemastine fumarate
clonidine
cyclothiazide
cyproheptadine
desipramine
dexbrompheniramine
dexchlorpheniramine
diethazine

dimethindene
diphenhydramine
diphenylpyraline
disopyramide
doxylamine
dronabinol
ether
ethopropazine
etretinate
fluphenazine
hashish
hexamethonium
homatropine
hydrochlorothiazide
hydroflumethiazide
imipramine
indapamide

isotretinoin
lithium carbonate
marihuana
mesoridazine
methdilazine
methotrexate
methotrimeprazine
methoxsalen
methscopolamine
methyclothiazide
methyldopa
methylthiouracil
metolazone
metoprolol
morphine
nadolol
niacin(?)
niacinamide(?)
nicotinyl alcohol(?)

nitrous oxide
nortriptyline
opium
oxprenolol
perazine
periciazine
perphenazine
pheniramine
pimozide
pindolol
piperacetazine
polythiazide
practolol
prochlorperazine
promazine
promethazine
propiomazine
propranolol
protriptyline

pyrilamine
quinethazone
scopolamine
tetrahydrocannabinol
thiethylperazine
thiopropazate
thioproperazine
thioridazine
timolol
tolterodine
tartrate
trichlormethiazide
trichloroethylene
trifluoperazine
triflupromazine
trimeprazine
trioxsalen
tripelennamine
triprolidine

(7) Felty syndrome (uveitis–rheumatoid arthritis syndrome)
(8) Gougerot-Sjögren syndrome (oligophrenia–ichthyosis–spastic diplegia syndrome)
(9) Heerfordt syndrome (uveoparotitis)
(10) Lubarsch–Pick syndrome (primary amyloidosis)
(11) Mikulicz syndrome—acryoadenitis and parotitis
    a. Hodgkin disease
    b. Leukemia
    c. Lymphoma
    d. Lymphosarcoma
    e. Mumps
    f. Sarcoidosis syndrome (Schaumann syndrome)
    g. Syphilis
    h. Tuberculosis
    i. Waldenstrom macroglobulinemia
(12) Pancreatitis
(13) Pheochromocytoma, medullary thyroid carcinoma, and multiple mucosal neuromas
(14) Polyarteritis nodosa (Kussmaul disease)
(15) Relapsing polychondritis
(16) Rheumatoid arthritis (adult)
(17) Scleroderma (progressive systemic sclerosis)

Fraunfelder FT, Fraunfelder FW. *Drug-induced ocular side effects.* Woburn, MA: Butterworth-Heinemann, 2001.

Geier SA. Sicca syndrome in patients infected with the human immunodeficiency virus. *Ophthalmology* 1995;102:1319–1324.

Newell FW. *Ophthalmology, principles and concepts,* 7th ed. St. Louis: CV Mosby, 1992.

Roy FH. *Ocular syndromes and systemic diseases,* 3rd ed. Philadelphia: Lippincott Williams & Wilkins, 2002.

DACRYOCYSTITIS (INFECTION OF THE LACRIMAL SAC)

1. Acute dacryocystitis
   *A. Beta-hemolytic streptococcus
   B. *Corynebacterium diphtheriae*
   C. Dacryolith
   D. Erysipelothrix insidiosa
   E. Friedlander bacillus
   F. Fusobacterium (canaliculitis and dacryocystitis)
   G. Granulomatous "pseudotumor"
   *H. Haemophilus aegyptius (Koch–Weeks bacillus)
   I. Infectious mononucleosis
   J. Influenza
   K. Lymphocytic neoplasia
   L. *Neisseria catarrhalis*
   M. *Pasteurella multocida*
   *N. Pneumococcus
   *O. *Pseudomonas aeruginosa*
   P. Rhinosporidiosis
   Q. Rubeola (measles)
   R. Serratia marcescens—gram-negative coccobacillus
   *S. Staphylococcus
   T. Streptococcus
   U. Tularemia
   V. Variola

2. Chronic dacryocystitis
   A. Associated with osteopoikilosis
   B. *Actinomyces israelii*
   C. Aspergillus
   D. *Bacillus fusiformis*
   E. *Candida albicans*
   F. *Escherichia coli*
   G. Lymphoma of the lacrimal sac
   H. *Mycobacterium fortuitum* and *Mycobacterium chelonei*
   I. *Nocardia asteroides*
   J. *Francisella tularensis*
   K. *Mycobacterium leprae*
   L. *Proteus vulgaris*
   M. Sporotrichosis
   N. Syphilis (acquired lues)
   O. Systemic sarcoidosis
   P. Thermal burns
   Q. Trachoma
   R. *Treponema vincentii*
   S. Tuberculosis (*Mycobacterium tuberculosis*)
   T. Wegener granulomatosis

* = most important

Artenstein AW, et al. Chronic dacryocystitis caused by *Mycobacterium fortuitum. Ophthalmology* 1993;100: 666–668.

Gunal I, et al. Dacryocystitis associated with osteopoikilosis. *Clin Genet* 1993;44:211–213.

Haynes BF, et al. The ocular manifestations of Wegener's granulomatosis: fifteen year's experience and review of the literature. *Am J Med* 1977;63:131.

Karesh JW, et al. Dacryocystitis associated with malignant lymphoma of the lacrimal sac. *Ophthalmology* 1993; 100:669–673.

Roy FH. *Ocular syndrome and systemic diseases*, 3rd ed. Philadelphia: Lippincott Williams & Wilkins, 2002.

Extraocular Muscles

CONTENTS

PSEUDOESOTROPIA (OCULAR APPEARANCE OF ESOTROPIA WHEN NO MANIFEST DEVIATION OF VISUAL AXIS IS PRESENT)

*1. Abnormal shape of skull or abnormal thickness of skin surrounding the orbits
2. Enophthalmos
3. Entropion (p. 79)
4. Hypotelorism with narrow interpupillary distance
5. Lateral displacement of the concavity of the upper eyelid margin from the center of the pupil
*6. Negative-angle kappa—pupillary light reflex displaced temporally (see Decentered Pupillary Light Reflex, p. 361)
*7. Prominent epicanthal fold
8. Telecanthus—the orbits are normally placed, but the medial canthi are far apart secondary to lateral displacement of the soft tissues

Shaterian ET, Weismann IL. An unusual case of pseudostrabismus. *Am Orthop J* 1973;23:68–70.

Urist MJ. Pseudostrabismus caused by abnormal configuration of the upper eyelid margins. *Am J Ophthalmol* 1973; 75:455–456.

ESOPHORIA AND ESOTROPIA (VISUAL AXIS DEVIATED INWARD; MAY BE LATENT OR MANIFEST)

1. Comitant (nonparalytic)—angle of deviation is constant in all directions of gaze
  A. Accommodative—hyperopic refractive error
  B. Nonaccommodative—refractive error not cause of deviation
    (1) Anomalous insertion of horizontally acting muscles
    (2) Abnormal check ligaments
    (3) Faulty innervational development
    (4) Autosomal recessive trait

* = most important

      (5) Idiopathic
      (6) Tumor of the brain
         a. Cerebellar astrocytoma
         b. Pontine glioma
2. Noncomitant—the angle of deviation varies in different directions of gaze
   A. Abducens palsy (p. 161)
   B. Accommodative spasm
   C. Blowout fracture
   D. Divergence paralysis
   E. Drug use (marihuana)
   F. Duane syndrome
   G. Myasthenia gravis
   H. Thyroid myopathy
3. "V" pattern esotropia—deviation greater in downward gaze
   A. Underaction—superior oblique muscles
   B. Overaction—inferior oblique muscles
4. "A" pattern esotropia
   A. Underaction—inferior oblique muscles
5. Monocular esotropia—one eye may be used to the exclusion of the other; amblyopia is usual in the deviating eye
6. Esotropia—near/distance disparity
   A. High accommodation convergence–accommodation (AC/A) ratio—greater convergence for near than for distance, causing greater esodeviation for near than for distance
   B. Convergence excess—greater esodeviation for near than for distance
   C. Divergence insufficiency—greater esodeviation for distance than for near

Helveston EM. The origins of congenital esotropia. *J Pediatr Ophthalmol Strabismus* 1993;30:215–232.

von Noorden GK. *Binocular vision and ocular motility: theory and management of strabismus.* St. Louis: CV Mosby, 1995.

Wright KW. *Pediatric ophthalmology and strabismus.* St. Louis: CV Mosby, 1995.

Williams AS, Hoyt CS. Acute comitant esotropia in children with brain tumors. *Arch Ophthalmol* 1989;107:376.

PSEUDOEXOTROPIA (OCULAR APPEARANCE OF EXOTROPIA WHEN NO MANIFEST DEVIATION OF VISUAL AXIS IS PRESENT)

1. Displaced macula (heterotopia of the macula; see p. 451)
2. Heterochromia when the lighter-colored eye appears to diverge (see p. 368–372)
3. Hypertelorism with wide interpupillary distance
4. Exophthalmos
5. Positive-angle kappa—pupillary light reflex displaced nasally (see decentered pupillary light reflex, p. 361)
6. Narrow lateral canthus
7. Wide palpebral fissure

Beyer-Machule C, von Noorden GK. *Atlas of ophthalmic surgery,* Vol 1: *Lids, orbits, extraocular muscles.* New York: Thieme Medical, 1984.

Shaterian ET, Weissman IL. An unusual case of pseudostrabismus. *Am Orthopt J* 1973;23:68–70.

EXOPHORIA AND EXOTROPIA (VISUAL AXIS DEVIATED OUTWARD; MAY BE LATENT OR MANIFEST)

1. Comitant
    A. Refractive—myopic refractive error cause of deviation (low AC/A ratio)
    B. Nonrefractive—refractive error not cause of deviation
    C. Anomalous insertion of horizontally acting muscles
    D. Abnormal check ligaments
    E. Faulty innervational development
    F. Autosomal-dominant trait
    G. Idiopathic
2. Noncomitant
    A. Convergence insufficiency
    B. Divergence excess
    C. Duane type II, III
    D. Internuclear ophthalmoplegia
    E. Myasthenia gravis
    F. Third nerve palsy
    G. Thyroid myopathy
3. Pattern exotropia
    A. V exotropia—deviation greater in upward than in downward gaze
        (1) Underaction superior oblique
        (2) Overaction inferior oblique
    B. Exotropia—deviation greater in downward than in upward gaze
        (1) Underaction inferior oblique muscle
        (2) Overaction superior oblique muscle

von Noorden GK. *Binocular vision and ocular motility: theory and management of strabismus.* St. Louis: CV Mosby.

Wright KW. *Pediatric ophthalmology and strabismus.* St. Louis: CV Mosby, 1995.

PSEUDOHYPERTROPIA

1. Facial asymmetry with one eye placed higher than the other
2. Unilateral coloboma of lid
3. Unilateral ptosis

Shaterian ET, Weissman IL. An unusual case of pseudostrabismus. *Am Orthop J* 1973;23:68–70.

Wright DW. *Pediatric ophthalmology and strabismus.* St. Louis: CV Mosby, 1995.

HYPERPHORIA AND HYPERTROPIA (VISUAL AXIS DEVIATED UPWARD; MAY BE MANIFEST OR LATENT)

1. Nonparalytic hypertropia
    A. Abnormal insertion of muscles
    B. Abnormal fascial attachments
    C. Complications of systemic diseases, such as myasthenia gravis, thyrotoxicosis, and orbital tumors
2. Paralytic hypertropia—isolated cyclovertical muscle palsy
    A. Brainstem disease
    B. Fourth nerve palsy
    C. Multiple sclerosis

    D. Skew deviation

    E. Third nerve palsy

3. Double hyperphoria (alternating circumduction)—fuses, but cover test shows alternating hyperphoria

4. Apparent paralysis of elevation of one eye

    A. Local neuromuscular and orbital causes

        (1) Dysthyroid ophthalmoplegia (noncongestive and congestive form)

        (2) Myasthenia gravis (Erb–Goldflam syndrome)

        (3) Orbital floor fracture

        (4) Progressive supra nuclear ophthalmoplegia

        (5) Oculomotor nerve paresis superior division

        (6) Unilateral double-elevator palsy, congenital dysfunction of superior rectus and inferior oblique muscles

        (7) Myositis

            a. "Collagen diseases"

            b. Infectious myositis

            c. Trichinosis

        (8) Orbital tumors

            a. Dermoid cyst

            b. Hemangioma

            c. Lymphoma

            d. Meningioma

            e. Optic nerve glioma

            f. Previous strabismus surgery

            g. Rhabdomyosarcoma

        (9) Systemic amyloidosis with ocular muscle infiltration

       (10) Vertical retraction syndrome (Parinaud syndrome)

       (11) Superior oblique tendon sheath syndrome (Brown syndrome)

    B. Skew deviation due to a central nervous system lesion—one eye is above the other; may be the same for all directions of gaze or vary in different directions of gaze

        (1) Unilateral labyrinthine disease

        (2) Cerebellar tumors, such as astrocytomas and medulloblastomas

        (3) Acoustic neuromas

        (4) Vascular accidents of pons and cerebellum, such as thrombosis of cerebellar and pontine arteries

        (5) Unilateral internuclear ophthalmoplegia and less frequently bilateral internuclear ophthalmoplegia

        (6) Compressive lesions, such as platybasia and Arnold–Chiari malformation

        (7) Brain-stem arteriovenous malformations

        (8) Aberrant regeneration of third nerve

    C. Central nervous system lesions

        (1) Arteriosclerosis, thrombosis, arteritis (syphilitic), or embolus of fine vessels to midbrain

5. Apparent paralysis of elevation of both eyes

    A. Physiologic in older persons

    B. Parinaud syndrome (divergence paralysis)

    C. Chronic progressive external ophthalmology (CPEO)

    D. Progressive supranuclear palsy

    E. Myasthenia gravis
    F. Midbrain lesion
       (1) Upgaze center
       (2) Bilateral third nerve palsy
       (3) Dorsal midbrain syndrome
    G. Congenital fibrous syndrome
    H. Thyroid myopathy
    I. Metastatic tumor (breast cancer)
6. Paralysis of downward gaze
    A. Reverse Parinaud syndrome
    B. Associated with choreoathetotic syndromes
    C. Parkinsonian syndromes
    D. Myasthenia gravis
    E. Miscellaneous

Flaherty MP, et al. Congenital fibrosis of the extraocular muscles associated with cortical dysplasia and maldevelopment of the basal ganglia. *Ophthalmology* 2001;108:1313–1322.

Keane JR. Ocular skew deviation. *Arch Neurol* 1975;32:185.

Metz HS. Double elevator palsy. *J Ped Ophthal Strab* 1981;18:31–36.

Kushner BJ. Errors in the three-step test in the diagnosis of vertical strabismus. *Ophthalmol* 1989;96:127–132.

BROWN SUPERIOR OBLIQUE TENDON SHEATH SYNDROME (LIMITATION OF ELEVATION IN ADDUCTION THAT RESEMBLES AN UNDERACTION OF INFERIOR OBLIQUE MUSCLE)

1. Congenital onset
    A. Congenital Brown syndrome
    B. Inelastic muscle-tendon complex
2. Anomalies of Superior Oblique Tendon fibers
3. Congenital pseudo–Brown Syndrome—anomalous inferior orbital adhesions
4. Posterior orbital bonds
5. Acquired onset
    A. Acquired Brown syndrome
    B. Peritrochlear scarring and adhesions
    C. Chronic sinusitis
6. Trauma—superior temporal orbit
7. Blepharoplasty and fat removal
8. Lichen sclerosis at astrophicus and morpheae
9. Tendon–trochlear inflammation and edema
10. Idiopathic inflammatory (pain and click)
11. Trochleitis with superior oblique myositis
12. Acute sinusitis
13. Adult rheumatoid arthritis
14. Juvenile rheumatoid arthritis
15. Systemic lupus erythematosus
16. Possibly distant trauma (CPR [cardiopulmonary resusitation] and long-bone fractures)
17. Possibly postpartum hormonal change
18. Superior nasal orbital mass
19. Glaucoma implant
20. Neoplasm

21. Tight or inelastic superior oblique muscles
22. Thyroid disease (inelastic muscles)
23. Peribulbar anesthesia (inelastic tendon)
24. Hurler Scheie syndrome (inelastic tendon)
25. Superior oblique tuck (short tendon)
26. Idiopathic
27. Acquired pseudo-Brown syndrome
28. Orbital fracture
29. Retinal band around inferior oblique muscle
30. Inferior temporal adhesion
31. Following double plate Molteno implantation

Dobler-Dixon AA, et al. Prospective evaluation of extraocular motility following double-plate molteno implantation. *Arch Ophthalmol* 1999;117:1155–1160.

Kaban JT, et al. Natural history of presumed congenital Brown's syndrome. *Arch Ophthalmol* 1993;111:102.

Wang FM, et al. Brown's syndrome in children with juvenile rheumatoid arthritis. *Ophthalmology* 1984;91:23–26.

Wilson ME, et al. Brown's syndrome. *Surv Ophthal* 1989;34:153.

DUANE SYNDROME

Congenital ocular motility disorder is characterized by limited abduction or limited adduction. The palpebral fissure narrows on attempted adduction.

1. Type 1 characteristics
     a. A or V phenomena
     b. Defective abduction
     c. Palpebral fissure narrowing on adduction
     d. Retraction of the globe
     e. Updrift or downdrift of the affected eye on adduction or attempted abduction
2. Type 2 characteristics
     a. Abduction appears to be normal or only slightly limited
     b. Distinct narrowing of the palpebral fissure and retraction of the globe on attempted adduction.
     c. Limitation or complete palsy of adduction with exotropia of the paretic eye.
3. Type 3 characteristics
     a. Limitation or absence of both abduction and adduction of the affected eye
     b. Globe retraction and narrowing of the palpebral fissure on attempted adduction

Duane A. Congenital deficiency of abduction associated with impairment of adduction, retraction movements, contraction of the palpebral fissure, and oblique movements of the eye. *Arch Ophthalmol* 1996;114:1255–1256.

Duane TD, et al. Pseudo-Duane's retraction syndrome. *Trans Am Ophthalmol Soc* 1977;74:122–132.

OCULOMOTOR APRAXIA

Oculomotor apraxia is defined as defective or absent horizontal voluntary eye movements and includes head thrusting to look at objects to the side.

1. Ataxia–telangiectasia syndrome

2. Brain tumor
    A. Astrocytoma
    B. Lipoma
3. Isolated
4. Male predominance
5. Neurofibromatosis
6. Oral–facial–digital syndrome type II
7. Post cardiac surgery

Isenberg SJ. *The eye in infancy*. Chicago: Year Book Medical, 1989.

Moschner C, et al. Comparison of oculomotor findings in the progressive ataxia syndromes. *Brain* 1995;117:15–25.

Zackon DH, Noel L. Ocular motor apraxia following cardiac surgery. *Can J Ophthal* 1991;26:102.

Zaret C, et al. Congenital ocular motor apraxia and brainstem tumor. *Arch Ophthalmol* 1980;98:328–330.

MONOCULAR LIMITATION OF ELEVATION OF ADDUCTED EYE WITH FORCED DUCTION TEST [IN ELEVATION AND ADDUCTION (SEE CHART) STRABISMUS WITH RESTRICTED MOTILITY]

1. Acquired
    A. Thyroid myopathy
    *B. Excessive recession or resection of muscle
    C. Orbital fracture
    D. Retinal detachment operation
    E. Strabismus surgery complicated by adhesions
    F. CPEO
2. Congenital
    A. Congenital fibrous syndrome
    B. Neurogenic paralysis with secondary contracture of antagonist muscle
    C. Duane retraction syndrome
    D. Brown superior oblique tendon sheath syndrome
    E. Strabismus fixus

Harley RD, et al. Congenital fibrosis of the extraocular muscles. *Trans Am Ophthal Soc* 1978;76:197.

Wright KW. *Pediatric ophthalmology and strabismus*. St. Louis: CV Mosby, 1995.

CYCLIC, RECURRENT, REPETITIVE, EPISODIC DISORDERS OF EXTRAOCULAR MUSCLES

1. Cyclic strabismus
    A. Associated with frontoorbital fibrous dysplasia
    B. Associated with Graves disease
    C. Associated with optic atrophy
    D. Cyclic superior oblique palsy
    E. Cyclic third nerve palsy
    F. Esotropia, vertical
        (1) Comitant
        (2) Noncomitant
2. Cyclic vertical deviation
3. Diabetic nerve palsies
4. Myasthenia gravis

* = most important

5. Oculogyric crisis (see p. 152)
6. Periodic alternating gaze deviation
7. Periodic alternating nystagmus
8. Periodic vertical nystagmus
    A. Associated with potassium abnormality
    B. Familial
9. Petit mal epilepsy
    A. Exotropia
    B. Upward deviation
10. Ping-pong gaze
11. Recurrent sixth nerve paralysis in children (see p. 169)
12. Spasmus nutans
13. Twitch of lids (orbicularis)

Hamed L. *Cyclic periodic disorders in diagnostic problems in clinical ophthalmology.* Margo CL, ed. Philadelphia: WB Saunders, 1994.

Hoyt WF, Keane JR. Superior oblique myokymia. *Arch Ophthalmol* 1970;84:461–467.

Windsor CE, Berg EF. Circadian heterotropia. *Am J Ophthalmol* 1969;67:565–571.

SYNDROMES AND DISEASES ASSOCIATED WITH STRABISMUS

1. Esotropia syndrome
2. Exotropia syndrome
3. Aarskog syndrome (facial–digital–genital syndrome)
4. Aberfeld syndrome (congenital blepharophimosis associated with generalized myopathy)
5. Achondroplasia
6. Addison pernicious anemia
7. African eyeworm disease
8. Albinism
9. Albright hereditary osteodystrophy (pseudohypoparathyroidism)
10. Amyloidosis
11. Apert syndrome (acrocephalosyndactylism syndrome)
12. Arnold–Chiari syndrome (platybasia syndrome)
13. Arylsulfatase A deficiency syndrome
14. Aspergillosis
15. Axenfeld–Schurenberg syndrome (cyclic oculomotor paralysis)
16. Bacterial endocarditis
17. Bang disease (brucellosis)
18. Behçet syndrome (oculobuccogenital syndrome)
19. Benedikt syndrome (tegmental syndrome)
20. Best disease (vitelliform dystrophy)
21. Bielschowsky–Lutz–Cogan syndrome (internuclear ophthalmoplegia)
22. Bing–Neel syndrome (associated with macroglobulinemia and central nervous system symptoms)
23. Bloch–Sulzberger disease (incontinentia pigmenti)
24. Blocked nystagmus syndrome (nystagmus blockage syndrome)
25. Bonnet–Dechaume–Blanc syndrome (neuroretinoangiomatosis syndrome)
26. Bonnevie–Ullrich syndrome (pterygolymphangiectasia)
27. Botulism

28. Brown–Marie syndrome (hereditary ataxia syndrome)
29. Canine tooth syndrome (class VII superior oblique palsy)
30. Cerebral palsy
31. Chediak–Higashi syndrome (anomalous leukocytic inclusions with constitutional stigmata)
32. Chromosome partial deletion (short-arm) syndrome (Wolf syndrome)
33. Chromosome 13q partial deletion (long-arm) syndrome (thirteen Q syndrome)
34. Chromosome partial deletion (long-arm) syndrome (DeGrouchy syndrome)
35. Chromosome partial (short-arm) partial deletion syndrome
36. Congenital syphilis
37. Convergence insufficiency syndrome
38. Craniocarpotarsal dysplasia (Freeman–Sheldon syndrome; whistling face syndrome)
39. Craniostenosis
40. Cri-du-chat syndrome (Cry of the cat syndrome)
41. Crohn disease (granulomatous ileocolitis)
42. Crouzon disease (craniofacial dysostosis)
43. Cushing syndrome (II) (cerebellopontine angle syndrome)
44. Cysticercosis
45. Cytomegalic inclusion disease, congenital
46. Dawson disease (subacute sclerosing panencephalitis)
47. De Lange syndrome (congenital muscular hypertrophy—cerebral syndrome)
48. Dengue fever
49. Devic syndrome (ophthalmoencephalomyelopathy)
50. Diabetes mellitus
51. Diphtheria
52. Diamond–Blackfan syndrome
53. Down disease (mongolism, trisomy 21)
54. Drugs, including the following:

alcohol
baclofen
calcitriol
chloramphenicol(?)
chloroform
cholecalciferol
ergocalciferol
insulin
iothalamate meglumine and
　sodium iothalamic acid
isocarboxazid

measles and rubella virus
　vaccine (live)
measles, mumps, and rubella
　virus vaccine (live)
measles virus vaccine (live)
metoclopramide
metrizamide
mumps virus vaccine (live)
nialamide
pemoline
pentylenetetrazol

phenelzine
rubella and mumps virus
　vaccine (live)
rubella virus vaccine (live)
tranylcypromine
tripelennamine
vitamin A
vitamin D_2
vitamin D_3

54. Drummond syndrome (idiopathic hypercalcemia)
55. Duane syndrome (retraction syndrome)
56. Ectrodactyly–ectodermal dysplasia clefting syndrome (EEC syndrome)
57. Ehlers–Danlos disease (fibrodysplasia elastica generalisata)
58. Electrical injury
59. Ellis–van Creveld syndrome (chondroectodermal dysplasia)
60. Encephalitis, acute
61. Engelmann syndrome (osteopathia hyperostotica scleroticans multiplex infantalis)
62. Epidermal nevus syndrome (ichthyosis hystrix)

63. Erb–Goldflam disease
64. Fetal alcohol syndrome
65. Fibrosarcoma
66. François dyscephalic syndrome
67. Gaucher syndrome (glucocerebroside storage disease)
68. Gangliosidosis
    A. Infantile (GM1)
    B. Juvenile (GM2)
69. Goltz syndrome (focal dermal hypoplasia syndrome)
70. Gorlin–Goltz syndrome (multiple basal cell nevi syndrome)
71. Greig syndrome (ocular hypertelorism syndrome)
72. Grönblad–Strandberg syndrome (systemic elastodystrophy)
73. Hemangiomas
74. Hemifacial hyperplasia with strabismus (Bencze syndrome—autosomal dominant)
75. Hemifacial microsomia (otomandibular dysostosis)
76. Homocystinuria
77. Hurler disease (mucopolysaccharidoses type I)
78. Hutchinson syndrome (adrenal cortex neuroblastoma with orbital metastasis)
79. Hydrocephalus, congenital
80. Hydrophobia (rabies)
81. Hyperthyroidism
82. Hypocalcemia
83. Hypomelanosis of Ito syndrome (incontinentia pigmenti achromians)
84. Hypothermal injury
85. Hysteria
86. Infectious mononucleosis
87. Influenza
88. Jacobs syndrome (triple X syndrome)
89. Johnson syndrome (adherence syndrome)
90. Klippel–Feil syndrome (congenital brevicollis)
91. Koerber–Salus–Elschnig syndrome (nystagmus retractorius syndrome)
92. Kohn–Romano syndrome (telecanthus, ptosis, epicanthus inversus, blepharophimosis)
93. Krause syndrome (congenital encephaloophthalmic dysplasia)
94. Kugelberg–Welander syndrome (progressive muscle atrophy)
95. Kussmaul disease (necrotizing angiitis)
96. Larsen syndrome (hypertelorism, microtia, and facial clefting)
97. Laurence–Moon–Bardet–Biedl syndrome (retinitis pigmentosa-polydactyly-adiposo-genital syndrome)
98. Leigh disease (subacute necrotizing encephalomyelopathy)
99. Leukemia
100. Linear nevus sebaceous of Jadassohn
101. Lowe syndrome (oculocerebrorenal syndrome)
102. Lymphangioma
103. Lymphedema
104. Lymphoid hyperplasia (Burkitt lymphoma)
105. Malaria
106. Malignant hyperpyrexia syndrome
107. Malignant hyperthermia syndrome
108. Maple syrup urine disease

109. Marcus Gunn syndrome (jaw-winking syndrome)
110. Marfan syndrome (arachnodactyly–dystrophia mesodermalis congenita)
111. Measles
112. Melnick–Needles syndrome (osteodysplasty)
113. Mieten syndrome (corneal opacity, nystagmus, flexion contracture, growth failure)
114. Millard-Gubler syndrome (abducens—facial hemiplegia alternans)
115. Möbius syndrome (congenital paralysis of sixth or seventh nerves)
116. Monofixation syndrome (blind-spot syndrome)
117. Morning glory syndrome (hereditary central glial anomaly of the optic disk)
118. Mucocele
119. Mucormycosis
120. Mulibrey nanism syndrome (Perheentupa syndrome)
121. Multiple lentigines syndrome (leopard syndrome)
122. Multiple sclerosis
123. Mumps
124. Myasthenia gravis (Erb–Goldflam syndrome)
125. Naegeli syndrome (melanophoric nevus syndrome)
126. Nematode ophthalmia syndrome (toxocariasis)
127. Neonatal hemolytic disease of hyperbilirubinemia
128. Neuroblastoma
129. Nevus sebaceous of Jadassohn
130. Nevoid basal cell carcinoma syndrome
131. Nielsen syndrome (exhaustive psychosis syndrome)
132. Noonan syndrome (male Turner syndrome)
133. Noone–Milroy–Meige disease (congenital trophedema)
134. Nothnagel syndrome (ophthalmoplegia cerebellar ataxia syndrome)
135. Nystagmus compensation syndrome
136. Obesity–cerebrolocular–skeletal anomalies syndrome
137. Ocular vaccinia
138. Oculocerebellar tegmental syndrome
139. Oculo–oto–ororenoerythropoietic syndrome
140. Ophthalmoplegic retinal degeneration syndrome
141. Orbital floor syndrome (Dejean syndrome)
142. Paget syndrome (osteitis deformans)
143. Pallister–Killian syndrome
144. Papillon–Léage and Psaume syndrome (orodigital facial syndrome)
145. Parkinson syndrome
146. Parry–Romberg disease (progressive facial hemiatrophy)
147. Periocular and ocular metastatic tumors
148. Pertussis (whooping cough)
149. Pierre Robin syndrome (micrognathia–glossoptosis syndrome)
150. Polymyalgia rheumatica
151. Postvaccinial ocular syndrome
152. Pseudoophthalmoplegia syndrome (Roth–Bielschowsky syndrome)
153. Prader–Willi syndrome (hypotonia–obesity syndrome)
154. Pseudohypoparathyroidism (Seabright–Bantam syndrome)
155. Reiter syndrome (conjunctivourethrosynovial syndrome)
156. Relapsing fever

157. Retinoblastoma
158. Ring chromosome 18
159. Ring D chromosome
160. Ring dermoid syndrome
161. Rocky Mountain spotted fever
162. Rubella, congenital
163. Rubinstein–Taybi syndrome (broad-thumb syndrome)
164. Sabin–Feldman syndrome
165. Sandifer syndrome (hiatus hernia-torticollis syndrome)
166. Schilder syndrome (encephalitis periaxialis diffusa)
167. Seckel bird-headed dwarfism
168. Skew deviation syndrome
169. Smallpox
170. Smith–Lemli–Opitz syndrome (cerebrohepatorenal syndrome)
171. Spongy degeneration of the white matter
172. Streptococcus
173. Superior oblique tendon sheath syndrome (Brown syndrome)
174. Supravalvular aortic stenosis syndrome (infantile hypercalcemia with mental retardation)
175. Tay–Sachs syndrome (familial amaurotic idiocy)
176. Temporal arteritis syndrome (cranial arteritis syndrome)
177. Terson syndrome (subarachnoid hemorrhage syndrome)
178. Thomsen syndrome (congenital myotonia syndrome)
179. Trichinosis

Fraunfelder FT, Fraunfelder FW. *Drug-induced ocular side effects*. Woburn, MA: Butterworth-Heinemann, 2001.

Hayashi N, et al. Ocular histopathologic study of a patient with the T 8993-G point mutation in Leigh's syndrome. *Ophthalmology* 2000;107:1397–1402.

McKusick VA. *Mendelian inheritance in man*, 12th ed. Baltimore: Johns Hopkins University Press, 1998.

Roy FH. *Ocular syndromes and systemic diseases*, 3rd ed. Philadelphia: Lippincott Williams & Wilkins, 2002.

HORIZONTAL GAZE PALSY

Horizontal gaze palsy comprises an inability to look horizontally in a given direction; analysis includes optically induced movement, voluntary or command movement, pursuit movement, or vestibular movement.

1. Horizontal palsy of voluntary and command movement—frontal lobe gaze center (second frontal gyrus, Brodmann area 8) or in the corresponding internal capsule gaze palsy of side opposite lesion; it may be associated with facial palsy as well as hemiparesis or hemiplegia toward the side of the gaze palsy, caloric ocular movement intact, and doll's head intact.
2. Horizontal palsy of command and pursuit movements, optically induced movements, and vestibular movements—pons and posterior longitudinal bundle; the gaze palsy is toward the side of the lesion, facial palsy often present, caloric and doll's head responses are absent.

Huber A. *Eye symptoms in brain tumors*, 2nd ed. St. Louis: CV Mosby, 1971:44–47.

OSCILLATIONS OF EYES (INVOLUNTARY, RAPID, TO-AND-FRO MOVEMENT OF EYES HAVING NO RHYTHM OR REGULARITY)

1. Ocular dysmetria—"overshooting" of the eyes with attempted fixation; horizontal ocular dysmetria is associated with lesions of the cerebellum or its pathways as in Friedreich ataxia, Huntington chorea, spinocerebellar degeneration, internuclear ophthalmoplegia, manic depression, alcoholism, schizophrenia, severe diffuse brain damage, cerebellopontine angle tumors, hereditary ectodermal dysplasia with olivopontocerebellar degeneration, Fabry disease (glycosphingolipid lipidosis), vestibulocerebellar ataxia, and toluene abuse

2. Ocular flutter—flutter-like oscillations that are intermittent, rapid, to-and-fro motions, or motions of equal amplitude, interrupt maintained fixation; horizontal ocular flutter is associated with lesions of the cerebellum or its pathways as in limb ataxia, multiple sclerosis, poliomyelitis, neoplasms, or vascular accident

3. Opsoclonus—irregular, hyperkinetic, multidirectional, spontaneous eye movement that persists in sleep
   A. Infections
      (1) Coxsackie B3
      (2) Encephalitis—mild, severe, viral or post infections (including St. Louis encephalitis)
      (3) *Haemophilus influenzae*
      (4) Meningitis
      (5) Paratyphi A
      (6) Psittacosis
      (7) Salmonella
   B. Tumors
      (1) Breast malignancy
      (2) Bronchogenic carcinoma
      (3) Glioblastoma
      (4) Neuroblastoma
      (5) Thyroid carcinoma
      (6) Uterine carcinoma
   C. Toxins and drugs
      (1) Amitriptyline
      (2) Chlordecone
      (3) Lithium–haloperidol (Haldol)
      (4) Thallium
      (5) Toluene abuse
   D. Other
      (1) Acute cerebellar ataxia
      (2) Friedreich ataxia
      (3) Multiple sclerosis (disseminated sclerosis) (rare)
      (4) Nonketotic coma
      (5) Sign of "myoclonic encephalopathy of infancy"
      (6) Vascular accidents
      (7) Vertebrobasilar insufficiency

4. Lightning eye movements (ocular myoclonus)—rapid to-and-fro movements of small conjugate saccades; probably because of bilateral abnormality of a pontine paramedial

zone and pretectal lesions, such as vascular, inflammatory, neoplastic, demyelinating, or trauma of tegmentum as thyroid, lung or uterus carcinoma, neuroblastoma, Menzel hereditary ataxia, pontine myelinolysis, coxsackie B infection, cherry-red spot myoclonus syndrome, Ramsay–Hunt syndrome, and L-tryptophan

Dropcho E, Payne R. Paraneoplastic opsoclonus myoclonus: association with medullary thyroid carcinoma and review of the literature. *Arch Neurol* 1986;43:410–415.

Farris BK, et al. Neuro-ophthalmologic findings in vestibulocerebellar ataxia. *Arch Neurol* 1986;43:1050–1053.

Lazar RB, et al. Multifocal central nervous system damage caused by toluene abuse. *Neurology* 1983;33:1337–1340.

Matsumura K, et al. Syndrome of opsoclonus-myoclonus in hyperosmolar nonketotic coma. *Ann Neurol* 1985;18:623–624.

COGWHEEL EYE MOVEMENTS (JERKY INACCURATE PURSUIT MOVEMENTS)

1. Basal ganglia disease
   A. Anoxia
   B. Carbon disulfide poisoning
   C. Carbon monoxide poisoning
   D. Drugs, including:

acetophenazine	etidocaine	prazepam
alcohol	fluphenazine	prilocaine
allobarbital	flurazepam	primidone
alprazolam	halazepam	probarbital
alseroxylon	heptabarbital	procaine
amitriptyline	hexethal	prochlorperazine
amobarbital	hexobarbital	promazine
aprobarbital	imipramine	promethazine
barbital	lidocaine	propiomazine
bromide	lithium carbonate	propoxycaine
bupivacaine	lorazepam	protriptyline
butabarbital	mephobarbital	rauwolfia serpentina
butalbital	mepivacaine	rescinnamine
butallylonal	mesoridazine	reserpine
butaperazine	metharbital	secobarbital
butethal	methdilazine	syrosingopine
carphenazine	methitural	talbutal
chloral hydrate	methohexital	temazepam
chlordiazepoxide	methotrimeprazine	thiamylal
chloroprocaine	midazolam	thiethylperazine
chlorpromazine	nitrazepam	thiopental
clonazepam	nortriptyline	thiopropazate
clorazepate	oxazepam	thioproperazine
cyclobarbital	pentobarbital	thioridazine
cyclopentobarbital	perazine	triazolam
deserpidine	periciazine	trifluoperazine
desipramine	perphenazine	triflupromazine
diazepam	phencyclidine	trimeprazine
diethazine	phenobarbital	vinbarbital
ethopropazine	piperacetazine	

E. Exposure to manganese
F. Idiopathic
G. Parkinsonism (shaking palsy)
H. Trauma

2. Cerebellar tumors
    A. Astrocytomas
    B. Hemangioblastomas
    C. Medulloblastomas

3. With homonymous hemianopia, indicates parietal or occipital lobe involvement

Fraunfelder FT, Fraunfelder FW. *Drug-induced ocular side effects*. Woburn, MA: Butterworth-Heinemann, 2001.

Huber A. *Eye symptoms in brain tumors*, 2nd ed. St. Louis: CV Mosby, 1971.

Walsh FB, Hoyt WF. *Clinical neuro-ophthalmology*, 4th ed. Baltimore: Williams & Wilkins, 1985.

PENDULAR NYSTAGMUS

Pendular nystagmus comprises oscillations that are approximately equal in rate in two directions; they may be horizontal or vertical.

1. Albinism in which the macula does not develop
2. Aniridia (see p. 364–365)
3. Bilateral chorioretinal lesions involving the macula in early infancy (congenital toxoplasmosis)
4. Brainstem or cerebellar dysfunction
*5. Congenital—cause unknown, may be inherited as autosomal dominant recessive or X-linked recessive trait; not infrequently associated with astigmatism and convergent strabismus
*6. Congenital cataracts
7. Congenital glaucoma
8. Corneal scars
9. Demyelinating disease
10. High myopia of early life
11. Internuclear ophthalmoplegia
12. Laurence–Moon–Bardet–Biedl syndrome (retinitis pigmentosa–polydactyly–adiposogenital syndrome)
13. Leber congenital amaurosis
14. Monocular or binocular visual deprivation
15. Optic nerve hypoplasia, coloboma
*16. Total color blindness (monochromatism)
17. Work in poor illuminations (e.g., mining) (rare)

Cogan DG. *Neurology of the ocular muscles*, 4th ed. Springfield, IL: Charles C Thomas, 1978.

Roy FH. *Ocular syndrome and systemic diseases*, 3rd ed. Philadelphia: Lippincott Williams & Wilkins, 2002.

Walsh FB, Hoyt WF. *Clinical neuro-ophthalmology*, 4th ed. Baltimore: Williams & Wilkins, 1985.

HORIZONTAL JERK NYSTAGMUS (HORIZONTAL OSCILLATORY MOVEMENT OF EYES WITH A FAST AND SLOW PHASE)

1. Albinism
2. Amblyopia (manifest latent nystagmus)

* = most important

3. Cerebellar disease, acute or chronic; fast component to side of lesion
4. Chediak–Higashi syndrome (anomalous leukocytic inclusions with constitutional stigmata)
5. Congenital achromatopsia
6. Congenital cataracts
7. Congenital stationary night-blindness
8. Congenital X-linked, dominant, recessive
9. Leber congenital amaurosis
10. Lesions of labyrinth (e.g., Meniere syndrome) or when one labyrinth has been removed
11. Neoplastic angioendotheliomatosis
12. Optic nerve hypoplasia, coloboma
13. Vestibular nuclei involvement as in persons with multiple sclerosis

Barton JJ, Sharpe JA. Oscillopsia and horizontal nystagmus with accelerating slow phases following lumbar puncture in the Arnold-Chiari malformation. *Ann Neurol* 1993;33:418–421.

Cogan DG. *Neurology of the ocular muscles*, 4th ed. Springfield, IL: Charles C Thomas, 1978.

Elner VM, et al. Neoplastic angioendotheliomatosis. *Ophthalmology* 1986;93:1237–1245.

Spaeth GL. Ocular manifestations of the lipidoses. In: Tasman WC, ed. *Retinal disease in children*. New York: Harper & Row, 1971:187–188.

VERTICAL NYSTAGMUS (SPONTANEOUS VERTICAL OSCILLATIONS OF EYES)

1. Upbeat nystagmus—nystagmus in which the fast component is upward and usually most marked when the gaze is directed upward; usually due to a lesion in the posterior fossa
   A. Brainstem lesion, such as that of the vestibular nuclei
   B. Cerebellar disease—acute or chronic, especially in the vermis
   C. Cerebellar degeneration
   D. Drugs—barbiturates and Dilantin (phenytoin)
   E. Encephalitis
   F. Labyrinth disease—rare; has no lateralizing value
   G. Multiple sclerosis
   H. Idiopathic
2. Downbeat nystagmus—nystagmus in which the fast component is downward and usually most marked when the gaze is directed downward; probably due to a lesion in the lower end of the brain stem or cerebellum
   A. Alcoholic cerebellar disease
   B. Aneurysm of the supraclinoid part of left carotid siphon
   C. Arnold–Chiari malformation—herniation of cerebellar tonsils and part of medulla through foramen magnum
   D. Cerebellar atrophy/degeneration
   E. Carbamazepine
   F. Deformities of cervical spine
   G. Diabetes mellitus
   H. Encephalopathy
   I. Ependymoma of posterior part of the fourth ventricle
   J. Idiopathic
   K. Insufficiency of basilar artery
   L. Klippel-Feil anomaly—upward displacement of odontoid process into foramen magnum

M. Meningioma extending into pontine cistern
N. Morphine poisoning
O. Multiple sclerosis (disseminated sclerosis)
P. Neurogenic muscular atrophy
Q. Platybasia (cerebellomedullary malformation syndrome)

Burde RM, Henkind P. Downbeat nystagmus. *Surv Ophthalmol* 1981;25:263.

Chrousos GA. Downbeat nystagmus and oscillopsia associated with carbamazepine. *Am J Ophthalmol* 1957;103: 221–224.

Holmes GL, et al. Primary position upbeat nystagmus following meningitis. *Ann Ophthalmol* 1981;13:935.

Monteiro ML, Sampaio CM. Lithium-induced downbeat nystagmus in a patient with Arnold-Chiari malformation. *Am J Ophthal* 1993;116:648–649.

ROTARY NYSTAGMUS (ROTARY OSCILLATORY MOVEMENT OF EYES)

1. Benign paroxysmal positional nystagmus—fast component toward lower ear
*2. Cerebellar disease—acute or chronic
3. Cerebrotendinous xanthomatosis
4. Encephalitis
5. Lesion of vestibular nuclei in floor of fourth ventricle associated with multiple sclerosis, syringobulbia, or thrombosis of posteroinferior cerebellar artery or its branches
*6. Superior oblique myokymia—benign, intermittent, uniocular
7. Vestibular involvement (e.g., labyrinthitis, Meniere syndrome)

Leigh RJ, et al. Loss of ipsidirectional quick phases of torsional nystagmus with a unilateral midbrain lesion. *J Vestib Res* 1993;3:115–121.

Rosengart A, et al. Intermittent downbeat nystagmus due to vertebral artery compression. *Neurology* 1993;43: 216–218.

SEE-SAW NYSTAGMUS

One eye moves up as other eye moves down; in addition, there is torsion of eyes—eye moving up intorts, and eye moving down extorts. This nystagmus probably is due to lesions located in mesodiencephalic region, hypothalamus, and thalamus; it may be associated with bitemporal hemianopsia and reduced vertical optokinetic nystagmus.

1. Brainstem vascular disease
*2. Chiasmal glioma
*3. Chromophobe adenoma of the pituitary gland involving the optic chiasm and third ventricle
4. Congenital
*5. Craniopharyngioma, involving the optic chiasm and hypothalamus
6. Head injury with fracture of frontal
7. Idiopathic
8. Multiple sclerosis
9. Oligodendroglioma involving the pons and third ventricle
10. Postoperative after strabismus surgery
11. Retinitis pigmentosa
12. Septooptico dysplasia
13. Suprasellar epidermoid tumor involving optic chiasm and hypothalamus
14. Syringomyelia and syringobulbia

15. Toxoplasmosis of the brainstem

Fein JM, Williams RDB. See-saw nystagmus. *J Neurol Neurosurg Psychiatry* 1969;32:202–207.

Walsh FB, Hoyt WF. *Clinical neuro-ophthalmology*, 4th ed. Baltimore: Williams & Wilkins, 1985.

RETRACTION NYSTAGMUS

Spasmodic retraction of eyes can occur when an attempt is made to move them in any direction; it is caused by lesions of midbrain, especially lesions in the vicinity of aqueduct of Sylvius).

1. Arteriovenous aneurysm
2. Brucellosis (Bang disease)
3. Cysticercus cyst
4. Ependymoma
5. Koerber–Salus–Elschnig syndrome (sylvian aqueduct syndrome)
*6. Parinaud syndrome (paralysis of vertical movement)
7. Vascular lesions

Duke-Elder S, Scott GI. *System of ophthalmology*, Vol XII. St. Louis: CV Mosby, 1971.

Huber A. *Eye symptoms in brain tumors*, 2nd ed. St. Louis: CV Mosby, 1971.

MONOCULAR NYSTAGMUS

1. Horizontal
   A. Lesions of optic nerve, chiasm, midbrain, or brainstem
   B. Nervous system disease, such as multiple sclerosis, epidemic meningitis, and congenital syphilis
   C. Seizures
   D. Superior oblique myokymia—benign, intermittent, uniocular
   E. Spasmus nutans—most common cause in children
   F. Tumors of brainstem
   G. Unilateral amblyopia
   H. Unilateral astigmatism or high refractive error
   I. Unilateral opacity of the ocular media
2. Vertical
   A. Multiple sclerosis
   B. Myokymia of lower eyelid
   C. Sleep
   D. Spasmus nutans
   E. Unilateral amblyopia

Farmer J, Hoyt CS. Monocular nystagmus in infancy and early childhood. *Am J Ophthalmol* 1984;98:504–509.

Gottlob I, et al. Signs distinguishing spasmus nutans from infantile nystagmus. *Ophthalmology* 1990;97:1166.

Jacome DE, Fitzgerald R. Monocular ictal nystagmus. *Arch Neurol* 1982;39:653.

Smith JL, et al. Monocular vertical oscillations of amblyopia. *J Clin Neurol* 1982;39:653.

PERIODIC ALTERNATING NYSTAGMUS

Periodic alternating nystagmus is central vestibular nystagmus with rhythmic jerk type of nystagmus that undergoes phasic or cyclic changes in amplitude and direction.

* = most important

1. Arnold–Chiari malformation
2. Cerebral trauma or fractured skull
3. Chiasmal lesion, such as craniopharyngioma
4. Chronic otitis media
5. Congenital
6. Diabetes mellitus
7. Encephalitis
8. Friedreich hereditary ataxia
9. Meningioma of tentorium cerebelli, cerebellar glioma, and cholesteatoma of the cerebellopontine angle
10. Head trauma
11. Mesencephalic brainstem and cerebellar disease
12. Multiple sclerosis (disseminated sclerosis)
13. Syringobulbia (Passow syndrome)
14. Syphilitic optic atrophy
15. Tumor of the corpus callosum
16. Vertebrobasilar artery insufficiency
17. Vestibular nuclei lesions
18. von Recklinghausen syndrome (neurofibromatosis)

Davis DG, Smith JL. Periodic alternating nystagmus. *Am J Ophthalmol* 1971;72:757–762.

Walsh FB, Hoyt WF. *Clinical neuro-ophthalmology*, 4th ed. Baltimore: Williams & Wilkins, 1985.

POSITIONAL NYSTAGMUS

Positional nystagmus is nystagmus that appears or changes in form or intensity after certain positional changes of the head indicate vestibular stimulation.

1. After general anesthesia
2. After head injury
3. Drugs, including the following:

acetophenazine	bromide	cefazolin
alcohol	bromisovalum	cefonicid
allobarbital	broxyquinoline	cefoperazone
alprazolam	bupivacaine	ceforanide
amiodarone	butabarbital	cefotaxime
amitriptyline	butalbital	cefotetan
amobarbital	butallylonal	cefoxitin
amodiaquine	butaperazine	cefsulodin
amoxapine	butethal	ceftazidime
aprobarbital	calcitriol	ceftizoxime
aspirin	carbamazepine	ceftriaxone
auranofin	carbinoxamine	cefuroxime
aurothioglucose	carbon monoxide	cephalexin
aurothioglycanide	carbromal	cephaloglycin
baclofen	carisoprodol	cephaloridine
barbital	carphenazine	cephalothin
Bacille Calmette–Guérin	cefaclor	cephapirin
(BCG) vaccine	cefadroxil	cephradine
bleomycin(?)	cefamandole	chloral hydrate

chloramphenicol(?)
chlordiazepoxide
chloroform
chloroprocaine
chloroquine
chlorpromazine
cholecalciferol
clemastine
clomipramine
clonazepam
clorazepate
colistimethate
colistin
cyclobarbital
cyclopentobarbital
cytarabine
desipramine
diazepam
diethazine
digitalis(?)
diiodohydroxyquin
dimethyl tubocurarine
   iodide
diphenhydramine
diphenylhydantoin
diphenylpyraline
disulfiram
divalproex sodium
doxepin
doxylamine
dronabinol
ergocalciferol
ergot(?)
ethacrynic acid
ethchlorvynol
ethopropazine
ethotoin
etidocaine
fenfluramine
flecainide
floxuridine
fluorouracil
fluphenazine
flurazepam
glutethimide
gold Au 198
gold sodium thiomalate
gold sodium thiosulfate
halazepam

hashish
heptabarbital
hexethal
hexobarbital
hydroxychloroquine
ibuprofen
imipramine
influenza virus vaccine(?)
insulin
iodochlorhydroxyquin
iodoquinol
iophendylate
isoniazid
ketamine
lidocaine
lithium carbonate
lorazepam
marijuana
meperidine
mephenesin
mephentermine
mephenytoin
mephobarbital
mepivacaine
meprobamate
mesoridazine
metaraminol
methaqualone
metharbital
methdilazine
methitural
methocarbamol
methohexital
methotrimeprazine
methoxamine
methyl alcohol
methylpentynol
methylthiouracil
methyprylon
metoclopramide
metocurine iodide
metrizamide
mexiletine
midazolam
nalidixic acid
nifedipine
nitrazepam
nitrofurantoin
norepinephrine

nortriptyline
oral contraceptives
oxazepam
paramethadione
pemoline
penicillamine
pentazocine
pentobarbital
perhexiline
pericyazine
perphenazine
phenelzine
phenobarbital
phenylpropanolamine
phenytoin
piperacetazine
piperazine
polymyxin B
prazepam
prilocaine
primidone
probarbital
procaine
procarbazine
prochlorperazine
promazine
promethazine
propiomazine
propoxycaine
protriptyline
quinine
scopolamine
secobarbital
sodium salicylate
streptomycin
talbutal
temazepam
tetanus immune globulin
tetanus toxoid
tetrahydrocannabinol
thiamylal
thiethylperazine
thiopental
thioperazine
thiopropazate
thioproperazine
thioridazine
tobramycin
tocainide

tranylcypromine	tripelennamine	vinblastine(?)
triazolam	tubocurarine	vincristine(?)
trichloroethylene	urea(?)	vitamin A
trifluoperazine	urethan	vitamin D
triflupromazine	valproate sodium	vitamin D_2
trimeprazine	valproic acid	vitamin D_3
trimethadione	verapamil	
trimipramine	vinbarbital	

4. Inner ear pathologic changes, including hemorrhage, inflammation, thrombosis, emboli, circulatory and secretory conditions
5. "Normal" persons
6. Other causes include neuritis, meningitis, tumors, vascular anomalies, degeneration, atrophy, syphilis, arteriosclerosis, hypertonia, vasomotor disturbance, allergic and toxic conditions, cranial trauma, hemorrhage, emboli, or thrombosis

Fraunfelder FT, Fraunfelder FW. *Drug-induced ocular side effects.* Woburn, MA: Butterworth-Heinemann, 2001.

Fuijimoto M, et al. A study into the phenomenon of head-shaking nystagmus: its presence in a dizzy population. *J Otolaryngol* 1993;22:376–379.

Solmon SD. Positional nystagmus. *Arch Otolaryngol* 1969;90:58–63.

OPTOKINETIC NYSTAGMUS

Normal physiologic nystagmus is obtained by watching moving targets; slow components in direction targets are moving, and fast component move in the opposite direction. Abnormal optokinetic nystagmus can be seen in the following:

1. Aberrant regeneration of third nerve—absent vertical optokinetic nystagmus, normal horizontal optokinetic nystagmus
2. Internuclear palsies—horizontal targets bring out dissociation of ocular response movements
3. Lesions of optic tract, geniculate body, temporal and occipital lobes show no asymmetry of horizontal optokinetic responses
4. Lesions of parietal lobe give asymmetric horizontal optokinetic responses
5. Occipital lobe lesions with homonymous hemianopia and asymmetrical horizontal optokinetic responses suggests a mass lesion extending into parietal lobe rather than a vascular lesion
6. Parinaud syndrome—vertical optokinetic nystagmus with targets moving downward enhances the retraction nystagmus seen on attempted upgaze.
7. Parkinsonism (shaking palsy)—vertical optokinetic nystagmus may be reduced
8. See-saw nystagmus—vertical optokinetic nystagmus may be reduced either upward or downward (see p. 144)
9. Test for malingering in "blind" eye or eyes with normal optokinetic responses

Smith JL. *Optokinetic nystagmus: its use in topical neuro-ophthalmologic diagnosis.* Springfield, IL: Charles C Thomas, 1963.

Walsh FB, Hoyt WF. *Clinical neuro-ophthalmology,* 4th ed. Baltimore: Williams & Wilkins, 1985.

SYNDROMES AND DISEASES ASSOCIATED WITH NYSTAGMUS

1. African eye-worm disease
2. Albers–Schönberg syndrome (osteosclerosis fragilis generalisata)

3. Albinism, ocular
4. Alexander disease
5. Anterior spinal artery syndrome
6. Apert syndrome (acrocephalosyndactylism syndrome)
7. Arnold–Chiari syndrome (platybasia syndrome)
8. Arylsulfatase A deficiency syndrome
9. Babinski–Nageotte syndrome (medullary tegmental syndrome)
10. Bacterial endocarditis
11. Bassen–Kornzweig syndrome (abetalipoproteinemia)
12. Behçet syndrome (dermatostomatoophthalmic syndrome)
13. Behr disease (optic atrophy–ataxia syndrome)
14. Bielschowsky–Lutz–Cogan syndrome (internuclear ophthalmoplegia)
15. Bloch–Sulzberger disease (incontinentia pigmenti)*
16. Blocked nystagmus syndrome (nystagmus blockage syndrome)
17. Bonnet–Dechaume–Blanc syndrome (neuroretinoangiomatosis syndrome)
18. Botulism
19. Brown–Marie syndrome (hereditary ataxia syndrome)
20. Caisson syndrome (bends)
21. Canavan disease (spongy degeneration of the white matter)
22. Cerebral palsy
23. Cestan–Chenais syndrome (combination of Babinski–Nageotte and Avellis syndrome)
24. Charcot–Marie–Tooth disease (progressive peroneal muscular atrophy)
25. CHARGE syndrome (colomba, heart disease, atresia, choanae, retarded growth and retarded development or central nervous system anomalies, genital hypoplasia, and ear anomalies or deafness syndrome)
26. Chediak–Higashi syndrome (anomalous leukocytic inclusions with constitutional stigmata)
27. Cherry-red spot myoclonus syndrome
28. Chromosome 6p12
29. Chromosome 18, partial deletion (long-arm) syndrome
30. Cockayne syndrome (dwarfism with retinal atrophy and deafness)
31. Cogan syndrome (II) (oculomotor apraxia syndrome)
*32. Cone dysfunction syndrome (achromatopsia)
33. Costen syndrome (temporomandibular joint syndrome)
34. Craniocervical syndrome (whiplash syndrome)
35. Craniopharyngioma
36. Craniostenosis
37. Creutzfeldt–Jakob syndrome (spastic pseudosclerosis)
38. Crouzon disease (craniofacial dysostosis)
39. Curtius syndrome (ectodermal dysplasia with ocular malformations)
40. Cushing syndrome (II) (angle tumor syndrome)
41. Cytomegalic inclusion disease, congenital
42. Dawson disease (subacute sclerosing panencephalitis)
43. de Lange syndrome (congenital muscular hypertrophy-cerebral syndrome)
44. Diencephalic syndrome (autonomic epilepsy syndrome) (Russell syndrome)
45. Disseminated lupus erythematosus (Kaposi–Libman–Sacks syndrome)
*46. Disseminated sclerosis (multiple sclerosis)
47. Down disease (mongolism, trisomy 21)
48. Drummond syndrome (idiopathic hypercalcemia)

* = most important

49. Eclampsia and preeclampsia
50. Electrical injury
51. Encephalitis, acute
52. Epidermal nevus syndrome (ichthyosis hystrix)
53. Epiphysial dysplasia, microcephaly, and nystagmus—autosomal recessive
54. Extreme hydrocephalus syndrome
55. Fanconi–Turler syndrome (familial ataxic diplegia)
56. Fetal hydantoin syndrome
57. Forsius–Eriksson syndrome (Aland disease)
58. François dyscephalic syndrome
59. Gangliosidosis (generalized gangliosidosis, infantile)
60. General fibrosis syndrome
61. Goltz syndrome (focal dermal hypoplasia syndrome)
62. Gorlin–Chaudhry–Moss syndrome
63. Guillain–Barré syndrome (acute infectious neuritis)
64. Hallervorden–Spatz syndrome (pigmentary degeneration of globus pallidus)
65. Hallgren syndrome (retinitis pigmentosa–deafness–ataxia syndrome)
66. Hand–Schüller–Christian syndrome (histiocytosis X)
67. Hanhart syndrome (recessive keratosis palmoplantaris)
68. Hartnup syndrome (niacin deficiency)
69. Hennebert syndrome (luetic–otitic–nystagmus syndrome)
70. Hermansky–Pudlak syndrome (oculocutaneous albinism and hemorrhagic diathesis)
71. Hurler syndrome (mucopolysaccharidoses I-H)
72. Hypervitaminosis D
73. Hypomelanosis of Ito syndrome (incontinentia pigmenti achromians)
74. Hypothyroidism (cretinism)
75. Hysteria
76. Infantile globoid cell leukodystrophy (Krabbe disease)
77. Infantile neuroaxonal dystrophy
78. Infectious mononucleosis
79. Japanese River fever (typhus)
80. Jeune disease (asphyxiating thoracic dystrophy)
81. Kernicterus—high levels of bilirubin in the blood
82. Klippel–Feil syndrome (congenital brevicollis)
83. Koerber–Salus–Elschnig syndrome (sylvian aqueduct syndrome)
84. Kohn–Romano syndrome (blepharophimosis, ptosis, epicanthus inversus, telecanthus) (Blepharophimosis syndrome)
85. Kugelberg–Welander syndrome (progressive proximal muscle atrophy)
86. Laurence–Moon–Bardet–Biedl syndrome (retinitis pigmentosa-polydactyly-adiposo-genital syndrome)*
87. Leber congenital amaurosis syndrome (retinal aplasia)
88. Leigh disease (subacute necrotizing encephalomyelopathy)
89. Lenoble–Aubineau syndrome (nystagmus-myoclonia syndrome)
90. Lermoyez syndrome (form of Meniere disease)
91. Linear nevus sebaceous of Jadassohn
92. Lockjaw (tetanus)
93. Louis–Bar syndrome (ataxia-telangiectasia syndrome)
94. Lowe disease (oculocerebrorenal syndrome)
95. Malignant hyperthermia syndrome

96. Maple syrup urine disease
97. Marfan syndrome (acrachnadactyly–dystrophia mesodermalis congenita)
98. Marinesco–Sjögren syndrome (congenital spirocerebellar ataxia–congenital cataract–oligophrenia syndrome)
98. Meniere syndrome (vertigo, tinnitus, nystagmus)
99. Meningococcemia (meningitis)
100. Mietens syndrome
101. Morning glory syndrome (optic nerve dysplasia, encephalocele)
102. Moyamoya disease (multiple progressive intracranial arterial occlusion)
103. Multiple lentigines syndrome (Leopard syndrome)
104. Naegeli syndrome (melanophoric nevus syndrome)
*105. Nystagmus, congenital
106. O'Donnell–Pappas syndrome (dominant foveal hypoplasia and presenile cataracts)* optic nerve hypoplasia, coloboma
107. Papillon-Lefèvre syndrome (hyperkeratosis palmoplantaris with periodontosis)
108. Parkinson disease
109. Passow syndrome (status dysraphicus syndrome)
110. Pelizaeus–Merzbacher disease (aplasia axialis extracorticalis congenita)—x-linked
111. Photomyoclonus, diabetes mellitus, deafness, neuropathy, and cerebellar dysfunction—autosomal dominant
112. Poliomyelitis
113. Posthypoxic encephalopathy syndrome
114. Pyle disease (familial metaphyseal dysplasia)
115. Quincke disease (angioedema)
116. Rubella, congenital
117. Reimann syndrome (hyperviscosity syndrome)
118. Relapsing polychondritis
119. Scaphocephaly syndrome
120. Schilder disease (encephalitis periaxialis diffusa)
121. Seckel syndrome (bird-headed dwarf syndrome)*
122. Septooptic dysplasia (de Morsier syndrome)
123. Smith–Lemli–Opitz syndrome (cerebrohepatorenal syndrome)
124. Sorsby syndrome (hereditary macular coloboma syndrome)
125. Spastic paraplegia—x-linked
126. Split hand with congenital nystagmus, fundal changes, cataracts—autosomal dominant
127. Stannus cerebellar syndrome (riboflavin deficiency)
128. Subclavian steal syndrome
129. Tay–Sachs disease (familial amaurotic idiocy)
130. Traumatic encephalopathy syndrome (punch-drunk syndrome)
131. Tremor, nystagmus, and duodenal ulcer—autosomal dominant
132. Tuomaala–Haapanen syndrome (similar to pseudohypoparathyroidism)
133. Vermis syndrome
134. Vertebral basilar artery syndrome
135. von Economo syndrome (encephalitis lethargica)
136. von Reuss syndrome (galactosemic syndrome)
137. Wagner syndrome (hyaloideoretinal degeneration)
138. Wallenberg syndrome (lateral bulbar syndrome)
139. Werner syndrome (progeria of adults)
140. Wernicke syndrome (superior hemorrhagic polioencephalopathic syndrome)

* = most important

141. Wildervanck syndrome (cervicooculoacoustic syndrome)
142. Wilson disease (hepatolenticular degeneration)
143. Wolf syndrome (monosomy partial syndrome)
144. Zellweger syndrome (cerebrohepatorenal syndrome of Zellweger)

Hayashi N, et al. Ocular histopathologic study of a patient with the T 8993-G point mutation in Leigh's syndrome. *Ophthalmology* 2000;107:1397–1402.

McKusick VA. *Mendelian inheritance in man*, 12th ed. Baltimore: Johns Hopkins University Press, 1998.

Roy FH. *Ocular syndromes and systemic diseases*, 3rd ed. Philadelphia: Lippincott Williams & Wilkins, 2002.

OCULOGYRIC CRISIS (SPASMODIC AND INVOLUNTARY DEVIATION OF EYES, USUALLY UPWARD, LASTING FROM A FEW MINUTES TO SEVERAL HOURS)

1. Cerebellar disease
2. Drugs, including the following:

acetophenazine	flurazepam	phencyclidine
alprazolam	halazepam	pimozide
alseroxylon	haloperidol	piperacetazine
amantadine	hydroxychloroquine	prazepam
amitriptyline	imipramine	prochlorperazine
amodiaquine	influenza virus vaccine	promazine
butaperazine	levodopa	promethazine
carbamazepine	lithium carbonate	propiomazine
carphenazine	lorazepam	protriptyline
chlordiazepoxide	loxapine	rauwolfia serpentina
chloroquine	mesoridazine	rescinnamine
chlorpromazine	methdilazine	reserpine
chlorprothixene	methotrimeprazine	syrosingopine
cisplatin	metoclopramide	temazepam
clonazepam	metronidazole	thiethylperazine
clorazepate	midazolam	thiopropazate
deserpidine	nitrazepam	thioproperazine
desipramine	nortriptyline	thioridazine
diazepam	oxazepam	thiothixene
diethazine	pemoline	triazolam
doxepin	pentazocine	trifluoperazine
droperidol	perazine	trifluperidol
ethopropazine	pericyazine	triflupromazine
fluphenazine	perphenazine	trimeprazine

3. Late manifestations of encephalitis
4. Lesions of fourth ventricle and cerebellum, especially lesions of the flocculus
5. Multiple sclerosis (disseminated sclerosis)
6. Parkinsonism syndrome (shaking palsy)
7. Syphilis (acquired lues)
8. Trauma

Burstein AH, Fullerton T. Oculogyric crisis possibly related to pentazocine. *Ann Pharmacotherapy* 1993;27:874–876.

Fraunfelder FT, Fraunfelder FW. *Drug-induced ocular side effects*. Woburn, MA: Butterworth-Heinemann, 2001.

OCULAR BOBBING

Both globes move synchronously in vertical plane by spontaneously and intermittently dipping downward through an arc of a few millimeters and then return to primary position; reverse ocular bobbing also has been described. Ocular bobbing differs from vertical nystagmus by virtue of absence of a fast and a slow component in movements; it is due to advanced pontine disease.

1. Acute organophosphate poisoning (Diazinon)
2. Associated with palatal myoclonus
*3. Encephalitis
4. Fibrocartilaginous embolism to the anterior spinal artery
5. Hypertensive pontine hemorrhage
6. Leigh encephalopathy (gangliosidosis GM type 3)
7. Locked-in syndrome
8. Phenothiazine and benzodiazepine poisoning (combined; reverse)
9. Ruptured giant distal posterior inferior cerebellar artery aneurysm
10. Thrombosis of basilar, middle cerebral, or vertebral arteries with posterior fossa infarction

Hata S, et al. Atypical ocular bobbing in acute organophosphate poisoning. *Arch Neurol* 1986;43:185–186.

Larmoude P, et al. Ocular bobbing: abnormal eye movement. *Ophthalmology* 1983;187:161–165.

Osenbach RK, et al. Ocular bobbing with ruptured giant distal posterior interior cerebellar artery aneurysm. *Surg Neurol* 1986;25:149–152.

Tijssen CC, Terbruggen JP. Locked-in syndrome associated with ocular bobbing. *Acta Neurol Scand* 1986;73: 444–446.

PARALYSIS OF THIRD NERVE (OCULOMOTOR NERVE)

This type of paralysis includes ptosis, an inability to rotate the eye upward or inward, a dilated unreactive pupil (iridoplegia), and paralysis of accommodation (cycloplegia).

1. Intracerebral
   A. Lesion of red nucleus (Benedikt syndrome)—homolateral oculomotor paralysis with contralateral intention tremor
   B. Myasthenia Gravis and Mesencephalic Cavernous Angioma
   C. Nuclear types—pareses of a single or a few extraocular muscles supplied by the oculomotor nerve in one or both eyes; there may or may not be pupillary disturbances (mydriasis, sluggish pupillary reaction) and paresis of accommodation; in tumors within or near the midbrain (pinealomas), there is a combination of isolated muscle pareses with vertical gaze palsy, possibly a disturbance of convergence, and nystagmus retractorius (Parinaud syndrome, sylvian aqueduct syndrome, pineal syndrome); includes Axenfeld–Schurenberg syndrome (cyclic oculomotor paralysis), Bruns syndrome (postural change syndrome), Claude syndrome (inferior nucleus ruber syndrome), congenital vertical retraction syndrome, and Nothnagel syndrome (ophthalmoplegia-cerebellar ataxia syndrome)
   D. Occlusion of basilar artery—due to emboli especially but also to hemorrhage or aneurysm
   E. Recurrent third nerve palsy secondary to vascular spasm of migraine
   F. Syndrome of cerebral peduncle (Weber syndrome)—homolateral oculomotor paralysis and cross-hemiplegia
   G. Tumors

* = most important

Paralysis of third nerve

	Intracerebral						Intracranial								Cranial Cavity Exit			
	Benedikt Syndrome	Weber Syndrome	Basilar Artery Emboli	Migraine	Tumors as Pinealoma	Parinaud Syndrome	Aneurysm Rupture Base Brain	Neuritis as Diabetes Mellitus	Poliomyelitis	Meningitis	Multiple Sclerosis	Temporal Arteritis	Post Coronary Artery Aneurysm	Post Viral	Cavernous Sinus Syndrome as Carotid-Cavernous Fistula	Superior Orbital Fissure Syndrome as Sphenoid Ridge Meningioma	Orbital Apex Syndrome	Isolated
History																		
1. All age groups				U									U					U
2. Children, 2 to 8 years				S										S				
3. Common—seventh decade	S	S						S				U				U		
4. Congenital									S									
5. Familial				U														
6. Head trauma	U	U	U				U									S	S	S
7. Hemorrhage/neoplasm/inflammation	U	U	U		U	U	U								U	U	U	
8. Unilateral	U	U	U	U			U								U	U		U
9. Unilateral transient visual loss				U														
10. Usually more than 40 years	U	U	U				U	U				U				U		
11. Viral infection									U					U				
12. Visual loss				S			S			S		S				S		R
Physical Findings																		
1. Acute decreased intraocular pressure				U								S						
2. Anterior ischemic optic neuropathy								S				S						
3. Cataract								U										
4. Central retinal artery occlusion												U						
5. Central retinal vein occlusion					S													
6. Convergence abnormal	U				U	U	S											U
7. Corneal anesthesia												S			S	S	S	
8. Corneal opacity															S			
9. Corneal ulcer															S			
10. Cotton wool exudates								U										
11. Disk hemorrhage													U					
12. Elevation and depression of eyes limited	U	U				S												R
13. Fixed/dilated pupil	U	U	U	S	U	U	S	S					U	U	U	U	U	U
14. Glaucoma														S				
15. Hard exudates								U										
16. Horner syndrome															S	S		R
17. Keratitis														U	S			
18. Lid edema																U	U	
19. Macular edema								S		S								
20. Microaneurysms of retina								S										
21. Miosis															R			
22. Nystagmus		S									U							
23. Ocular bruit															U			

Paralysis of third nerve (Continued)

	Intracerebral						Intracranial								Cranial Cavity Exit			
	Benedikt Syndrome	Weber Syndrome	Basilar Artery Emboli	Migraine	Tumors as Pinealoma	Parinaud Syndrome	Aneurysm Rupture Base Brain	Neuritis as Diabetes Mellitus	Poliomyelitis	Meningitis	Multiple Sclerosis	Temporal Arteritis	Post Coronary Artery Aneurysm	Post Viral	Cavernous Sinus Syndrome as Carotid-Cavernous Fistula	Superior Orbital Fissure Syndrome as Sphenoid Ridge Meningioma	Orbital Apex Syndrome	Isolated
Physical Findings																		
24. Ocular pain			U				U						S	S	S	U	U	S
25. Optic nerve atrophy								S					U	R	R	S	S	S
26. Optic neuritis									S	S	U				S			S
27. Orbital hemorrhage							R								S		S	
28. Papilledema						U	R	S		R					S	U	S	
29. Proptosis												U	U	S	U			S
30. Ptosis		U																
31. Retinal hemorrhage							S	U		R					S			
32. Uveitis											U					S		
33. Visual field defects						S	S					S						
34. Vitreous hemorrhage							S	S										
Laboratory Data																		
1. Cerebrospinal fluid abnormal					S		S						S					
2. Computed tomographic scan/MRI	U	U	U		U	U	U					U				U	U	U
3. Elevated blood sugar								U										
4. Erythrocyte sedimentation rate elevated												U						
5. Red blood cell count, white blood cell count, hemoglobin, and hematocrit									U	U					U	U		
6. Selective cerebral angiography	S	S	U			S	U											

R = rarely; S = sometimes; and U = usually.

2. Intracranial
   A. Amebic dysentery
   B. Aneurysm rupture at base of brain—third nerve paralysis, pain around the face (fifth nerve), and headache
   C. Botulism
   D. Chickenpox
   E. Craniopharyngioma
   F. Dengue fever
   G. Devic syndrome (optical myelitis)
   H. Diphtheria
   I. Encephalitis, acute
   J. Hepatic failure
   K. Hepatitis
   L. Influenza
   M. Lockjaw (tetanus)
   N. Lymphoma
   O. Malaria
   P. Measles immunization
   Q. Meningococcal meningitis
   R. Multiple sclerosis (disseminated sclerosis)
   S. Ophthalmic migraine
   T. Periarteritis nodosa
   U. Poliomyelitis
   V. Polyneuritis because of toxins such as alcohol, lead, arsenic, and carbon monoxide; dinitrophenol or carbon disulfide poisoning; or diabetes mellitus, herpes zoster, or mumps
   W. Rabies
   X. Relapsing polychondritis
   Y. Smallpox vaccination
   Z. Subdural hematoma
   AA. Syphilis (acquired lues)
   BB. Temporal arteritis syndrome (Hutchinson–Horton–Magrath–Brown syndrome)
   CC. Tuberculosis
3. Lesions affecting exit from cranial cavity
   A. Cavernous sinus syndrome—paralysis of third, fourth, and sixth nerves with proptosis
      (1) Aneurysm (arteriovenous fistula syndrome)
      (2) Carotid-cavernous fistula
      (3) Cavernous sinus thrombosis
      (4) Extension from lateral sinus thrombosis
      (5) Extension of nasopharyngeal tumor
      (6) Pituitary adenoma—lateral extension
      (7) Tolosa–Hunt syndrome (painful ophthalmoplegia)
   B. Superior orbital fissure syndrome—same as for cavernous sinus syndrome except exophthalmos is less likely to occur and optic nerve involvement and miotic pupil are more likely
      (1) Aneurysm of internal carotid artery syndrome (foramen lacerum syndrome)
      (2) Occlusion of superior ophthalmic vein

(3) Skull fractures or hemorrhage

(4) Sphenoid sinus suppuration (sphenocavernous syndrome)

(5) Temporal syndrome (Gradenigo syndrome)

(6) Tumors, such as sphenoid ridge meningioma (Rochon–Duvigneaud syndrome), nasopharyngeal tumor, metastatic carcinoma, rhabdomyosarcoma, chordoma, and sarcoma

   C. Orbital apex—involvement of third, fourth, sixth, and first division of fifth cranial nerves and optic nerve proptosis is common

4. Other

   A. Alber–Schönberg syndrome (marble bone disease, osteopetrosis)

   B. Associated with aspirin poisoning

   C. Congenital

   D. Hodgkin disease

   E. Lupus erythematosus (Kaposi–Libman–Sacks syndrome)

   F. Myasthenia gravis (masquerade)

   G. Passow syndrome (status dysraphicus syndrome)

   H. Porphyria cutanea tarda

   I. Sarcoid (Schaumann syndrome)

Harrison AR, Wirtschafter JD. Isolated inferior rectus paresis secondary to a mesencaphalic cavernous angioma. *Am J Ophthalmol* 1999;127,5:617–620.

Holmes JM, et al. Pediatric third, fourth, and sixth nerve palsies: a population-based study. *Am J Ophthalmol* 1999; 127:388–392.

Ing EB, et al. Oculomotor nerve palsies in children. *J Pediatr Ophthal Strabismus* 1992;29:331–336.

Purvin V. Third cranial nerve palsy. In: Margo CE, ed. *Diagnostic problems in clinical ophthalmology*. Philadelphia: WB Saunders, 1994:678.

Roy FH. *Ocular syndromes and systemic diseases*, 3rd ed. Philadelphia: Lippincott Williams & Wilkins, 2002.

Childhood Causes of Third Nerve (Oculomotor) Palsy

1. Trauma
2. Neoplasm
3. Undetermined
4. Ophthalmoplegic migraine
5. Postoperative cause
6. Meningitis/encephalitis
7. Subdural hematoma
8. Viral or post-upper respiratory tract infection
9. Varicella-zoster virus
10. Aneurysm
11. Orbital cellulitis
12. Sinus disease
13. Mesencephalic cyst
14. Cyclic oculomotor nerve palsy
15. Poison

Holmes JM, et al. Pediatric third, fourth, and sixth nerve palsies: a population-based study. *Am J Ophthalmol* 1999; 127:388–392.

Kodsi SR, Younge BR. Acquired oculomotor, trochlear, and abducent cranial nerve palsies in pediatric patients. *Am J Ophthalmol* 1992;114:568–574.

PARALYSIS OF FOURTH NERVE (TROCHLEAR NERVE)

This type of paralysis produces palsy of superior oblique muscle resulting in limitation of downward movement of eye when it is in adducted position; it is frequently associated with third cranial nerve palsy.

1. Intracerebral
    A. Thrombosis of nutrient vessels, including median penetrating branch of basilar artery to fourth nucleus
    B. Hemorrhage in the roof of the midbrain
    C. Aneurysm, including direct involvement by posterior cerebral and superior cerebellar arteries
    D. Tumors (rare if isolated fourth palsy)
        (1) Primary
            a. Gliomas, such as astrocytomas, ependymomas, and medulloblastomas
            b. Other primary tumors, including meningiomas, pinealomas, craniopharyngiomas, and hemangiomas
        (2) Unilateral trochlear nerve palsy
    E. Metastatic lesions, such as those from the nasopharynx, rhabdomyosarcomas, and neuroblastomas
    F. Neonatal hypoxia
    G. Nuclear type—trochlear paresis combined with a homolateral oculomotor paresis, occasionally in association with vertical gaze palsies, convergence spasm or convergence palsy, and pupillary disturbances seen in tumors of the roof of the midbrain or pinealomas (pineal syndrome)
    H. Claude syndrome (inferior nucleus ruber syndrome)
    I. Passow syndrome (syringomyelia)
    J. Inflammatory lesions, such as meningoencephalitis, cerebellitis, and abscess
    K. Pseudotumor cerebri
2. Intracranial
    A. Aneurysms, such as that of the posterior communicating artery or foramen lacerum syndrome (aneurysm of internal carotid artery syndrome)
    B. Hematomas, traumatic
    C. Hydrocephalus
    D. Meningitis, encephalitis, polyneuritis—diabetes mellitus, herpes zoster, multiple sclerosis, myasthenia gravis, chickenpox, diphtheria, hydrophobia, Gradenigo syndrome, influenza, malaria, poliomyelitis
    E. Trauma
    F. Tumors, including cerebellopontine angle tumor and pituitary adenoma
3. Lesions affecting exit from cranial cavity
    A. Cavernous sinus syndrome (Foix syndrome)
    B. Superior orbital fissure syndrome (Rochon–Duvigneaud syndrome)
    C. Orbital apex syndrome (Rollet syndrome)
4. Orbital lesions
    A. Fracture of superior orbital rim
    B. Sinusitis
    C. Operations on the frontal sinus in which there is trochlear displacement
    D. Trochlear disturbance, such as in Paget disease or hypertrophic arthritis
    E. Adherence syndrome—adhesions between the superior rectus and superior oblique muscles

Paralysis of fourth nerve

	Intracerebral			Intracranial			Exit from Cranial Cavity		Orbital		
	Thrombosis Basilar Artery	Aneurysm Posterior Cerebral/Superior Cerebellar Arteries	Tumor as Pinealoma	Aneurysm Posterior Communicating Artery	Tumor as Cerebellopontine Angle	Polyneuritis	Cavernous Sinus Syndrome	Orbital Apex Syndrome	Superior Orbital Rim Fracture	Isolated	Isolated Congenital
History											
1. Bacterial infection							S	S			
2. Hemorrhagic, neoplasic, or inflammation cause							U	U	U		
3. Metabolic disorder							U				
4. More than 40 years	R	R	R	R	R	S	R	S	R	U	U
5. Rare incidence											S
6. Bilateral											
Physical Findings											
1. Conjunctival hemorrhage							S		S		
2. Convergence insufficiency				U	R						
3. Cotton-wool spots							S				
4. Fixed and dilated pupil	S			U			R	U		R	R
5. Keratitis							S				
6. Limitation of adduction	S	U	S	U	R	S			S	R	R
7. Limitation of downward/upward gaze	S	U	U	U	R	S		U	S	R	R
8. Ocular/periocular pain	U	R		S			S	S	S	R	R
9. Ophthalmoplegia, third and sixth nerves	U	S		S			S	S	S	R	R
10. Optic nerve atrophy							R	S	S		
11. Optic neuritis								S	S		
12. Palsy—fifth, sixth, seventh, eighth, ninth, and tenth cranial nerves					U						
13. Papilledema							S	S	S		
14. Progressive proptosis				U				U	S		
15. Ptosis	S			U				U	S		
16. Pupil afferent defect								S	S		
17. Retinal hemorrhages							S				
18. Retinal neovascularization/microaneurysms							U				
19. Subdural/orbital bleeding									U		
20. Temporary homonymus field defect		S									
Laboratory Data											
1. Blood sugar elevated/SED rates							U				
2. Cerebral arteriography	U	U		U				U			
3. Cerebrospinal fluid abnormal			U	U							
4. Computed tomographic brain scan	U	U	U	U	U			U	U	U	S
5. Magnetic resonance imaging		S									S
6. Orbit roentgenogram										U	
7. Skull roentgenogram	U	S	S		U				S	U	S
8. Visual field test		S									

R = rarely; S = sometimes; and U = usually.

F. Abnormal insertion of superior oblique muscle or abnormal fascial attachments
G. Rochon–Duvigneaud syndrome (superior orbital fissure syndrome)
H. Idiopathic

Feinberg AS, Newman NJ. Schwannoma in patients with isolated unilateral trochlear Nerve palsy. *Am J Ophthalmol* 1999;127:183–188.

Holmes JM, et al. Pediatric third, fourth, and sixth nerve palsies: a population-based study. *Am J Ophthalmol* 1999; 127:388–392.

Keane JR. Fourth nerve palsy: historical review and study of inpatients. *Neurology* 1993;43:2439–2433.

Peterman SH, Newman NJ. Pituary macroadenoma manifesting as an isolated fourth nerve palsy. *Am J Ophthalmol* 1999;127,2:235–236.

Roy FH. *Ocular syndromes and systemic diseases*, 3rd ed. Philadelphia: Lippincott Williams & Wilkins, 2002.

Speer C, et al. Four cranial nerve palsy in pediatric patients with pseudotumor cerebri. *Am J Ophthalmol* 1999;127:236–237.

Childhood Causes of Fourth Nerve (Trochlear) Palsy

1. Trauma
2. Neoplasm
3. Undetermined
4. Postoperative cause
5. Meningitis
6. Hydrocephalus
7. Ophthalmoplegic migraine
8. Viral infection
9. Aneurysm
10. Other

Holmes JM, et al. Pediatric third, fourth, and sixth nerve palsies: a population-based study. *Am J Ophthalmol* 1999; 127:388–392.

Kodsi SR, Younge BR. Acquired oculomotor, trochlear, and abducent cranial nerve palsies in pediatric patients. *Am J Ophthalmol* 1992;114:568–574.

PSEUDOABDUCENS PALSY

1. Accommodative spasm
2. Blowout fracture (medial rectus entrapment)
3. Cross fixation (congenital esotropia)
4. Duane syndrome (retraction syndrome)
5. Fibrosis of medial rectus
6. Horizontal gaze palsy (bilateral)—with or without contraction
7. Lack of effort involved in abducting a habitually adducted eye patch on other eye differentiates from abducens palsy
8. Myasthenia gravis
9. Myositis
10. Orbital cellulitis (abscess)
11. Overambitious (large) resection of medial rectus
12. Thyroid myopathy (Graves disease, hyperthyroidism)
13. Unwillingness to cooperate—doll's head phenomenon (sudden passive turning of head) differentiates from abducens palsy

Beyer-Machule C, von Noorden GK. *Atlas of ophthalmic surgery,* Vol 1: *Lids, orbits, extraocular muscles.* New York: Thieme Medical, 1984.

Goldhammer Y. Pseudopalsy of the abducens nerve. In: Smith JL, ed. *Neuro-ophthalmology update.* New York: Masson, 1977.

PARALYSIS OF SIXTH NERVE (ABDUCENS PALSY)

This type of paralysis produces palsy of the lateral rectus muscle with esotropia increasing when the eye is moved laterally. The course of the sixth nerve makes it more vulnerable to injury than other cranial nerves.

1. Intracerebral
   A. Foville syndrome (Foville peduncular syndrome)
   B. Gaucher disease (cerebroside lipidosis)
   C. Hydrocephalus
   D. Inflammatory lesions, such as meningoencephalitis, cerebellitis, and abscess
   E. Lateral ventricular cyst
   F. Leukemia
   G. Millard–Gubler syndrome (abducens–facial hemiplegia alternans)
   H. Mycoplasma pneumoniae
   I. Nuclear aplasia—autosomal dominant
   J. Platybasia (cerebellomedullary malformation syndrome)
   K. Spontaneous subdural hematoma
   L. Thrombosis or aneurysm of nutrient vessels to sixth nucleus—basilar artery
   M. Tumors—intracranial, pontine glioma, or metastatic tumor from breast, thyroid glands, or nasopharynx
      (1) Primary
         a. Gliomas, such as astrocytomas, ependymomas, and medulloblastomas
         b. Other primary tumors, including meningiomas, pinealomas, craniopharyngiomas, and hemangiomas
      (2) Metastatic lesions, such as those from the nasopharynx, rhabdomyosarcomas, and neuroblastomas
   N. Wernicke encephalopathy—thiamine deficiency in alcoholics with sixth nerve palsy, paresis of horizontal conjugate gaze, nystagmus, ataxia, and Korsakoff psychosis
2. Intracranial
   A. Carotid artery aneurysm (foramen lacerum syndrome)
   B. Cerebellopontine angle tumor, such as acoustic neuroma, producing unilateral deafness, facial paralysis, diplopia, and papilledema
   C. Chickenpox
   D. Coccidioidomycosis
   E. Congenital absence of sixth nerve
   F. Cushing syndrome (II) (angle tumor syndrome)
   G. Dandy–Walker syndrome (atresia of the foramen Magendie)
   H. Diphtheria
   I. Gradenigo syndrome—osteitis of petrous tip of pyramid following homolateral mastoid or middle ear infection; facial pain (fifth nerve involvement)
   J. Greig syndrome (ocular hypertelorism syndrome)
   K. Hydrophobia (rabies)
   L. Hydrocephalus (decreased intracranial pressure)

Paralysis of sixth nerve

	Intracerebral					Intracranial						Cranial Cavity Exit				
	Basilar Artery Aneurysm	Wernicke Encephalopathy	Millard-Grubler Syndrome	Foville Syndrome	Cerebellomedullary Malformation Syndrome	Meningitis	Carotid Artery Aneurysm	Gradenigo Syndrome	Cerebellopontine Angle Tumor as Acoustic Neuroma	Neuritis as Diabetes Mellitus	Myasthenia Gravis	Cavernous Sinus Syndrome	Superior Orbital Fissure Syndrome	Orbital Apex Syndrome	Isolated	Pseudo Tumor Cerebai
History																
1. Bilateral					U											
2. Children								U								S
3. Common in alcoholics		U													U	S
4. Common—20 to 40 years																
5. Common—more than 40 years	U		U	U						U						S
6. Common—more than 60 years	U					U								U	R	R
7. Extradural abscess of petrous portion temporal bone								U								
8. Lack of vitamin B₁ (thiamine)		U														
9. More in females											U					
10. More in males							U									U
11. Pain, periocular							U					U	S	S		
12. Severe pain in ophthalmic branch of fifth cranial nerve								U							ı	
13. Vascular/infectious/tumor at the pons base			U													
14. Vascular/inflammatory/tumor in cranial cavity												U	U	U		
15. Vascular/thrombosis/tumor of pyramidal tract				U												
16. Vestibular nerve tumor									U							
Physical Findings																
1. Anesthesia of face				U												
2. Associated hydrocephalus	S				S				S							U
3. Blepharitis		S														
4. Cataract																
5. Central scotoma		S														S
6. Conjunctivitis		S			U											
7. Cortical blindness					S											
8. Cotton-wool spots										U						
9. Deviation of eyes to the side opposite lesion and inability to move toward side lesion when unilateral			U													
10. Esotropia	U	S	U	U	S	S	S	S	S	S	S	U	U	U	U	
11. Hard exudates										S						
12. Involvement—other cranial nerves	S		U	U			U	U	S	R		U	U	U		S
13. Keratitis				U	U								S			
14. Lacrimation								U								
15. Nystagmus		S				S			S							
16. Ophthalmoplegia		S										S				

Paralysis of sixth nerve (Continued)

Column groups: **Intracerebral** (Basilar Artery Aneurysm – Cerebellomedullary Malformation Syndrome); **Intracranial** (Meningitis – Myasthenia Gravis); **Cranial Cavity Exit** (Cavernous Sinus Syndrome – Pseudo Tumor Cerebai).

	Basilar Artery Aneurysm	Wernicke Encephalopathy	Millard-Grubler Syndrome	Foville Syndrome	Cerebellomedullary Malformation Syndrome	Meningitis	Carotid Artery Aneurysm	Gradenigo Syndrome	Cerebellopontine Angle Tumor as Acoustic Neuroma	Neuritis as Diabetes Mellitus	Myasthenia Gravis	Cavernous Sinus Syndrome	Superior Orbital Fissure Syndrome	Orbital Apex Syndrome	Isolated	Pseudo Tumor Cerebai
Physical Findings																
17. Optic nerve atrophy		S					U			R		S	S	S		S
18. Optic neuritis		S				S	S	R						S		
19. Papilledema		S		U			S		S				U	S		U
20. Paralysis lateral conjugate gaze			U									U		U		
21. Ptosis		S											U	U		S
22. Pupillary afferent defects		S														
23. Pupillary paralysis		S														
24. Reduced corneal sensitivity								S								
25. Retinal hemorrhages		S								S						
26. Retinal microaneurysms										U						
27. Retinal neovascularization										U						
28. Uveitis							U									
29. Vertical nystagmus in upgaze and downgaze					U											
30. Visual field defects							U					S	S	S		U
Laboratory Data																
1. Cerebral arteriography												U		S		U
2. Cerebrospinal fluid abnormalities			U	U												U
3. Computed tomographic scan	U		U	U		U	U	U				U	U	U		U
4. Blood sugar (glycemia)										U						
5. MRI	U		U	U	U		U	U	U				U	U		U
6. Red blood cell count, white blood cell count, hemoglobin, and hematocrit						U						U				
7. Tensilon test											U					
8. Twenty-four-hour urine—thiamine		U														
9. Ultrasonography (oculorbital)													U	U		

R = rarely; S = sometimes; and U = usually.

Paralysis of third, fourth, and sixth cranial nerves

	Cavernous Sinus Thrombosis	Pituitary Adenoma	Aneurysm	Carotid-Cavernous Fistula	Nasopharyngeal Tumor	Lateral Sinus Thrombosis	Skull Fracture	Tumor as Sphenoid Ridge Meningioma	Superior Ophthalmic Vein Occlusion	Orbital Mass
History										
1. Common during fourth to seventh decades		U	S	S	U			U		
2. Common in females				S					U	
3. Common in males					U		S		U	
4. Congenital				S	R					S
5. Following head trauma	R			S	U		U			
6. Infectious etiology (septic thrombus)	U								U	S
7. Ocular pain				S	S		U			S
8. Unilateral	U			U	S		U		U	U
9. Visual loss		S		S	R		S			S
Physical Findings										
1. Anisocoria	U		U						U	
2. Central retinal vein occlusion				S						
3. Corneal ulcer	S			S						
4. Choroidal folds	S			S		S				S
5. Dilated conjunctival vessels	S			U		S				S
6. Dilation of episcleral veins	U			U					S	
7. Facial nerve involvement							U			
8. Glaucomatous cupping	S			S						
9. Hyperopia								S		
10. Increased intraocular pressure	S			U						S
11. Infections face/nose/forehead									U	
12. Ipsilateral horizontal gaze paresis						U				
13. Ischemic neuritis	S								S	
14. Keratopathy	U							U		
15. Leakage of blood/spinal fluid from external ear canal							U			
16. Lid edema	U					U				S
17. Mastoid ecchymosis (Battle sign)							U			
18. Miosis		S								
19. Nasolacrimal obstruction					U		S			
20. Ocular bruit				U						
21. Ocular hypotony		S								
22. Optic nerve atrophy		S	S				S	S		
23. Orbital hemorrhage		R					R			S
24. Papilledema	S	R	R				S	S		S
25. Pulsating exophthalmos				U						
26. Pupil, afferent defect	U		U							
27. Proptosis	U							U	U	S
28. Ptosis	U	S		S			U	S		U
29. Retinal hemorrhages	S	S								S
30. Trigeminal aesthesia	S			S			S		S	
31. Visual field defects		S				U		U		

Paralysis of third, fourth, and sixth cranial nerves (Continued)

	Cavernous Sinus Thrombosis	Pituitary Adenoma	Aneurysm	Carotid-Cavernous Fistula	Nasopharyngeal Tumor	Lateral Sinus Thrombosis	Skull Fracture	Tumor as Sphenoid Ridge Meningioma	Superior Ophthalmic Vein Occlusion	Orbital Mass
Laboratory Data										
1. Arteriography, cerebral			U	U				S		
2. Biopsy/culture of paranasal sinus	S									S
3. Biopsy nasopharynx lesions					U					
4. Blood culture	U								S	S
5. Cerebrospinal fluid abnormal			U							
6. Computed tomographic orbit scan				U						U
7. Culture lesions face/nose/forehead	U								U	S
8. Paranasal sinus roentgenogram	U						S			S
9. Pituitary panel—serum prolactin, growth hormone, adrenocorticotropic hormone, follicle-stimulating hormone, luteinizing hormone, thyroid-stimulating hormone		S								
10. Selective catheterization of external carotid arteries				U						
11. Selective cerebral angiography			U	U						
12. Visual field test		U							S	

R = rarely; S = sometimes; and U = usually.

   M. Increased intracranial pressure
   N. Malaria
   O. Massive pituitary adenoma
   P. Measles
   Q. Meningitis
   R. Möbius syndrome (congenital paralysis of sixth and seventh nerves)
   S. Neuritis because of diseases such as diabetes mellitus, herpes zoster, poliomyelitis, lead or arsenic poisoning, multiple sclerosis, syphilis, brucellosis
   T. Ophthalmoplegic migraine syndrome
   U. Osteosarcoma
   V. Passow syndrome (status dysraphicus syndrome)
   W. Pseudotumor cerebri (Symonds syndrome)
   X. Raymond syndrome (pontine syndrome)
   Y. Relapsing polychondritis
   Z. Skeletal dysplasia (mental retardation, abducens palsy)—x-linked
 AA. Skull fractures—usually crush injury
 BB. Spontaneous dissection of the internal carotid artery
 CC. Subdural hematoma
 DD. Trichinellosis
 EE. Tumor extension as chordoma
 FF. Vascular lesions, because of congenital aneurysm, arteriovenous fistulas, diabetes, hypertension
 GG. Water-soluble contrast myelography

3. Lesions affecting exit of sixth nerve from cranial cavity
   A. Cavernous sinus syndrome (Foix syndrome)
   B. Le Fort I maxillary osteotomy
   C. Optic nerve sheath fenestration
   D. Orbital apex lesion
   E. Percutaneous thermal ablation of trigeminal nerve rootlet
   F. Sphenocavernous syndrome
   G. Sphenopalatine fossa lesion—loss of tearing and paresis of second division of fifth nerve, most frequently because of malignant tumor
   H. Superior orbital fissure syndrome
   I. Tolosa–Hunt syndrome (painful ophthalmoplegia)
   J. Transient in newborns

4. Other
   A. Cluster headache
   B. Cretinism (hypothyroid goiter)
   C. Duane syndrome (retraction syndrome)
   D. Engelmann syndrome (hereditary multiple diaphyseal sclerosis)
   E. Following lumbar puncture, lumbar anesthesia, or Pantopaque injection for myelography
   F. Kahler disease (multiple myeloma)
   G. Lupus erythematosus (Kaposi–Libman–Sacks syndrome)
   H. Myasthenia gravis
   I. Optic nerve sheath fenestration (rare)
   J. Preeclampsia
   K. Sarcoidosis
   L. Secondary to immunization or viral illness

M. Toxic substances, such as arsenic, carbon tetrachloride, dichloroacetylene, Dilantin, gold salts, isoniazid, nitrofuran, thalidomide, trichloroethylene, furaltadone (Altafur), lithium

Holmes JM, et al. Pediatric third, fourth, and sixth nerve palsies: a population-based study. *Am J Ophthalmol* 1999; 127:388–392.

McKusick VA. *Mendelian inheritance in man*, 12th ed. Baltimore: Johns Hopkins University Press, 1998.

Mullaney PB, et al. Ophthalmic involvement as a presenting feature of nonorbital childhood parameningeal embryonal rhabdomyosarcoma. *Ophthalmology* 2001;108:179–182.

Roy FH. *Ocular syndromes and systemic diseases*, 3rd ed. Philadelphia: Lippincott Williams & Wilkins, 2002.

Rucker CW. The causes of paralysis of the third, fourth, and sixth cranial nerves. *Am J Ophthalmol* 1966;61:1293.

Childhood Causes of Sixth Nerve (Abducans) Palsy

1. Trauma
2. Neoplasm
3. Undetermined
4. Viral/benign
5. Gradenigo syndrome
6. Meningitis/encephalitis
7. Pseudotumor cerebri
8. Leukemia
9. Hydrocephalus
10. Arteriovenous malformation, brain
11. Multiple sclerosis
12. Miscellaneous

Holmes JM, et al. Pediatric third, fourth, and sixth nerve palsies: a population-based study. *Am J Ophthalmol* 1999; 127:388–392.

Kodsi SR, Younge BR. Acquired oculomotor, trochlear, and abducent cranial nerve palsies in pediatric patients. *Am J Ophthalmol* 1992;114,5:568–574.

Childhood Causes of Third, Fourth, and Sixth Nerve Palsy

1. Trauma
2. Neoplasm
3. Undetermined
4. Postoperative cause
5. Meningitis
6. Hydrocephalus
7. Ophthalmoplegic migraine
8. Viral infection
9. Aneurysm
10. Other

Holmes JM, et al. Pediatric third, fourth, and sixth nerve palsies: a population-based study. *Am J Ophthalmol* 1999; 127:388–392.

Kodsi SR, Younge BR. Acquired oculomotor, trochlear, and abducent cranial nerve palsies in pediatric patients. *Am J Ophthalmol* 1992;114:568–574.

ACUTE OPHTHALMOPLEGIA (ACUTE ONSET OF EXTRAOCULAR MUSCLE PALSY)

1. Infranuclear
    A. Aneurysm of internal carotid artery or circle of Willis
    B. Trauma
        (1) Orbital fracture
        (2) Orbital hematoma
    C. Orbital cellulitis secondary to acute paranasal sinusitis including mucormycosis in a diabetic
    D. Ophthalmoplegic migraine
    E. Myasthenia gravis
    F. Orbital pseudotumor
    G. Orbital tumors
        (1) Lymphoma
        (2) Metastatic
        (3) Rhabdomyosarcoma
2. Nuclear
    A. Acute and subacute infections
        (1) Infectious encephalitis
            a. Viral encephalitis
                (i) Anterior poliomyelitis
                (ii) Encephalitis lethargica and other epidemic viral encephalitides
                (iii) Fisher syndrome (ophthalmoplegia, ataxia, areflexia)
                (iv) Rabies
                (v) Vaccinal encephalitis
                (vi) Varicella, variola, measles, mumps, influenza, infectious mononucleosis
                (vii) Zoster
            b. Organismal encephalitic infections
                (i) Typhoid
                (ii) Scarlet fever
                (iii) Whooping cough
                (iv) Gas gangrene
                (v) Septicemia
                (vi) Pneumonia
                (vii) Typhus
                (viii) Malaria
            c. Acute central nervous system diseases
                (i) Acute demyelinating diseases—acute disseminated encephalomyelitis, acute multiple sclerosis
                (ii) Neuritic infections
                    (a) Polyradiculoneuritis
                    (b) Epidemic paralyzing vertigo
                    (c) Acute infectious (rheumatic) polyneuritis
                    (d) Interstitial neuritis—meningitis, cranial sinusitis, petrositis, nasal sinusitis, orbital periostitis, orbital abscess
                (iii) Widespread infections
                    (a) Meningovascular syphilis

        (b) Mucormycosis (diabetes, immunosuppressed, AIDS)
        (c) Tuberculosis
        (d) Torula and cryptococcosis
     (iv) Toxic conditions
        (a) Diphtheria
        (b) Tetanus
        (c) Botulism
     (v) Allergic conditions
        (a) Sarcoidosis syndrome (Schaumann syndrome)
        (b) Recurrent multiple cranial nerve palsies
  B. Metabolic diseases
    (1) Deficiency diseases
      a. Thiamine deficiency (Wernicke–Korsakoff syndrome)
      b. Nicotinic acid deficiency—pellagra
      c. Ascorbic acid deficiency—scurvy
    (2) Diabetes
    (3) Anemias
      a. Primary anemia—leukemia
      b. Secondary anemia (loss of blood)
    (4) Exophthalmic ophthalmoplegia
    (5) Porphyria
  C. Poisoning such as lead, carbon monoxide, snake poisons, wasp stings, ergot, sulfuric acid, phosphorus, triorthoceresylphosphate, and dichloroacetylene
  D. Drugs, including the following:

vaccine (adsorbed)	butalbital	desipramine
acebutolol	butallylonal	desoxycorticosterone
acetohexamide	butaperazine	dexamethasone
acetophenazine	butethal	dextrothyroxine
adrenal cortex injection	calcitriol(?)	diazepam(?)
alcohol	carbamazepine	dibucaine
aldosterone	carisoprodol	diethazine
allobarbital	carphenazine	digitalis
amitriptyline	chloral hydrate	digitoxin
amobarbital	chlorambucil	dimethyl tubocurarine iodide
amodiaquine atenolol	chlordiazepoxide	diphenhydramine
amoxapine	chloroform	diphenylhydantoin
amphotericin B	chloroprocaine	diphtheria and tetanus
aprobarbital	chloroquine	toxoids (adsorbed)
aspirin	chlorpromazine	diphtheria and tetanus
auranofin	chlorpropamide	toxoids and pertussis
aurothioglucose	cisplatin	diphtheria toxoid (adsorbed)
aurothioglycanide	clomipramine	disulfiram
barbital	clonazepam	doxepin
beclomethasone	clorazepate	DPT vaccine
betamethasone	colchicine	ergocalciferol(?)
botulin A toxin	cortisone	ethambutol
butallylonal	cyclobarbital	ethopropazine
bupivacaine	cyclopentobarbital	etidocaine
butabarbital	cytarabine	

fludrocortisone
fluphenazine
fluprednisolone
flurazepam
glyburide
gold Au 198
gold sodium thiomalate
gold sodium thiosulfate
halazepam
griseofulvin
heptabarbital
hexachlorophene
hexethal
hexobarbital
hydrocortisone
hydroxychloroquine
imipramine
indomethacin
influenza virus vaccine
insulin
iodide and iodine solutions
   and compounds(?)
iophendylate
isoniazid
ketoprofen
labetalol
levodopa
levothyroxine
lidocaine
liothyronine
liotrix
lorazepam
measles and rubella virus
   vaccine (live)
measles, mumps, and rubella
   virus vaccine
measles virus vaccine
mephenesin
mephobarbital
mepivacaine
meprobamate
mesoridazine
metharbital

methdilazine
methitural
methohexital
methotrexate
methotrimeprazine
methoxiflurane
methyl alcohol
methyldopa
methylene blue
methylprednisolone
metoclopramide
metocurine iodide
metoprolol
metrizamide
midazolam
mumps virus vaccine (live)
nadolol
nalidixic acid
naproxen
nitrazepam
nitrofurantoin
nortriptyline
oral contraceptives
oxazepam
oxyphenbutazone
paramethadione
paramethasone
pentobarbital
periciazine
perphenazine phenytoin
pindolol
piperacetazine
phenobarbital
phenylbutazone
piperazine
piperocaine
poliovirus vaccine
prazepam
prednisolone
prednisone
prilocaine
primidone
probarbital

procaine
prochlorperazine
promazine
promethazine
propiomazine
propoxycaine
proprandol
protriptyline
quinacrine
radioactive iodides(?)
rubella and mumps virus
   vaccine (live)
rubella virus vaccine (live)
secobarbital
sodium salicylate
succinylcholine
talbutal
temazepam
tetracaine
thiamylal
thiethylperazine
thiopental
thiopropazate
thioproperazine
thioridazine
thyroglobulin
thyroid trifluoperazine
triflupromazine
trimeprazine
trimethadione
trimipramine
tolazamide
tolbutamide
triamcinolone
trichloroethylene
tubocurarine
vinbarbital
vinblastine
vincristine
vitamin A
vitamin D
vitamin D_2
vitamin D_3

E. Neoplasms and cysts
F. Trauma affecting the midbrain, base of the skull, and orbit
G. Vascular lesions as arteriosclerosis, hemorrhage and thrombosis in the midbrain, sub-
   arachnoid, hemorrhage, aneurysms, congenitally dilated arteries, giant-cell arteritis
H. Idiopathic—etiologic basis undetermined

Fraunfelder FT, Fraunfelder FW. *Drug-induced ocular side effects*. Woburn, MA: Butterworth-Heinemann, 2001.

Pacifici L, et al. Acute third cranial nerve ophthalmoplegia: possible pathogenesis from alpha-II-interferon treatment. *Ital J Neurol Sci* 1993;14:579–580.

Roy FH. *Ocular syndromes and systemic diseases*, 3rd ed. Philadelphia: Lippincott Williams & Wilkins, 2002.

CHRONIC OPHTHALMOPLEGIA (SLOW ONSET OF EXTRAOCULAR MUSCLE PALSY)

1. Degenerative conditions
   A. Amyotrophic lateral sclerosis—progressive bulbar palsy
   B. Chronic progressive external ophthalmoplegia
   C. Hereditary ataxias—Friedreich ataxia, Sanger–Brown ataxia
   D. Progressive supranuclear palsy
   E. Syringomyelia (syringobulbia)
   F. Thyroid myopathy (Graves disease)
2. Infective conditions
   A. Diffuse sclerosis
   B. Disseminated sclerosis (multiple sclerosis)
   C. Syphilis

Duke-Elder S, Scott GI. *System of ophthalmology*, Vol XII. St. Louis: CV Mosby, 1971.

Roy FH. *Ocular syndromes and systemic diseases*, 3rd ed. Philadelphia: Lippincott Williams & Wilkins, 2002.

BILATERAL COMPLETE OPHTHALMOPLEGIA (BILATERAL PALSY OF OCULAR MUSCLES, PTOSIS, WITH PUPIL AND ACCOMMODATION INVOLVEMENT)

1. Arteriosclerotic hemorrhage and occlusion
2. Cerebellopontine angle tumors (Cushing syndrome II)
3. Encephalitis, acute
4. Fisher syndrome (ophthalmoplegia–ataxia areflexia syndrome)
5. Giant-cell arteritis (Hutchinson–Horton–Magath–Brown syndrome)
6. Kiloh–Nevin syndrome (ocular myeomyopathy)
7. Midbrain tumors
8. Multiple sclerosis (rare)
9. Mucormycosis
10. Ohaha syndrome (ophthalmoplegia, hypotonia, ataxia hypacusis, athetosis)
11. Orbital abscess
12. Parinaud syndrome (conjunctiva-adenitis syndrome)
13. Retrobulbar block complication
14. Rochon–Duvigneaud syndrome (superior orbital fissure syndrome)
15. Rollet syndrome (orbital apex-sphenoidal syndrome)
16. Syphilis (acquired lues)
17. Trauma
18. Wernicke encephalopathies (thiamine deficiency)
19. Whipple disease (intestinal lipodystrophy)

Kaufman LM, et al. Invasive sinonasal polyps causing ophthalmoplegia, exophthalmos, and visual field loss. *Ophthalmology* 1989;96:1667–1672.

McKusick VA. *Mendelian Inheritance in Man*, 12th ed. Baltimore: Johns Hopkins Hospital Press, 1998.

Roy FH. *Ocular syndromes and systemic diseases*, 3rd ed. Philadelphia: Lippincott Williams & Wilkins, 2002.

Sergott RC, et al. Simultaneous, bilateral diabetic ophthalmoplegia. *Ophthalmology* 1984;91:18–22.

EXTERNAL OPHTHALMOPLEGIA (PARALYSIS OF OCULAR MUSCLES INCLUDING PTOSIS WITH SPARING OF PUPIL AND ACCOMMODATION)

1. Abiotrophy—specific for one particular tissue, bilateral, symmetric
2. Amyloidosis (Lubarsch–Pick syndrome)
3. Aneurysm of internal carotid artery (foramen lacerum syndrome)
4. Bassen–Kornzweig syndrome (familial hypolipoproteinemia)
5. Bee sting
6. Chronic progressive external ophthalmoplegia
7. Congenital and familial
8. Diabetes mellitus (Willis disease)
9. Diphtheria
10. Epidemic encephalitis
11. Friedreich ataxia
12. Garcin syndrome (Schmincke tumor unilateral cranial paralysis)
13. Graves disease (hyperthyroidism)
14. Jacod syndrome (petrosphenoidal space syndrome)
15. Kearns–Sayre syndrome (ophthalmoplegic retinal degeneration syndrome)
16. Mumps
17. Myasthenia gravis (Erb–Goldflam syndrome)
18. Myotonic dystrophy (Curschmann–Steinert syndrome)
19. Myositis
20. Nevus sebaceous of Jadassohn
21. Nothnagel syndrome (ophthalmoplegia-cerebellar ataxia syndrome)
22. Oculopharyngeal syndrome (progressive muscular dystrophy with ptosis and dysphagia)
23. Olivopontocerebellar atrophy III (with retinal degeneration)—dominant
24. Ophthalmoplegia, progressive external, and scoliosis (horizontal gaze paralysis, familial)—recessive
25. Pernicious anemia
26. Polyradiculoneuronitis (Guillain–Barré and Fisher syndromes)
27. Progressive facial hemiatrophy (Parry–Romberg syndrome)
28. Pseudotumor (orbital)
29. Refsum syndrome (heredopathia atactica polyneuritiformis syndrome)
30. Scleroderma (progressive systemic sclerosis)
31. Shy–Drager syndrome (orthostatic hypotension syndrome)
32. Shy–Gonatas syndrome (accumulation of lipids in muscles simulates gargoylism)
33. Tick paralysis (Lyme disease, Rocky Mountain spotted fever)
34. Vincristine—may have fifth and seventh nerve and peripheral neuropathies
35. Wernicke encephalopathies (beriberi, thiamine deficiency)

Fassati A, et al. Chronic progressive external ophthalmoplegia: a correlative study of quantitative molecular data and histochemical and biochemical profile. *J Neurol Sci* 1994;123:140–146.

Marsch SC, Schaefer HG. External ophthalmoplegia after total intravenous anaesthesia. *Anaesthesia* 1994;49: 525–527.

McKusick VA. *Mendelian inheritance in man*, 12th ed. Baltimore: Johns Hopkins University Press, 1998.

Roy FH. *Ocular syndromes and systemic diseases*, 3rd ed. Philadelphia: Lippincott Williams & Wilkins, 2002.

INTERNUCLEAR OPHTHALMOPLEGIA

This condition comprises paralysis of the medial rectus muscles on attempted conjugate lateral gaze without other evidence of third nerve paralysis due to involvement of medial longitudinal fasciculus. Jerk nystagmus of abducting eye and vertical nystagmus, usually on upward gaze, may be present.

1. Bilateral
    - A. Arnold–Chiari malformation (cerebellomedullary malformation syndrome)
    - B. "Crack" cocaine
    - C. Fabry disease (glycosphingolipid lipidosis)
    - D. Inflammation, such as upper respiratory infection
    - E. Midbrain infarction
    - *F. Multiple sclerosis (disseminated sclerosis)
    - G. Myasthenia gravis (Erb–Goldflam syndrome)
    - H. Occlusive vascular disease
    - I. Oculocerebellar tegmental syndrome
    - J. Pontine hematoma
    - K. Syphilis (acquired lues)
    - L. Temporal arteritis
    - M. Vertebral basilar artery syndrome (whiplash injury)
    - N. Webino syndrome (wall-eyed exotropia bilateral internuclear ophthalmoplegia)
    - O. Wernicke encephalopathy
2. Unilateral
    - A. Bielschowsky–Lutz–Cogan syndrome (internuclear ophthalmoplegia)
    - B. Cryptococcosis (torulosis)
    - C. Multiple sclerosis (disseminated sclerosis)
    - D. Myasthenia gravis (Erb–Goldflam syndrome)
    - E. Neuro-Behçet Disease
    - F. Tumors of the brainstem
    - *G. Vascular lesion—infarct of small branch of basilar artery

Atabay C, et al. Eales disease with internuclear ophthalmoplegia. *Ann Ophthalmol* 1992;24:267–269.

Glaser JS. *Neuro-ophthalmology*, 3rd ed. Philadelphia: JB Lippincott, 1990.

Okuda B, et al. Bilateral internuclear ophthalmoplegia, ataxia, and tremor from a midbrain infarction. *Stroke* 1993; 24:481–482.

Zee DS. Internuclear ophthalmoplegia: pathophysiology and diagnosis. *Baillieres Clin Neurol* 1992;1:455–470.

PAINFUL OPHTHALMOPLEGIA (PALSY OF OCULAR MUSCLES WITH PAIN)

1. Adenocarcinoma metastatic to the orbit
2. Atypical facial neuralgia
3. Cavernous sinus syndrome (Foix syndrome)
4. Collier sphenoidal palsy
5. Diabetic ophthalmoplegia
6. Intracavernous carotid aneurysm
7. Myositis (orbital)
8. Nasopharyngeal tumor
9. Ophthalmoplegic migraine
10. Orbital abscess (mucormycosis-diabetes, immunosuppressed, AIDS)
11. Orbital apex sphenoidal syndrome (Rollet syndrome)

* = most important

Internuclear ophthalmoplegia

	Multiple Sclerosis	Inflammation as Upper Respiratory Infection	Neoplasm as Medulloblastoma	Myasthenia Gravis	Arnold Chiari Malformation	Fabry Disease	Ischemia (Vasolar)
History							
1. Age 20 to 40 years	U			U	S		
2. Over 60							U
3. First decade of life		U	U				
4. Hereditary						U	
5. More in females				U			
6. More in males			U				
7. Usually viral infection		U					
Physical Findings							
1. Associated hydrocephalus			S		S		
2. Central retinal artery occlusion						U	
3. Cogan lid twitch				U			
4. Conjunctivitis		U					
5. Cornea verticillata						U	
6. Corneal opacities						U	
7. Corneal ulcer		S					
8. Dacryoadenitis		S					
9. Dacryocystitis		S					
10. Esotropia, sudden onset			U				
11. Keratitis		S					
12. Lid edema						U	
13. Myokimia of lids	S						
14. Nystagmus	U		S		U		
15. Optic nerve atrophy	S						S
16. Optic neuritis	U	S					
17. Oscillopsia	S						
18. Panophthalmitis		S					
19. Papilledema			U		U	U	
20. Ptosis	S			U			
21. Pupillary afferent defect	U						
22. Reduced visual acuity with exercise/hyperthermia	S						S
23. Uveitis	S	S					
24. Varicosities palpebral/bulbar conjunctiva						U	
25. Visual field defects	S		S				S
Laboratory Data							
1. Cerebral anteriography						S	
2. Chest roentgenogram		S					
3. Cerebrospinal fluid abnormal	U	S	S		S		
4. Computed tomographic scan			U	U	U	U	
5. MRI	U	S	U	R	U	U	U
6. Peripheral blood test (Sadate, CBC, etc)		S					U
7. Throat culture		U					

R = rarely; S = sometimes; and U = usually.

Painful ophthalmoplegia

	Rhabdomyosarcoma	Thyroid Myopathy	Diabetes Mellitus (Third in Palsy)	Myositis	Orbital Cellulitis	Tolosa-Hunt Syndrome	Superior Orbital Fissure Syndrome	Nasopharyngeal Tumor	Pseudotumor (orbital)	Metastatic Adenocarcinoma	Neuralgia as Tic Doloreaux of First Division Trigeminal	Cavernous-Sinus Syndrome	Carotid/Dural Sinus Fistula
History													
1. Bilateral	R	S		S	R				R	U			S
2. Chronic inflammatory disease						U							
3. Familial			U										
4. Idiopathic inflammation				U		U			U				
5. Inflammatory, traumatic, tumor, or vascular lesion							U					U	
6. Ipsilateral lacrimation during pain											U		
7. Loss of vision	S	S	S	R	S	R			S	S		S	S
8. More in females											U		
9. More in males								U					
10. More than 40 years old		S											U
11. Only in children	U					U							
12. Periorbital pain	S	S		S		U			U		U		U
13. Scintillating scotoma						U							
Physical Findings													
1. Cataract			U										
2. Central retinal artery thrombosis										R			
3. Cotton-wool spots			U										
4. Chemosis, conjunctiva		S	S		S							U	U
5. Diminished corneal sensitivity							U	U	S			S	
6. Glaucoma			U							U	R		
7. Hard exudates			U										
8. Intraorbital bleeding										U			
9. Keratitis		S	S									U	S
10. Lid edema		S					U	U	S	U			
11. Mild conjunctivitis							U		S	U			
12. Nasolacrimal obstruction							R		U				
13. Ocular bruit												U	U
14. Optic neuritis						U				S	R		
15. Optic nerve atrophy			R					U		S		S	
16. Papilledema			S					U		S			
17. Periorbital edema and tenderness	S	S			U					S			S
18. Proptosis	U	U		S	S	U	U	S	U	U		U	U
19. Ptosis			U					U	S				
20. Sluggish pupil reaction to light			S				U	U					
21. Uveitis											S		
Laboratory Data													
1. Arteriography, cerebral												U	U
2. Biopsy								U	U	S			
3. Blood sugar elevated			U										
4. Computed tomographic scan of orbit	U	U		U	U	U	S	U	U	U		U	R
5. MRI	R	R	U	R	R	S	R	S	R	S	S		R
6. Ultrasonography (oculo-oribital)		S		S	S		U	U	U	U		S	S

12. Orbital periostitis
13. Postherpetic neuralgia
14. Pseudotumor of orbit
15. Superior orbital fissure syndrome (Rochon–Duvigneaud syndrome, including superior orbital fissuritis)
16. Temporal arteritis
17. Tic douloureux of the first trigeminal division
18. Tolosa–Hunt syndrome (inflammatory lesion of cavernous sinus)

Mannor GE, et al. Outcome of orbital myositis. *Ophthalmology* 1997;104:409–414.

Roy FH. *Ocular syndromes and systemic diseases*, 3rd ed. Philadelphia: Lippincott Williams & Wilkins, 2002.

Sananman ML, Weintroub MI. Remitting ophthalmoplegia due to rhabdomyosarcoma. *Arch Ophthalmol* 1971;86: 6:459–461.

TRANSIENT OPHTHALMOPLEGIA (EXTRAOCULAR MUSCLE PARALYSIS OF SHORT DURATION)

1. Cranial irradiation and intrathecal chemotherapy
2. Cyclic esotropia
3. Cyclic oculomotor palsy
4. Following internal carotid artery ligation for treatment of intracavernous giant aneurysm
5. Lethargic encephalitis
6. Multiple sclerosis (disseminated sclerosis—usually the lateral rectus)
7. Myasthenia gravis (ocular, early)
8. Oculomotor nuclear complex infarction
9. Ophthalmoplegia migraine
10. Post lumbar puncture abducens palsy
11. Syphilis (acquired lues)
12. Tabes dorsalis
13. Treatment of arteriovenous fistulas with Debrun balloon technique
14. Wilson disease (hepatolenticular degeneration)

Gadoth N, Liel Y. Transient external ophthalmoplegia in Wilson's disease. *Metab Pediatr. Ophthalmol* 1980; 4:71–72.

Lepore FE, Nissenblatt MJ. Bilateral internuclear ophthalmoplegia after intrathecal chemotherapy and cranial irradiation. *Am J Ophthalmol* 1981;92:851–853.

Nakao S, et al. Transient ophthalmoplegia following internal carotid artery ligation for treatment of intracavernous giant aneurysm. *Surg Neurol* 1982;17:458–463.

PAINFUL OCULAR MOVEMENTS (PAIN WITH MOVEMENT OF THE EYES)

1. Bone-break fever (dengue fever) (rare)
2. Influenza
3. Myositis
    A. "Collagen diseases"
    B. Infectious myositis
    C. Trichinosis

4. Orbital cellulitis
5. Orbital periostitis
6. Retrobulbar neuritis

Jampel RS, Fells P. Monocular elevation paresis caused by a central nervous system lesion. *Arch Ophthalmol* 1968; 80:45.

POOR CONVERGENCE (INABILITY OF BOTH EYES TO FIXATE SIMULTANEOUSLY ON A NEAR OBJECT)

1. Functional
   A. Convergence insufficiency
   B. Exophoria
   C. Exotropia
   D. Hysteria
   E. Poor attention span
2. Organic
   A. Brain lesion, to include bilateral occipital lobe lesions, superior colliculi, and anterior internuclear ophthalmoplegia, such as in hemorrhage, trauma, or tumors
   B. Dorsal midbrain syndrome
   C. Encephalitis
   D. Exophthalmic goiter—Möbius sign
   E. Exophthalmos
   F. Multiple sclerosis
   G. Myotonic dystrophy
   H. Narcolepsy
   I. Poor visual acuity in one or both eyes
   J. Postencephalitis
   K. Syphilis and tabes
   L. Third nerve paralysis (see p. 153)
   M. Whiplash injury
3. Drugs, including the following:

alcohol
allobarbital
amobarbital
amphetamine
aprobarbital
barbital
bromide
bromisovalum
butabarbital
butalbital
butallylonal
butethal
carbamazepine
carbon dioxide
chloral hydrate
cyclobarbital
cyclopentobarbital
dextroamphetamine
dimethyl tubocurarine iodide
diphenylhydantoin
floxuridine
fluorouracil
heptabarbital
hexethal
hexobarbital
mephobarbital
methamphetamine
metharbital
methitural
methohexital
metocurine iodide
morphine
opium
penicillamine
pentobarbital
phenmetrazine
phenobarbital
phenytoin
primidone
probarbital
secobarbital
talbutal
thiamylal
thiopental
tubocurarine
vinbarbital

Fraunfelder FT, Fraunfelder FW. *Drug-induced ocular side effects*.Woburn, MA: Butterworth-Heinemann, 2001.

Walsh FB, Hoyt WF. *Clinical neuro-ophthalmology*, 4th ed. Baltimore: Williams & Wilkins, 1985.

SPASM OF CONVERGENCE

Spasm of convergence occurs with spasm of accommodation and miosis (i.e., spasm of the near reflex).

1. Encephalitis—accompanied with nystagmus
2. Hysteria—may be confused with lateral rectus palsy
3. Labyrinthine fistulas
4. Kenny syndrome
5. Oculogyric crisis in myasthenia gravis
6. Paralysis of horizontal gaze with compensatory spasm of near reflex
7. Parinaud syndrome (divergence paralysis)
8. Tabes dorsalis
9. Trauma
10. Wernicke syndrome (avitaminosis B_1)

Feiler-Ofry V, et al. Lipoid proteinosis (Urbach–Wiethe Syndrome). *Br J Ophthalmol* 1979;63:694–698.

Thompson RA, Zynde RH. Convergence spasm associated with Wernicke's encephalopathy. *Neurology* 1969;19: 711–712.

DIVERGENCE PARALYSIS

Divergence paralysis is defined as having a supranuclear cause with sudden onset of comitant esotropia and uncrossed diplopia at distance, fusion at near (usually 1–2 m) normal ductions and versions, and gross impairment of fusional amplitudes of divergence.

*1. Brainstem lesions
    A. Cerebellar cyst
    B. Hemangioma
    C. Tumors, such as cerebellar and acoustic neuromas and pontine glioma
2. Cerebral hemorrhage
3. Diazepam
4. Diphtheria
5. Dorsal midbrain syndrome
6. Epidemic encephalitis
7. Functional
8. Head injuries
9. Increased intracranial pressure
10. Influenza
11. Lead poisoning
12. Multiple sclerosis (disseminated sclerosis)
13. Poliomyelitis
14. Syphilis
15. Unknown
16. Vascular disease
    A. Diabetes mellitus
    B. Hypertension

    C. Occlusion of subclavian artery with reversal of flow in vertebral artery

    D. Vertebral basilar insufficiency

Arai M, Fujii S. Divergence paralysis *Neurology* 1990;237:45–46.

Brown SM, Iacuone JJ. Intact sensory fusion in a child with divergence paresis caused by a pontine glioma. *Am J Ophthalmol* 1999;128:528–530.

Krohel GB, et al. Divergence paralysis. *Am J Ophthalmol* 1982;94:506.

Walsh FB, Hoyt WF. *Clinical neuro-ophthalmology*, 4th ed. Baltimore: Williams & Wilkins, 1985.

OCULOCARDIAC REFLEX

Bradycardia, nausea, and faintness occur and are dependent on trigeminal sensory stimulation evoked by pressure on or within the eyeball or from sensory impulses by stretching of ocular muscles.

1. Acute glaucoma
2. Anophthalmic socket
3. During ophthalmoscopy examination of premature infants
4. Exaggerated in epidemic encephalitis
5. Intermittent exophthalmos due to congenital venous malformations of the orbit
6. Intraocular injections
7. Orbital hematoma
*8. Pressure on globe
9. Retinal detachment operation
10. Severe injury to eye or orbit
*11. Traction on extraocular muscles including levator palpebrae superioris

Arnold RW, et al. Lack of global vagal propensity in patients with oculocardiac reflex. *Ophthalmology* 1994;101:1347–1352.

Clarke WN, et al. The oculocardiac reflex during ophthalmoscopy in premature infants. *Am J Ophthalmol* 1985;99:649–651.

Ginsburg RN, et al. Oculocardiac reflex in the anophthalmic socket. *Ophthalmic Surg* 1992;23:135–137.

Walsh FB, Hoyt WF. *Clinical neuro-ophthalmology*, 4th ed. Baltimore: Williams & Wilkins, 1985.

RETRACTION OF THE GLOBE (ON HORIZONTAL CONJUGATE GAZE)

*1. Duane syndrome (retraction syndrome)—cocontraction of horizontal rectus muscles, lateral rectus, and both vertical muscles, or medial and inferior rectus muscles or fibrotic lateral rectus
    A. Acrorenoocular syndrome
    B. Goldenhar syndrome
    C. Hanhart syndrome
    D. Isolated
    E. Okihiro syndrome
    F. Wildervanck syndrome (Klippel–Feil anomaly with Duane syndrome)
2. Fibrosis secondary to strabismus surgery
3. Medial wall fracture with incarceration of orbit contents—retraction of globe with attempted abduction
4. Orbital mass
    A. Dermoid cyst
    B. Hemangioma

* = most important

    C. Lymphangioma

    D. Osteofibroma

5. Retraction of convergent nonfixating eye associated with loss of conjugate lateral gaze and occurrence of the near reflex on attempted lateral gaze

6. Thyroid myopathy

Holtz SJ. Congenital ocular anomalies associated with Duane's retraction syndrome, the nevus of ota, and axial anisometropia. *Am J Ophthalmol* 1974;74:729–731.

Isenberg SJ. *The eye in infancy.* Chicago: Year Book Medical, 1989.

FORCED DUCTION TEST

The eyeball is moved away from the muscle being tested; this is accomplished by grasping with a forceps the conjunctiva and episclera close to the limbus.

1. Supraduction–infraduction
   A. Resistance
      (1) Abnormal fascial or muscle attachments
      (2) Congenital fibrosis syndrome
      (3) Double elevator palsy
      (4) Orbital floor fracture
      (5) Orbital mass
      (6) Thyroid myopathy of inferior rectus muscle
   B. Unrestricted
      (1) Elevator paresis
      (2) Paresis of inferior superior rectus muscle
2. Supraduction in adduction
   A. Brown superior oblique tendon sheath syndrome—resistance (see p. 132)
   B. Paresis of inferior oblique muscle—unrestricted
3. Adduction
   A. Resistance
      (1) Chronic third nerve palsy with contracture lateral rectus
      (2) Congenital fibrosis syndrome
      (3) Duane retraction syndrome because of fibrosis of lateral rectus muscle
      (4) Orbital mass
      (5) Tight lateral rectus following excessive resection operation
      (6) Thyroid myopathy
   B. Unrestricted
      (1) Extensive medial rectus recession
      (2) Duane retraction syndrome because of central or peripheral cocontraction of medial and lateral rectus on attempted adduction
4. Abduction
   A. Resistance
      (1) Abnormal fascial or muscle attachments including strabismus fixus
      (2) Blowout fracture
      (3) Chronic sixth nerve palsy with contracture medial rectus
      (4) Myositis
      (5) Orbital mass
      (6) Thyroid myopathy

Tight medial rectus following excessive resection operation

B. Unrestricted
  (1) Extensive lateral rectus recession
  (2) Paralysis of lateral rectus muscle

Beyer-Machule C, von Noorden GK. *Atlas of ophthalmic surgery*, Vol 1: *Lids, orbits, extraocular muscles*. New York: Thieme Medical, 1984.

DOUBLE ELEVATOR PALSY (APPARENT PARALYSIS OF GLOBE ELEVATORS [I.E., SUPERIOR RECTUS AND INFERIOR OBLIQUE MUSCLES])

1. Inferior rectus muscle restriction
   A. Anomalous insertion of inferior rectus muscle
   B. Blow-out fracture
   C. Congenital orbital fibrosis syndrome
   D. Thyroid ophthalmopathy
2. Monocular elevation paresis secondary to central nervous system lesions
   A. Monocular elevation paresis
   B. Skew deviation
3. Neurogenic or myogenic superior rectus muscle weakness
   A. Myasthenia gravis (Erb–Goldflam syndrome)
   B. Postoperative Berke–Motais surgery
   C. Superior oblique tendon sheath syndrome (see p. 132)
   D. Third cranial nerve palsy (see p. 153)
   E. Trauma

Callahan M.A. Surgically mismanaged ptosis associated with double elevator palsy. *Arch Ophthalmol* 1981;99:108.

OCULAR NEUROMYOTONIA (PAROXYSMAL MONOCULAR DEVIATIONS ASCRIBABLE TO INVOLUNTARY CONTRACTION OF MUSCLES INNERVATED BY THIRD, FOURTH, OR SIXTH CRANIAL NERVES)

1. Aneurysmal compression of third nerve
2. Chondrosarcoma
3. Cystic craniopharyngioma
4. Following radiation therapy
5. Rhabdomyosarcoma

Bateman DE, Saunders M. Cyclic oculomotor palsy. *J Neurol Neurosurg Psychiatry* 1983;46:451.

Lessell S, et al. Ocular neuromyotonia after radiation therapy. *Am J Ophthalmol* 1986;102:766–770.

EXTRAOCULAR MUSCLE ENLARGEMENT ON ORBITAL COMPUTERIZED AND TOMOGRAPHIC SCAN

1. Diffuse
   A. Acromegaly
   B. Amyloidosis
   *C. Graves disease as thyroid ophthalmopathy
   *D. Infection
   E. Parasitic infiltration
   F. Trauma

* = most important

    G. Tumors, including pseudotumor

    H. Vascular abnormalities as arteriovenous fistula

    I. Collagen vascular disease

  2. Focal

    A. Cysticercosis

    B. Hemorrhagic cyst

    C. Primary or metastatic carcinoma

    D. Trichinella

Albert DM, Jakobiec FA. *Principles and practice of ophthalmology*. Philadelphia: WB Saunders, 1994:1881–2095.

Howard GR, et al. Orbital dermoid located within lateral rectus muscle. *Ophthalmology* 1994;101:767–778.

Kaltreider SA, et al. Destructive cysts of the maxillary sinus affecting the orbit. *Arch Ophthalmol* 1988;106: 1398–1402.

Maurrello JA, Flanagan JC. Management of orbital inflammatory disease: a protocol. *Surv Ophthalmol* 1984;29: 104–116.

5

Conjunctiva

CONTENTS

CELLULAR RESPONSES

1. Basophilic reaction—significant only when seen in large numbers; immunoglobulin E (Ig-E) mediated allergic conditions; key role in asthma, atopy, and hypersensitivity responses; present in vernal (eosinophils) and giant papillary conjunctivitis (GPC) conjunctivitis.

2. Eosinophilic reaction—GPC (giant papillary conjunctivitis); Charcot–Leyden crystals are more prominent than intact eosinophils in chronic allergy; parasitic conjunctivitis.
   *A. Vernal conjunctivitis—characteristic with fragmentation of eosinophil
   B. Hay fever conjunctivitis—rarely fragmentation of eosinophil
   C. Allergic conjunctivitis from various drugs, cosmetics, and other antigens
   D. Atropine sensitivity—not present when eserine or pilocarpine is used
3. Mononuclear reaction
   A. Viral disease—100% without secondary infection; usually lymphocytic
      *(1) Epidemic keratoconjunctivitis—adenovirus type 8
      (2) Pharyngoconjunctival fever—adenovirus type 3
      *(3) Herpetic keratoconjunctivitis
      (4) Acute follicular conjunctivitis of Beal
   B. Chronic ocular infections
4. Neutrophilic reaction—early stage of severe viral conjunctivitis
   A. All bacteria but two—*Neisseria catarrhalis* and *Haemophilus duplex* (Morax–Axenfeld diplobacillus)
   B. Viruses of the family *Chlamydiaceae* [trachoma inclusion conjunctivitis (TRIC) agent]
      (1) Trachoma
      *(2) Inclusion conjunctivitis
      (3) Lymphogranuloma venereum
   C. Fungal disease
      (1) Streptothrix conjunctivitis secondary to canaliculitis
      (2) Nocardial corneal ulcers
      (3) Monilial corneal ulcers
   D. Unknown cause
      *(1) Erythema multiforme (Stevens–Johnson syndrome)
      (2) Conjunctivitis of Reiter disease
   E. Vernal conjunctivitis—eosinophilic and neutrophilic reaction
   F. Epidemic keratoconjunctivitis and herpetic keratoconjunctivitis have a shift from mononuclear to polymorphonuclear reaction when a membrane is formed
5. Plasma-cell reaction—trachoma—especially with spontaneous rupturing of follicles; chlamydial conjunctivitis
6. Epithelial changes
   A. Keratinization of conjunctival epithelial cells
      *(1) Alkali burn
      (2) Vitamin A deficiency
      (3) Exposure
      (4) Cicatrization (such as pemphigoid and Stevens–Johnson syndrome)
      (5) Keratoconjunctivitis sicca—partially keratinized epithelial cells, specific
      (6) Epithelial plaque
      (7) Superior limbic keratoconjunctivitis (SLK)
   B. Large, multipointed epithelial cells
      (1) Characteristic of viral infection
      *(2) Most often found in herpetic keratitis
   C. Intracellular granules
      (1) Pseudoinclusion bodies—extension of nuclear material into cytoplasm
      (2) Intracellular-free green pigment in cytoplasm—present in persons with dark complexion

        (3) Intracellular-free blue granules—present in cytoplasm in about 12% of normal individuals

        (4) Sex chromatin—present in nuclei of females only

7. Cellular inclusions

    A. Trachoma and inclusion conjunctivitis have identical inclusions—basophilic, cytoplasmic (Halberstaedter–Prowazek)

  *B. Molluscum contagiosum—eosinophilic, cytoplasmic (Henderson/Patterson)

    C. Lymphogranuloma venereum—eosinophilic

  *D. Herpes simplex and herpes zoster—eosinophilic, internuclear (Lipschütz)

    E. Measles—multinucleated giant cells with eosinophilic internuclear inclusion bodies and cytoplasmic, eosinophilic masses

  *F. Chickenpox—eosinophilic, internuclear

    G. Smallpox—eosinophilic, cytoplasmic

Brinser JH, Burd EM. Principles of diagnosis ocular microbiology. In: Tabbara KF, Hyndiuk RA, eds. *Infections of the eye*. Boston: Little, Brown, 1986:73–92.

Fedukowicz HB. *External infections of the eye: bacterial, viral, mycotic*, 3rd ed. New York: Appleton-Century-Crofts, 1984.

Soparkar, Charles NS, et al. *Arch Opthalmol* 1997;115:34–38.

Spencer WH. *Ophthalmic pathology*, Vol 1. Philadelphia: WB Saunders, 1985.

PURULENT CONJUNCTIVITIS

Purulent conjunctivitis is characterized as violent acute conjunctival inflammation, great swelling of lids, copious secretion of pus, and a marked tendency to corneal involvement and even possible loss of the eye.

1. Gram-positive group

    A. Bacillus of Doderlein (*Lactobacillus* sp.)

    B. *Listeria monocytogenes*

  *C. Pneumococcus

    D. Staphylococcus

  *E. Streptococcus

2. Gram-negative group

    A. *Aerobacter aerogenes*

    B. Enterobacteriaceae

    C. *Escherichia coli*

  *D. *Haemophilus influenzae* biotype III

    E. *Klebsiella pneumoniae*

    F. *Moraxella lacunata*

  *G. *Neisseria gonorrhoeae*

    H. *Neisseria meningitidis*

    I. *Proteus* species

    J. *Pseudomonas* species

    K. *Serratia marcescens*

3. Vaccinia virus

4. Fungus

    A. *Actinomyces* species

    B. *Candida* species

  *C. *Nocardia* species

* = most important

5. Wiskott–Aldrich syndrome—x-linked

Fedukowicz HB. *External infections of the eye: bacterial, viral, mycotic*, 3rd ed. New York: Appleton-Century-Crofts, 1984.

Roy FH. *Ocular syndromes and systemic diseases*, 3rd ed. Philadelphia: Lippincott Williams & Wilkins, 2002.

Snead JW, et al. Listeria monocytogenes endophthalmitis. *Am J Ophthalmol* 1977;84:337–344.

ACUTE MUCOPURULENT CONJUNCTIVITIS

This type of conjunctivitis is epidemic pink eye, marked hyperemia and a mucopurulent discharge, which tends toward spontaneous recovery.

1. Gram-positive group
   *A. Pneumococcus
   B. Staphylococcus—eyelid lesions and punctate staining of the lower cornea may occur
2. Gram-negative group
   *A. *Haemophilus aegyptius* (Koch–Weeks bacillus)
   B. *H. influenzae*
3. Associated with exanthems and viral infections
   A. German measles (Greig syndrome)
   B. Measles (rubeola)
   C. Mumps
   *D. Reiter syndrome (conjunctivourethrosynovial syndrome)
   E. Scarlet fever
4. Fungus
   A. *Candida albicans*
   B. Leptothrix
5. Lyell disease—toxic epidermal necrolysis or scalded-skin syndrome
6. Relapsing polychondritis
7. Sjögren syndrome (secretoinhibitor syndrome)
8. Etiology obscure in many cases

Fedukowicz HB. *External infections of the eye: bacterial, viral, and mycotic*, 3rd ed. New York: Appleton-Century-Crofts, 1984.

Okumoto M, Smolin G. Pneumococcal infections of the eye. *Am J Ophthalmol* 1974;77:346–352.

Roy FH. *Ocular syndromes and systemic diseases*, 3rd ed. Philadelphia: Lippincott Williams & Wilkins, 2002.

CHRONIC MUCOPURULENT CONJUNCTIVITIS (MUCOPURULENT DISCHARGE, MODERATE HYPEREMIA WITH A CHRONIC COURSE)

1. Infective element—lids or lacrimal apparatus
   A. *Monilia* species
   B. Morax–Axenfeld diplobacillus (angular conjunctivitis)
   *C. Pneumococcus
   D. Pubic lice
   E. Staphylococcus
   F. *Streptothrix foersteri*
2. Allergic—cosmetic
3. Irritative
   A. Associated infections or irritation of lids, lacrimal apparatus, nose, or skin
   B. Deficiency of lacrimal secretions

C. Direct irritants—foreign body, mascara, dust, wind, smog, insecticides, chlorinated water, and many others

D. Exposure—ectropion, facial paralysis, exophthalmos, and others

E. Eyestrain

F. Metabolic conditions—gout, alcoholism, or prolonged digestive disturbances

G. Overtreatment by drugs—antibiotics, miotics, mydriatics

Fedukowicz HB. *External infections of the eye: bacterial, viral, and mycotic*, 3rd ed. New York: Appleton-Century-Crofts, 1984.

Geyer O, et al. Phenylephrine prodrug. *Ophthalmology* 1991;98:1483.

Okumoto M, Smolin G. Pneumococcal infections of the eye. *Am J Ophthalmol* 1974;77:346–352.

Roy FH. *Ocular syndromes and systemic diseases*, 3rd ed. Philadelphia: Lippincott Williams & Wilkins, 2002.

MEMBRANOUS CONJUNCTIVITIS

Exudate permeates epithelium to such an extent that removal of membrane is difficult and a raw bleeding surface results. Membranous conjunctivitis can lead to symblepharon, ankyloblepharon, and entropion with trichiasis.

1. Chemical irritants
    A. Acids, such as acetic or lactic
    *B. Alkalis, such as ammonia or lime
    C. Metallic salts, such as silver nitrate or copper sulfate
2. *Corynebacterium diphtheriae*
3. Ligneous conjunctivitis—chronic, cause unknown
4. Pneumococcus
5. Streptococcus
6. Uncommon—actinomyces, glandular fever, measles, *Neisseria catarrhalis*, variola, *Pseudomonas aeruginosa*, herpes simplex, *Leptothrix*, and epidemic keratoconjunctivitis (type adenovirus)

Fedukowicz HB. *External infections of the eye: bacterial, viral, and mycotic*, 3rd ed. New York: Appleton-Century-Crofts, 1984.

Roy FH. *Ocular syndromes and systemic diseases*, 3rd ed. Philadelphia: Lippincott Williams & Wilkins, 2002.

PSEUDOMEMBRANOUS CONJUNCTIVITIS

In pseudomembranous conjunctivitis, the fibrin network is easily peeled off, leaving the conjunctiva intact; it forms on the conjunctiva.

1. Bacteria
    A. *C. diphtheriae*
    *B. Gonococcus
    *C. Meningococcus
    D. Pneumococcus
    E. Staphylococcus
    *F. Streptococcus
    G. Uncommon—*H. aegyptius, H. influenzae, N. catarrhalis, Pseudomonas aeruginosa, E. coli, Bacillus subtilis,* Shigella, *Bacillus faecalis* alcaligenes, *Salmonella paratyphi* B, *Mycobacterium tuberculosis,* and *Treponema pallidum*
2. Viral
    *A. Epidemic keratoconjunctivitis (type adenovirus)
    *B. Herpes simplex

* = most important

C. Herpes zoster
D. Reiter syndrome (conjunctivourethrosynovial syndrome)
E. Vaccina
3. Fungal— *C. albicans*
*4. Allergic—vernal conjunctivitis
5. Toxic
*A. Stevens–Johnson syndrome can be caused by drugs, including the following:

acetaminophen
acetanilid
acetazolamide
acetohexamide
acetophenazine
allobarbital
allopurinol
amidone
aminosalicylate(?)
aminosalicylic acid(?)
amithiozone
amobarbital
amodiaquine
amoxicillin
ampicillin
antipyrine
aprobarbital
aspirin
auranofin
aurothioglucose
aurothioglycanide
barbital
belladonna
bendroflumethiazide
benzathine penicillin G
benzthiazide
bromide
bromisovalum
butabarbital
butalbital
butallylonal
butaperazine
butethal
captopril
carbamazepine
carbenicillin
carbromal
carisoprodol
carphenazine
cefaclor
cefadroxil

cefamandole
cefazolin
cefonicid
cefoperazone
ceforanide
cefotaxime
cefotetan
cefoxitin
cefsulodin
ceftazidime
ceftizoxime
ceftriaxone
cefuroxime
cephalexin
cephaloglycin
cephaloridine
cephalothin
cephapirin
cephradine
chloroquine
chlorothiazide
chlorpromazine
chlorpropamide
chlortetracycline
chlorthalidone
cimetidine
clindamycin
cloxacillin
cyclobarbital
cyclopentobarbital
cyclothiazide
danazol
demeclocycline
dichlorphenamide
dicloxacillin
diethazine
diphenylhydantoin
doxycycline
enalapril
erythromycin
ethopropazine

ethosuximide
ethotoin
ethoxzolamide
fenoprofen
fluphenazine
furosemide
gentamicin
glyburide
gold Au 198
gold sodium thiomalate
gold sodium thiosulfate
heptabarbital
hetacillin
hexethal
hexobarbital
hydrabamine penicillin V
hydrochlorothiazide
hydroflumethiazide
hydroxychloroquine
ibuprofen
indapamide
indomethacin
isoniazid
lincomycin
mephenytoin
mephobarbital
meprobamate
mesoridazine
methacycline
metharbital
methazolamide
methdilazine
methicillin
methitural
methohexital
methotrimeprazine
methsuximide
methyclothiazide
methylphenidate
metolazone
minocycline

minoxidil
moxalactam
nafcillin
naproxen
oxacillin
oxyphenbutazone
oxytetracycline
paramethadione
pentobarbital
perazine
pericyazine
perphenazine
phenacetin
phenobarbital
phenoxymethyl penicillin
phensuximide
phenylbutazone
phenytoin
piperacetazine
piproxen
polythiazide
potassium penicillin G
potassium penicillin V
potassium phenethicillin
potassium phenoxymethyl
  penicillin

primidone
probarbital
procaine penicillin G
prochlorperazine
promazine
promethazine
proparacaine
propiomazine
propranolol
quinethazone
quinine
rifampin
secobarbital
smallpox vaccine
sodium salicylate
sulfacetamide
sulfachlorpyridazine
sulfacytine
sulfadiazine
sulfadimethoxine
sulfamerazine
sulfameter
sulfamethazine
sulfamethizole
sulfamethoxazole
sulfamethoxypyridazine

sulfanilamide
sulfaphenazole
sulfapyridine
sulfasalazine
sulfathiazole
sulfisoxazole
sulindac
sulthiame
talbutal
tetracycline
thiabendazole
thiamylal
thiethylperazine
thiopental
thiopropazate
thioproperazine
thioridazine
tolazamide
tolbutamide
trichlormethiazide
trifluoperazine
triflupromazine
trimeprazine
trimethadione
vancomycin
vinbarbital

*B. Benign mucous membrane pemphigoid can be caused by drugs, including the
following:

carbamazepine
carbimazole
diphenylhydantoin
ethosuximide
griseofulvin
hydralazine

isoniazid
methimazole
methsuximide
methylthiouracil
paramethadione
phensuximide

practolol
propylthiouracil
streptomycin
trimethadione

C. Lyell disease (toxic epidermal necrolysis or scalded-skin syndrome) can be caused
by drugs, including the following:

acetaminophen
acetanilid
acetazolamide
acid bismuth sodium tartrate
adrenal cortex injection
aldosterone
allobarbital
amoxapine
amoxicillin
amobarbital
ampicillin

antipyrine
aprobarbital
aurothioglucose
aurothioglycanide
barbital
bendroflumethiazide
benzthiazide
benzathine penicillin G
betamethasone
bismuth oxychloride
bismuth sodium tartrate

bismuth sodium
  thioglycollate
bismuth sodium
  triglycollamate
busulfan
butabarbital
butalbital
butallylonal
butethal
carbamazepine
carbenicillin

* = most important

carbimazole
chlorambucil
chlorothiazide
chlortetracycline
chlorthalidone
clomipramine
cloxacillin
cortisone
cyclobarbital
cyclopentobarbital
cyclothiazide
cyclophosphamide
dapsone
demeclocycline
desoxycorticosterone
dexamethasone
dichlorphenamide
dicloxacillin
diltiazem
diphenylhydantoin
doxepin
doxycycline
erythromycin
ethambutol
ethotoin
ethoxzolamide
fludrocortisone
fluprednisolone
gold Au 198
gold sodium thiomalate
heptabarbital
hetacillin
hexethal
hexobarbital
hydrabamine penicillin V
hydrochlorothiazide
hydrocortisone
ibuprofen
indapamide

indomethacin
isoniazid
kanamycin
mechlorethamine
melphalan
mephenytoin
mephobarbital
meprednisone
methacycline
metharbital
methazolamide
methicillin
methitural
methohexital
methotrexate
methyclothiazide
methylprednisolone
metolazone
minocycline
nafcillin
nitrofurantoin
oxacillin
oxyphenbutazone
oxytetracycline
paramethadione
paramethasone
penicillamine
pentobarbital
phenobarbital
phenylbutazone
phenytoin
piroxicam
poliovirus vaccine
polythiazide
phenoxymethyl penicillin
phenylbutazone
potassium penicillin G
potassium penicillin V
potassium phenethicillin
prednisolone
prednisone

primidone
probarbital
procaine penicillin G
procarbazine
quinethazone
secobarbital
smallpox vaccine
sodium salicylate
streptomycin
sulfacetamide
sulfachlorpyridazine
sulfadiazine
sulfadimethoxine
sulfamerazine
sulfameter
sulfamethazine
sulfamethizole
sulfamethoxazole
sulfamethoxypyridazine
sulfanilamide
sulfaphenazole
sulfapyridine
sulfasalazine
sulfathiazole
sulfisoxazole
sulindac
talbutal
tetracycline
thiabendazole
thiamylal
thiopental
triamcinolone
trichlormethiazide
triethylene-melamine
trimethadione
trimipramine
uracil mustard
vinbarbital

    D. Pemphigus vulgaris
    E. Hereditary epidermolysis bullosa
  6. Chemical irritants
    A. Acids, such as acetic or lactic
   *B. Alkalis, such as ammonia or lime
    C. Metallic salts, such as silver nitrate or copper sulfate
    D. Vegetable and animal irritants
  7. Acute graft-versus-host disease
  8. Foot-and-mouth disease

9. Koch–Weeks bacillus
10. Ligneous conjunctivitis—chronic, cause unknown
11. Lipoid proteinosis (Urbach–Wiethe disease)
*12. Superior limbic keratoconjunctivitis
13. Traumatic or operative healing of wounds
14. Wegner granulomatosis

Barthelemy H, et al. Lipoid proteinosis with pseudomembranous conjunctivitis. *J Am Acad Dermatol* 1986;14: 367–371.

Fraunfelder FT, Fraunfelder FW. *Drug-induced ocular side effects.* Woburn, MA: Butterworth-Heinemann, 2001.

Pau H. *Differential diagnosis of eye diseases,* 2nd ed. New York: Thieme Medical, 1988.

OPHTHALMIA NEONATORUM (CONJUNCTIVITIS OCCURRING IN NEWBORNS)

*1. Chemical conjunctivitis, such as from silver nitrate instillation
*2. Chlamydial trachomatis
3. Bacteria
   A. Gram positive
     (1) *C. diphtheriae*
     (2) *Staphylococcus aureus*
     (3) *Staphylococcus epidermidis*
     (4) Streptococcus group D
     (5) *Streptococcus pneumoniae*
     (6) *Streptococcus viridans*
   B. Gram negative
     (1) Coliform bacillus, such as *E. coli*
     (2) *Enterobacter cloacae*
     (3) *Haemophilus influenzae*
     (4) *Haemophilus parainfluenzae*
     (5) *K. pneumoniae*
     (6) Meningococcus
     (7) Mima polymorpha—gram negative
     (8) *N. gonorrhoeae* and *N. catarrhalis*
     (9) *Neisseria* organisms
     (10) Pneumonococcus
     (11) *Proteus mirabilis*
     (12) *P. aeruginosa*
     (13) *Pseudomonas pyocyanea*
     (14) *S. marcescens*
4. Virus
   A. Herpes simplex
   B. *Streptococcus viridans*
   C. Coxsackie A
   D. TRIC virus
5. Other
   A. *Acinetobacter* species
   B. *Branhamella catarrhalis*
   C. *C. albicans*

* = most important

    D. *Citrobacter feundi*
    E. *Clostridium perfringes*
    F. Inclusion blennorrhea
    G. Listeriosis (*L. monocytogenes*)
    H. *Moraxella* species
    I. *Mycoplasma* organisms
    J. *Peptococcus prevotii*
    K. *Propionibacterium* species
    L. *Trichomonas vaginalis*

Cohen KL, McCarthy LR. Haemophilus influenzae ophthalmia neonatorum. *Arch Ophthalmol* 1980;98:1214.

Isenberg SJ. *The eye in infancy.* Chicago: Year Book Medical, 1989.

Rapoza PA, et al. Epidemiology of neonatal conjunctivitis. *Ophthalmology* 1986;94:461.

Stenson S, et al. Conjunctivitis in the newborn: observations on incidence, cause, and prophylaxis. *Ann Ophthalmol* 1981;13:329.

ACUTE FOLLICULAR CONJUNCTIVITIS LYMPHOID FOLLICLES (COBBLESTONING) OF CONJUNCTIVA WITH RAPID ONSET

*1. Inclusion conjunctivitis—adult inclusion conjunctivitis (AIC) (begins 2 days after exposure to organism, may be bilateral, no systemic symptoms, and a unilateral or bilateral preauricular node is often present.

*2. Adenovirus conjunctivitis—EKC has been reported worldwide from virus serotypes (the most common are 8, 11, and 19); pharyngoconjunctival fever (PCF) is usually caused by serotypes 3, 4, and 7.
    A. Pharyngoconjunctival fever—usually because of type adenovirus; common in swimming-pool epidemics in the summer and fall
    B. Epidemic keratoconjunctivitis because of adenovirus type (rarely occurs in children)

*3. Primary herpetic keratoconjunctivitis—conjunctival reaction may be follicular or pseudomembranous

4. Newcastle disease (fowlpox) conjunctivitis—usually seen in poultry handlers, veterinarians (caused by a paramyxovirus: single-stranded RNA virus that causes respiratory infections)

5. Influenza virus A

6. Herpes zoster

*7. Cat-scratch fever (Parinaud oculoglandular syndrome)—fever caused by two types of rickettsia: *Rochalimaea henselae* and *Afipia felis*)

8. Echovirus keratoconjunctivitis

9. Trachoma (sometimes)

10. Bacterial *Streptococcus, Moraxella,* and *Treponema* organisms

11. Mesantoin use

12. *Chlamydia epizootic* (feline pneumonitis)

13. Ophthalmomyiasis

14. Acute hemorrhagic conjunctivitis

15. Neonatal inclusion conjunctivitis

16. Unknown types—a case that resists etiologic classification is encountered occasionally; it is probable that other viruses occasionally produce acute follicular conjunctivitis

17. Associated with regional adenitis
    A. Angelucci syndrome (critical allergic conjunctivitis syndrome)

B. Anoxic overwear syndrome

C. Benjamin–Allen syndrome (brachial arch syndrome)

D. Floppy eyelid syndrome

*E. Giant papillary conjunctivitis syndrome

*F. Inclusion conjunctivitis in adults—acute mucopurulent follicular inflammation, persisting as long as several months, sometimes with scarring

G. Syndrome of Beal—transient unilateral disease, usually resolving in weeks

Allansmith MR. *The eye and immunology.* St. Louis: CV Mosby, 1982.

Kowalski RP, Harwick JC. Incidence of Moraxella conjunctival infection. *Am J Ophthalmol* 1986;101:437–440.

Roy FH. *Ocular syndromes and systemic diseases*, 3rd ed. Philadelphia: Lippincott Williams & Wilkins, 2002.

Uchio E, et al. Acute follicular conjunctivitis caused by adenovirus type 34. *Am J Ophthalmol* 1990;128:680–686.

CHRONIC FOLLICULAR CONJUNCTIVITIS (LYMPHOID FOLLICLES COBBLESTONING) OF CONJUNCTIVA WITH LONG-TERM COURSE)

1. Chronic follicular conjunctivitis—Axenfeld's type (orphan's) frequently found in institutionalized children; almost asymptomatic; long duration (to months or longer); no keratitis; cause unknown

*2. Chronic follicular conjunctivitis, toxic type

A. Bacterial origin, such as that due to a diplobacillus or other microorganism

B. Drugs, including the following:

acyclovir	DPE	neomycin
adenine arabinoside	echothiophate	neostigmine
amphotericin B	eserine	physostigmine
apraclonidine	F3T	pilocarpine
atropine	framycetin	scopolamine
carbachol	gentamicin	sulfacetamide
clonidine	homatropine	sulfamethizole
demecarium	hyaluronidase	sulfisoxazole
diatrizoate meglumine and	idoxuridine	trifluorothymidine
sodium	isoflurophate	trifluridine
diisopropyl fluorophosphate	ketorolac tromethamine	vidarabine
dipivefrin	methscopolamine	

3. Chronic follicular conjunctivitis with epithelial keratitis; differentiated from Axenfeld type by shorter duration (to months) and by epithelial keratitis involving upper third of cornea; epidemic in schools; can be transmitted by mascara pencil; cause unknown

4. Ectodermal syndrome (Rothmund syndrome)

5. Folliculosis—associated general lymphoid hypertrophy

*6. Molluscum contagiosum conjunctivitis

7. Neurocutaneous syndrome (ectodermal dysgenesis)

8. Parinaud syndrome—chronic fever and regional lymphadenopathy, frequently cat-scratch fever

*9. Postoperative penetrating keratoplasty or cataract surgery sutures

10. Sebaceous carcinoma with papillary conjunctivitis

11. Trachoma—stages to 3

12. Use of hard and soft contact lens

*14. Use of ocular prostheses

* = most important

15. With generalized lymphadenopathy

Cunningham ET, Koehler JE. Ocular bartonellosis. *Am J Ophthalmol* 2000;130:340–349.

Fedukowicz HB. *External infections of the eye: bacterial, viral, and mycotic*, 3rd ed. New York: Appleton-Century-Crofts, 1984.

Fraunfelder FT, Fraunfelder FW. *Drug-induced ocular side effects.* Woburn, MA: Butterworth-Heinemann, 2001.

Gloor P, et al. Sebaceous carcinoma presenting as a unilateral papillary conjunctivitis. *Am J Ophthalmol* 1999;124, 4:458–459.

Mondino BJ, et al. Allergic and toxic reactions in soft contact lens wearers. *Surv Ophthalmol* 1982;26:337.

Roy FH. *Ocular syndromes and systemic diseases*, 3rd ed. Philadelphia: Lippincott Williams & Wilkins, 2002.

CICATRICIAL CONJUNCTIVITIS (SCARRING OF CONJUNCTIVA)

*1. General: a postinfectious type of membranous conjunctivitis such as *C. diphtheriae*, streptococcal conjunctivitis, autoimmune or presumably autoimmune sarcoidosis, scleroderma, Stevens–Addison, pemphigoid, lichen planus, atopic blepharoconjunctivitis, miscellaneous causes and linear IgA dermatosis.

2. Upper lid
   A. Trachoma

3. Lower lid
   *A. Acne rosacea (ocular rosacea)
   B. Chemical (especially alkali)
   C. *Chlamydia* organisms (psittacosis–lymphogranuloma group)
   D. Chronic cicatricial conjunctivitis—occurs in the elderly; has a chronic course; may have concurrent skin and mucous membrane lesions
   *E. Congenital syphilis
   F. Dermatitis herpetiformis
   G. Epidemic keratoconjunctivitis
   H. Epidermolysis acuta toxica (Lyell syndrome)
   I. Epidermolysis bullosa
   *J. Erythema multiforme (Stevens–Johnson disease)
   K. Erythroderma ichthyosiforme
   L. Exfoliative dermatitis
   M. Fuchs–Lyell syndrome
   N. Hydroa vacciniforme
   O. Impetigo
   P. Lamellar ichthyoses
   *Q. Ocular pemphigoid
   R. Paraneoplastic lichen planus
   S. Radium burns
   T. Reiter syndrome (conjunctivourethrosynovial syndrome)
   U. Sjögren syndrome (secretoinhibitor syndrome)
   V. Staphylococcal granuloma
   W. Syphilis (acquired lues)
   X. Systemic scleroderma (progressive systemic sclerosis)
   Y. Vaccinia

*4. Drugs
   A. Demecarium bromide
   *B. Echothiophate iodide
   C. Idoxuridine

   D. Penicillamine
   E. Pilocarpine
   F. Practolol
   G. Thiabendazole
   H. Timolol
 *I. Topical ocular epinephrine

Chan LS, et al. Ocular cicatricial pemphigoid occurring as a sequela of Stevens-Johnson syndrome. *JAMA* 1991; 266:1543–1546.

Chiou AG, et al. Management of conjunctival cicatrizing diseases and severe ocular surface dysfunction. *Surv Ophthalmol* 1998;43:19–46.

Cruz AV, et al. Eyelid abnormalities in lamellar ichthyoses. *Ophthalmology* 2000;107:1895–1898.

Fraunfelder FT, Fraunfelder FW. *Drug-induced ocular side effects.* Woburn, MA: Butterworth-Heinemann, 2001.

Hahn JM, et al. Cicatrizing conjunctivitis associated with paraneoplastic lichen planus. *Am J Ophthalmol* 2000;129: 98–99.

Hoang-Xuan T, et al. Epidermolysis bullosa acquisita diagnosed by direct immunoelectron microscopy of the conjunctiva. *Ophthalmology* 1997;104:1414–1420.

Hoang-Xuan T, et al. Pure ocular cicatricial pemphigoid. *Ophthalmology* 1999;106:355–362.

ANGULAR CONJUNCTIVITIS (INFLAMMATION AT ANGLE OF EYE, USUALLY LATERAL)

  1. *C. albicans*
 *2. *M. lacunata* (Morax–Axenfeld diplobacillus)
  3. Stannus cerebellar syndrome (riboflavin deficiency)
  4. *S. aureus*

Fedukowicz HB. *External infections of the eye: bacterial, viral, and mycotic*, 3rd ed. New York: Appleton-Century-Crofts, 1984.

Scheie HG. *Textbook of ophthalmology*, 10th ed. Philadelphia: WB Saunders, 1986.

CONJUNCTIVAL DISORDERS ASSOCIATED WITH DERMATOLOGIC DISORDERS

 1. Dermatoses
   A. Acanthosis nigricans
   B. Acne rosacea
   C. Acrodermatitis chronica atrophicans
   D. Acrodermatitis enteropathica
 *E. Atopic eczema dermatitis
   F. Diffuse cutaneous mastocytosis
   G. Erythroderma exfoliativa (Wilson–Brocq disease)
   H. Ichthyosis
   I. Keratosis follicularis
   J. Keratosis follicularis spinulosa decalvans
   K. Lichen planus
   L. Pityriasis rubra pilaris; lichen acuminatus
   M. Porokeratosis
   N. Psoriasis vulgaris
   O. Seborrhea
   P. Xeroderma pigmentosum

* = most important

2. Mucocutaneous eruptions
   *A. Behçet disease (dermatostomatoophthalmic syndrome)
   B. Benign mucous membrane pemphigoid
   C. Dermatitis herpetiformis (Duhring–Brocq disease)
   *D. Erythema multiforme (Stevens–Johnson disease)
   E. Epidermolysis bullosa
   F. Hydroa vacciniforme (recurrent summer eruption)
   G. Pemphigus-vulgaris, vegetans, foliaceus
   H. Pyostomatitis vegetans
   I. Reiter disease (polyarthritis enterica)

Roy FH. *Ocular syndromes and systemic diseases*, 3rd ed. Philadelphia: Lippincott Williams & Wilkins, 2002.

Wilson LA. *External diseases of the eye*. New York: Harper & Row, 1979.

CONJUNCTIVAL DISORDERS ASSOCIATED WITH GENITAL DISORDERS

1. Bacteria
   A. *Bacteroides* species
   B. *Calymmatobacterium granulomatis* (granuloma inguinale)
   C. *E. coli*
   D. *Haemophilus ducreyi*
   E. *Haemophilus vaginalis*
   F. *Mimeae* species
   G. *Mycobacterium leprae*
   H. *M. tuberculosis*
   *I. *N. gonorrhoeae*
   J. *Proteus* species
   *K. *P. aeruginosa*
   L. *Staphylococcus* species
   M. *Streptococcus* species
2. Fungi
   A. *Candida* species
   B. Other
3. Viruses
   A. Cytomegalovirus
   *B. Herpes virus hominis 2
   *C. *Molluscum contagiosum* virus
   D. Rubella
   E. Varicella zoster
   F. Verruca virus
4. Spirochetes
   A. *T. pallidum*
5. *Chlamydiae*
   A. *Chlamydia lymphogranuloma*
   *B. *Chlamydia oculogenitalis*
   C. Unclassified *Chlamydia* from Reiter disease
6. Parasites
   A. Beetles
   B. Fly larvae
   C. Moths

D. *Phthirus pubis*
E. *T. vaginalis*

Roy FH. *Ocular syndromes and systemic diseases*, 3rd ed. Philadelphia: Lippincott Williams & Wilkins, 2002.
Vergnami RJ, Smith RS. Reiter syndrome in a child. *Arch Ophthalmol* 1974;91:165–166.

CONGESTION OF CONJUNCTIVA (NONINFECTIOUS HYPEREMIA OF THE CONJUNCTIVA)

*1. Acute lupus erythematosus (Kaposi–Libman–Sacks syndrome)
 2. Alcoholism
*3. Allergic conjunctivitis, such as contact with cosmetics or plastic
 4. Avitaminosis
 5. Carcinoid syndrome
*6. Carotid–cavernous fistula or arteriovenous aneurysm
 7. Cavernous sinus thrombosis (Foix syndrome)
 8. Conjunctivitis caused by air pollution (smog, dust, or smoke)
*9. Drugs causing conjunctival hyperemia, including the following:

acetohexamide
acetylcholine
acyclovir
adrenal cortex injection
adsorbed
alcohol
aldosterone
allobarbital
allopurinol
alprazolam
alseroxylon
alseroxylon
amithiozone
amobarbital compounds and
  pertussis vaccine
antazoline
apraclonidine
aprobarbital
aspirin
atropine
auranofin
aurothioglucose
aurothioglycanide
barbital
bischloroethylnitrosourea
  (BCNU)
beclomethasone
belladonna
bendroflumethiazide
benzalkonium
benzthiazide

betamethasone
brimonidine tartrate
bupivacaine
butalbital
butallylonal
butethal
carbachol
carmustine
cefaclor
cefadroxil
cefamandole
cefazolin
cefonicid
cefoperazone
ceforanide
cefotaxime
cefotetan
cefoxitin
cefsulodin
ceftazidime
ceftizoxime
ceftriaxone
cefuroxime
cephalexin
cephaloglycin
cephaloridine
cephalothin
cephapirin
cephradine
chloral hydrate
chloramphenicol

chlordiazepoxide
chloroform
chloroprocaine
chlorothiazide
chlorpropamide
chlortetracycline
chlorthalidone
chrysarobin
cimetidine
cisplatin
clindamycin
clindamycin
clofibrate
clonazepam
clorazepate
colchicine
colloidal silver
cortisone
cyclobarbital
cyclopentobarbital
cycloserine
cyclosporine
cyclothiazide
cytarabine
deferoxamine
deserpidine
desoxycorticosterone
dexamethasone
dextran
dextrothyroxine
diacetylmorphine

* = most important

diatrizoate meglumine and
  diazepam
dicumarol
diethylcarbamazine
diltiazem
dimercaprol
diphenadione
diphtheria and tetanus
  toxoids
disodium clodronate
disodium etidronate
disodium pamidronate
  emedastine
difumarate
disopyramide
doxorubicin
emetine
ephedrine
erythromycin
ether
ethotoin
ethyl biscoumacetate
etidocaine
F3T
fenoprofen
fludrocortisone
fluorescein
fluorometholone
fluprednisolone
flurazepam
flurbiprofen
gentamicin
glyburide
gold Au
gold sodium thiomalate
gold sodium thiosulfate
griseofulvin
halazepam
heparin
heptabarbital
hexethal
hexobarbital
homatropine
hydralazine
hydrochlorothiazide
hydrocortisone
hydroflumethiazide
ibuprofen
idoxuridine (IDU)

indapamide
indomethacin
interferon
iodide and iodine solutions
iothalamate meglumine and
  iothalamic acid
ketoprofen
levothyroxine
lidocaine
lincomycin
liothyronine
liotrix
lithium carbonate
lorazepam
maprotiline
measles and rubella virus
measles virus vaccine (live)
medrysone
meperidine
mephentermine
mephenytoin
mephobarbital
mepivacaine
meprednisone
mercuric oxide
metaraminol
methacholine
metharbital
methimazole
methitural
methocarbamol
methohexital
methoxamine
methoxsalen
methyclothiazide
methyldopa
methylprednisolone
methylthiouracil
metolazone
metoprolol
metronidazole
mianserin
midazolam
minoxidil
morphine
moxalactam
mumps virus vaccine (live)
naproxen
nifedipine

nitrazepam
nitromersol
norepinephrine
olopatadine HCl
paramethasone
phenoxybenzamine
opium
oxazepam
oxprenolol
oxyphenbutazone
oxyphenonium
pentazocine
pentobarbital
phenacetin
phenindione
phenobarbital
phenprocoumon
phenylbutazone
phenylephrine
phenylmercuric acetate
phenylmercuric nitrate
pilocarpine
piroxicam
piroxicam
polythiazide
practolol
prazepam
prazosin
prednisolone
prednisone
prilocaine
primidone
probarbital
procaine
propoxycaine
propranolol
propylthiouracil
quinethazone
radioactive iodides
ranitidine
rauwolfia serpentina
rescinnamine
reserpine
rifampin
rubella and mumps virus
rubella virus vaccine (live)
scopolamine
secobarbital
sildenafil citrate

silver nitrate
silver protein
sodium chloride
sodium salicylate
streptomycin
sulfacetamide
sulfachlorpyridazine
sulfacytine
sulfadiazine
sulfadimethoxine
sulfamerazine
sulfameter
sulfamethazine
sulfamethizole
sulfamethoxazole
sulfamethoxypyridazine
sulfanilamide

sulfaphenazole
sulfapyridine
sulfasalazine
sulfathiazole
sulfisoxazole
syrosingopine
talbutal
temazepam
tetanus immune globulin
tetanus toxoid
tetracycline
thiabendazole
thiacetazone
thiamylal
thimerosal
thiopental
thiotepa

thyroglobulin
thyroid
tolazamide
tolazoline
tolbutamide
triamcinolone
triazolam
trichlormethiazide
trichloroethylene
trifluridine
trioxsalen vaccine (live)
vancomycin
verapamil
vidarabine
vinbarbital
vitamin A

10. Gout (hyperuricemia)
11. Hormone deficiency (estrogenic)
12. Hypothyroidism
13. Irritative follicular conjunctivitis (see p. 193)
    *A. Chemical conjunctivitis because of drugs, including the following:

acenocoumarol
acetaminophen
acetanilid
acetohexamide
allobarbital
allopurinol
alprazolam
amobarbital
anisindione
antazoline
antipyrine
aprobarbital
aspirin
barbital
bendroflumethiazide
benzalkonium
benzthiazide
butabarbital
butalbital
butallylonal
butethal
carbamazepine
carbimazole
cefaclor
cefadroxil
cefamandole

cefazolin
cefonicid
cefoperazone
ceforanide
cefotaxime
cefotetan
cefoxitin
cefsulodin
ceftazidime
ceftizoxime
ceftriaxone
cefuroxime
cephalexin
cephaloglycin
cephaloridine
cephalothin
cephapirin
cephradine
chloramphenicol
chlordiazepoxide
chlorothiazide
chlorpropamide
chlortetracycline
chlorthalidone
chrysarobin
cimetidine

cisplatin
clofibrate
clonazepam
clorazepate
colloidal silver
cyclobarbital
cyclopentobarbital
cycloserine
cyclosporine
cyclothiazide
cytarabine
dextran
diazepam
dicumarol
diethylcarbamazine
diltiazem
dimercaprol
diphenadione
diphtheria and tetanus
    toxoids and pertussis
    vaccine
disopyramide
doxorubicin
emetine
ephedrine
ethotoin

* = most important

ethyl biscoumacetate
fenoprofen
flurazepam
flurbiprofen
halazepam
heparin
heptabarbital
hexethal
hexobarbital
hydralazine
hydrochlorothiazide
hydroflumethiazide
ibuprofen
indapamide
indomethacin
interferon
iodide and iodine solutions
   and compounds
iothalamate
meglumine and sodium
   iothalamic acid
ketoprofen
lithium carbonate
lorazepam
maprotiline
measles and rubella virus
   vaccine (live)
measles virus vaccine (live)
meperidine
mephenytoin
mephobarbital
metharbital
methimazole
methitural
methocarbamol
methohexital
methyclothiazide
methyldopa
methylthiouracil

metolazone
metronidazole
mianserin
midazolam
minoxidil
morphine
moxalactam
mumps virus vaccine (live)
naproxen
nifedipine
nitrazepam
opium
oxazepam
oxprenolol
oxyphenbutazone
oxyphenonium
pentazocine
pentobarbital
phenacetin
phenindione
phenobarbital
phenprocoumon
phenylbutazone
phenylephrine
piroxicam
polythiazide
practolol
prazepam
prazosin
primidone
probarbital
propranolol
propylthiouracil
quinethazone
radioactive iodides
ranitidine
rubella and mumps virus
   vaccine (live)
rubella virus vaccine (live)

secobarbital
silver nitrate
silver protein
sodium salicylate
streptomycin
sulfacetamide
sulfachlorpyridazine
sulfacytine
sulfadiazine
sulfadimethoxine
sulfamerazine
sulfameter
sulfamethazine
sulfamethizole
sulfamethoxazole
sulfamethoxypyridazine
sulfanilamide
sulfaphenazole
sulfapyridine
sulfasalazine
sulfathiazole
sulfisoxazole
talbutal
temazepam
tetanus immune globulin
tetanus toxoid
tetracycline
thiamylal
thiopental
thiotepa
tolazamide
tolbutamide
triazolam trichlormethiazide
trichloroethylene
verapamil
vinbarbital
vitamin A
warfarin

   B. Topical drugs that are hypotonic, hypertonic, or in which the pH is above or below
      6.9 or a drug degradation causing chemical irritation
   C. Toxic conjunctivitis because of drugs such as miotics or cycloplegics
   D. Vegetable irritants (e.g., caster bean)
*14. Malignant lymphoma
 15. Ophthalmic vein thrombosis
 16. Photosensitive conjunctivitis
*17. Polycythemia vera (Vaquez disease)
 18. Sjögren syndrome (secretoinhibitor syndrome)

19. Vascular changes
   A. Facial paralysis (see p. 66–68)
   *B. Hereditary hemorrhagic telangiectasis (Rendu–Osler–Weber disease)
   C. Petechial hemorrhage of conjunctiva (see p. 206)

Collins JF. *Handbook of clinical ophthalmology.* New York: Masson, 1982.

Fraunfelder FT, Fraunfelder FW. *Drug-induced ocular side effects.* Woburn, MA: Butterworth-Heinemann, 2001.

CILIARY FLUSH

Ciliary flush involves circumcorneal congestion and congestion of ciliary vessels immediately surrounding the cornea; individual vessels are not seen; color is violaceous; redness fades toward the fornices; and vessels do not move with conjunctiva.

1. Corneal disease, such as with inflammations and erosions
2. Glaucoma, especially acute glaucoma
3. Iridocyclitis
4. Iris irritation, such as with corneal foreign bodies
5. Iritis

Vaughan D, et al. *General ophthalmology,* 14th ed. Los Altos, CA: Lange Medical, 1995.

CONJUNCTIVAL ANEURYSMS, VARICOSITIES, TORTUOUSITIES, AND TELANGIECTASIS

1. Local causes
   *A. Acne rosacea
   B. Chronic congestive glaucoma
   C. Delayed mustard gas keratitis
   D. Idiopathic anomaly
   E. Irradiation of the eye
   F. Long-standing ocular inflammation
   *G. Metastatic primary tumor
   *H. Pterygium
   *I. Underlying choroidal or ciliary body melanomas
2. Systemic causes
   A. Acquired immunodeficiency syndrome (AIDS)
   B. Arteriosclerosis
   C. Associated with familial amyloidotic polyneuropathy, type 1
   D. Ataxic telangiectasia (Louis–Bar syndrome)
   *E. Degos syndrome (malignant atrophic papulosis)
   F. Diabetes
   G. Dysproteinemia as in Waldenström macroglobulinemia, cryoglobulinemia, and multiple myeloma
   H. Endangiitis obliterans
   I. Fabry disease (diffuse angiokeratosis)
   J. Hereditary hemorrhagic telangiectasia (Rendu–Osler–Weber disease)
   K. Hypertension
   L. Klippel–Trenaunay–Weber syndrome (angioosteohypertrophy syndrome)
   M. Normal individuals
   *N. Pulmonary insufficiency

* = most important

O. Reimann syndrome (hyperviscosity syndrome)
P. Renal failure
Q. Rheumatic fever or rheumatic heart disease
R. Scleroderma (progressive systemic sclerosis)
S. Sturge–Weber syndrome (meningocutaneous syndrome)
*T. Syphilis (acquired lues)
U. Varicose veins—generalized

Ando E, et al. Ocular microangiopathy in familial amyloidotic polyneuropathy, type 1. *Graefes Arch Clin Exp Ophthalmol* 1992;230:1–5.

Baumann S, et al. Conjunctival microvasculopathy and Kaposi's sarcoma in patients with AIDS. *AIDS* 1994;8:134–135.

Roy FH. *Ocular syndromes and systemic diseases*, 3rd ed. Philadelphia: Lippincott Williams & Wilkins, 2002.

CONJUNCTIVAL SLUDGING AND SEGMENTATION

1. Local
   A. Aging
   B. Hypothermia
   C. Sympathetic irritation
   D. Vasodilator drugs that are applied locally
2. Systemic or hyperviscosity with increase in serum proteins
   A. Cryoglobulinemia
   B. Hyperglobulinemia
   C. Hypertension
   D. Macroglobulinemia (Waldenström syndrome)
   *E. Multiple myeloma (Kahler disease)
   *F. Sickle cell disease (Herrick syndrome)

Lu LM, et al. Sjögren's syndrome and benign hyperglobulinemic purpura of Waldenstrom. *Ann Ophthalmol* 1981;13:1285–1287.

Maisel JM, et al. Multiple myeloma presenting with ocular inflammation. *Ann Ophthalmol* 1987;19:170–174.

Roy FH. *Ocular syndromes and systemic diseases*, 3rd ed. Philadelphia: Lippincott Williams & Wilkins, 2002.

CONJUNCTIVAL EDEMA (CHEMOSIS)

1. Acquired blockage of orbital lymphatics following orbital surgery (lateral orbitotomy) or because of erysipelas or lymphogranuloma venereum
*2. Chronic hereditary lymphedema (Nonne–Milroy–Meige disease)
*3. Drugs, including the following:

acetohexamide	aminosalicylate	antipyrine
acetophenazine	aminosalicylic acid	aprobarbital
acetyldigitoxin	amobarbital	aspirin
actinomycin C	amodiaquine	auranofin
adrenal cortex injection	amphotericin B	aurothioglucose
albuterol	antimony lithium thiomalate	aurothioglycanide
aldosterone	antimony potassium tartrate	barbital
allobarbital	antimony sodium tartrate	benoxinate
amantadine	antimony sodium	benzathine penicillin G
aminopterin	thioglycollate	betamethasone

* = most important

benzalkonium
bleomycin
brinzolamide
bupivacaine
butabarbital
butacaine
butalbital
butallylonal
butaperazine
butethal
cactinomycin
captopril
carbachol
carbamazepine
carbenicillin
carphenazine
cefaclor
cefadroxil
cefamandole
cefazolin
cefonicid
cefoperazone
ceforanide
cefotaxime
cefotetan
cefoxitin
cefsulodin
ceftazidime
ceftizoxime
ceftriaxone
cefuroxime
cephalexin
cephaloglycin
cephaloridine
cephalothin
cephapirin
cephradine
chloral hydrate
chlorambucil
chloramphenicol
chlorhexidine
chlorisondamine
chloroprocaine
chloroquine
chlorpromazine
chlorpropamide
chlortetracycline
chrysarobin
cisplatin

clofibrate
clomipramine
cloxacillin
cocaine
colistin
colloidal silver
cortisone
cyclobarbital
cyclopentobarbital
cyproheptadine
dactinomycin
danazol
dapsone
daunorubicin
demecarium
demeclocycline
desipramine
deslanoside
desoxycorticosterone
dexamethasone
dextrothyroxine
diacetylmorphine
diatrizoate meglumine and
    sodium
dibucaine
dicloxacillin
diethazine
diethylcarbamazine
digitoxin
dionin
dorzolamide
doxepin
doxorubicin
doxycycline
dromostanolone
dyclonine
echothiophate
emetine
enalapril
epinephrine
ergonovine
ergotamine
erythromycin
ethopropazine
etidocaine
etretinate
F3T
floxuridine
fludrocortisone

fluorouracil
fluoxymesterone
fluphenazine
fluprednisolone
gitalin
glyburide
gold Au 198
gold sodium thiomalate
griseofulvin
heptabarbital
hetacillin
hexachlorophene
hexamethonium
hexethal
hexobarbital
hydrabamine penicillin
hydralazine
hydrocortisone
hydroxychloroquine
ibuprofen
idoxuridine
IDU
imipramine
iodide and iodine solutions
    and compounds
iron dextran
isoflurophate
isosorbide
isotretinoin
ketoprofen
lanatoside C
levodopa
levothyroxine
lidocaine
lithium carbonate
mannitol
maprotiline
mecamylamine
medrysone
melphalan
mephobarbital
mepivacaine
meprednisone
mercuric oxide
mesoridazine
metharbital
methdilazine
methitural
methohexital

methotrimeprazine
methyldopa
methylergonovine
methylpentynol
methylprednisolone
methysergide
metoclopramide
metrizamide
metronidazole
mianserin
mild silver protein
minocycline
mitomycin
moxalactam
nafcillin
naproxen
neomycin
nitromersol
nortriptyline
oral contraceptives
ouabain
oxacillin
oxprenolol
oxyphenbutazone
oxytetracycline
paramethasone
pentobarbital
pentolinium
perazine
pericyazine
perphenazine
phenacaine
phenazine
phenobarbital
phenylbutazone

phenylephrine
pilocarpine
piperacetazine
piperazine
piperocaine
pipobroman
poliovirus vaccine
polynoxylin B
potassium penicillin G
potassium penicillin V
potassium phenethicillin
practolol
prazosin
prednisolone
prednisone
prilocaine
primidone
probarbital
procaine
procaine penicillin G
prochlorperazine
promazine
promethazine
propiomazine
propoxycaine
protriptyline
quinacrine
radioactive iodides
rifampin
rubella virus vaccine (live)
sanguinarine
secobarbital
silicone
silver nitrate
silver protein

sodium antimonylgluconate
sodium salicylate
stibocaptate
stibophen
streptomycin
succinylcholine
sulindac
suramin
talbutal
testolactone
testosterone
tetracaine
tetracycline
tetraethylammonium
thiamylal
thiethylperazine
thimerosal
thiopental
thiopropazate
thioproperazine
thioridazine
thiotepa
thyroid
tolazamide
tolbutamide
triamcinolone
trifluoperazine
triflupromazine
trimeprazine
trimethaphan
trimethidinium
urokinase
vidarabine
vinbarbital
vinblastine

   4. Glandular fever
   5. Hypersensitivity—local topical allergies
 *6. Increased bulk of orbital contents—orbital tumors, cysts, or endocrine exophthalmos
   7. Local inflammatory conditions
      *A. Cerebral cavity—acute meningitis
      *B. Eye—viral conjunctivitis, corneal ulcer, fulminating iritis, or panophthalmitis
       C. Lacrimal passages—dacryocystitis
       D. Lids—styes, vaccinia, acute meibomitis, insect bites, or vaccinal pocks
       E. Nasal cavity—sinusitis
      *F. Orbit—cellulitis, periostitis, dacryoadenitis, tenonitis
   8. Myxedema—infiltration with mucopolysaccharides
   9. Reduced plasma protein level—nephrotic state
  10. Systemic lupus erythematosus

*11. Vasomotor instability—angioneurotic edema or premenstrual phase of water retention
  12. Venous congestion—local obstruction of orbital apex, carotid–cavernous fistula, thrombosis of cavernous sinus, or right-sided heart failure
  13. Whipple disease

Disdier P, et al. Chemosis associated with Whipple's disease. *Am J Ophthalmol* 1991;112:217–219.

Fraunfelder FT, Fraunfelder FW. *Drug-induced ocular side effects.* Woburn, MA: Butterworth-Heinemann, 2001.

Leahey AB, et al. Chemosis as a presenting sign of systemic lupus erythematosus. *Arch Ophthalmol* 1992;110: 609–610.

CONJUNCTIVAL XEROSIS (DRYNESS OF CONJUNCTIVA)

  1. Absence of blinking
  2. Drugs, including the following:

acebutolol (?)
amiodarone
atenolol (?)
betaxolol
busulfan
chlorambucil
clonidine (?)
cyclophosphamide
doxepin
ibuprofen

ketoprofen
labetalol (?)
levobunolol
methyldopa
metoprolol (?)
nadolol (?)
naproxen (?)
oxprenolol (?)
perhexiline
pindolol (?)

practolol
primidone
propoxyphene
propanolol (?)
quinidine
sulindac
thiabendazole
timolol
vinblastine (?)

  3. Following cicatricial conjunctivitis (see p. 194)
  4. Illness or coma
 *5. Lack of closure of lids in sleep
  6. Result of exposure of conjunctiva to air
     A. Deficient closure of lids, such as with paralysis of orbicularis, as part of facial palsy, spasms of the levator, or ectropion
     B. Excessive proptosis, such as in exophthalmic goiter or orbital tumor
 *7. Vitamin A deficiency
     A. Dietary deficiencies, including malnutrition, cystic fibrosis, anorexia nervosa, and bulimia
     B. Digestive tract disorders
        (1) Colitis and enteritis
       *(2) In pancreas—chronic pancreatitis
        (3) In stomach—achlorhydria, chronic gastritis or diarrhea, peptic ulcer
     C. Hookworm disease
    *D. Liver disease, such as chronic cirrhosis
     E. Malaria
     F. Pregnancy
     G. Pulmonary tuberculosis
     H. Skin disorders, such as pityriasis rubra pilaris
    *I. Thyroid gland disorder, such as hyperthyroidism
     J. Uyemura syndrome (fundus albipunctatus with hemeralopia and xerosis)
  8. Decrease tear production
     A. Congenital alacrima

* = most important

B. Keratoconjunctivitis sicca
C. Riley-Day syndrome (familial dysautonomia)
D. Sjögren syndrome
E. Surgical excision of the lacrimal and accessory lacrimal glands
F. X-irradiation of the lacrimal gland
9. Following x-irradiation of the conjunctiva

Fraunfelder FT, Fraunfelder FW. *Drug-induced ocular side effects.* Woburn, MA: Butterworth-Heinemann, 2001.

Gilbert JM, et al. Ocular manifestations and impression cytology of anorexia nervosa. *Ophthalmology* 1990;97: 1001.

Newell FW. *Ophthalmology: principles and concepts,* 7th ed. St. Louis: CV Mosby, 1991.

Roy FH. *Ocular syndromes and systemic diseases,* 3rd ed. Philadelphia: Lippincott Williams & Wilkins, 2002.

BITOT SPOTS

Bitot spots are small gray or white, sharply outlined areas, cheeselike or foamy, occurring on either side of the limbus but especially in the temporal area.
1. Associated with coloboma of lid
2. Associated with corectopia, nystagmus, and absent foveal reflexes
3. Associated with Rieger anomaly
4. Congenital anomaly
5. Corneal snowflake dystrophy
6. Exposure
7. Idiopathic
*8. Keratosis follicularis (Darier–White disease) associated with retinitis pigmentosa
9. Pellagra or other poor nutritional states
10. Vitamin A deficiency

Daicker B. Ocular involvement in keratosis follicularis associated with retinitis pigmentosa. *Ophthalmologica* 1995; 209:47–51.

de Keizer RJ. Conjunctival xerosis, arcus lipoides, and Rieger's disease. *Doc Ophthalmol* 1991;78:365–371.

SUBCONJUNCTIVAL HEMORRHAGE (BLOOD UNDER CONJUNCTIVA)

1. Acute febrile systemic infections
    A. Bacteria, such as those responsible for meningococcal septicemia, subacute bacterial endocarditis, scarlet fever, diphtheria, typhoid fever, or cholera
    B. Parasites, such as plasmodia (malaria)
    C. Rickettsia, such as those causing typhus fever
    D. Unknown infective agents, such as those causing glandular fever
    E. Viruses, such as those responsible for influenza, smallpox, measles, yellow fever, sandfly fever, or Kaposi sarcoma
2. Associated with use of drugs, including the following:

acetylcholine
acid bismuth sodium tartrate
adrenal cortex injection
aldosterone
allopurinol
alseroxylon

aspirin
benoxinate
betamethasone
bismuth carbonate
bismuth oxychloride
bismuth salicylate

bismuth sodium tartrate
bismuth sodium
  thioglycollate
bismuth sodium
  triglycollamate
bismuth subcarbonate

bismuth subsalicylate
bupivacaine
butacaine
chloroprocaine
cobalt (?)
cocaine
combination products of
    estrogens and
    progestogens etidocaine
cortisone
deserpidine
desoxycorticosterone
dexamethasone
dibucaine
dyclonine
epinephrine
ethambutol
fludrocortisone
fluorometholone
fluorouracil
fluprednisolone
glycerin
heparin
hexachlorophene
hydrocortisone
indomethacin (?)
iodide and iodine solutions
    and compounds (?)
isosorbide
ketoprofen

leuprolide acetate
lincomycin
mannitol
medroxyprogesterone
medrysone
mepivacaine
meprednisone
methaqualone
methylphenidate
methylprednisolone
mithramycin
mitotane
oxyphenbutazone
paramethasone
penicillamine
phenacaine
phenytoin
phenylbutazone
piperocaine
plicamycin
pralidoxime
prednisolone
prednisone
prilocaine
procaine
proparacaine
propoxycaine
radioactive iodides (?)
rauwolfia serpentina
rescinnamine

reserpine
sodium chloride
sodium salicylate
sulfacetamide
sulfachlorpyridazine
sulfacytine
sulfadiazine
sulfadimethoxine
sulfamerazine
sulfameter
sulfamethazine
sulfamethizole
sulfamethoxazole
sulfamethoxypyridazine
sulfanilamide
sulfaphenazole
sulfapyridine
sulfasalazine
sulfathiazole
sulfisoxazole
sulindac
syrosingopine
tamoxifen
tetracaine
triamcinolone
trichloroethylene
urea
urokinase (?)
vitamin A

3. Blood dyscrasias
    A. Associated with thrombocytopenia
        *(1) Anemias, especially, aplastic anemia
        *(2) Drugs, including the following:

absorbed acebutolol
acebutolol
acenocoumarin
acenocoumarol
acetaminophen
acetanilid
acetazolamide
acetohexamide
acetophenazine
actinomycin C
acyclovir
allobarbital
allopurinol
alprazolam

aminopterin
aminosalicylic acid (?)
amithiozone
amitriptyline
amobarbital
amodiaquine
amphotericin B
ampicillin
anisindione
antimony lithium thiomalate
antimony potassium tartrate
antimony sodium
    thioglycollate
antipyrine

aprobarbital
atenolol
auranofin
aurothioglucose
aurothioglycanide
azatadine
azathioprine
barbital
bacillus Calmette Guérin
    (BCG) vaccine
BCNU
bendroflumethiazide
benzathine penicillin G
benzthiazide

* = most important

bishydroxycoumarin
bleomycin
brompheniramine
busulfan
butabarbital
butalbital
butallylonal
butaperazine
butethal
cactinomycin
calcifediol
calcitriol
captopril
carbamazepine
carbenicillin
carbimazole
carbinoxamine
carisoprodol
carmustine
carphenazine
chloroethyl-cyclohexyl-
    nitrosourea (CCNU)
cefaclor
cefadroxil
cefamandole
cefazolin
cefonicid
cefoperazone
ceforanide
cefotaxime
cefotetan
cefoxitin
cefsulodin
ceftizoxime
ceftriaxone
cefuroxime
cephalexin
cephaloglycin
cephaloridine
cephalothin
cephapirin
cephradine
chlorambucil
chloramphenicol
chlordiazepoxide
chloroquine
chlorothiazide
chlorpheniramine

chlorpromazine
chlorpropamide
chlorprothixene
chlortetracycline
chlorthalidone
cholecalciferol
cimetidine
cisplatin
clemastine
clindamycin
clofibrate
clonazepam
clorazepate
cloxacillin
colchicine
cyclobarbital
cyclopentobarbital
cyclophosphamide
cycloserine
cyclothiazide
cyproheptadine
cytarabine
dacarbazine
dactinomycin
dapsone
daunorubicin
deferoxamine
demeclocycline
desipramine
dexbrompheniramine
dexchlorpheniramine
diazepam
diazoxide
dimethyl imidazole
    carboxamide (DIC)
dichlorphenamide
dicloxacillin
dicumarol
diethazine
dihydrotachysterol
diltiazem
dimercaprol
dimethyl sulfoxide
diphtheria and tetanus
    toxoids and pertussis
    vaccine
dimethindene
diphenadione

diphenhydramine
diphenylhydantoin
diphenylpyraline
divalproex sodium
dimethyl sulfoxide (DMSO)
doxorubicin
doxycycline
doxylamine
dromostanolone
droperidol
enalapril
ergocalciferol
erythromycin
ethacrynic acid
ethopropazine
ethosuximide
ethotoin
ethoxzolamide
ethyl biscoumacetate
fenfluramine
fenoprofen
flecainide
floxuridine
fluorouracil
fluoxymesterone
fluphenazine
flurazepam
furosemide
ganciclovir
gentamicin
glutethimide
glyburide
gold Au 198
gold sodium thiomalate
gold sodium thiosulfate
    halazepam
griseofulvin
guanethidine
haloperidol
heparin
heptabarbital
hetacillin
hexethal
hexobarbital
hydracarbazine
hydralazine
hydrochlorothiazide
hydroflumethiazide

hydroxychloroquine
hydroxyurea
hydralazine
ibuprofen
imipramine
indapamide
indomethacin
interferon alpha, beta, or gamma
iopamidol
isocarboxazid
isoniazid
ketoprofen
labetalol
levodopa
lincomycin
lithium carbonate
lomustine
lorazepam
loxapine
maprotiline
measles virus vaccine
mechlorethamine
mefenamic acid
melphalan
mephenytoin
mephobarbital
meprobamate
mercaptopurine
mesoridazine
metolazone
methacycline
methaqualone
metharbital
methazolamide
methdilazine
methicillin
methimazole
methitural
methohexital
methotrexate
methotrimeprazine
methsuximide
methyclothiazide
methyldopa
methylene blue
methylphenidate
methylthiouracil

methyprylon
metrizamide
metronidazole
mexiletine
mianserin
minocycline
mitomycin
moxalactam
mumps virus vaccine (live)
nadolol
nafcillin
nalidixic acid
naproxen
nialamide
nifedipine
nitrazepam
nitrofurantoin
nitroglycerin
nortriptyline
oral contraceptives
orphenadrine
oxacillin
oxazepam
oxyphenbutazone
oxytetracycline
paramethadione
penicillamine
penicillin
pentobarbital
perazine
pericyazine
perphenazine
phenacetin
phenelzine
phenformin
phenindione
pheniramine
phenobarbital
phenoxymethyl
phenoxymethylpenicillin
phenprocoumon
phensuximide
phenylbutazone
phenytoin
pindolol
piperacetazine
piperazine
pipobroman

polio virus vaccine
polythiazide
potassium penicillin G
potassium penicillin V
potassium phenethicillin
potassium phenoxymethyl
prazepam
primidone
probarbital
procaine penicillin G
procarbazine
prochlorperazine
promazine
promethazine
propiomazine
propylthiouracil
protriptyline
pyrimethamine
quinacrine
quinethazone
quinidine
quinine
ranitidine
rifampin
rubella and mumps virus vaccine (live)
secobarbital
semustine
sodium antimonylgluconate
stibocaptate
stibophen
streptomycin
streptozocin
suramin
temazepam
sulfonamides
talbutal
testolactone
testosterone
tetracycline
thiabendazole
thiamylal
thiethylperazine
thioguanine
thiopental
thiopropazate
thioproperazine
thioridazine

thiotepa	trifluoperazine	vancomycin
thiothixene	trifluperidol	verapamil
tocainide	triflupromazine	vidarabine
tolazoline	trimeprazine	vinbarbital
tranylcypromine	trimethadione	vinblastine
trazodone	tripelennamine	vincristine
triazolam	triprolidine	vitamin A
tolazamide	uracil mustard	vitamin D
tolbutamide	urethan	vitamin D_2
trichlormethiazide	valproate sodium	vitamin D_3
triethylenemelamine	valproic acid	warfarin

*(3) Leukemia
 (4) Septicemias
 (5) Splenic disorders, such as Banti or Gaucher disease, Felty syndrome, and hemolytic icterus
*(6) Systemic lupus erythematosus (Kaposi–Libman–Sacks syndrome)
  B. Ehlers–Danlos syndrome (fibrodysplasia elastica generalisata)
  C. Hemochromatosis
  D. Schomberg disease
  E. Scurvy (avitaminosis C)
  F. Secondary, such as that because of nephritic, cardiac, or hepatic disease
  G. Thrombocytopenia purpura
4. Fragility of vessel walls because of systemic vascular disease
  A. Age
  B. Arteriosclerosis
  C. Diabetes
  D. Hypertension
  E. Nephritis
5. Gravity inversion
6. Injury to orbital or adjacent structures, such as sinus, basal skull fracture, subarachnoid hemorrhage
7. Local acute inflammation, including, acute pneumococcal conjunctivitis, leptospirosis ictero-hemorrhagica, epidemic typhus, and scrub typhus
8. Local trauma, including surgical trauma
9. Remote injury associated with fractured bones and fat emboli following angiography or open heart operation causing "splinter" subconjunctival hemorrhage
10. Spontaneous during menstruation
11. Spontaneous rupture of telangiectasis, varicosities, aneurysm, or angiomatous tumor (see p. 201)
*12. Sudden severe venous congestion of head, including that because of coughing, vomiting, epileptic fit, strangulation, or an orbital tumor (neuroblastoma)
13. Without apparent cause—most common

Fraunfelder FT, Fraunfelder FW. *Drug-induced ocular side effects.* Woburn, MA: Butterworth-Heinemann, 2001.

Friberg TR, Weinreb RN. Ocular manifestations of gravity inversion. *JAMA* 1985;253.

Tasman W, Jaeger E, eds. *Duane's clinical ophthalmology.* Philadelphia: JB Lippincott, 1990.

Werblin TP, Peiffer RL. Persistent hemorrhage after extracapsular surgery associated with excessive aspirin ingestion. *Am J Ophthalmol* 1987;104:426.

TUMORS OF THE CONJUNCTIVA

1. Epithelial tumors
    A. Keratoacanthoma
    B. Dyskeratosis
        (1) Epithelial plaques—leukoplakia, hereditary benign intraepithelial dyskeratosis
        (2) Intraepithelial epithelioma (Bowen disease) (61N)
    C. Metastatic uveal melanoma
    *D. Papilloma—including virus types 11, 16, and 18
    E. Epithelioma
    F. Adenoma
        (1) Papillary cystadenoma lymphomatosum (Warthin tumor)
        (2) Oncocytoma (oxyphil-cell adenoma)
        (3) Pleomorphic adenoma of Krause glands
2. Mesoblastic tumors
    A. Inflammatory hyperplasias
        (1) Granuloma
        (2) Plasmoma
    B. Connective tissue tumors
        (1) Fibroma
        (2) Lipoma
        (3) Myxoma
3. The reticuloses
    *A. Lymphoma
    B. Lymphosarcoma
    *C. Mycosis fungoides
4. Vascular tumors—angiomas
    A. Polymorphous hemangioma, telangiectatic granuloma, granuloma pyogenicum
    B. Lymphangioma
    C. Angiosarcoma monomorphous angioma, Kaposi (hemorrhagic) sarcoma
5. Pigmented tumors
    *A. Nevus
    B. Malignant melanoma
    C. Intraepithelial melanoma–precancerous melanosis
6. Peripheral nerve tumors
    A. Neurofibroma
        *(1) Neurilemmoma (neurinoma, schwannoma)
        (2) Malignant schwannoma (neurogenic sarcoma; neurofibrosarcoma)
        (3) Plexiform neurofibromatosis
    B. Tuberous sclerosis (Bourneville disease)
    *C. Intrascleral nerve loops
7. Amyloidosis
8. Metastatic renal cell carcinoma
9. Trematode-induced granulomas
10. Hypertrophic discoid lupus erythematosus

Crawford JB, et al. Combined nevi of the conjunctiva. *Arch Ophthalmol* 1999;117:1121–1127.

Grossniklaus HE, et al. Hemangiopericytoma of the conjunctiva. *Ophthalmology* 1986;93:265–267.

Jay V, Font RL. Conjunctival amelanotic malignant melanoma arising in primary acquired melanosis sine pigmento. *Ophthalmology* 1998;105:191–194.

* = most important

Marsh WM, et al. Localized conjunctival with amyloidosis associated with extranodal lymphoma. *Ophthalmology* 1987;94:61–64.

Odrich MG, et al. A spectrum of bilateral squamous conjunctival tumors associated with the human papillomavirus type 16. *Ophthalmology* 1991;98:628–635.

Peter J, Hidayat AA. Myxomas of the conjunctiva. *Am J Ophthalmol* 1986;102:80–86.

Rathinam S, et al. An outbreak of trematode-induced granulomas of the conjunctiva. *Ophthalmology* 2001;108: 1223–1229.

Sagerman RH, Abramson DH. *Tumors of the eye and ocular adnexae.* New York: Pergamon Press, 1982.

Uy HS, et al. Hypertrophic discoid lupus erythematosus of the conjunctiva. *Am J Ophthalmol* 1999;127:604–605.

Ware GT, et al. Renal cell carcinoma with involvement of iris and conjunctiva. *Am J Ophthalmol* 1999;127,4: 458–459.

Winward KE, Curtin VT. Conjunctival squamous cell carcinoma in a patient with human immunodeficiency virus infection. *Am J Ophthalmol* 1989:554–556.

CONJUNCTIVAL CYSTS

1. Congenital corneoscleral cyst (rare)
2. Epibulbar dermoids with cystic form
*3. Epithelial cyst
   A. Apposition of folds of conjunctival mucosa (common)
   *B. Downgrowth of epithelium—chronic inflammatory conditions, such as that following inflammation of pterygium
   C. Glandular retention—involvement of Krause glands in chronic inflammatory conditions, including trachoma and pemphigus
   D. Pigmented cyst appearing after prolonged topical use of cocaine or epinephrine
4. Limbal wounds with iris prolapse
5. Lymphatic cyst
*6. Muscle inclusion cyst/complication of strabismus surgery
7. Parasitic cyst such as filarial cyst
8. Traumatic cyst (epithelial implantation)

Cibis GW, Waeltermann JM. Muscle inclusion cyst as a complication of strabismus surgery. *Am J Ophthalmol* 1985;100:740–741.

Jahnle RL, et al. Conjunctival inclusion cyst simulating malignant melanoma. *Am J Ophthalmol* 1985;100:483–484.

Soong HK, et al. Corneal astigmatism from conjunctival cysts. *Am J Ophthalmol* 1982;93:118.

LIMBAL MASS

1. Allergic reaction
   *A. Phlyctenules
   B. Vernal limbal lesions
2. Amyloid—perilimbal
3. Associated with skin disease
   *A. Acne rosacea (ocular rosacea)
   B. Hereditary benign intraepithelial dyskeratosis
   *C. Hodgkin disease
   D. Limbal squamous carcinoma in xeroderma pigmentosa
   E. Pityriasis rubra pilaris
   F. Psoriasis (psoriasis vulgaris)
   *G. Reticulum cell sarcoma—raised, pink, smooth lesions
4. Benign nodular fascitis

*5. Dermoids
6. Ectopic lacrimal gland tissue
7. Epithelial hyperplasia
8. Fibrous histiocytoma
9. Fibroxanthoma
10. Granular cell tumor
11. Granulomas
12. Hemangioma
13. Intraepithelial epitheliomas (Bowen disease)
14. Lymphomas
15. Malignant melanomas
16. Mononucleosis (infectious)
*17. Nevi
18. Papillomas
19. Pterygia
20. Sarcomas
21. Salmon patch associated with relapsing polychondritis
22. Squamous cell carcinoma
23. Subconjunctival nodules associated with Crohn disease
24. Synthetic fiber granuloma

Charles NC, et al. Epibulbar granular cell tumor. *Ophthalmology* 1997;104:1454–1456.

Engelbrecht NE, et al. Combined intraepithelial squamous neoplasia and atypical fibroxanthoma of the cornea and limbus. *Am J Ophthalmol* 2000;129:94–95.

Ferry AP. Synthetic fiber granuloma 'teddy bear' granuloma of the conjunctiva. *Arch Ophthalmol* 1994;112: 1339–1341.

Grewal RK, et al. Subconjunctival nodules: an unusual ocular complication of Crohn's disease. *Can J Ophthalmol* 1994;29:238–239.

Urback SF. Infectious mononucleosis presenting as a unilateral conjunctival tumor. *Acta Ophthalmol Scand* 1993; 72:133–135.

LARGE, FLAT, FLESHY LESIONS OF PALPEBRAL CONJUNCTIVA

1. Accidental or surgical injuries
2. Carthy disease (pyorhinoblepharostomatitis vegetans)
*3. Chalazion
*4. Embryonal rhabdomyosarcoma of children
*5. Granuloma pyogenicum
6. Ligneous conjunctivitis
7. Lymphogranuloma venereum
8. Meibomian cell carcinoma
9. Myopic infection
10. Papillary hyperplasia of vernal conjunctivitis
*11. Syphilis
12. Tuberculosis
13. Tularemia

Friedman AH, Henkind P. Granuloma pyogenicum of the palpebral conjunctiva. *Am J Ophthalmol* 1971;71:868–872.

Pau H. *Differential diagnosis of eye diseases*, 2nd ed. New York: Thieme Medical, 1988.

* = most important

CHRONIC OR RECURRENT ULCERS OF THE CONJUNCTIVA

1. Behçet disease
2. Crohn disease
3. Drugs, including the following:

allopurinol	ferrous succinate	iron sorbitex
amphotericin B	ferrous sulfate	phenytoin
aspirin	floxuridine	polysaccharide–iron complex
ferrocholinate	fluorouracil	sodium salicylate
ferrous fumarate	gentamicin	
ferrous gluconate	iron dextran	

  4. Fungi
*5. Herpes simplex
  6. Mucous membrane pemphigoid
  7. Pseudomonas ulcer in patients with AIDS
  8. Soft chancre
*9. Syphilis (acquired lues)
10. Tuberculosis
11. Wegener granulomatosis

Fraunfelder FT, Fraunfelder FW. *Drug-induced ocular side effects.* Woburn, MA: Butterworth-Heinemann, 2001.

Fraunfelder FT, Roy FH. *Current ocular therapy*, 5th ed. Philadelphia: WB Saunders, 2000.

Hegab SM, et al. Conjunctival ulcer in patients with Crohn's disease. *Ophthalmic Surg Lasers* 1994;25:638–639.

Jordan DR, et al. Wegener's granulomatosis: eyelid and conjunctival manifestations as the presenting feature in two individuals. *Ophthalmology* 1994;101:602–607.

PHLYCTENULAR KERATOCONJUNCTIVITIS

This condition involves a localized conjunctival, limbal, or corneal nodule measuring about 1 to 3 mm.
*1. Delayed hypersensitivity to bacterial protein, particularly tuberculoprotein and staphylococci; lymphopathia venereum and coccidioidomycosis may also be allergens
  2. Malnutrition
  3. Secondary infection of the conjunctiva, especially from *S. aureus*, pneumococcus, and Koch–Weeks bacillus
  4. Systemic infection
    A. Bang disease (brucellosis)
    B. Candidiasis
    C. Neurodermatitis
    D. Mikulicz–Radecki syndrome (dacryosialoadenopathy)
    E. Trachoma
    F. Sjögren syndrome (secretoinhibitor syndrome)

Davis PL, Watson JI. Experimental conjunctival phlyctenulosis. *Can J Ophthalmol* 1969;4:183–190.

Newell FW. *Ophthalmology: principles and concepts*, 7th ed. St. Louis: CV Mosby, 1991.

PIGMENTATION OF THE CONJUNCTIVA (SEE PIGMENT SPOTS OF SCLERA AND EPISCLERA, P. 237)

1. Blood pigment
    *A. After subconjunctival hemorrhage—red or later fine brown spots (see p. 206)
    B. Yellow tinge of malaria, blackwater fever, or yellow fever
    C. Pigmentary limbal ring associated with senile, traumatic, or diseased conditions
2. Bile pigments (yellow)—obstructive or hemorrhagic jaundice
3. Melanin pigmentation
    A. Acanthosis nigricans
    *B. Addison disease (adrenal cortical insufficiency)
    C. Alcaptonuric ochronosis
    D. Chlorpromazine (Thorazine)
    E. Endogenous ochronosis
    F. Keratomalacia
    G. Trachoma
    *H. Use of epinephrine or epinephrine bitartrate, borate, and hydrochloride
    I. Vernal conjunctivitis
    J. Vitiligo (leukoderma)—increased conjunctival pigmentation
    K. Xeroderma pigmentosum
4. Drugs, including the following:

acid bismuth sodium tartrate	captopril	iron dextran
Alcian blue	chloroquine	iron sorbitol
amiodarone	chlortetracycline	ketoprofen
amodiaquine	chrysarobin	methacycline
amphotericin B	clofazimine	minocycline
antimony lithium thiomalate	colloidal silver	minoxidil
antimony potassium tartrate	demeclocycline	methylene blue
antimony sodium tartrate	diethazine	oxytetracycline
antimony sodium	doxycycline	penicillamine
thioglycollate	enalapril	rifabutin
antipyrine	ethopropazine	rifampin silver nitrate silver
bismuth carbonate(?)	ferrocholinate	protein
bismuth oxychloride(?)	ferrous fumarate	trypan blue
bismuth salicylate(?)	ferrous gluconate	polysaccharide iron complex
bismuth sodium tartrate	ferrous succinate	quinacrine
bismuth sodium	ferrous sulfate	rose bengal
thioglycollate (?)	fluorescein	sodium antimonylgluconate
bismuth sodium	gold AU 198	stibocaptate
triglycollamate(?)	gold sodium thiomalate	stibophen
bismuth subcarbonate	gold sodium thiosulfate	tetracycline
bismuth subsalicylate	hydroxychloroquine	vitamin A

5. Foreign substances such as silver (argyrosis), iron (siderosis), copper (chalcosis), arsenic (arsenic melanosis), gold (chrysiasis), aluminum, quinones, aniline dyes, and eye cosmetics containing carbon black
    *6. Benign melanosis—overactivity of melanocytes
    A. Epithelial—congenital or acquired, for example., following radiation or use of

chemicals (arsenic); in Addison disease; because of chronic conjunctivitis (trachoma, vernal conjunctivitis, onchocerciasis, keratomalacia)

    B. Subepithelial—congenital or in association with melanosis oculi or nevus of Ota

7. Neoplasms

    *A. Nevus—most common in children, localized stationary, elevated, cystic, may or may not have pigmentation

    *B. Malignant melanoma arising from preexisting nevus, apparently normal conjunctiva, or from an area of acquired pigmentation (intraepithelial melanoma); occurs primarily in middle age; diffuse, flat, pigmentation; progressive; no cysts

    C. Secondary melanotic tumors

    D. Incidentally pigmented tumors, such as a melanocarcinoma

    E. Secondary metastatic tumors from lung or breast

8. Ocular causes, including the following:

    A. Apocrine adenocarcinomas

    B. Foreign bodies

    C. Hematic cysts

    D. Moll gland cystadenomas

    E. Staphylomas

    F. Subconjunctival hematomas

Cheskes J, et al. Ocular manifestations of alkaptonuric ochronosis. *Arch Ophthalmol* 2000;118:724–727.

Fraunfelder FT, Fraunfelder FW. *Drug-induced ocular side effects.* Woburn, MA: Butterworth-Heinemann, 2001.

Linebarger EJ, et al. Conjunctival aluminum deposition following pneumatic cryopexy. *Arch Ophthalmol* 1999;117:692.

Roy FH. *Ocular syndromes and systemic diseases,* 3rd ed. Philadelphia: Lippincott Williams & Wilkins, 2002.

Seregard S. Conjunctival melanoma. *Surv Ophthalmol* 1998;42:321–350.

DISCOLORATION OF CONJUNCTIVA

1. Red

    A. Subconjunctival hemorrhage

2. Yellow

    A. Bilirubinemia—obstructive or hemorrhagic jaundice

    B. Picric acid

    C. Leptospirosis

    D. Brucellosis (Barg disease or Mediterranean fever)

    E. Aromatic nitro and amino compounds

    F. Conjunctival fat—occurs primarily in older and black patients

    G. Blood pigment tinge of malaria, blackwater fever, and yellow fever

3. Gray (black)

    *A. Argyrosis (silver)

    B. Drugs, including the following:

acetyomilid	phenols, specifically
atabrine	phenylic acid and carbon
nitrochlorobenzene	disulfide

    C. Chrysiasis (gold)—grayish green effect

    D. Arsenicals—ash white

    E. Mascara

4. Brown

    A. Subconjunctival hemorrhage—fine brown spots

B. Pigmentary limbal ring associated with senile, traumatic, or diseased conditions

*C. Benign melanosis—overactivity of melanocytes
    (1) Epithelial—congenital or acquired, following radiation or use of chemicals (arsenic); in Addison disease (adrenal cortical insufficiency); because of chronic conjunctivitis (trachoma, vernal conjunctivitis, onchocerciasis, keratomalacia)
    (2) Subepithelial—congenital or in association with melanosis oculi or nevus of Ota

D. Neoplasms
    *(1) Nevus—most common in children, localized, stationary, elevated, cystic, may or may not have pigmentation
    *(2) Malignant melanoma arising from preexisting nevus, apparently normal conjunctiva, or from an area of acquired pigmentation (intraepithelial melanoma); occurs primarily in middle age; diffuse, flat, pigmentation; progressive; no cysts

E. Drugs, including the following:

anilquinoline combinations (benzoquinone, paraquinone, hydroquinone)	aniline dyes bromides chromic acid and chromates phenol derivatives	phenothiazine sympathomimetics (adrenalin, Eppy)

F. Metabolic or vitamin disturbance, including alkaptonuria

5. Blue pigmentation
    A. Ink tattoo from pens
    B. Manganese dust

Crawford JB, et al. Combined nevi of the conjunctiva. *Arch Ophthalmol* 1999;117:1121–1127.

Fraunfelder FT, Fraunfelder FW. *Drug-induced ocular side effects.* Woburn, MA: Butterworth-Heinemann, 2001.

Roy FH. *Ocular syndromes and systemic diseases*, 3rd ed. Philadelphia: Lippincott Williams & Wilkins, 2002.

SYMBLEPHARON

Symblepharon involves fusing of the eyelid to an opposing surface, such as the tarsal and bulbar conjunctiva.

1. Physical trauma with denuded epithelium, including purulent, membranous, bullous, or ulcerative conjunctivitis and trauma

*2. Chemical burns—especially lime or caustic burns

*3. Inflammation—especially from drug reactions, including:

allobarbital	carbachol (?)	gold sodium thiomalate
amobarbital	clonidine (?)	gold sodium thiosulfate
aprobarbital	colloidal silver	heptabarbital
auranofin	cyclobarbital	hexethal
aurothioglucose	demecarium	hexobarbital
aurothioglycanide	diethylpropanediol (DEP)	idoxuridine
barbital	dipiperidinoethane (DPE)	idoxuridine (IDU)
benzalkonium	dipivefrin	isoflurophate
butabarbital	echothiophate	mephobarbital
butalbital	epinephrine	metharbital
butallylonal	F3T	methitural
butethal	gold Au 198	methohexital

* = most important

mild silver protein	sulfacetamide	sulfapyridine
mitomycin	sulfachlorpyridazine	sulfasalazine
oxyphenbutazone	sulfacytine	sulfathiazole
penicillamine	sulfadiazine	sulfisoxazole
pentobarbital	sulfadimethoxine	talbutal (?)
phenobarbital	sulfamerazine	thiamylal
phenylbutazone	sulfameter	thiopental (?)
pilocarpine	sulfamethazine	timolol
primidone	sulfamethizole	trifluridine
probarbital	sulfamethoxazole	vidarabine
secobarbital	sulfamethoxypyridazine	vinbarbital (?)
silver nitrate	sulfanilamide	
silver protein	sulfaphenazole	

4. Long-standing acute inflammation
   A. Pemphigus (Cazenave disease)
   B. Stevens–Johnson disease (dermatostomatitis)
5. Congenital
6. Associated with cyanoacrylate tissue adhesive
7. Epidemic keratoconjunctivitis

Fraunfelder FT, Fraunfelder FW. *Drug-induced ocular side effects.* Woburn, MA: Butterworth-Heinemann, 2001.

Leahey AB, Gottsch JD. Symblepharon associated with cyanoacrylate tissue adhesive. *Am J Ophthalmol* 1993;115: 46–49.

Meyer SJ, et al. Conjunctival involvement in paraneoplastic pemphigus. *Am J Ophthalmol* 1992;114:621–624.

CONJUNCTIVAL CONCRETIONS

Conjunctival concretions are small yellow spots that are most common in tarsal conjunctiva.
1. Chronic inflammatory conditions, including atopic keratoconjunctivitis, vernal conjunctivitis, and posttrachomatous degenerations
2. Elderly
3. Calcium deposits in patients with chronic renal failure treated with maintenance hemodialysis

Chin GN, et al. Ultrastructural and histochemical studies of conjunctival concretions. *Arch Ophthalmol* 1980;98: 720.

Pahor D, et al. Conjunctival and corneal changes in chronic renal failure patients treated with maintenance hemodialysis. *Ophthalmologica* 1995;209:14–16.

LESIONS OF CARUNCLE

  1. Apocrine hydrocystoma
 *2. Basal cell carcinoma
  3. Capillary hemangioma
  4. Chronic inflammation
  5. Dermoid
  6. Ectopic lacrimal gland
  7. Epithelial inclusion cyst
  8. Foreign-body granuloma
  9. Granular cell myeloblastoma
 10. Histiocytic lymphoma

11. Lipogranuloma
12. Lymphangiectasis
13. Malignant melanoma
14. Nevus
15. Normal caruncle
*16. Oncocytoma
17. Papilloma
18. Pilar cyst
19. Plasmacytoma
20. Pyogenic granuloma
21. Reactive lymphoid hyperplasia
22. Sebaceous gland hyperplasia
*23. Sebaceous gland adenoma
24. Seborrheic keratosis
25. Squamous cell carcinoma

Rennie IG. Oncocytomas of the lacrimal caruncle. *Br J Ophthalmol* 1980;64:935.

Shields CL, et al. Types and frequency of lesions of the caruncle. *Am J Ophthalmol* 1986;102:771–778.

Shields CL, Shields JA. Tumors of the caruncle. *Int Ophthalmol Clin* 1993;33:31–36.

6

Globe

CONTENTS

MICROPHTHALMIA (SMALL GLOBE)

1. Microphthalmia associated with the following:
   A. Cataract—dominant inheritance
   B. Coloboma—dominant and sex-linked inheritance
   C. Congenital spastic diplegia—x-linked
   D. Ectopic pupils—dominant inheritance
   E. Glaucoma—recessive inheritance
   F. Harelip and cleft palate—autosomal recessive
   G. High hypermetropia—recessive inheritance
   H. Malformation of hands and feet—autosomal recessive
   I. Polydactyly—autosomal recessive
   J. Retinitis pigmentosa and glaucoma—dominant inheritance
2. Colobomatous microphthalmia
   A. X-linked
      (1) Aicardi syndrome
      (2) Bloch–Sulzberger syndrome (incontinentia pigmenti)
      (3) Goltz syndrome (focal dermal hypoplasia)
      (4) Lenz microphthalmia syndrome
   B. Autosomal recessive
      (1) Cohen syndrome
      (2) Ellis–van Creveld syndrome
      (3) Hepatic fibrosis, polycystic kidneys, colobomas, and encephalopathy
      (4) Humeroradial synostosis
      (5) Kartagener syndrome

       (6) Laurence–Moon–Biedl syndrome

       (7) Marinesco–Sjögren syndrome

       (8) Meckel syndrome

       (9) Micro syndrome

     (10) Sjögren–Larsson syndrome

     (11) Warburg syndrome

  C. Autosomal dominant

       (1) Basal cell nevus syndrome

       (2) Congenital contractural arachnodactyly

       (3) Crouzon syndrome

       (4) Stickler syndrome

       (5) Treacher Collins syndrome

       (6) Tuberous sclerosis

       (7) Zellweger syndrome

  D. Chromosomal abnormalities

       (1) Deletions 4p, 4r, 11q, 13q, 18q, 18r, XO

       (2) Duplications 3q, 4p, 4q, 7q, 9p, 9q, 13q, 22q

       (3) Ring B syndrome

       (4) Triploidy

       (5) Trisomy 8, 9, 13, 17, 18, XXX, XYY

  E. Unknown cause

       (1) Amniogenic band syndrome (Streeter dysplasia)

       (2) Cat's-eye syndrome (Schmid–Fraccaro syndrome)

       (3) CHARGE (colomba, heart disease, atresia choanae, retarded growth and re-
tarded growth development or central nervous system anomalies, genital hypoplasia, and ear anomalies, or deafness) syndrome

       (4) Dyscraniopygophalangea (Ullrich syndrome)

       (5) Facial-clefting syndromes

       (6) Frontonasal dysplasia (median cleft face syndrome)

       (7) Goldenhar syndrome (oculoauriculovertebral syndrome)

       (8) Hemifacial microsomia syndrome

       (9) Linear sebaceous nevus syndrome

     (10) Rubinstein–Taybi syndrome

3. Noncolobomatous microphthalmia

  A. X-linked

       (1) Anderson–Warburg syndrome

       (2) Forsius–Eriksson syndrome (Aland disease)

       (3) Lowe syndrome (oculocerebrorenal syndrome)

  B. Autosomal recessive

       (1) Cerebrooculofacioskeletal syndrome

       (2) Conradi syndrome

       (3) Cross syndrome

       (4) Diamond–Blackfan syndrome

       (5) Fanconi

       (6) Obesity–cerebral–ocular-skeletal anomalies syndrome

  C. Autosomal dominant

       (1) Blatt syndrome

       (2) Gansslen syndrome

       (3) Hypomelanosis of Ito syndrome

(4) Leri syndrome

(5) Myotonic dystrophy

(6) Rieger syndrome

D. Chromosomal abnormalities

(1) Duplication 10q

(2) Trisomy 21Q syndrome

(3) Chromosome deletion Xp22.1

E. Unknown cause

(1) Arachnoidal cyst

(2) Gorlin–Chaudhry–Moss syndrome

(3) Hallerman–Streiff syndrome

(4) Hutchinson–Gilford syndrome (progeria)

(5) Krause syndrome (encephaloophthalmic)

(6) Meyer–Schwickerath and Weyers syndrome

(7) Pierre Robin syndrome

(8) Retinal disinsertion syndrome

(9) Sabin–Feldman syndrome

(10) Weyers syndrome

F. Infectious etiology

(1) Congenital rubella (Gregg syndrome)

(2) Congenital spherocytic anemia

(3) Congenital toxoplasmosis

(4) Cytomegalovirus

(5) Epstein–Barr syndrome

(6) Herpes virus

(7) Mumps

(8) Varicella

G. Intoxicants

(1) Fetal alcohol effects

(2) Maternal phenylketonuria fetal effects

4. Idiopathic

5. Nanophthalmos

Eng A, et al. Linear facial skin defects associated with microphthalmia and other malformations, with chromosome deletion Xp22.1. *J Am Acad Dermatol* 1994;31:680–682.

McKusick VA. *Mendelian inheritance in man*, 12th ed. Baltimore: Johns Hopkins University Press, 1998.

Roy FH. *Ocular syndromes and systemic diseases*, 3rd ed. Philadelphia: Lippincott Williams & Wilkins, 2002.

BUPHTHALMOS (LARGE GLOBE)

Buphthalmos usually is associated with corneal abnormalities such as opacities and rupture of Descemet membrane; the transition from cornea to sclera is unclear, and a thin, bluish sclera may be present.

1. Associated with anterior chamber cleavage syndrome (Reese–Ellsworth syndrome)

2. Autosomal recessive inheritance

3. Cerebrohepatorenal syndrome (Smith–Lemli–Opitz syndrome)

4. Chondrodystrophia calcificans congenita (Conradi syndrome)

5. Congenital glaucoma

6. Congenital rubella syndrome (Gregg syndrome)

7. Cryptophthalmia syndrome (cryptophthalmos–syndactyly)
8. Hurler syndrome
9. Krabbe syndrome
10. Lowe syndrome (oculocerebrorenal syndrome)
11. Milroy disease (chronic hereditary edema; Noone–Milroy–Meige disease)
12. Neurofibromatosis (von Recklinghausen disease)
13. Oculodentodigital dysplasia
14. Rieger syndrome (hypodontia and iris dysgenesis)
15. Sporadic occurrence
16. Sturge–Weber syndrome (encephalotrigeminal syndrome)

McKusick VA. *Mendelian inheritance in man*, 12th ed. Baltimore: Johns Hopkins University Press, 1998.

Roy FH. *Ocular syndromes and systemic diseases*, 3rd ed. Philadelphia: Lippincott Williams & Wilkins, 2002.

PSEUDOENDOPHTHALMITIS (CONDITIONS THAT SIMULATE ENDOPHTHALMITIS)

*1. Chemical reactions from irritating chemicals (irrigating solutions or medications) introduced into the anterior chamber
2. Foreign material in the anterior chamber
3. Metastatic carcinoma
4. Retained lenticular material
5. Severe postoperative iridocyclitis
6. Toxic anterior segment syndrome (TASS)

Levine RA, Williamson DE. Metastatic carcinoma simulating a post-operative endophthalmitis. *Arch Ophthalmol* 1970;83:59–60.

Mamalis N. Inflammation. In: Charlton JF, Weinstein GW. *Ophthalmic surgery complications: prevention and management*. Philadelphia: JB Lippincott, 1995:313–338.

Monson MC, et al. Toxic anterior segment inflammation following cataract surgery. *J Cataract Ref Surg* 1992;18: 184–189.

ENDOPHTHALMITIS (INTRAOCULAR INFECTION)

1. Bacterial agents
   A. Gram positive
      (1) Bacillus subtilis, megaterium, anthracis, cereus
      (2) *Clostridium perfringens* (*B. welchii*)
      (3) *Clostridium tetani*
      (4) *Coryneform bacterium*
      (5) *Diplococcus pneumoniae* (*Pneumococcus*)
      (6) Diphtheroids
      (7) *Listeria monocytogenes*
      *(8) *Propionibacterium acnes*
      *(9) *Staphylococcus aureus, albus*, and *epidermidis*
      (10) *Streptococcus viridans, S. hemolytic, S. pneumoniae*, and *Pyogenes salivarius*
   B. Gram negative
      (1) *Aerobacter aerogenes*
      (2) *Enterobacter cloacae*
      (3) *Escherichia coli*

* = most important

(4) *Fusobacterium* organisms
(5) *Klebsiella pneumoniae* (Friedlander bacillus)
(6) Meningococci
(7) *Morganella* species
(8) *Mycobacterium* organisms
(9) *Neisserias catarrhalis*
(10) *Ochrobactrum anthropi*
(11) *Pasteurella multocida* and *tularensis*
(12) *Proteus vulgaris* (*B. proteus*) and *mirabilis*
*(13) *Pseudomonas aeruginosa* (*B. pyocyaneus*)
(14) *Serratia marcescens*
(15) *Yersinia enterocolitica* or *Y. pseudotuberculosis*

2. Fungal agents
   A. Acanthamoeba
   B. *Actinomyces* species, including *Nocardiosis*
   C. *Aspergillus* species
   D. *Blastomyces dermatitidis*
   E. *Candida* species
   F. *Cephalosporium* species, hyphas
   G. *Coccidioides immitis*
   H. *Crytococcus neoformans*
   I. Hormodendrum
   J. *Hyalopus bogolepofi*
   K. Hyalosporus
   L. *Mucormycosis* species
   M. *Neurospora sitophila*
   N. *Sporothrix schenkii*
   O. *Sporotrichum schenkii*
   P. *Volutella* species

3. Viral agents
   A. Behçet syndrome (dermatostomatoophthalmic syndrome)
   B. Cytomegalovirus
   C. Myxovirus (influenza)
   D. *Nocardia asteroides*
   E. Vaccinia
   F. Variola

4. Nematode agents
   A. *Taenia solium*
   B. *Toxocara canis* and *T. cati*

5. Other agents
   A. Mycosis fungoides
   B. *Exophiala jeanselmei* (yeast)

Blackman DM, et al. Bacillus cereus endopthalmitis secondary to self-inflicted periocular injections. *Arch Ophthalmol* 2000;118:1585–1586.

Chen JC, Roy M. Epidemic bacillus endophthalmitis after cataract surgery II. *Ophthalmology* 2000;107:1038–1041.

Clark WL, et al. Treatment strategies and visual acuity outcomes in chronic postoperative propionibacterium acnes endophthalmitis. *Ophthalmology* 1999;106:1665–1670.

Hofling-Lima AL, et al. *Exophiala jeanselmei* causing late endophthalmitis after cataract surgery. *Am J Ophthalmol* 1999;128,4:512–514.

Li Suhui, et al. Unilateral blastomyces dermatitidis endophthalmitis and orbital cellulitis. *Ophthalmology* 1998;105: 1466–1470.

Okada AA, et al. Endogenous bacterial endophthalmitis: report of a ten-year retrospective study. *Ophthalmology* 1994;101:832–888.

Roy FH. *Ocular syndromes and systemic diseases*, 3rd ed. Philadelphia: Lippincott Williams & Wilkins, 2002.

Weishaar PD, et al. Endogenous aspergillus endophthalmitis. *Ophthalmology* 1998;105:57–68.

INTRAOCULAR CARTILAGE

1. Angiomatosis of the retina
2. Chromosome deletion
3. Chronic inflammation
4. Facial nevus of Jadassohn (linear sebaceous nevus syndrome)
5. Incidental findings in microphthalmic eye, microphthalmos with cyst, microphthalmic eye from a cyclopic orbit, in eyes with coloboma of the choroid and retina or ciliary body
6. Incontinentia pigmenti (Bloch–Sulzberger disease)
7. Persistent hyperplastic primary vitreous
8. Retinal dysplasia
9. Teratoid medulloepithelioma (dictyomas)
10. Trisomy (13-Patau syndrome) (globe less than 10 mm in diameter)

Roy FH. *Ocular syndromes and systemic diseases*, 3rd ed. Philadelphia: Lippincott Williams & Wilkins, 2002.

Wilkes SR, et al. Ocular malformation in association with ipsilateral facial nevus of Jadassohn. *Am J Ophthalmol* 1981;92:344–352.

INTRAOCULAR CALCIFICATIONS

1. Choroidal osteoma
2. Facial nevus of Jadassohn (linear sebaceous nevus syndrome)
3. Intraocular calcifications
   A. Congenital deformity
   B. Gitelman syndrome
   C. Recurrent iritis and keratitis
   D. Retinal detachment
   E. Trauma (perforating, nonperforating, or surgical)
4. Intraocular sarcoma
*5. Retinoblastoma
6. Retinopathy of prematurity (end stage)
7. Sites of intraocular calcification
   A. Calcific emboli of retinal and ciliary arteries
   B. Cyclitic membrane
   C. Lens
   D. Peripapillary choroid
   E. Posterior pole to ora serrata in region of choroid and pigment epithelium
   F. Retina
   G. Vitreous

Bourcier T, et al. Sclerochoroidal calcification associated with Gitelman syndrome. *Am J Ophthalmol* 1999;128: 767–768.

* = most important

Trimble SN, et al. Spontaneous decalcification of a choroidal osteoma. *Ophthalmology* 1988;95:631–634.

Wolter JR. The message of a bony lens. *Ophthalmic Surg Lasers* 1981;12:332.

INTRAOCULAR ADIPOSE TISSUE

1. Congenital malformations
   A. Dermoid or dermolipoma extending from the cornea or limbus into the globe
   B. Malformed optic nerve
   C. Persistent hyperplastic vitreous (PHPV) and other related ocular malformations, such as microphthalmia, persistent hyaloid vessels, cataract, and abnormal differentiation of the angle of the anterior chamber
2. Embolic phenomenon secondary to crush wounds of the thorax and abdomen or fracture of long bones of the extremities
3. Formation of fatty tissue within the marrow spaces of metaplastic bone
4. Missile passing through orbit carrying orbital fat into the eye

Font RL, et al. Intraocular adipose tissue and persistent hyperplastic primary vitreous. *Arch Ophthalmol* 1969;82:43–59.

Willis R, et al. Heterotropic adipose tissue and smooth muscle in the optic disc: association with isolated colobomas. *Arch Ophthalmol* 1972;86:139–146.

SOFT GLOBE (DECREASED INTRAOCULAR PRESSURE)

*1. Fistula from intraocular source, including penetrating intraocular trauma or surgery and ruptured wall of the globe
*2. Laser or cryotherapy ciliodestructive procedure
 3. *Phthisis bulbi*
 4. Choroidal detachment
 5. Injury to the cervical sympathetic nerve
 6. Serous detachment of the retina
 7. Myotonic dystrophy (Curschmann–Steinert syndrome)
 8. Systemic disturbances
    A. Cardiac edema
    B. Diabetic coma
    C. Extreme or rapid dehydration because of malnutrition, cholera, or diarrhea
    D. Decrease in ocular blood pressure due to hypotension, ligation of the carotid artery, carotid occlusion, or pulseless disease (Takayasu syndrome)
    E. Giant cell arteritis (temporal arteritis syndrome)
    F. Leprosy (Hansen disease)
    G. Parkinson disease (shaking palsy)
    H. Postencephalitic syndrome following severe cerebral trauma, barbiturate poisoning, in deep anesthesia, following leukotomy, or on the paralyzed side in cases of cerebral hemiplegia
    I. Severe abdominal disturbances, such as intestinal perforation or obstruction
    J. Profound anemias
    K. Uremic coma

* = most important

9. Drugs, including the following:

acebutolol
aceclidine
acetazolamide
acetylcholine
acetyldigitoxin
adrenal cortex injection
aldosterone
albuterol
alcohol
allobarbital
alseroxylon
amobarbital
amyl nitrite
antazoline
aprobarbital
acebutolol
aspirin
atenolol
barbital
beclomethasone
bendroflumethiazide
benzthiazide
betamethasone
betaxolol
bupivacaine
butabarbital
butalbital
butallylonal
butethal
carbachol
carisoprodol (?)
chlordiazepoxide
chlorisondamine
chloroform
chlorothiazide
chlorthalidone
cidofovir
clofibrate (?)
clonidine
cortisone
cyclobarbital
cyclopentobarbital
cyclothiazide
demecarium
diethylpropanediol (DEP)
deserpidine
deslanoside

desoxycorticosterone
dexamethasone
diacetylmorphine
diazepam
dichlorphenamide
digitoxin
digoxin
dimethyl tubocurarine iodide
diphenylhydantoin
dipivefrin
dipiperidinoethane (DPE)
dronabinol
droperidol
echothiophate
ephedrine
epinephrine
ergotamine
ergonovine
erythrityl tetranitrate
ether
ethoxzolamide
etidocaine
fludrocortisone
fluorometholone
fluprednisolone
flurazepam
furosemide
gitalin
glycerin
guanethidine
haloperidol
hashish
heparin
heptabarbital
hexamethonium
hexethal
hexobarbital
hydrochlorothiazide
hydrocortisone
hydroflumethiazide
indapamide
insulin
isoflurophate
isosorbide
isosorbide dinitrate
labetalol
lanatoside C

levobunolol
lidocaine
mannitol
mannitol hexanitrate
marijuana
mecamylamine
medrysone
meperidine
mephenesin
mephobarbital
mepivacaine
meprednisone
meprobamate(?)
methacholine
metharbital
methazolamide
methitural
methohexital
methoxyflurane
methyclothiazide
methyldopa
methylergonovine
methylprednisolone
methysergide
metipranolol
metocurine iodide
metolazone
metoprolol
morphine
nadolol
naphazoline
neostigmine
nitroglycerin
nitrous oxide
norepinephrine
opium
oral contraceptives
ouabain
oxprenolol
oxygen
paramethasone
phenylephrine
pindolol
prednisone
procaine
pyrilamine tripelennamine
pargyline

pentaerythritol tetranitrate	quinethazone	thiopental
pentobarbital	rauwolfia serpentina	timolol
pentolinium	rescinnamine	tolazoline
phenobarbital	reserpine	trichloroethylene
phenoxybenzamine(?)	secobarbital	trichlormethiazide
physostigmine	sodium salicylate	trifluperidol
pilocarpine	spironolactone	trimethaphan
polythiazide	succinylcholine	trimethidinium
practolol	syrosingopine	trolnitrate
prednisolone	talbutal	tubocurarine
primidone	tetraethylammonium	urea
probarbital	tetrahydrocannabinol	urokinase
propranolol	tetrahydrozoline	vinbarbital
protriptyline	thiamylal	vitamin A

10. Detachment of the ciliary body, planned or inadvertent
11. Hyperosmotic agents, such as mannitol or urea
12. Iritis or iridocyclitis
13. After central retinal vein occlusion
14. Myopia—low scleral rigidity may give false low readings with Schiötz tonometer, but normal readings with applanation intraocular pressure
15. Herpes zoster
16. Following irradiation by roentgenograms or beta rays
17. Congenital lesions, including microphthalmos, aniridia, and coloboma
18. Concussion trauma
19. Necrosis of anterior segment of the eye
20. Idiopathic, including normal variation

Fraunfelder FT, Fraunfelder FW. *Drug-induced ocular side effects.* Woburn, MA: Butterworth-Heinemann, 2001.

Maus M, Katz JL. Choroidal detachment flat anterior chamber and hypotony as complications of YAG laser cyclocoagulation. *Ophthalmology* 1990;97:69–71.

Roy FH. *Ocular syndromes and systemic diseases,* 3rd ed. Philadelphia: Lippincott Williams & Wilkins, 2002.

PHTHISIS BULBI (DEGENERATIVE SHRINKAGE OF EYEBALL WITH HYPOTONY)

1. Ciliodestructive procedures such as cyclocryotherapy or laser
2. Endophthalmitis
3. Following cataract surgery, especially with rubella syndrome (German measles)
4. Panophthalmitis
5. Severe ocular injury with loss of tissue
6. Severe uveitis
7. Sympathetic ophthalmia
8. Tumor, such as retinoblastoma or malignant melanoma

Cyclin MN, et al. Ciliodestructive procedures in glaucoma: clinical signs. *Ophthalmology* 1991;12:1–15.

Newell FW. *Ophthalmology, principles and concepts,* 7th ed. St. Louis: CV Mosby, 1991.

CLINICAL ANOPHTHALMOS (APPARENT ABSENCE OF GLOBE)

1. Anencephaly

2. Gross midline facial defects (median cleft face syndrome)
3. Dyscraniopygophalangea
4. Goldenhar syndrome (oculoauriculovertebral syndrome)
5. Goltz syndrome (focal dermal hypoplasia syndrome)
6. Hallermann–Streiff syndrome (dyscephalic mandibulo-oculofacial syndrome)
7. Hypervitaminosis A
8. Idiopathic
9. Klinefelter syndrome (gynecomastia-aspermatogenesis)
10. Lanzieri syndrome (craniofacial malformations)
11. Leri syndrome (carpal tunnel syndrome)
12. Meckel syndrome (dysencephalia splanchnocystica syndrome)
13. Oculovertebral dysplasia (Weyers–Thier syndrome)
14. Otocephaly
15. Trisomy 13–15
16. Sex-linked or recessive hereditary
17. Waardenburg anophthalmia syndrome (anophthalmos with limb anomalies)—recessive

Graham CA, et al. X-linked clinical anophthalmos: localization of the gene to Xq27-Xq28. *Ophthal Paediatrics Genetics* 1991;12:43–48.

Roy FH. *Ocular syndromes and systemic diseases*, 3rd ed. Philadelphia: Lippincott Williams & Wilkins, 2002.

OCULODIGITAL STIMULATION

The patient presses on the globe through the lids with the index finger or hand; the patient has poor visual acuity.

1. Bilateral congenital cataracts
2. Combined retinal detachment and congenital cataract
3. Congenital glaucoma
4. Congenital rubella syndrome (German measles)
5. Leber amaurosis congenita or other congenital retinal degeneration (Leber tapetoretinal dystrophy syndrome)
6. Norrie disease (fetal iritis syndrome)
7. Total corneal leukoma

Franklin AH. Norrie's disease. *Am J Ophthalmol* 1971;72:947–948.

Roy FH. Ocular autostimulation. *Am J Ophthalmol* 1967;63:1776–1777.

ANTERIOR SEGMENT ISCHEMIA

This condition involves hypoxia with involvement of the cornea, iris, anterior chamber, lens, and ciliary body.

1. Damage to normal intact anterior vessels
   A. Pressure
      (1) Scleral buckle
      (2) Suture (Jensen procedure)
   B. Thermal
      (1) Cryotherapy
      (2) Diathermy
2. Disinsertion of normal vessels (Hummelsheim or Knapp procedure)
3. Fuchs syndrome (I) (heterochromic cyclitis syndrome)
4. Hematologic abnormality

A. Extreme leukocytosis
B. Extreme thrombocytosis
C. Hyperglobulinemia
D. Red blood cell dysfunction including sickle cell trait
    (1) Hemoglobinopathy
    (2) Polycythemia vera (Vaquez–Osler syndrome)
5. Vessel wall abnormality (arteriosclerosis)
  A. Arteriosclerosis
  B. Giant cell arteritis

Birt CM, et al. Anterior segment ischemia in giant cell arteritis. *Can J Ophthalmol* 1994;29:93–94.

Roy FH. *Ocular syndromes and systemic diseases*, 3rd ed. Philadelphia: Lippincott Williams & Wilkins, 2002.

Saunder RA, et al. Anterior segment ischemia after strabismus surgery. *Surv Ophthalmol Lasers* 1995;38:456–466.

7
Sclera

CONTENTS

BLUE SCLERA

Blue sclera is characterized by localized or generalized blue coloration of sclera because of thinness and loss of water content, which allow underlying dark choroid to be seen.

1. Associated with high urine excretion
    A. Folling syndrome (phenylketonuria)
    B. Hypophosphatasia (phosphoethanolaminuria)
    C. Lowe syndrome (oculocerebrorenal syndrome; chondroitin-4-sulfate-uria)
2. Associated with skeletal disorders
    A. Brachmann–de Lange syndrome
    B. Brittle cornea syndrome (blue sclera syndrome)—recessive
    C. Crouzon disease (craniofacial dysostosis)
    D. Hallermann–Streiff syndrome (dyscephalia mandibulooculofacial syndrome)
    *E. Marfan syndrome (dystrophia mesodermalis congenita)
    F. Marshall–Smith syndrome
    G. McCune–Albright syndrome (fibrosus dysplasia)
    H. Mucopolysaccharidosis VI (Maroteaux–Lamy syndrome)
    I. Osteogenesis imperfecta (van der Hoeve syndrome)
    J. Paget syndrome (osteitis deformans)
    K. Pierre Robin syndrome (micrognathia–glossoptosis syndrome)
    L. Robert syndrome
    M. Silver–Russell syndrome
    N. Werner syndrome (progeria of adults)
3. Chromosome disorders
    A. Trisomy syndrome
    B. Turner syndrome
4. Ocular
    *A. Congenital glaucoma
    B. Myopia

    * = most important

*C. Repeated surgeries
   D. Scleromalacia (perforans)
*E. Staphyloma
   F. Trauma
5. Miscellaneous
   A. Ehlers–Danlos syndrome (fibrodysplasia elastica generalisata)
   B. Goltz syndrome (focal dermal hypoplasia syndrome)
   C. Incontinentia pigmenti (Bloch–Sulzberger syndrome)
   D. Lax ligament syndrome
   E. Minocycline-induced
   F. Oculodermal melanocytosis (nevus of Ota)
   G. Pseudoxanthoma elasticum (Grönblad–Strandberg syndrome)
   H. Relapsing polychondritis

Cameron JA, et al. Epikeratoplasty for keratoglobus associated with blue sclera. *Ophthalmology* 1991;98:446–452.
Fraunfelder FT, Randall JA. Minocycline-induced sclera pigmentation. *Ophthalmology* 1997;104:936–938.
Roy FH. *Ocular syndromes and systemic diseases*, 3rd ed. Philadelphia: Lippincott Williams & Wilkins, 2002.

Blue sclera

	McCune-Albright syndrome	Brittle cornea syndrome	Cruson's syndrome	Brachmann de Lange syndrome	Ehlers-Danlos syndrome	Hallerman-Streiff-François syndrome	Hypophosphatasia	Marfan syndrome	Osteogenesis imperfecta	Turner's syndrome	Werner's syndrome
History											
1. Chromosomal abnormality										U	
2. Common in females	U									U	
3. Familial occurrence and consanguinity						R					S
4. Hereditary	U	U	U	U	U			U	U		U
5. Inborn error of metabolism							U				
6. Male and female equal						U					
7. Occurs during second to third decades											U
8. Present from birth	U		U		U						
Physical Findings											
1. Abnormal deep recess in angle of anterior chamber									U		
2. Absence of eyelashes and scanty eyebrows											U
3. Angioid streaks					S						
4. Aniridia								R			
5. Anisocoria				S							
6. Antimongoloid obliquity (downward displacement of temporal canthus)			U	U		S					
7. Astigmatism											S
8. Bilateral exophthalmos			U	S		S	U			S	
9. Blepharophimosis				S							
10. Bullous keratitis											S
11. Cataract	S		S			S	S	R	U	S	
12. Chorioretinal hemorrhages					S						
13. Conjunctival calcification							S				
14. Corneal dystrophy			R								S
15. Corneal nebulae										S	
16. Corneal spontaneous perforation	S	S									
17. Corneal subepithelial calcification							U				
18. Epicanthal folds										S	
19. Exposure keratitis			S								
20. Extraocular muscles hypotony					S						
21. Glaucoma						S			S	S	
22. High myopia			S	S				U			
23. Hydrophthalmos								R			
24. Hyperelasticity of palpebral skin					U						
25. Hypertelorism	S		U							U	
26. Hypertrichosis of eyebrows				U							
27. Iris atrophy						S					
28. Iris coloboma						S		R			
29. Iris heterochromia								R			
30. Keratitis	S										
31. Keratoglobus						S					
32. Lens coloboma								R			
33. Lens subluxation					S			U			
34. Lid retraction							S				
35. Lid telangiectasia											S

Blue sclera (Continued)

	McCune-Albright syndrome	Brittle cornea syndrome	Cruson's syndrome	Brachmann-e Lange syndrome	Ehlers-Danlos syndrome	Hallerman-Streiff-François syndrome	Hypophosphatasia	Marfan syndrome	Osteogenesis imperfecta	Turner's syndrome	Werner's syndrome
Physical Findings											
36. Long eyelashes				U							
37. Macula and optic nerve coloboma								R			
38. Macular degeneration					S						
39. Megalocornea								R			
40. Microcornea					S	S					
41. Microphthalmos						U			R		
42. Miosis								U			
43. Nystagmus			S	S		S				S	
44. Optic disc and choroid coloboma						S					
45. Optic nerve atrophy			S	S		S	U				
46. Papilledema	S		S				U				
47. Paramacular retinal degeneration											S
48. Persistent pupillary membrane						S					
49. Pigmentary retinal degeneration								R			
50. Presbyopia, early											S
51. Prominent iris processes								U			
52. Ptosis			S	S	U					S	
53. Retinal detachment					S			U			
54. Retinitis proliferans					S						
55. Sclera and choroidal calcifications	S										
56. Strabismus	S		S	S	S	S					
57. Telecanthus				S							
58. Thinning of cornea with keratoconus					S				R	S	
59. Upper lid easy eversion					U						
60. Uveitis											S
Labaratory Data											
1. Blood phosphate							U				
2. Chromosome studies										U	
3. Hearing test									S		
4. Hyperglycemia											S
5. Skeletal roentgenogram									U	S	
6. Skull roentgenogram			U	S					U		

R = rarely; S = sometimes; and U = usually.

DILATED EPISCLERAL VESSELS

1. Carotid–cavernous fistula
2. Cavernous sinus thrombosis (Foix syndrome)
*3. Chronic respiratory diseases
*4. Glaucoma, untreated
5. Increased viscosity of circulating blood
    A. Leukemia (early)
    B. Polycythemia vera (erythema, Vaquez–Osler syndrome)
6. Occlusion of orbital veins of the apex of the orbit
    A. Endocrine exophthalmos of rapid development
    B. Inflammatory lesions
    C. Orbital thrombophlebitis
    D. Tumor (rare)
7. Ophthalmic vein thrombosis
8. Tricuspid Incompetence
9. Uveal neoplasm with localized engorgement

Boniuk M. The ocular manifestations of ophthalmic vein and aseptic cavernous sinus thrombosis. *Trans Am Acad Ophthalmol Otolaryngol* 1972;76:1519–1534.

Minas TF, Podos SM. Familial glaucoma associated with elevated episcleral venous pressure. *Arch Ophthalmol* 1968;80:202–213.

EPISCLERITIS

Episcleritis is a benign, self-limited, nodular or diffuse disease that usually resolves spontaneously within weeks but has a tendency to recur. Inflammation of episcleral tissues causes discomfort rather than pain; it does not affect visual acuity. Even recurrent attacks do not produce scleritis. Complications are minimal and include areas of scleral transparency and localized keratitis)

*1. Idiopathic (single, short episode that does not recur)
2. Associated with the following diseases (recurrent attacks)
    A. Addison syndrome (adrenal cortical insufficiency)
    B. Arthritides
        (1) Involving small and medium-sized vessels
            a. Necrotizing granulomatous arthritis; Wegener granulomatosis (Wegener syndrome)
            b. Polyarteritis nodosa (Kussmaul disease)
        (2) Involving small, medium, and large vessels
            a. Arteritis in collagen vascular diseases
                (i) Progressive systemic sclerosis (PSS; scleroderma)
                (ii) Rheumatoid arthritis
                (iii) Rheumatic fever
    C. Cogan syndrome
    D. Crohn disease (granulomatous ileocolitis)
    E. Goodpasture syndrome (pulmonary hemosiderosis)
    F. Heerfordt disease (uveoparotid fever)
    G. Inflammatory pseudotumor
    H. Initial manifestation of uveal melanoma (ciliary body)

* = most important

I. Myeloproliferative diseases
   (1) Hodgkin disease
   (2) T-cell leukemia
J. Paraneoplastic syndromes
   (1) Dermatomyositis
   (2) Sweet syndrome (cutaneous paraneoplastic syndrome)
K. Paraproteinemia
   (1) Familial Mediterranean fever
   (2) Necrobiotic xanthogranuloma [increased immunoglobulin G (IgG)/IgA]
L. Parry–Romberg syndrome (progressive hemifacial atrophy)
M. Relapsing polychondritis
N. Skin diseases
   (1) Chronic cutaneous lupus erythematosus (CCLE)
   (2) Erythema elevatum diutinum
   (3) Lichen planus
   (4) PSS; scleroderma
   (5) Psoriasis
   (6) Reiter syndrome (polyarteritis enterica)
   (7) Wiskott–Aldrich syndrome
O. Terrien marginal corneal disease
P. Ulcerative colitis (regional enteritis)
Q. Weber–Christian disease (systemic panniculitis)
R. Pseudoepiscleritis (lesions resembling episcleritis)
   (1) Conjunctivitis
   (2) In-growing lash
  *(3) Inflamed pinguecula
   (4) Punctate keratitis
   (5) Sclerosing keratitis
   (6) Wegener granulomatosis

3. Drugs
  A. Pamidronate disodium

4. Infectious
  A. Brucellosis (Bang disease, undulant fever)
  B. Coccidioidomycosis
  C. Influenza
  D. Leprosy (Hansen disease)
  E. Leptospirosis (Weil disease)
  F. Lyme disease (borreliosis, relapsing fever)
  G. Lymphogranuloma venereum (Nichols–Favre disease)
  H. Nematode (*Angiostrongylus cantonensis*)
  I. Q fever

5. Trauma
 *A. Episcleral foreign body
  B. Following transscleral fixation of posterior chamber IOL (intraocular lens)
  C. Insect bite granuloma
  D. Malpositioned (Jones) tube

Akpek EK, et al. Severity of episcleritis and systemic disease association. *Ophthalmology* 1999;106:729–731.

Marcarol V, Fraunfelder FT. Pamidronate disodium and possible ocular adverse drug reactions. *Am J Ophthalmol* 1994;118:220–224.

Read RW, et al. Episcleritis in childhood. *Ophthalmology* 1999;106:2377–2379.

Roy FH. *Ocular syndromes and systemic diseases*, 3rd ed. Philadelphia: Lippincott Williams & Wilkins, 2002.

PIGMENT SPOTS OF SCLERA AND EPISCLERA

*1. Acquired melanosis
2. Cysts
3. Drugs, including the following:

acetophenazine	iron dextran	promethazine
butaperazine	iron sorbitex	propiomazine
carphenazine	mesoridazine	thiethylperazine
chlorpromazine	methdilazine	thiopropazate
diethazine	methotrimeprazine	thioproperazine
ethopropazine	perazine	thioridazine
ferrocholinate	pericyazine	trifluoperazine
ferrous fumarate	perphenazine	triflupromazine
ferrous gluconate	piperacetazine	trimeprazine
ferrous succinate	polysaccharide iron complex	vitamin D
ferrous sulfate	prochlorperazine	vitamin D_2
fluphenazine	promazine	vitamin D_3

4. Extension of adjacent or underlying malignant melanoma
5. Foreign body
6. Intrascleral nerve loops with uveal pigment (painful to touch)
*7. Nevus
8. Ochronosis with melanin deposition
*9. Resolving hemorrhage
10. Staphyloma
11. Transscleral migration of pigment following cryotherapy of intraocular tumor or trauma
12. Uveal melanocytes carried by the scleral emissaria into the episclera (most often in eyes, with dark irides in superior, inferior temporal, and nasal quadrants in descending frequency; conjunctiva freely movable over them)

Fraunfelder FT, Fraunfelder FW. *Drug-induced ocular side effects*. Woburn, MA: Butterworth-Heinemann, 2001.

Kampik A, et al. Ocular ochronosis. *Arch Ophthalmol* 1980;98:1411.

Shields JA, et al. Uveal pseudomelanoma due to post-traumatic pigmentary migration. *Arch Ophthalmol* 1973;89: 519–522.

SCLERITIS

Scleritis involves a potentially destructive inflammatory process that may accompany severe systemic disease. Ocular pain occasionally radiates to the temple, jaw, or sinuses. Women are more frequently affected than men. Most cases begin with bilateral involvement. Early perforation of sclera is possible. The anterior portion of the eye is affected most severely. Posterior scleritis may be a diagnostic challenge.

1. Associated with systemic disease
   A. Collagen diseases
      *(1) Dermatomyositis (Wagner–Unverricht syndrome)
      *(2) Felty syndrome
      *(3) Giant cell (temporal) arteritis

* = most important

    (4) Juvenile rheumatoid arthritis (Still disease)
    (5) Polyarteritis nodosa (Kussmaul disease)
    (6) PSS; scleroderma
    (7) Relapsing polychondritis
    (8) Reiter syndrome (polyarteritis enterica)
    (9) Rheumatoid arthritis
  (10) Sjögren syndrome
  (11) Systemic lupus erythematosus (SLE)
  (12) Wegener granulomatosis (Wegener syndrome)

B. Metabolic diseases
    (1) Cretinism (hypothyroidism)
    (2) Gout
    (3) Porphyria cutanea tarda

C. Myeloproliferative diseases
    (1) Hodgkin disease (lymph node disease)
    (2) Mycosis fungoides syndrome (Sézary syndrome)

2. Infectious

A. Bacterial
    (1) Leprosy
    (2) Lymphogranuloma venereum (Nichols–Favre disease)
    (3) Syphilis (acquired lues)
    (4) Tuberculosis

B. Viral infections
    (1) Herpes simplex
    (2) Herpes zoster
    (3) Influenza
    (4) Mumps

C. Fungal—aspergillosis

D. Helminth infection—acanthamoeba

E. Protozoan—toxoplasmosis

F. Infections
    (1) Associated with skin disease or immunosuppressive status
    (2) Spreading directly from conjunctiva, cornea, uvea, periorbital tissues, nose, or sinuses

3. Miscellaneous

A. Cogan syndrome

B. Crohn disease (granulomatous ileocolitis)

C. Goodpasture syndrome (pulmonary hemosiderosis)

D. Erythema nodosum

E. Exogenous infection via penetration through conjunctiva

F. Hashimoto thyroiditis

G. Heerfordt disease (uveoparotid fever)

H. Necrobiotic xanthogranuloma (increased IgG/IgA)

I. Terrien marginal corneal disease

J. Uveitis

4. Drugs

A. Pamidronate disodium

*5. Trauma—following cataract or strabismus surgery

Heiligenhaus A, et al. Ultrasound biomicroscopy in scleritis. *Ophthalmology* 1998;105:527–534.

Knox C, Michele MD, et al. Brief reports. *Am J Opthalmol* 1997;123:5,713–714.

Maza MS, et al. Scleritis-associated uveitis. *Ophthalmology* 1997;104:58–63.

Perry SR, et al. The clinical and pathologic constellation of Wegener granulomatosis of the orbit. *Ophthalmology* 1997;104:683–694.

Riono WP, et al. Scleritis. *Ophthalmology* 1999;106:1328–1333.

Roy FH. *Ocular syndromes and systemic diseases*, 3rd ed. Philadelphia: Lippincott Williams & Wilkins, 2002.

Tuft SJ, Shah P, et al. Posterior scleritis—an unusual manifestation of Cogan's syndrome. *Br J Rheumatol* 1994; 33:774–775.

STAPHYLOMA (STRETCHING AND THINNING OF THE SCLERA WITH INCARCERATION OF UVEAL TISSUE)

1. Collagen diseases
    A. Felty syndrome
    B. Rheumatoid arthritis (adult)
    C. Wegener syndrome (Wegener granulomatosis)
2. Following trauma
    A. Beta radiation
    B. Deep scleral resection for episcleral malignancies
    C. Pterygium excision and mitomycin therapy
    *D. Scleral buckle removal
    E. Subconjunctival injection of corticosteroids
    F. Ultrasound treatment for glaucoma
3. Infectious
    A. Aspergillosis
    B. Herpes zoster (rare)
    C. Plague (bubonic plague)
    D. Syphilis
    E. Tuberculosis
4. Ocular cause
    A. Buphthalmos associated with increased intraocular pressure
    B. Corneoscleral ectasia
    C. Myopia with increased anteroposterior diameter
    D. Scleritis (e.g., secondary to rheumatoid arthritis)
    E. Uveitis
5. Miscellaneous
    A. Ehlers–Danlos syndrome (fibrodysplasia elastica generalisata)
    B. Endarteritis
    C. Epidermolysis bullosa
    D. Hyperparathyroidism
    E. Meckel syndrome (dysencephalia syndrome)
    F. Oculodental syndrome (Peter syndrome)
    G. Porphyria cutanea tarda

Dunn JP, et al. Development of scleral ulceration and calcification after pterygium excision and mitomycine therapy. *Am J Ophthalmol* 1991;112:344.

Fraunfelder FT, Roy FH. *Current ocular therapy*, 5th ed. Philadelphia: WB Saunders, 2000.

Roy FH. *Ocular syndromes and systemic diseases*, 3rd ed. Philadelphia: Lippincott Williams & Wilkins, 2002.

* = most important

EPISCLERAL AND SCLERAL TUMORS

1. Carcinomas
2. Choroidal melanomas
*3. Epibulbar tumor
4. Fibromas
5. Hemangiomas
6. Histiocytosis
7. Lymphomas
8. Leiomyoma (transscleral)
9. Melanoblastoma (spread from choroid)
10. Retinoblastoma

Ireland KC, et al. Sinus histiocytosis presenting as bilateral epibulbar masses. *Am J Ophthalmol* 1999;127,3:360–361.

Pau H. *Differential diagnosis of eye diseases*, 2nd ed. New York: Thieme Medical, 1988.

Perry HD. Isolated episcleral neurofibroma. *Ophthalmology* 1982;89:1095.

8

Cornea

CONTENTS

CRYSTALS OF THE CORNEA (DEPOSITION OF CRYSTALLINE SUBSTANCES IN THE CORNEA)

1. Bietti marginal crystalline dystrophy
2. Calcium oxalate—dieffenbachia and other plants
3. Cholesterol crystals—primary or secondary with corneal neovascularization
*4. Crystalline dystrophy of Schnyder
5. Crystalline retinopathy
6. Cystinosis syndrome (Lignac–Fanconi syndrome)
    A. Benign adult
    B. Congenital
7. Drugs, such as indomethacin (Indocin), chloroquine, thioridazine (Mellaril), and clofazimine
8. Dysproteinemia
    A. Cryoglobulinemia
    *B. Multiple myeloma
9. Elevated bilirubin with crystalline dystrophy
10. Fine, multicolored glittering crystals following successful transplant that later underwent graft rejection and was treated with steroids
11. Gout (hyperuricemia)
12. Hyperparathyroidism
13. Immunoglobulin G (IgG) K monoclonal gammopathy
*14. Infectious crystalline retinopathy, usually with more indolent streptococcal and staphylococcal species

* = most important

15. Post keratoplasty (Kaye dots)
16. Renal failure
17. Subconjunctival 5-fluorouracil
18. Uremia
19. Waldenström syndrome (macroglobulinemia syndrome)

Font RL, et al. Polychromatic corneal and conjunctival crystals secondary to clofazimine therapy in a leper. *Ophthalmology* 1989;96:311–315.

Ormerod LD, et al. Paraproteinemic crystalline keratopathy. *Ophthalmology* 1988;95:202–212.

Rothman RF, et al. Noninfectious crystalline keratopathy after postoperative subconjunctival 5-fluorouracil. *Am J Ophthalmol* 1999;128,2:236–237.

Roy FH. *Ocular syndromes and systemic diseases*, 3rd ed. Philadelphia: Lippincott Williams & Wilkins, 2002.

Vesaluoma MH, et al. In vivo confocal microscopy of a family with Schnyder crystalline corneal dystrophy. *Ophthalmology* 1999;106:944–951.

Crystals of the cornea (deposition of crystalline substance in the cornea)	Cystinosis (i.e., Congenital)	Crystalline Dystrophy of Schnyder	Multiple Myeloma	Bietti Marginal Crystalline Dystrophy	Gout	Drugs (i.e., Chloroquine)	Hyperparathyroidism	Porphyria Cutanea Tarda	Cholesterol Crystals	Infectious Crystalline Keratopathy
History										
1. Amaurosis fungax			S							
2. Between 50 and 70 years			S							
3. Common in 40s								U		
4. Corneal trauma including chemical burns; infections including herpes simplex and zoster; interstitial kerstitis									U	
5. Crystals appear 6 to 24 months	U	U								
6. Disseminated malignancy of plasma cells			U							
7. Excessive alcohol intake								U		
8. Fatal disease	U									
9. Genetic metabolic disease	S			S	U					
10. Glare						U				
11. Hereditary	U	U		U						
12. Thyroid surgery							S			
13. Photophobia	U									
14. Prior Corneal Surgery										U
Physical Findings										
1. Attenutated retinal vessels						S				
2. Bull's eye or doughnut retinal lesion						U				
3. Bushy eyebrows								S		
4. Cicatricial ectropion								S		
5. Conjunctival calcification								S	R	
6. Conjunctivitis					U					S
7. Corneal arcus		S								
8. Corneal neovascularization									S	
9. Corneal infiltrate										U
10. Cotton wool spots			S					S		
11. Crystals in conjunctiva	S		S				S			
12. Crystals in aqueous humor	U									
13. Choroidal detachment			S							
14. Dilated retina veins			S							
15. Episcleritis					S					
16. Lacrimal obstruction									S	
17. Macula edema									S	
18. Occlusion of central artery vein			S							
19. Ocular motor disturbances including sixth nerve palsy			S		S			S		
20. Optic nerve atrophy							U	S		
21. Pigmentary retinopathy	U					S				
22. Posterior scleritis					S					
23. Proptosis			S							
24. Ptosis							S			
25. Retinal hemorrhages			S							
26. Retinal microaneurysms			S							
27. Retinitis punctata albescens				U						
28. Retrobulbar neuritis			S							
29. Scleromalacia								S	R	

Crystals of the cornea (deposition of crystalline substance in the cornea) Continued

	Cystinosis (i.e., Congenital)	Crystalline Dystrophy of Schnyder	Multiple Myeloma	Bietti Marginal Crystalline Dystrophy	Gout	Drugs (i.e., Chloroquine)	Hyperparathyroidism	Porphyria Cutanea Tarda	Cholesterol Crystals	Infectious Crystalline Keratopathy
Physical Findings										
30. Silverwire or chalky-white arterioles						S				
31. Tumor of orbit			S							
32. Vascular engorgement of retina							S			
33. Vitreous hemorrhage			S							
34. Vogt limbal girdle		S								
35. Xanthelasma		S								
Laboratory Data										
1. Blood hyperviscosity			U							
2. Color vision abnormal						U				
3. Conjunctival biopsy	U								S	
4. Corneal cholesterol		U							U	
5. Electro-oculogram						S	S			
6. Corneal cholesterol		U							U	
7. Corneal scraping										U
8. Electro-oculogram						S	S			
9. Electroretinogram	U					U				
10. Fluorescein angiography	U					U				
11. High porphyria level in urine								U		
12. Hypercalcemia			U				U			
13. Hyperuricemia			S							
14. Hypophosphatemia							U	U		
15. Parathyroid hormone increased							U			
16. Proteinuria			U							
17. Serum lipid elevated									U	
18. Uricemia					U					
19. Visual field abnormal										
(blind spot enlarged and								U		
central scotoma)						U				

R = rarely; S = sometimes; and U = usually.

ANESTHESIA OF THE CORNEA (HYPESTHESIA OR DIMINISHED CORNEAL SENSATION IN TRIGEMINAL DISTRIBUTION)

1. Cornea
   * *A. Cerebellopontine angle tumors
   * B. Congenital
   * C. Corneal dystrophy—granular, lattice, macular, and crystalline
   * D. Dysautonomia
   * *E. Infections, including herpes zoster, herpes simplex, leprosy, and malaria
   * F. Inflammations, including that occurring after electrocautery of Bowman membrane, stromal edema, vascularized scars, congestive glaucoma, exposure keratitis, radiation damage, and vitamin A deficiency
   * G. Trauma, including constant wearing of contact lenses and postoperatively, including cataract extraction and within corneal transplant, following operation for detached retina—from an encircling band or, less frequently, a circumscribed buckle; from refractive surgery
2. Maxillary division
   * A. Congenital
   * B. Facial trauma
   * C. Interruption of trigeminal nerve or gasserian ganglion, including cerebellopontine angle tumor or other space-occupying lesion in the region of the superior orbital fissure
   * D. Maxillary antrum carcinoma
   * E. Neoplasm, foramen rotundum, sphenopterygoid fossa
   * F. Orbital floor fracture
   * G. Perineural spread of skin carcinoma
   * H. Surgery for trigeminal neuralgia
3. Ophthalmic division
   * A. Aneurysm, cavernous sinus
   * B. Neoplasm, cavernous sinus
   * C. Neoplasm, middle fossa
   * D. Neoplasm, orbital apex
   * E. Neoplasm, superior orbital fissure
4. Syndromes and diseases
   * A. Adie syndrome
   * B. Anhidrotic ectodermal dysplasia
   * C. Barré Lieou syndrome (posterior cervical sympathic syndrome)
   * D. Diabetes mellitus—youth onset, more marked with age
   * E. Eaton–Lambert syndrome (myasthenic syndrome)
   * F. Familial corneal hypesthesia
   * G. Foix syndrome (cavernous sinus syndrome)
   * H. Gradenigo syndrome (temporal syndrome)
   * I. Hereditary fleck dystrophy of the cornea
   * J. Herpes zoster
   * K. Hunt syndrome (herpes zoster auricularis)
   * L. Hydroa vacciniforme (lower cornea)
   * M. Multiple sclerosis
   * N. Oculoauriculovertebral dysplasia (Goldenhar–Gorlin syndrome)
   * O. Nephropathic cystinosis

P. Passow syndrome (Bremer status dysraphicus)
Q. Psoriasis (lower cornea)
R. Riley–Day syndrome (congenital familial dysautonomia)
S. Rochon–Duvigneaud syndrome (superior orbital fissure syndrome)
T. Rollet syndrome (orbital apex–sphenoidal syndrome)
U. Scholz subacute cerebral sclerosis (arylsulfatase A deficiency syndrome)
V. Temporal arteritis syndrome (cranial arteritis syndrome)
W. Tolosa–Hunt syndrome (painful ophthalmoplegia)
X. Vitamin A deficiency

5. Toxins and drugs, including oleoresin capsicum (pepper spray)

amiodarone
amitriptyline
amodiaquine
atenolol (?)
betaxolol
bromide
carbon dioxide
carbon disulfide
carisoprodol
chloroquine
clorazepate
desipramine

diazepam
gentamicin (?)
glutethimide
hydrogen sulfide
hydroxychloroquine
imipramine
levobunolol
meprobamate
methyprylon
metoprolol (?)
nadolol (?)
nortriptyline

paraldehyde
phencyclidine
pindolol (?)
propanolol
steladex
trifluoperazine (Stelazine)
timolol
trichloroethylene
vinblastine
vincristine

Fraunfelder FT, Fraunfelder FW. *Drug-induced ocular side effects*. Woburn, MA: Butterworth-Heinemann, 2001.

Glaser JS. *Neuro-ophthalmology*, 2nd ed. Philadelphia: JB Lippincott, 1989.

Katz B, et al. Corneal sensitivity in nephropathic cystinosis. *Am J Ophthalmol* 1987;104:413–416.

Roy FH. *Ocular syndromes and systemic diseases*, 3rd ed. Philadelphia: Lippincott Williams & Wilkins, 2002.

Zollman TM, et al. Clinical effects of oleoresin capsicum (pepper spray) on the human cornea and conjunctiva. *Ophthalmology* 2000;107:2186–2189.

HYPERPLASTIC CORNEAL NERVES

This condition involves overgrowth of corneal nerves up to 20 times the normal number. This nonspecific change may occur in association with the following conditions:

1. Deep filiform dystrophy of Maeder and Danis
*2. Herpes simplex
*3. Herpes zoster
*4. Multiple endocrine neoplasia—type II B
5. Neurofibromatosis (von Recklinghausen syndrome)
6. Neuroparalytic keratitis
7. Normal eyes at advanced age
8. Ocular pemphigus foliaceus (Cazenave disease)
9. Opaque corneal grafts
10. Phthisis bulbi
11. Posterior polymorphous dystrophy

Charlin R. Neoplasia endocrina multiple type II-B. *Arch Chil Oftal* 1981;38:21–27.

Menshen JH. Corneal nerves. *Surv Ophthalmol* 1974;19:1–18.

Roy FH. *Ocular syndromes and systemic diseases*, 3rd ed. Philadelphia: Lippincott Williams & Wilkins, 2002.

* = most important

INCREASED VISIBILITY OF CORNEAL NERVES

1. "Colloidin" skin syndrome (bullous ichthyosiform erythroderma)
2. Congenital
3. Ectodermal dysplasia (Rothmund syndrome)
4. Fuchs dystrophy
5. Ichthyosis
6. Idiopathic
*7. Keratoconus
8. Leprosy (Hansen disease)
9. Neurofibromatosis (von Recklinghausen syndrome)
*10. Neurofibromatosis associated with pheochromocytoma and thyroid carcinoma (Sipple syndrome)
11. Posterior polymorphous dystrophy
12. Primary amyloidosis
13. Refsum syndrome (phytanic acid storage disease)
14. Siemens disease (keratosis follicularis spinulosa decalvans)

Arffa RC. *Grayson's diseases of the cornea*, 3rd ed. St. Louis: Mosby–Year Book, 1991.

Pau H. *Differential diagnosis of eye diseases*, 2nd ed. New York: Thieme Medical, 1988.

Roy FH. *Ocular syndromes and systemic diseases*, 3rd ed. Philadelphia: Lippincott Williams & Wilkins, 2002.

PIGMENTATION OF THE CORNEA

1. Melanin pigmentation
   A. Epithelial melanosis
      (1) Congenital
      (2) Presence of limbal malignant melanoma
      (3) Sequela of trachoma and other inflammations
      (4) Melanocytic migration in heavily pigmented persons
   B. Stromal pigmentation such as that in ochronosis
   C. Endothelial melanosis
      (1) Congenital
      (2) Senile
      (3) Degenerative, including atrophic and inflammatory conditions (such as cornea guttata, herpes simplex, zoster keratitis, myopia, diabetes mellitus, senile cataract, chronic glaucoma, and melanoma)
      *(4) Krukenberg spindle, with or without pigmentary glaucoma, may be present in association with diabetes mellitus
      (5) Trauma—from contusions, wounds, or intraocular operations
      (6) Turks line—fine vertical line in the lower portion of the cornea
2. Hematogenous pigmentation
   *A. Blood staining of the cornea, most often because of total hyphema associated with elevated intraocular pressure
   B. Hemorrhage into cornea—following subconjunctival hemorrhage and intracorneal hemorrhage from newly formed vessels, as in interstitial keratitis or mustard gas keratitis
   C. Epithelial deposit associated with spherocytic anemia
   D. Hemachromatosis
3. Metallic pigmentation

A. Copper (chalcosis)
  *(1) Kayser–Fleischer ring—limbal ring associated with Wilson disease
  (2) Copper foreign body in cornea or intraocular region
  (3) Occupational exposure or topical therapeutic use of copper-containing substance
  (4) Advanced cirrhosis of the liver, such as that associated with parasitic infestation (schistosomiasis)
B. Silver (argyrosis)—from topical, local, or systemic use; also occupational use
C. Gold (chrysiasis)—from topical, local, or systemic use
D. Iron (siderosis)
  (1) Foreign body in cornea or intraocular area
  (2) Iron lines
    *a. Fleischer ring—associated with keratoconus around base of the cone
    b. Hudson–Stähli line—horizontal line at the junction of the middle and lower one third of the cornea, believed to be related to exposure, trauma of lid closure, and chronic corneal infection
    c. Stocker line—line running parallel with head of the pterygium
    d. Ferry line—associated with filtering blebs, believed to result from minute, repeated, localized trauma caused by eyelid striking the elevated bleb
    e. Circular lesion associated with congenital spherocytosis
    f. Iron lines following refractive corneal surgery, such as radial keratotomy and photorefractive keratectomy, and laser in situ keratomileusis (hyperopic and myopic)
E. Bismuth (bismuthiasis)—from therapeutic use
F. Arsenic melanosis
4. Drugs, discoloration, including the following:

acetophenazine
acid bismuth sodium tartrate
alcohol
amiodarone
amodiaquine
antimony potassium tartrate
antimony sodium tartrate
antimony sodium
  thioglycolate
auranofin
aurothioglucose
aurothioglycanide
bismuth carbonate
bismuth oxychloride
bismuth salicylate
bismuth sodium tartrate
bismuth sodium
  thioglycollate
bismuth sodium
  triglycollamate
bismuth subcarbonate
bismuth subsalicylate
butaperazine

calcitriol
carphenazine
chloroquine
chlorpromazine
chlorprothixene
chlortetracycline
colloidal silver
diethazine
echothiophate
epinephrine
ergocalciferol
ethopropazine
ferrocholinate
ferrous fumarate
ferrous gluconate
ferrous succinate
ferrous sulfate
fluphenazine
gold Au 198
gold sodium thiomalate
gold sodium thiosulfate
hydroxychloroquine
indomethacin

iodide
iodine solution
iron dextran
iron sorbitex
meperidine(?)
mercuric oxide
mesoridazine
methdilazine
methotrimeprazine
methylene blue
mild silver protein
perazine
perhexiline
pericyazine
perphenazine
phenylmercuric nitrate
piperacetazine
polysaccharide–iron complex
prazosin
prochlorperazine
promazine
promethazine
propiomazine

* = most important

quinacrine
quinidine
radioactive solution
silver nitrate
silver protein
sodium antimonylgluconate
stibocaptate
stibogluconate

stibophen
tetracycline
thiethylperazine
thimerosal
thiopropazate
thioproperazine
thioridazine
thiothixene

trifluoperazine
triflupromazine
trimeprazine
vitamin A(?)
vitamin D
vitamin D$_2$
vitamin D$_3$

5. Other color changes
   A. White discoloration—scars, fatty degeneration or infiltration, calcified areas
   B. Yellow, discoloration—hyaline or colloid degeneration, and Tangier disease (familial deficiency of high-density lipoprotein)
   C. Black discoloration—coal powder, dirt, epinephrine, or ink (tattooing)
   D. Yellow–brown discoloration—Kyrle disease (hyperkeratosis follicularis et parafollicularis in cutem penetrans)
   E. Grey–black discoloration—chronic phenol exposure as carbolic acid
   F. Grey–white discoloration—anesthetic cornea
   G. Brown discoloration—aniline (amidobenzole), including benzoquinone and hydroquinine

Brodrick JD. Pigmentation of the cornea. *Ann Ophthalmol* 1979;11:855–861.

Fraunfelder FT, Fraunfelder FW. *Drug-induced ocular side effects*. Woburn, MA: Butterworth-Heinemann, 2001.

Krueger R, et al. Corneal iron line associated with steep central islands after photorefractive keratectomy. *J Refract Surg* 1997;13:401–403.

Lazzaro DR, et al. Corneal findings in hemochromatosis. *Arch Ophthalmol* 1998;116:1531–1532.

Probst LE. Ocular copper deposition associated with benign monoclonal gammopathy and hypercupremia, keratoconus in identical twins. *Cornea* 1996;15,1:94–98.

Probst LE, et al. Pseudo-Fleischer ring after hyperopic laser in situ keratomileusis. *J Cataract Refract Surg* 1999; 25:866–870.

CORNEAL EDEMA

1. Drugs, including the following:

acetophenazine
acetylcholine
alpha-chymotrypsin
amodiaquine
amphotericin B
bacitracin
benoxinate
benzalkonium chloride
benzathine penicillin G
butacaine
butaperazine
carbachol
carphenazine
chloramphenicol
chlorhexidine
chloroquine
chlorpromazine

chlortetracycline
cocaine
colistin
deslanoside
dibucaine
diethazine
digitoxin
digoxin
dyclonine
epinephrine
erythromycin
ethopropazine
fluphenazine
hydrabamine penicillin
hydrogen peroxide
hydroxychloroquine
idoxuridine

idoxuridine (IDU)
lanatoside C
melphalan
mesoridazine
methdilazine
methicillin
methotrimeprazine
neomycin
perazine
pericyazine
perphenazine
phenacaine
phenoxymethyl penicillin
phenylephrine
piperacetazine
piperocaine
polymyxin B

potassium penicillin G
potassium penicillin V
potassium phenethicillin
potassium phenoxymethyl
  penicillin
procaine penicillin G
prochlorperazine
promazine
promethazine
proparacaine

propiomazine
quinacrine
silicone
streptomycin
tetracaine
tetracycline
thiethylperazine
thiopropazate
thioproperazine
thioridazine

thiotepa
trifluoperazine
triflupromazine
trifluridine
trimeprazine
urokinase
vidarabine
vinblastine

2. Endothelial decompensation
  A. Noninflammatory
    *(1) Acute hydrops with keratoconus
    (2) Congenital
        a. Anhidrotic ectodermal dysplasia
       *b. Birth trauma, typically a forceps injury
        c. Congenital glaucoma
        d. Congenital hereditary endothelial dystrophy
        e. Posterior polymorphous dystrophy
    (3) Environmental cold in trigeminal nerve palsy
    (4) Essential corneal edema
    (5) Failed corneal graft
    (6) Metabolic such as myxedema and hypercholesteremia
    (7) Neuropathic conditions
    (8) Postsurgical
        a. Anterior segment ischemia
        b. Anterior synechiae
        c. Direct mechanical damage to endothelium including argon laser iridotomy
        d. Epithelial or fibrous downgrowth
        e. Osmotic, such as irrigation of cornea or anterior chamber with distilled
           water
        f. Plasma gas sterilization
        g. Stripped Descemet membrane
        h. Vitreous touch
    *(9) Primary degenerative—Fuchs dystrophy
    (10) Traumatic
        a. Anoxia of epithelium, such as from excessive wearing of contact lens
           (Sattler veil)
        b. Brown–McLean Syndrome
        c. Chemical, such as tear gas, hydrogen peroxide and Hibiclens
        d. Exposure as in exophthalmos
        e. Large epithelial defect
        f. Nonpenetrating including after air bag inflation injury
        g. Penetrating
        h. Radiation injury such as from ultraviolet, roentgenograms, gamma rays
        i. Retained foreign body-anterior chamber
        j. Sympathectomy including jugular vein catheterization and Parry–Robson
           syndrome
        k. Trigeminal nerve palsy with cold exposure

* = most important

  B. Inflammatory
    (1) Any severe iritis
    (2) Acute graft rejection
    (3) Chandler syndrome (iridocorneal endothelial syndrome)
    *(4) Herpes simplex keratitis or keratouveitis
    *(5) Herpes zoster keratouveitis
    (6) Retinal tacks
3. Increased intraocular pressure
  *A. Acute glaucoma
  B. Chronic glaucoma
    (1) Minimal to moderate pressure elevations in the presence of abnormal endothelium
    (2) Prolonged moderately high elevations in the presence of normal or near-normal endothelium
4. Hypotony

Duffy RE, et al. An epidemic of corneal destruction caused by plasma gas sterilization. *Arch Ophthalmol* 2000; 118:1167–1176.

Fraunfelder FT, Fraunfelder FW. *Drug-induced ocular side effects.* Woburn, MA: Butterworth-Heinemann, 2001.

Herse P, Hooker B. Corneal edema recovery dynamics in diabetes: is the alloxan induced diabetic rabbit a useful model? *Invest Ophthalmol Vis Sci* 1994;35:310–313.

Lesher MP, et al. Corneal edema, hyphema, and angle recession after air bag inflation. *Arch Ophthalmol* 1993;111: 1320–1322.

Mietz H, et al. Acute corneal necrosis after excimer laser keratectomy for hyperopia. *Ophthalmology* 1999;106: 490–497.

Reed JW, et al. Clinical and pathologic findings of aphakic peripheral corneal edema: Brown-McLean syndrome. *Cornea* 1992;11:577–583.

Wilhelmus KR. Corneal edema following argon laser iridotomy. *Ophthalmic Surg Lasers* 1992;23:533–537.

Zamir E, et al. Neurotrophic corneal endothelial failure complicating acute Horner syndrome. *Ophthalmology* 1999; 106:1692–1696.

CORNEAL HYDROPS (RUPTURES OF DESCEMET MEMBRANE WITH CORNEA INTRALAMELLAR DISSECTION AND COLLECTION OF AQUEOUS HUMOR)

1. Congenital glaucoma
2. Forceps injury
*3. Keratoconus
4. Pellucid marginal degeneration
5. Terrien marginal degeneration
6. Trauma, blunt

Soong HK, et al. Corneal hydrops in Terrien's marginal degeneration. *Ophthalmology* 1986;93:340–343.

Taglia DP, Sugar J. Case reports and small case series. *Arch Opthalmol* 1997;115:274–275.

MICROCORNEA (CORNEA WITH A HORIZONTAL DIAMETER OF LESS THAN 10 MM)

1. Associated ocular findings
  A. Aniridia and subluxated lenses
  B. Autosomal-dominant cataract and myopia

C. Autosomal-dominant cataract, nystagmus, and glaucoma
D. Axenfeld syndrome (posterior embryotoxon)
E. Colobomatous microphthalmia
F. Congenital glaucoma
G. Corectopia and macular hypoplasia
H. Hyperopia
I. Meckel syndrome (dysencephalia splanchnocystica syndrome)
J. Nanophthalmos
K. Narrow-angle glaucoma
L. Sclerocornea

2. Aberfeld syndrome (congenital blepharophimosis associated with generalized myopathy)
3. Autosomal recessive or dominant trait
4. Carpenter syndrome (acrocephalopolysyndactyly II)
5. Cataract microcornea syndrome
6. Chromosome partial deletion (long-arm) syndrome
7. Deafness retardation, arched palate syndrome
8. Ehlers–Danlos syndrome (fibrodysplasia elastica generalisata)
9. Gansslen syndrome (familial hemolytic icterus)
10. Hallermann–Streiff syndrome (dyscephalic mandibulooculofacial syndrome)
11. Hemifacial microsomia syndrome (Francois Haustrate syndrome)
12. Hutchinson–Gilford syndrome (progeria)
13. Laurence–Moon–Biedl syndrome (retinitis pigmentosa–polydactylyadiposogenital syndrome)
14. Lenz microphthalmia syndrome
15. Little syndrome (nail patella syndrome)
16. Marchesani syndrome (mesodermal dysmorphodystrophy)
17. Marfan syndrome (arachnodactyly dystrophica mesodermalis congenita)
18. Meckel syndrome (dysencephalia splanchnocystica syndrome)
19. Meyer–Schwickerath–Weyers syndrome (oculodentodigital dysplasia)
20. Microcornea, glaucoma, absent frontal sinuses
21. Micro syndrome
22. Rieger syndrome (hypodontia and iris dysgenesis)
23. Ring chromosome
24. Roberts pseudothalidomide syndrome
25. Rubella syndrome (Gregg syndrome)
26. Sabin–Feldman syndrome
27. Schwartz syndrome (glaucoma associated with retinal detachment)
28. Smith–Magenis syndrome
29. Triploidy
30. Trisomy 13 (D trisomy, Patau syndrome)
31. Trisomy syndrome
32. Waardenburg syndrome (interoculoiridodermatoauditive dysplasia)

Mamdal AK, et al. Roberts pseudothalidomide syndrome. *Arch Ophthalmol* 2000;118:1462–1465.

Mollica F, et al. Autosomal dominant cataract and microcornea associated with myopia in a Sicilian family. *Clin Genet* 1985;28:42–46.

Roy FH. *Ocular syndromes and systemic diseases*, 3rd ed. Philadelphia: Lippincott Williams & Wilkins, 2002.

Warburg M, et al. Autosomal recessive microcephaly, microcornea, congenital cataract, mental retardation, optic atrophy, and hypogenitalism. *Arch Dis Child* 1993;147:1309–1312.

Microcornea

	Ehlers-Danlos Syndrome	Meyer-Schnickerath-Weyers Syndrome	Riegler Syndrome	Azenfeld Syndrome	Laurence-Moon-Biedl Syndrome	Weill-Marchesani Syndrome	Rubella*	Gansslen Syndrome	Hallerman-Strieff Syndrome	Hemifacial Microsomia Syndrome	Trisomy 13-15 (Patau Syndrome)
History											
1. Death during first month											
2. Hereditary											U
3. More in males	U		U	U	U	R		U	U		U
4. Onset in childhood		U			U			U		S	
Physical Findings											
1. Angioid streaks	S										
2. Aniridia											
3. Blue sclera									R		
4. Cataracts									S		
5. Chamber angle iris strands					R	S	U		S	S	S
6. Choroidal/vitreous hemorrhage	S										
7. Coloboma of iris											
8. Corectopia					S					S	S
9. Corneal opacification			U								
10. Ectopia lentis			S	S				S			S
11. Epicanthus	S					S					
12. Exophthalmos	S								S		
13. Glaucoma	S										R
14. Hypertelorism		S	U	U		R	U				
15. Hypoplasia anterior iris stroma				S					S		S
16. Iritis		S	U								
17. Keratoconus						S					
18. Lacrimal duct defects	S				S						
19. Lid skin laxity	S								R		
20. Macular pigment degeneration	S										
21. Microphthalmos	S	S			S	R	S				
22. Microspherophakia						S		S	U	S	S
23. Myopia						S					
24. Nystagmus	S	S			S	S		S			
25. Optic atrophy						S			S		
26. Optic nerve hypoplasia					S						
27. Persistent hyperplastic primary vitreous											R
28. Ptosis											S
29. Pupillary membrane	S				S						
30. Retinal detachment		S							S		
31. Retinal hemorrhage	S						R				
32. Retinitis pigmentosa							S	S			
33. Sclerocornea					S						
34. Soft retinal exudate									R		
35. Strabismus								S			
36. Subretinal neovascularization					S	S	S		S	U	
Laboratory Data											
1. Immunoglobuin M antibody							U				
2. Chromosomal studies											U

R = rarely; S = sometimes; and U = usually.

MEGALOCORNEA (CORNEA WITH A HORIZONTAL DIAMETER OF MORE THAN 14 MM)

1. Aarskog syndrome (faciodigitogenital syndrome)
2. Autosomal dominant or recessive trait
3. Congenital glaucoma (rare)
4. Craniosynostosis
5. Down syndrome
6. Facial hemiatrophy
7. Isolated
8. Marchesani syndrome (brachymorphia with spherophakia)
9. Marfan syndrome (arachnodactyly dystrophia mesodermalis congenita)
10. MMR (megalocornea–mental retardation) syndrome
11. MMMM (megalocornea, macrocephaly, mental and motor retardation) syndrome
12. Mucopolysaccharidoses I-S (Scheie syndrome)
13. Neuhauser syndrome (megalocornea–mental retardation syndrome)
14. Oculocerebrorenal syndrome (Lowe syndrome)
15. Oculodental syndrome (Peter syndrome)
16. Osteogenesis imperfecta (van der Hoeve syndrome)
17. Oxycephaly (dysostosis craniofacial dyostosis)
18. Pierre Robin syndrome (micrognathia–glossoptosis syndrome)
19. Posterior embryotoxon
20. Rieger syndrome (hypodontia and iris syndrome)
21. Rubella syndrome (Gregg syndrome)
22. Sex-linked recessive trait
23. Sturge–Weber syndrome (meningocutaneous syndrome)

Arffa RC. *Grayson's diseases of the cornea*, 3rd ed. St. Louis: Mosby–Year Book, 1991.

Frydman M, et al. Megalocornea, macrocephaly, mental and motor retardation (MMMM). *Clin Genet* 1990;38: 149–154.

Roy FH. *Ocular syndromes and systemic diseases*, 3rd ed. Philadelphia: Lippincott Williams & Wilkins, 2002.

Verloes A, et al. Heterogeneity versus variability in megalocornea-mental retardation (MMR) syndromes: report of new cases and delineation of probable types. *Am J Med Genet* 1993;46:132–137.

Megalocornea (cornea having a horizontal diameter of more than fourteen millimeters)

	Aarksog Syndrome	Autosomal Dominant or Recessive Trait	Congenital Glaucoma	Marfan Syndrome	Scheie Syndrome (Mucopolysaccharidoses I-S)	Lowe Syndrome	Osteogenesis Imperfecta	Posterior Embryotoxon	Rieger Syndrome	Sex-linked Recessive Trait
History										
1. Autosomal dominant trait		U		U			U	U	U	
2. Autosomal recessive trait		S			U					
3. Congenital			U					U		
4. Early childhood			U							
5. Hereditary			U							
6. Night blindness	U	U		U	U	U	U		U	U
7. Sex-linked recessive					U					
8. Tearing	U		S			U				U
Physical Findings										
1. Aniridia of iris										
2. Anisocoria										
3. Anterior displaced Schwalbe line								U	U	
4. Anterior embryotoxon								U	U	
5. Anterior synechiae										U
6. Antimongoloid lid slants (temporal canthus lower)		U								
7. Blepharoptosis	U									
8. Blue sclera										
9. Breaks in Descemet membrane							U			
10. Buphthalmos			U							
11. Cataracts			U			U				
12. Coloboma of iris			U	U	S	U	U			
13. Corneal clouding				R	U	U			S	
14. Corneal epithelial and stromal edema			U							
15. Epicanthal folds		U								
16. Glaucomatous cupping			U							
17. High astigmatism			U		S					
18. Hyperopic astigmatism	S									U
19. Hypertelorism	U									
20. Increased intraocular pressure			U							
21. Iris hypoplasia					S	U	U		U	
22. Keratoconus		S							U	
23. Krukenberg spindle				U						
24. Lens dislocation				U					R	U
25. Malformed anterior chamber angle/iris				U						
26. Microphakia						U				
27. Microphthalmos						U				
28. Myopia						U				
29. Nystagmus			S	U						U
30. Optic atrophy				S		U				
31. Proptosis			S		S			S		
32. Pupillary reaction absent					S					
33. Ring scotoma						U				
34. Spherophakia				U						
35. Strabismus	S			S		U				

Megalocornea (cornea having a horizontal diameter of more than fourteen millimeters)
Continued

	Aarksog Syndrome	Autosomal Dominant or Recessive Trait	Congenital Glaucoma	Marfan Syndrome	Scheie Syndrome (Mucopolysaccharidoses I-S)	Lowe Syndrome	Osteogenesis Imperfecta	Posterior Embryotoxon	Rieger Syndrome	Sex-linked Recessive Trait
Physical Findings										
36. Tapetoretinal degeneration					S					
37. Telecanthus	U									
Laboratory Data										
1. Bone roentgenogram				U			U			
2. Cardiovascular studies				U						
3. Genetic studies	U	U		U	U	U	U		U	U
4. Urine tests										
Aminoaciduria/phosphaturia						U				
Chondroitin sulfate B elevated						U				
Hematuria/proteinuria						U				
5. Visual field test				U	U				S	

R = rarely; S = sometimes; and U = usually.

CORNEAL OPACIFICATION IN INFANCY (SEE CONDITIONS SIMULATING CONGENITAL GLAUCOMA, P. 305)

*1. Birth trauma, such as Descemet membrane rupture
 2. Chromosomal aberrations
  A. Mongolism (Down syndrome)—trisomy 21
  B. Trisomy 13 (Patau syndrome)
 3. Congenital malformations
  A. Amyloidosis (Lubarsch–Pick syndrome)
  B. Anterior chamber cleavage syndromes
   (1) Axenfeld anomaly
   (2) Congenital central anterior synechiae
   (3) Congenital anterior staphyloma
   *(4) Peter anomaly
   (5) Rieger anomaly
  C. Bilateral corneal dermis-like choristomas
  D. Congenital glaucoma
  E. De Barsy syndrome
  *F. Dermoid tumors
  *G. Sclerocornea
  H. Xanthomas
 4. Corneal dystrophy
  *A. Congenital hereditary endothelial dystrophy
  B. Congenital hereditary stromal dystrophy
  C. Posterior polymorphous dystrophy
 5. Idiopathic
 6. Inborn errors of metabolism
  *A. Mucopolysaccharidoses (MPS)
   (1) Hurler syndrome (MPS IN)
   (2) Maroteaux–Lamy syndrome (MPS VI)
   (3) Morquio–Brailsford syndrome (MPS IV)
   (4) Scheie syndrome (MPS IS)
  B. Lowe syndrome (oculocerebrorenal syndrome)
  C. von Gierke disease (glycogen disease)
  D. Corneal lipoidosis—later
  E. Mucolipidosis
   (1) Generalized gangliosidosis (GM1-gangliosidosis I and II)
   (2) ML I (lipomucopolysaccharidosis)
   (3) ML III (pseudo-Hurler polydystrophy)
  F. Riley–Day syndrome (congenital familial dysautonomia)
 7. Inflammatory processes
  A. Corneal ulceration
  B. Herpes simplex and herpes zoster
  C. Interstitial keratitis
  D. Rubella syndrome (German measles)
  E. Savin syndrome

Kolker AE, Hetherington I. *Becker-Shaffer's diagnosis and therapy of glaucoma*, 6th ed. St. Louis: CV Mosby, 1989.

Roy FH. *Ocular syndromes and systemic diseases*, 3rd ed. Philadelphia: Lippincott Williams & Wilkins, 2002.

Topilow HW, et al. Bilateral corneal dermis-like choristomas. *Arch Ophthalmol* 1981;99:1387.

BAND-SHAPED KERATOPATHY

This type of corneal opacification extends horizontally over the cornea, at the level of the Bowman membrane, in the exposed part of the palpebral aperture.

1. Anterior mosaic dystrophy, primary type
    A. Episkopi (sex-linked recessive)
    B. Labrador keratopathy
2. Chemical fume related as mercury vapor or calcium bichromate vapor
3. Cyclosporine as eyedrops
4. De Barsy syndrome
5. Discoid lupus erythematosus
6. Dysproteinemia
7. Gout (hyperuricemia)
8. High levels of visible electromagnetic radiation, such as xenon arc photocoagulation and laser causing acute severe anterior uveitis
9. Hypercalcemia
    A. Excessive vitamin D as with oral intake, Boeck sarcoid with liver involvement, acute osteoporosis, Heerfordt syndrome, and Schaumann syndrome
    B. Hyperparathyroidism
    C. Hypophosphatasia (phosphoethanolaminuria)
    D. Idiopathic hypercalcemia
    E. Milk-alkali syndrome
    F. Paget syndrome (osteitis deformans)
    G. Renal failure, such as that associated with Fanconi syndrome (cystinosis)
10. Ichthyosis vulgaris
*11. Local degenerative diseases, including chronic uveitis, phthisis bulbi, absolute glaucoma, infantile polyarthritis (Still disease), rheumatoid arthritis, interstitial keratitis, Felty syndrome, and juvenile rheumatoid arthritis
12. Long-term miotic therapy
13. Long-term steroid phosphate preparations
14. Progressive facial hemiatrophy (Parry–Romberg syndrome)
15. Rothmund syndrome (ectodermal syndrome)
16. Silicone oil in anterior chamber
17. Traumatic—chronic exposure to irritants, such as mercury fumes, calomel, calcium bichromate vapor, and hair
18. Tuberous sclerosis (Bourneville syndrome)
19. Tumoral calcinosis
20. Viscoat usage
21. Wagner syndrome (hyaloideoretinal degeneration)
22. X-linked recessive ocular dystrophy

Aldave AJ, et al. Congenital corneal opacification in De Barsy syndrome. *Arch Ophthalmol* 2001;119:285–288.

Beekhuis WH, et al. Silicone oil in the anterior chamber of the eye. *Arch Ophthalmol* 1986;104:793.

Feist RM, et al. Transient calcific band-shaped keratopathy associated with increased serum calcium. *Am J Ophthalmol* 1992;113:459–461.

Gutt L, et al. Band keratopathy and calcific lid lesions in tumoral calcinosis. *Arch Ophthalmol* 1988;106:725–726.

Kachi S, et al. Unusual corneal deposit after the topical use of cyclosporine as eyedrops. *Am J Ophthalmol* 2000;130:667–670.

Roy FH. *Ocular syndromes and systemic diseases,* 3rd ed. Philadelphia: Lippincott Williams & Wilkins, 2002.

Schlotzer-Schrehardt U, et al. Corneal stromal calcification after topical steroid-phosphate therapy. *Arch Ophthalmol* 1999;117:1414–1416.

* = most important

CORNEAL KELOIDS

1. Lowe syndrome (oculocerebrorenal syndrome)
2. Trauma, usually with perforation of the iris

Cibis GW, et al. Corneal keloid in Lowe's syndrome. *Arch Ophthalmol* 1982;100:1795.

PUNCTATE KERATITIS OR KERATOPATHY

1. Alimentary disorders
   A. Mouth
      *(1) Dry mouth, as in Sjögren syndrome
      (2) Ulcers, such as primary herpes, ocular cicatricial pemphigoid, and erythema multiforme
   B. Lower alimentary tract
      (1) Ulcerative colitis as in Sjögren disease
      (2) Mild colitis, such as that due to an adenovirus
   C. Stomach
      (1) Indigestion as in Sjögren syndrome and acne rosacea
2. Articular diseases
   A. Psoriasis arthropathica
   B. Reiter disease (polyarthritis enterica)
   C. Riley–Day syndrome (congenital familial dysautonomia)
   D. Sjögren syndrome (secretoinhibitor syndrome)
3. Conjunctival discharge
   A. Mucoid
      (1) Other types of keratoconjunctivitis sicca
      (2) Sjögren disease (secretoinhibitor syndrome)
   B. Mucopurulent (see p. 186)
      (1) Angular blepharoconjunctivitis
      (2) Erythema multiforme (Stevens–Johnson syndrome)
      (3) Gonococcal
      (4) Inclusion conjunctivitis (acute stage)
      (5) Meningococcal
      (6) Reiter disease (polyarthritis enterica)
      (7) Trachoma
      (8) Vernal conjunctivitis
   C. Serous
      (1) Adenovirus
      (2) Herpes simplex
      (3) Herpes zoster
      (4) Inclusion conjunctivitis (later)
      (5) Molluscum contagiosum
      (6) Trachoma (later)
      (7) Warts
4. Conjunctival inflammation
   A. Cicatrizing (see p. 194)
      *(1) Ocular cicatricial pemphigoid
      (2) Chemical burns
      *(3) Erythema multiforme (Stevens–Johnson syndrome)
      (4) Diphtheria

(5) Fuchs–Salzmann–Terrien syndrome (allergic reactions from drugs)

(6) Radiation burns

*(7) Sjögren keratoconjunctivitis sicca

(8) Thermal burns

(9) Trachoma

B. Diffuse catarrhal

(1) Adenovirus

(2) Bacterial conjunctivitis

(3) Erythema multiforme (Stevens–Johnson syndrome)

(4) Onchocerciasis syndrome (river blindness)

(5) Reiter disease (polyarthritis enterica)

(6) Superior limbic keratoconjunctivitis

(7) Vaccinia

C. Follicular (see p. 192, 193)

(1) Adenovirus

(2) Herpes simplex

(3) Herpes zoster

(4) Inclusion conjunctivitis

(5) Molluscum contagiosum

(6) Trachoma

D. Giant papillary, such as in vernal and atopic conjunctivitis, and related to contact users, prosthesis, and exposed sutures

E. Papillary

(1) Sjögren syndrome (secretoinhibitor syndrome)

(2) Trachoma

5. Corneal conditions

A. Deep keratitis, disciform or irregular

*(1) Herpes simplex

(2) Herpes zoster and other viral diseases

(3) Corneal dystrophy (e.g., lattice)

(4) Harlequin syndrome

B. Thinned facets because of previous ulcerative or other lesions

(1) Acne rosacea (ocular rosacea)

(2) Erythema multiforme (Stevens–Johnson syndrome)

(3) Gorlin–Chaudhry–Moss syndrome

(4) Herpes simplex

(5) Sjögren keratoconjunctivitis sicca

C. Vascularization

(1) Acne rosacea (ocular rosacea)

(2) Molluscum contagiosum

(3) Ocular cicatricial pemphigoid

(4) Phlyctenular disease (see p. 214)

(5) Sjögren keratoconjunctivitis sicca

(6) Trachoma

(7) Vaccinia

D. Trauma

(1) Chemical injury

(2) Contact lens related

(3) Foreign body under upper eyelid

* = most important

(4) Mild, such as eye rubbing
(5) Ultraviolet photokeratopathy
    E. Thygeson superficial punctate keratitis (SPK)
6. Diseases of the lids
    A. Dermatitis
        (1) Psoriasis
        (2) Seborrheic blepharitis
    B. Ectropion (see p. 78–79)
        (1) Exposure keratopathy
        (2) Neuroparalytic keratopathy
    C. Folliculitis (see p. 94)
        (1) Blepharitis due to *Demodex folliculorum*
        (2) Seborrheic blepharitis
        (3) Staphylococcal blepharitis
    D. Lid retraction (see p. 62–64)
        (1) Endocrine exophthalmos
       *(2) Exposure keratopathy
    E. Madarosis, such as that associated with leprosy (stiff immobile lids)
    F. Nodules
        (1) Acne rosacea (ocular rosacea)
        (2) Molluscum contagiosum
        (3) Papilloma
        (4) Warts
    G. Trichiasis or entropion with traumatic keratitis
    H. Vesicles or ulcers
        (1) Herpes simplex
        (2) Herpes zoster
        (3) Ocular cicatricial pemphigoid
        (4) Vaccinia
    I. Floppy eyelid syndrome
7. Diseases of the skin associated with punctate keratitis
    A. Acne rosacea (ocular rosacea)
    B. CRST (calcinosis, cutis, Raynaud phenomenon, sclerodactyly, and telangiectasia syndrome (calcinosis)
    C. Erythema multiforme (Stevens–Johnson syndrome)
    D. Follicular hyperkeratosis of the palms and soles
    E. Hypertrichosis
    F. Ichthyosis
    G. Incontinentia pigmenti
    H. Leprosy (Hansen disease)
    I. Melkersson–Rosenthal syndrome (Melkersson idiopathic fibroedema)
    J. Ocular cicatricial pemphigoid
    K. Psoriasis
8. Genitourinary diseases associated with punctate keratitis
    A. Erythema multiforme (Stevens–Johnson syndrome)
    B. Inclusion blennorrhea
    C. Ocular cicatricial pemphigoid
    D. Reiter disease (polyarthritis enterica)
9. Keratitis associated with use of drugs, including the following:

* = most important

acebutolol
acetophenazine
acetyldigitoxin
acyclovir
adenine arabinoside
adrenal cortex injection
aldosterone
alcohol
allopurinol
amantadine
amphotericin B
antazoline
antipyrine
aspirin
atenolol
auranofin
aurothioglucose
aurothioglycanide
bacitracin
benoxinate
benzalkonium
betamethasone
betaxolol
botulinum A toxin
brimonidine tartrate
brinzolamide
brompheniramine
bupivacaine
butacaine
butaperazine
capecitabine
carbimazole
carphenazine
chloramphenicol
chlorambucil
chlorhexidine
chloroform
chloroprocaine
chlorpheniramine
chlorpromazine
chlorprothixene
chlortetracycline
chrysarobin
ciprofloxacin
cocaine
colchicine
cortisone
cyclopentolate

cytarabine
deslanoside
dexamethasone
dexbrompheniramine
dexchlorpheniramine
dextran
dibucaine
diclofenac
diethazine
diethylcarbamazine
digitoxin
digoxin
dimethindene
dipivefrin
dorzolamide
dipivalyl epinephrine (DPE)
dyclonine
emedastine difumarate
emetine
epinephrine
ether
ethopropazine
etidocaine
etretinate
F3T
firaxetine hydrochloride
floxuridine
fluprednisolone
flumethasone
fluorometholone
fluorouracil
fluphenazine
flurbiprofen
fluvoxamine maleate
framycetin
gold sodium thiosulfate
gentamicin
gitalin
gold Au 198
gold sodium thiomalate
guanethidine
hexachlorophene
hydrocortisone
idoxuridine
IDU
indomethacin
iodide and iodine solutions
    and compounds

isoniazid
isotretinoin
labetalol
lanatoside C
levobunolol
lidocaine
medrysone
mepivacaine
mesoridazine
methdilazine
methimazole
methotrexate
methotrimeprazine
methoxsalen
methylprednisolone
methylthiouracil
metipranolol
metoprolol
minoxidil
nadolol
naphazoline
neomycin
niacin
ofloxacin
oral contraceptives
ouabain
oxprenolol
oxyphenbutazone
paramethasone
penicillamine
perazine
pericyazine
perphenazine
phenacaine
pheniramine
phenylbutazone
phenylephrine
pilocarpine
pindolol
piperacetazine
piperocaine
polymyxin B
prednisolone
prilocaine
procaine
propofol
prochlorperazine
promazine

promethazine
proparacaine
propiomazine
propoxycaine
propylthiouracil
quinacrine
radioactive iodides
rubella virus vaccine (live)
smallpox vaccine
sodium salicylate
sulfacetamide
sulfachlorpyridazine
sulfacytine
sulfadiazine
sulfadimethoxine
sulfamerazine
sulfameter
sulfamethazine

sulfamethizole
sulfamethoxazole
sulfamethoxypyridazine
sulfanilamide
sulfaphenazole
sulfapyridine
sulfasalazine
sulfathiazole
sulfisoxazole
sulindac
suramin
tetracaine
tetracycline
tetrahydrozoline
thiethylperazine
thimerosal
thiopropazate
thioproperazine

thioridazine
thiotepa
thiothixene
timolol
tobramycin
trichloroethylene
trifluoperazine
trifluorothymidine
triflupromazine
trimeprazine
trimethoprim
trioxsalen
tripelennamine
triprolidine
tropicamide
vidarabine
vinblastine

10. Limbal conditions associated with punctate keratitis
    A. Focal necrotic lesions
        (1) Herpes simplex
        (2) Phlyctenular disease
        (3) Vaccinia
    B. Follicles
        (1) Acne rosacea (ocular rosacea)
        (2) Herpes simplex
        (3) Inclusion conjunctivitis
        (4) Molluscum contagiosum
        (5) Trachoma
        (6) Other viral infections
    C. Nodules and plaques
        (1) Avitaminosis A (Bitot spots)
        (2) Bowen disease (dyskeratosis)
        (3) Intraepithelial melanoma
        (4) Limbal vernal conjunctivitis
11. Punctate keratitis preceded by lymphadenopathy
    A. Adenovirus
    B. Herpes simplex
    C. Herpes zoster
    D. Inclusion conjunctivitis
    E. Trachoma
    F. Vaccinia
12. Respiratory diseases
    A. Adenovirus infections
    B. Myxovirus infections (influenza, Newcastle disease, mumps)
    C. Recurrent herpes complicating any fever

Ferreira RC, et al. Corneal abnormalities associated with incontinentia pigmenti. *Am J Opthalmol* 1997;123:549–551.

Fraunfelder FT, Fraunfelder FW. *Drug-induced ocular side effects.* Woburn, MA: Butterworth-Heinemann, 2001.

Jones BR. Differential diagnosis of punctate keratitis. *Int Ophthalmol Clin* 1962;2:591–611.

Roy FH. *Ocular syndromes and systemic diseases*, 3rd ed. Philadelphia: Lippincott Williams & Wilkins, 2002.

Sachs R. Corneal complications associated with the use of crack cocaine. *Ophthalmology* 1993;100:187–191.

Yang YF, et al. Epidemic hemorrhagic keratoconjunctivitis. *Am J Ophthalmol* 1975;30:192–197.

MORPHOLOGIC CLASSIFICATION OF PUNCTATE CORNEAL LESIONS (CLASSIFICATION BY ANATOMIC LOCATION)

1. Punctate epithelial erosions—fine, very slightly depressed spots scarcely visible without staining with fluorescein
   - A. Warts
   - B. Artificial—silk keratitis
   - C. Staphylococcal blepharoconjunctivitis (lower cornea)
   - *D. Keratoconjunctivitis sicca (interpalpebral area)
   - *E. Exposure keratitis (interpalpebral area)
   - F. Neuroparalytic keratitis (see p. 246)
   - G. Ocular medications (especially those with preservatives)
   - H. Trichiasis
   - I. Trauma, mild (e.g., eye rubbing)
2. Punctate epithelial keratitis—very small, whitish flecks on the surface of the epithelium
   - A. Fine
     - (1) Scattered—staphylococcal blepharitis; viral keratitis, especially trachoma and molluscum contagiosum, sometimes inclusion conjunctivitis, and not infrequently herpetic keratitis and rubeola and rubella
     - (2) Confluent—keratitis sicca, exposure keratitis, vernal conjunctivitis, topical steroid-induced, and early viral keratitis
   - B. Coarse
     - *(1) Thygeson superficial punctate keratitis (characteristic)
     - (2) Herpes zoster
     - (3) Adenovirus infections
     - (4) Early herpes simplex
     - (5) Acne rosacea (lower cornea)
     - (6) *Encephalitozoon hellum*
   - C. Areolar—spots have enlarged to occupy a large area
     - (1) Herpes simplex
     - (2) Thygeson superficial punctate keratitis
     - (3) Herpes zoster
     - (4) Vaccinia
3. Filamentary keratitis or keratopathy—formation of fine epithelial filaments that are attached at one end
   - *A. Keratoconjunctivitis sicca (frequent)
   - B. Infections, such as that due to adenovirus, herpes, vaccinia, acne rosacea, molluscum contagiosum, rubella, rubeola, and staphylococcus
   - C. Trauma, such as wounds, abrasions, exposure to shortwave diathermy, and prolonged eye patching
   - D. Edema of cornea, such as that due to recurrent erosions or wearing of contact lens
   - E. Sarcoid with infiltration of conjunctiva and lacrimal gland
   - F. Heerfordt syndrome and Mikulicz syndrome
   - G. After irradiation of the lacrimal gland

* = most important

    H. Keratoconus (see p. 288)

    I. Neuropathic keratopathy (anesthesia of cornea, p. 246)

    J. Conjunctival cicatrization, such as that associated with ocular cicatricial pemphigoid, erythema multiforme, ocular psoriasis, and advanced trachoma

    K. Degenerative condition of corneal epithelium, such as in advanced glaucoma

    L. Superior limbic keratoconjunctivitis

    M. Hereditary hemorrhagic telangiectasis (Rendu–Osler–Weber disease)

    N. Aerosol keratitis

    O. Diabetes mellitus

    P. Ectodermal dysplasia

    Q. Following cataract or corneal transplant surgery

    R. Following patching

    S. Use of diphenhydramine hydrochloride (Benadryl)

    T. Idiopathic

4. Punctate subepithelial keratitis—punctate epithelial keratitis may progress to combine epithelial and subepithelial lesions followed by healing of the epithelial component, leaving a punctate subepithelial keratitis typical of viral punctate keratitis

    A. Areolar or stellate lesions—grayish white

        (1) Herpes simplex (usually)

        (2) Herpes zoster

        (3) Vaccinia

        (4) Infectious mononucleosis

        (5) Epstein–Barr virus infection

        (6) Dimmer keratitis

        (7) Brucellosis

        (8) Onchocerciasis

    B. Fine or medium-sized lesions, typically

        (1) Adenovirus, especially types 3 and 7—grayish white

    C. Yellowish tinge—typical of trachoma, inclusion conjunctivitis, acne rosacea, and marginal "catarrhal infiltrates" associated with staphylococcal blepharitis, *Neisseria* conjunctivitis, and Reiter disease

5. Punctate opacifications of Bowman membrane—gray, homogeneous, thickened spots, often with irregular edges

    A. Salzmann degeneration

    B. Punctate lesion of trachoma, measles, or phlyctenular disease

Jones BR. Differential diagnosis of punctate keratitis. *Int Ophthalmol Clin* 1962;2:591–611.

Diesenhouse MC, et al. Treatment of microsporidial keratoconjunctivitis with topical fumagillin. *Am J Ophthalmol* 1993;115:293–298.

Roy FH. *Ocular syndromes and systemic diseases*, 3rd ed. Philadelphia: Lippincott Williams & Wilkins, 2002.

Seedor JA, et al. Filamentary keratitis associated with diphenhydramine hydrochloride. *Am J Ophthalmol* 1986;101: 376–377.

SICCA KERATITIS (DRY EYE WITH SECONDARY CORNEAL CHANGES)

1. Boeck sarcoid (Schaumann syndrome)
2. Dermatitis herpetiformis
3. Diabetes mellitus (Willis disease)
4. Herpes simplex
5. Lye burns

*6. Ocular cicatricial pemphigoid
7. Polychondritis
*8. Sjögren syndrome (secretoinhibitor syndrome)
9. Trachoma
10. Vitamin A deficiency (xerosis)
11. Stevens–Johnson syndrome

Arffa RC. *Grayson's diseases of the cornea*, 3rd ed. St. Louis: Mosby–Year Book, 1991.

WHITE RINGS OF THE CORNEA (COATS DISEASE)

These rings are made up of a series of tiny white dots that may coalesce at the level of Bowman membrane or just below it.

1. Congenital
2. Trauma
   *A. Foreign body, usually metal
   B. Occupational—in working with limestone, there may be deposition of some of the substance's components, especially calcium oxide, in the cornea
3. Intraocular disease
4. Iron deposition

Miller EM. Genesis of white rings of the cornea. *Am J Ophthalmol* 1966;61:904.

Nevins RC, Elliott JH. White ring of the cornea. *Arch Ophthalmol* 1969;82:457.

DRY SPOTS OF THE CORNEA (PRECORNEAL TEAR FILM DRYING IN SPOT-WISE FASHION)

The precorneal tear film is best examined by using fluorescein and cobalt-blue filtered light. Patients may have difficulty wearing contact lenses or may have corneal pain. Normal tear-film breakup time is greater than seconds and averages 25 to 30 seconds.

1. Associated with corneal dellen (see p. 280)
2. Chemical burns
3. Chronic bacterial or viral conjunctivitis
4. Congenital alacrima
5. Instillation of topical anesthetic
*6. Keratitis sicca
*7. Ocular cicatricial pemphigoid
8. Ocular pemphigus (chronic cicatricial conjunctivitis)
9. Sleep apnea syndrome
10. Sometimes in elderly persons without obvious pathology
11. Stevens–Johnson syndrome (erythema multiforme)
12. Vitamin A deficiency

Dohlman CH. The function of the corneal epithelium in health and disease. *Invest Ophthalmol* 1971;10:376–407.

Lemp MA, Hamill JR. Factors affecting tear film break-up in normal eyes. *Arch Ophthalmol* 1973;89:103–105.

Mojon DS, et al. Eyelid, conjunctival and corneal findings in sleep apnea syndrome. *Ophthalmology* 1999;106: 1182–1185.

ANTERIOR EMBRYOTOXON (ARCUS)

In this condition, white or gray substance is deposited at level of the Descemet membrane and Bowman membrane initially and then in the stroma with a clear limbal interval.

* = most important

*1. Age—may be present normally in a white patient older than 40 years of age or in a black patient older than 35 years of age
 2. Alagille syndrome
 3. Alport syndrome (hereditary nephritis)
 4. Associated with corneal disease, such as interstitial keratitis
*5. Contralateral carotid occlusive disease–when unilateral
 6. Familial hypercholesterolemia (type II, familial beta-lipoproteins and type III, familial hyper-beta and pre-beta lipoproteins [carbohydrate-induced hyperlipemia])
 7. Hereditary—autosomal dominant or autosomal recessive inheritance
 8. Isolated phenomenon
 9. Long exposure to irritating dust or chemicals
 10. Ocular anomaly association, such as blue sclera (see p. 231), megalocornea (see p. 255), or aniridia (see p. 364–365)
 11. Secondary to ocular disease, such as large corneal scars, sclerokeratitis, limbal dermoid, nevus, or epithelial cyst
 12. Schnyder crystalline dystrophy

Bagla SK, Golden RL. Unilateral arcus corneae senilis and carotid occlusive disease. *JAMA* 1975;233:450.

Chavis RM, Groshong T. Corneal arcus in Alport's syndrome. *Am J Ophthalmol* 1973;75:793–794.

Hingorani M, et al. Ocular abnormalities in Alagille syndrome. *Ophthalmology* 1999;106:330–337.

BOWMAN MEMBRANE FOLDS

 1. Bullous keratopathy
 2. Idiopathic
 3. Inflammation
 4. Lowering of intraocular pressure, such as occurs in association with phthisis bulbi

Duke-Elder S, Leigh AG. Diseases of the outer eye. *System of ophthalmology, Vol VIII, Part 2.* St. Louis: CV Mosby, 1965.

* = most important

Anterior corneal abnormalities

	Fabry Disease	Messman Dystrophy	Reis-Buckler Dystrophy	Drug-induced Cornea Vascularization	Post-traumatic Recurrent Erosion	Map-Dot Fingerprint Dystrophy
History						
1. Asymptomatic female carrier	U					
2. Bilateral	U	U	U	U		U
3. Common in adults					S	U
4. Common in women						U
5. Familial	S	U	U			S
6. Hereditary	S	U	U			S
7. History of corneal injury from fingernails, paper, photocoagulation or vitrectomy					U	
8. Ocular pain				S	U	R
9. Onset, first decade		U	U			
10. Patient taking chloroquine, amiodarone, phenotidzine, or indomethacin				U		
11. Photophobia		U	U		U	R
12. Recurrent erosions		R	U		U	S
Physical Findings						
1. Corneal bullae					S	
2. Corneal clouding			S			
3. Corneal irregularity		S	S		S	S
4. Decreased corneal sensation		R	S			
5. Diffuse opacities are geographic in nature at level of Bowman layer with peak-like projections into the epithelial layer			U			
6. Dot-like opacities, as gray-white intraepithelial opacities (round, oblong, or comma shaped)					S	U
7. Epithelial filament formation					U	S
8. Epithelial loss					U	S
9. Epithelial microcysts					U	U
10. Fingerprint lesions are concentric contoured lines						U
11. Fingerprints are formed by subepithelial sheets						U
12. Foreign body sensation					U	R
13. Gray-white interlacing lines resembling the architecture of a map or diffuse gray patches						S
14. Dendritiform lesions of cornea					S	
15. Lack of adherence of sheets of epithelium					U	S
16. Lacrimation			U	S	U	R
17. Pigmented whorl-shaped lines travel in the epithelial and superficial subepithelial tissue	U			U		
18. Small bleb-like lesions in epithelium appears as small white-gray punctate opcities diffusely distributed over corneal surface		U				
19. Subepithelial scarring				S	U	U
20. Superficial reticulated gray-white opacities and epithelial defects				U		
21. Superficial pseudomicrocysts						U
22. Visual acuity decreased with lesion in pupil				S	U	R

R = rarely; S = sometimes; and U = usually.

DELAYED CORNEAL WOUND HEALING

Delayed corneal wound healing because of drugs, including the following:

adenine	desoxycorticosterone	methylprednisolone
adrenal cortex injection	dexamethasone	paramethasone
aldosterone	dibucaine	penicillamine(?)
alpha chymotrypsin(?)	dyclonine	phenacaine
amphotericin B	F3T	phenylephrine(?)
arabinoside	floxuridine	piperocaine
azathioprine	fludrocortisone	prednisolone
bacitracin	fluorometholone	prednisone
beclomethasone	fluprednisolone	proparacaine
benoxinate	flurbiprofen	sulfacetamide
benzalkonium	fluorouracil	sulfamethizole
betamethasone	ganciclovir	sulfisoxazole
butacaine	gentamicin	tetracaine
chymotrypsin (?)	hydrocortisone	thiotepa
cocaine	idoxuridine	triamcinolone
colchicine	iodine solution	trifluorothymidine
cortisone	medrysone	trifluridine
cytarabine	meprednisone	vidarabine

Fraunfelder FT, Fraunfelder FW. *Drug-induced ocular side effects.* Woburn, MA: Butterworth-Heinemann, 2001.

ANTERIOR CORNEAL MOSAIC

A pattern of fluorescein pooling in corneal epithelial grooves can be induced in any normal eye by pressure on the cornea.
1. Exophthalmos as in dysthyroid eye disease with corneal compression against the eyelids
2. Exposure to a high-pressure fire extinguisher jet
3. Pressure on the cornea, either directly on the cornea or indirectly through the lids

Bron AJ. Anterior corneal mosaic. *Br J Ophthalmol* 1968;52:659.

Frazer DG, et al. Compression keratopathy. *Am J Ophthalmol* 1986;102:208–210.

LINEAR OPACITY IN SUPERFICIAL CORNEAL STROMA

1. Arc-like at superior limbus
    A. Poorly fit contact lens
    B. Well-fitting soft contact lens with tight eyelids
2. Central
    A. Amiodarone
    B. Chloroquine and hydroxychloroquine
    C. Microcystic epithelial dystrophy
    D. Phenothiazine

Arffa RC. *Grayson's diseases of the cornea*, 3rd ed. St. Louis: Mosby–Year Book, 1991.

Charles NC, et al. Band-shaped and whorled microcystic dystrophy of the corneal epithelium. *Ophthalmology* 2000; 107:1761–1764.

Horowitz GS, et al. An unusual corneal complication of soft contact lens. *Am J Ophthalmol* 1985;100:794–797.

SUPERFICIAL VERTICAL CORNEAL STRIATIONS—EPITHELIAL WRINKLES CAN BE ACCENTUATED WITH FLUORESCEIN

1. Corneal surgery with corneal indentation or low intraocular pressure
2. Graves disease
3. Scarred lids
4. Soft contact lens

Blue PW, Lapiana FG. Superficial vertical corneal striations: a new eye sign of Graves' disease. *Ann Ophthalmol* 1980;12:635.

Mobilia EF, et al. Corneal wrinkling induced by ultra-thin soft contact lenses. *Ann Ophthalmol* 1980;12:371.

DENDRITIC CORNEAL LESIONS (AREA OF STAINING OF CORNEA IN A BRANCHING PATTERN)

*1. Corneal erosions, in which the epithelium may become loose
*2. Herpes simplex
*3. Herpes zoster
 4. Use of soft contact lenses
*5. Acanthamoeba keratitis
 6. Latanoprost

Linquist TD, et al. Clinical signs and medical therapy of early acanthamoeba keratitis. *Arch Ophthalmol* 1988;106:73–76.

Margulies LJ, Mannis M. Dendritic corneal lesions associated with soft contact lenses wear. *Arch Ophthalmol* 1983;101:1551–1553.

Sudesh S, et al. Corneal toxicity associated with latanoprost. *Arch Ophthalmol* 1999;117:539–540.

BULLOUS KERATOPATHY (TERMINAL STAGES OF SEVERE OR PROLONGED EPITHELIAL EDEMA SECONDARY TO ENDOTHELIAL DAMAGE)

1. Anterior–posterior corneal incisions for myopia
2. Anterior synechiae
3. Associated with progressive facial hemiatrophy (Parry–Romberg syndrome)
4. Birth trauma (forceps injury)
5. Chronic uveitis, especially herpes simplex or herpes zoster
6. Congenital corneal dystrophy
7. Congenital glaucoma
8. Congenital hereditary endothelial dystrophy
9. Corneal hydrops (acute keratoconus)
10. Epithelial downgrowth
*11. Following cataract surgery with or without intraocular implantation
12. Following perforating wounds, especially when the lens capsule or vitreous is adherent to the cornea
*13. Fuchs epithelial–endothelial dystrophy
14. Immunologic reaction after keratoplasty or endothelial decompensation
15. Iridocorneal endothelial syndrome
16. Long-standing glaucoma
17. Posterior polymorphous dystrophy
18. Prolonged inflammation of corneal stroma, such as in disciform or interstitial keratitis (rare)

* = most important

19. Silicone oil in anterior chamber

Deekhuis WH, et al. Silicone oil in the anterior chamber of the eye. *Arch Ophthalmol* 1986;104:793.

Grayson M, Pieroni D. Progressive facial hemiatrophy with bullous and band-shaped keratopathy. *Am J Ophthalmol* 1970;70:42–44.

Yamaguchi T, et al. Bullous keratopathy after anterior posterior radial keratotomy for myopia and myopic astigmatism. *Am J Ophthalmol* 1982;93:600–606.

NUMMULAR KERATITIS (COIN-SHAPED LESIONS OF CORNEA)

1. Brucellosis
2. Dimmers nummular keratitis
3. Epidemic keratoconjunctivitis
4. Herpes zoster
5. Infectious mononucleosis—Epstein–Barr virus
6. Onchocerciasis (River blindness)
7. Varicella
8. Herpes simplex

Arffa RC. *Grayson's diseases of the cornea*, 3rd ed. St. Louis: Mosby–Year Book, 1991.

Pau H. *Differential diagnosis of eye diseases*, 2nd ed. New York: Thieme Medical, 1988.

DEEP KERATITIS

1. Behçet disease (dermatostomatoophthalmic syndrome)
2. Deep pustular keratitis
3. Disciform keratitis
4. Herpes zoster
5. Keratitis profunda
6. Stromal herpes
7. Vaccinia
8. Varicella

Arffa RC. *Grayson's diseases of the cornea*, 3rd ed. St. Louis: Mosby–Year Book, 1991.

INTERSTITIAL KERATITIS (CORNEAL STROMAL INFLAMMATION, NOT PRIMARILY ON ANTERIOR OR POSTERIOR SURFACES OF STROMA)

1. After burns
    A. Acid
    B. Alkali
2. Deep punctate
    A. Influenza
    B. Local trauma
    C. Mumps
    *D. Ophthalmic zoster
*3. Luetic (syphilis)
4. Nonluetic
    A. Acanthamoeba
    B. rosacea (ocular rosacea)
    C. Brucellosis (Bang disease)
    D. Cogan I syndrome (nonsyphilitic interstitial keratitis)

* = most important

    E. Epstein–Barr
    F. Filariasis
    G. Herpes simplex
    H. Hodgkin disease (lymph node disease)
    I. *Leishmania* species
    J. Measles
    K. Microsporida
    L. Mycosis fungoides
    M. Mumps
    N. Onchocerciasis
    O. Recurrent fever
    P. Roberts pseudothalidomide syndrome
    Q. Sarcoidosis (Schaumann syndrome)
    R. Sleeping sickness (von Economo syndrome)
    S. Steroid therapy
    T. Topical anesthetic abuse
    U. Trypanosomiasis
    V. Tuberculosis (scrofulous keratitis)
    W. Viral as metaherpetic keratitis
    X. Corneal opacification after forceps delivery
    Y. Human T-lymphotropic virus
5. Sclerosing keratitis
    A. Scleritis
        (1) Foci or some local process
        (2) Hennebert syndrome (luetic otitic nystagmus syndrome)
        (3) Sarcoidosis syndrome (Schaumann syndrome)
        (4) Syphilis (acquired lues)
        (5) Tuberculosis
    B. Sclerocornea
    C. Brawny (gelatinous) scleritis
6. With chemical poisons
    A. Arsenic
    B. Gold
7. With corneal ring abscess
    A. Anterior segment necrosis
        (1) After circular diathermy
        (2) After a ''string'' encircling procedure for retinal detachment
        (3) After multiple extraocular muscle surgery
    B. *Bacillus subtilis*
    C. *Bacterium pyocyaneum*
    D. Pneumococci
    E. *Proteus* species
8. With skin disease
    A. Herpes zoster
    B. Incontinentia pigmenti (Bloch–Sulzberger syndrome)
    C. Lichen planus
    D. Molluscum contagiosum
    E. Palmoplantar keratosis

    F. Pityriasis rubra pilaris
    G. Psoriasis

Arffa RC. *Grayson's diseases of the cornea*, 3rd ed. St. Louis: Mosby–Year Book, 1991.

Mandal AK, et al. Roberts pseudothalidomide syndrome. *Arch Ophthalmol* 2000;312–314.

Merle H, et al. A description of human T-lymphotropic virus type I–related chronic interstial keratitis in 20 patients. *Am J Ophthalmol* 2001;131:305–308.

Roy FH. *Ocular syndromes and systemic diseases*, 3rd ed. Philadelphia: Lippincott Williams & Wilkins, 2002.

PANNUS (SUPERFICIAL VASCULAR INVASION CONFINED TO A SEGMENT OF THE CORNEA OR EXTENDING AROUND THE ENTIRE LIMBUS)

 *1. Acne rosacea
 *2. Allergic marginal infiltration
 *3. Anoxic contact lens overwear syndrome
  4. Ariboflavinosis keratopathy
 *5. Contact lens usage
  6. Deerfly fever (tularemia)
  7. Degenerative-blind degenerative eyes; often associated with bullous keratopathy
  8. Dermatitis herpetiformis (Duhring–Brocq disease)
  9. Drugs including the following:

benoxinate	ibuprofen	proparacaine
benzalkonium	idoxuridine	silicone
butacaine	IDU	tetracaine
chlorhexidine	iodine solution	thimerosal
cocaine	oxyphenbutazone	trifluridine
dibucaine	phenacaine	urokinase(?)
dyclonine	phenylbutazone	vidarabine
F3T	piperocaine	

 10. Fuchs corneal dystrophy (degenerative pannus)
 11. Glaucoma (degenerative pannus)
 12. *Haemophilus influenzae*
 13. Histiocytosis X (Hand–Schüller–Christian syndrome)
 14. Hypoparathyroidism
 15. Inclusion conjunctivitis in infants and adults (micropannus) (chlamydia)
 16. Keratoconjunctivitis sicca
 17. Leishmaniasis
 18. Leprosy (Hansen disease)
 19. Linear nevus sebaceous of Jadassohn
 20. Lyell disease (toxic epidermal necrolysis or scalded skin syndrome)
 21. Lymphopathia venereum
 22. Molluscum contagiosum
 23. Ocular cicatricial pemphigoid
 24. Onchocerciasis (river blindness)
 25. Papilloma (wart)
 26. Pellagra (avitaminosis B_{12})
 27. Pemphigus foliaceus (Cazenave disease)
 28. Phlyctenular keratoconjunctivitis (see p. 280)
 29. Siemens disease (keratosis follicularis spinulosa decalvans)

*30. Staphylococcal keratoconjunctivitis (micropannus)
 31. Stevens–Johnson syndrome (mucocutaneous ocular syndrome)
*32. Superior limbic keratoconjunctivitis (micropannus)
 33. Terrien disease (senile marginal atrophy)
 34. Trachoma
 35. Tuberculosis
 36. Vaccinia
 37. Vernal conjunctivitis (micropannus)
 38. Vitamin B_{12} deficiency (Addison pernicious anemia syndrome)

Arffa RC. *Grayson's diseases of the cornea*, 3rd ed. St. Louis: Mosby–Year Book, 1991.

Dixon WS, Bron AJ. Fluorescein angiographic demonstration of corneal vascularization in contact lens wearers. *Am J Ophthalmol* 1973;75:1010–1015.

Fraunfelder FT, Fraunfelder FW. *Drug-induced ocular side effects*. Woburn, MA: Butterworth-Heinemann, 2001.

Roy FH. *Ocular syndromes and systemic diseases*, 3rd ed. Philadelphia: Lippincott Williams & Wilkins, 2002.

* = most important

Pannus (superficial invasion of blood vessels confined to segment of cornea or extending around limbus)

	Trachoma	Leprosy	Phlyctenular Keratoconjunctivitis	Acne Rosacea	Molluscum Contagiosum	Vernal Conjunctivitis	Contact Lens Use	Inclusion Conjunctivitis	Superior Limbic Keratoconjunctivitis	Fuchs Dystrophy	Glaucoma	Staphylococcal Keratoconjunctivitis	Hypoparathyroidism	Keratoconjunctivitis Sicca
History														
1. All age groups									U			U	S	
2. Allergic ocular disease			U			U								
3. Bilateral	U	U		S	S	U		U	U	U	U	U		U
4. Chronic skin disorder			U	U										
5. Common in children/young adults			U		S	U								
6. Common in females			U	U						U				U
7. Common in newborns								U						
8. Congenital											S			
9. Familial										U	U			
10. Hereditary										U				
11. More than 30 to 50 years old				U						U				
12. Ocular pain			U						U	S				S
13. Photophobia			U			U							U	
14. Poor sanitation and medical care	U	S												
15. Pruritis			U									S		S
Physical Findings														
1. Anisocoria		S												
2. Blepharospasm		U	U						U				S	
3. Bullous keratopathy										U				
4. Cataract										S	S		S	
5. Chalazion				U								U		
6. Chronic blepharoconjunctivitis			U	U								U		S
7. Chronic keratoconjunctivitis	U						U							
8. Closed anterior chamber angle											U			
9. Conjunctival follicies/papillae		U				U	U							
10. Conjunctival nodules			U									U	U	
11. Conjunctival Tranta spots						U								
12. Conjunctival ulcers			U									S		
13. Conjunctival vegetations onto cornea						S								
14. Conjunctivitis, cicatricial	U													
15. Conjunctivitis, follicular								U						
16. Conjunctivitis, mucopurulent												U		
17. Conjunctivitis, mucous						U			U					U
18. Corneal abscess												S		
19. Corneal cicatrization				R						U				
20. Corneal edema							U			U	U			
21. Corneal endothelium degeneration										U				
22. Corneal filaments										S				U
23. Corneal hypesthesia											U			
24. Corneal infiltration								U						
25. Corneal nodules			S										U	
26. Corneal opacities	U	U	S					U	S					
27. Corneal perforation				R										R

Pannus (superficial invasion of blood vessels confined to segment of cornea or extending around limbus) Continued

	Trachoma	Leprosy	Phlyctenular Keratoconjunctivitis	Acne Rosacea	Molluscum Contagiosum	Vernal Conjunctivitis	Contact Lens Use	Inclusion Conjunctivitis	Superior Limbic Keratoconjunctivitis	Fuchs Dystrophy	Glaucoma	Staphylococcal Keratoconjunctivitis	Hypoparathyroidism	Keratoconjunctivitis Sicca
Physical Findings														
28. Corneal phlyctenules			U									S		
29. Corneal plaques						U								S
30. Corneal thinning				S								S		S
31. Corneal ulcer			S	S			S	R				S		S
32. Dacryocystitis		S												
33. Decreased intraocular pressure		S												
34. Decreased tear secretion									S					U
35. Entropion	U													
36. Epiphora	U		U		U	U	U		U					
37. Episcleritis		S			U									
38. Folds in Descemet membrane										U	U			
39. Forward displacement of the iris											U			
40. Glaucomatous disc cupping											U			
41. Increased intraocular pressure										S	U			
42. Iris atrophy														
43. Keratitis	U	U	S	S		S		S		S		U	U	U
44. Lagophthalmos		U												
45. Madarosis		U										S	U	
46. Multiple pupils		S												
47. Myopia											U			
48. Optic nerve atrophy													S	
49. Optic neuritis													S	
50. Papilledema														
51. Paralysis of seventh nerve		S												
52. Peripheral anterior synechiae											U			
53. Pigment on posterior corneal surface									S				S	
54. Ptosis	U						S							
55. Punctal occlusion														
56. Uveitis		U								U				
57. Visual field defects														
Laboratory Data														
1. Biopsy of skin (acid fast stain)		U												
2. Calcium diminished in plasma														
3. Chest roentgenogram			R											
4. Conjunctival fluorescent antibody staining	U							S						
5. Conjunctival smears														
Geimsa stain	U					U		U				U		
Gram stain			U											
Hematoxylin-eosin stain					U								U	
6. Phosphate elevated in plasma														
7. Purified protein derivative skin test			R											

R = rarely; S = sometimes; and U = usually.

CORNEAL OPACITY—DIFFUSE

1. Acromesomelic dysplasia
*2. Birth trauma
3. Cockayne syndrome
*4. Congenital hereditary endothelial dystrophy
5. Congenital hereditary stromal dystrophy
6. Cystinosis
7. Fabry syndrome
8. Fetal rubella effects
9. GM gangliosidosis type 1
10. Hurler syndrome
11. Infection
12. Maroteaux–Lamy syndrome
13. Morquio syndrome
14. Mucolipidosis III
15. Mucolipidosis IV
16. Multiple sulfatase deficiency
17. MPS VII
18. Pachyonychia congenita syndrome
19. Pena–Shokeir type II syndrome [cerebrooculofacial–skeletal (COFS) syndrome]
20. Rutherford syndrome
21. Scheie syndrome
*22. Sclerocornea
23. Seip syndrome
24. Sialidosis, Goldberg type
25. Trisomy syndrome
26. 18q syndrome

Isenberg SJ. *The eye in infancy.* Chicago: Year Book Medical, 1989.

Roy FH. *Ocular syndromes and systemic diseases,* 3rd ed. Philadelphia: Lippincott Williams & Wilkins, 2002.

CORNEAL OPACITY—LOCALIZED, CONGENITAL

1. Acromegaloid changes, cutis verticis gyrata, and corneal leukoma
2. Aniridia
3. Autosomal dominant colomba
4. Cataract microcornea syndrome
*5. Dermoid limbal, central, and ring
6. Fetal alcohol syndrome
7. Fetal rubella effects
8. Fetal transfusion syndrome
9. Fucosidosis
10. Group 13—trisomy phenotype
11. Keratoconus posticus circumscriptus
12. Meesman syndrome
13. Peters anomaly and short stature
14. Pilay syndrome (ophthalmomandibulomelic dysplasia)

15. Radial aplasia, anterior chamber cleavage syndrome
16. Richner–Hanhart syndrome
17. Rieger syndrome
18. Trisomy syndrome
19. Waardenburg syndrome
20. Wedge-shaped stromal opacity
21. 4p syndrome
22. 11q syndrome
23. 18q syndrome

Isenberg SJ. *The eye in infancy.* Chicago: Year Book Medical, 1989.

Roy FH. *Ocular syndromes and systemic diseases*, 3rd ed. Philadelphia: Lippincott Williams & Wilkins, 2002.

DEEP CORNEAL STROMAL DEPOSITS

*1. Cornea farinata
 2. Deep filiform dystrophy
 3. Deep punctiform dystrophy associated with ichthyosis
 4. Fleck corneal dystrophy
 5. Gold (chrysiasis)
 6. Lattice corneal dystrophy
 7. Macular corneal dystrophy
 8. Polymorphic amyloid degeneration

Kincaid MC, et al. Ocular chrysiasis. *Arch Ophthalmol* 1982;100:1791.

Mannis MJ, et al. Polymorphic amyloid degeneration of the cornea. *Arch Ophthalmol* 1981;99:1217–1219.

INTRACORNEAL HEMORRHAGE

1. Associated with intraocular surgery
2. Diseases of cornea, such as corneal ulcers and chemical burns
3. Microbial keratitis
4. Migration from subconjunctival hemorrhage
5. Mooren ulceration
6. Ocular trauma
7. Spontaneous in contact lens wearers

Hurwitz BS. Spontaneous intracorneal hemorrhage caused by aphakic contact lens wear. *Ann Ophthalmol* 1981;13:57.

Ormerod LD, Egan KM. Spontaneous hyphaema and corneal haemorrhage as complications of microbial keratitis. *Br J Ophthalmol* 1988;71:933.

Wagoner MD, et al. Intracorneal hematoma in Mooren ulceration. *Am J Ophthalmol* 2000;129:251–253.

CENTRAL POSTERIOR STROMAL CORNEAL DEPOSITS

1. Bence Jones proteinuria
2. Dysproteinemia
3. Filiform corneal dystrophy
4. Immunoglobulin deposition
    A. Abnormal gamma globulin
    B. Benign monoclonal gammopathy

* = most important

5. Multiple myeloma

Barr CC, et al. Corneal crystalline deposits associated with dysproteinemia. *Arch Ophthalmol* 1980;98:884–889.

Yassa NH, et al. Corneal immunoglobulin deposition in the posterior stroma. *Arch Ophthalmol* 1987;105:99–103.

DELLEN

Dellen is characterized by shallow corneal excavation near the limbus, usually on the temporal side; the base of the lesion is hazy and dry.

1. Following the wearing of contact lens
2. In elderly persons—limbal vasosclerosis
3. Lagophthalmos
4. Lengthy administration of cocaine
5. Postcataract section
*6. Swelling of perilimbal tissues
   A. Allergic conjunctival edema
   B. Episcleritis
  *C. Filtering bleb
   D. Limbal tumor
  *E. Postoperative advancement of rectus muscle
   F. Postoperative retinal detachment
   G. Pinguecula
   H. Subconjunctival effusion or injection
7. With hemeralopia

Soong HK, Quigley HA. Dellen associated with filtering blebs. *Arch Ophthalmol* 1983;101:385–387.

PHLYCTENULAR KERATOCONJUNCTIVITIS

This condition is characterized by a localized conjunctival, limbal, or corneal nodule about 1 to 3 mm in size.

*1. Delayed hypersensitivity to bacterial protein, particularly tuberculoprotein and staphylococci; lymphopathia venereum and coccidioidomycosis may also be allergens
2. Malnutrition
3. Secondary infection of the conjunctiva, especially from *Staphylococcus aureus*, pneumococcus, Koch–Weeks bacillus, chlamydia, coccidioidomycosis, and gonorrhea
4. Systemic infection
   A. Bang disease (Brucellosis)
   B. Candidiasis
   C. Neurodermatitis
   D. Mikulicz–Radecki syndrome (dacryosialoadenopathy)
   E. Trachoma
   F. Sjögren syndrome (secretoinhibitor syndrome)

Newell FW. *Ophthalmology, principles and concepts*, 7th ed. St. Louis: CV Mosby, 1991.

CORNEAL RING LESION

1. Acanthamoebic keratitis
2. Associated with rheumatoid arthritis—inferior

3. Associated with Sjögren syndrome (secretoinhibitor syndrome)
4. *Capnocytophaga ochracea*
5. Double-ring formation—allergic keratitis
6. Marginal dystrophy—degenerative chronic corneal lesion with stromal thinning and intact epithelium
7. Marginal ulceration—secondary to massive granuloma of sclera or necrotizing nodular scleritis (see p. 237)
8. Mooren ulcer—deeply undermined central edges and chronic course with inflammation, painful
9. Ring abscess—rapidly destructive purulent lesion in the deepest parts of the cornea
10. Ring ulcer—see marginal corneal ulcers (p. 283–286)
11. Steroid use in furrow dystrophy
12. Terrien marginal degeneration—usually begins superiorly
13. Wegener granulomatosis (Wegener syndrome)

Daut PM, et al. Chronic exposure keratopathy complicating surgical correction of ptosis in patients with chronic progressive external ophthalmoplegia. *Am J Ophthalmol* 2000;130:519–521.

Heidemann DG, et al. Necrotizing keratitis caused by *Capnocytophaga ochracea*. *Am J Ophthalmol* 1988;105: 655–660.

Theodore FH, et al. The diagnostic value of a ring infiltrate in acanthamoebic keratitis. *Ophthalmology* 1985;92: 1471–1480.

CORNEOSCLERAL KERATITIS

1. Boeck sarcoid (Schaumann syndrome)
2. Gout (hyperuricemia)
3. Leprosy (Hansen disease)
4. Infections (e.g., pseudomonas)
5. Malformations, such as in sclerocornea (see p. 301)
6. Sarcoma
7. Syphilis (acquired lues)
8. Trisomy 13 (trisomy D)
9. Tuberculosis
10. Wegener granulomatosis

Arffa RC. *Grayson's diseases of the cornea*, 3rd ed. St. Louis: Mosby–Year Book, 1991.

CENTRAL CORNEAL ULCER

1. Bacterial origin
   *A. *Diplococcus pneumoniae* (pneumococcus)—infiltrated gray–white or yellow disc-shaped central ulcer typically associated with diffuse keratitis, severe iridocyclitis, and hypopyon; follows corneal abrasion; occurs especially in the presence of chronic dacryocystitis; enhanced by general debility
   *B. Beta-hemolytic streptococcus and other streptococcus species
   *C. *Pseudomonas aeruginosa* but may also have *Pseudomonas acidovorans*, *Pseudomonas stutzeri*, Pseudomonas mallei, and *Pseudomonas pseudomallei*—primary corneal involvement, rapid spread often to panophthalmitis, large hypopyon, thick, greenish pus; may be contaminant of eserine and fluorescein often is associated with contact use.

* = most important

    D. *Escherichia coli*
    E. *Moraxella liquefaciens* (diplococcus of Petit)—morphologically resembles diplobacillus of Morax–Axenfeld, which is never seen in central corneal ulcers
    F. *Klebsiella pneumoniae*
    G. *Proteus vulgaris*
    H. Actinomyces
    I. Tuberculous—secondary to conjunctival or uveal infections
    J. *Serratia marcescens*—gram-negative coccobacillus
  *K. *Staphylococcus aureus, S. epidermidis,* and other *Staphylococcus* species
    L. Mima polymorpha
    M. Dysgonic fermenter-2
    N. Others
  2. Viral origin
   *A. Herpes simplex virus
    B. Herpes zoster
    C. Vaccinia virus
    D. Variola
    E. Others
  3. Mycotic origin—follows corneal trauma, such as foreign bodies in the cornea or corneal abrasions caused by vegetable matter, or diseases, such as radiation keratitis, exposure keratitis, herpes zoster, and ocular pemphigus; chronic course; shallow crater; absent corneal vascularization; may follow treatment with antibiotics or, more likely, treatment with steroid–antibiotic combinations
    A. *Absidia corymbifera*
   *B. *Aspergillus* species
    C. *Blastomyces dermatitidis*
   *D. *Candida albicans*
    E. *Cephalosporium* species
   *F. *Fusarium solani*
    G. *Nocardia* species
    H. Others
  4. Acquired immune deficiency syndrome (AIDS) related
  5. Atopic
  6. Basement membrane abnormalities as microcysts, evidence of map, dot fingerprints, or anterior stromal dystrophies, trauma history, other dystrophy
  7. Brittle cornea syndrome
  6. Chemical—latex keratitis, alkali/acid burn
 *8. Dry eyes, including Sjögren syndrome
  9. Exposure as lagophthalmos, lid abnormalities, inadequate blink, facial palsy, proptosis, thyroid disease
10. Extrusion of anterior chamber intraocular lens
11. Factitious
12. Hypogammaglobulinemia
13. Medicamentosus as drops
14. Neurotrophic
15. Thermal/radiation burns
16. Sjögren syndrome
17. Soluble tyrosine aminotransferase (STAT) deficiency

Akpek EK, et al. Bilateral consecutive central corneal perforations associated with hypogammaglobulinemia. *Ophthalmology* 2000;107:123–126.

Alexandrakis G, et al. Capnocytophaga keratitits. *Ophthalmology* 2000;107:1503–1506.

Kiel RJ, et al. Corneal perforation caused by dysgonic fermenter-2. *JAMA* 1987;257:3269–3270.

Marshall DH, et al. Post-traumatic corneal mucormycosis caused by *Absidia corymbifera. Ophthalmology* 1997; 104:1107–1111.

McKnight GT, et al. Transcorneal extrusion of anterior chamber intraocular lenses. *Arch Ophthalmol* 1987;105: 1656–1664.

Roy FH. *Ocular syndromes and systemic diseases*, 3rd ed. Philadelphia: Lippincott Williams & Wilkins, 2002.

Santos C, et al. Bilateral fungal corneal ulcers in a patient with AIDS-related complex. *Am J Ophthalmol* 1986; 102:108–109.

MARGINAL CORNEAL ULCERS

1. Ring ulcers—often bilateral, circumcorneal injection, and continuous ring or confluent multiple lesions
    A. Acute leukemia
    B. Bacillary dysentery
    C. Brucellosis (Bang disease)
    *D. Coalescence of several marginal ulcers
    E. Dengue fever
    F. Gold poisoning
    G. Gonococcal arthritis
    H. Following penetrating keratoplasty
    I. Hookworm infestation
    J. Influenza
    K. Last stages of trachoma, secondary to small circumferential pannus
    *L. Mooren ulcer
    M. Polyarteritis nodosa (Kussmaul disease)
    N. Porphyria
    *O. Rheumatoid arthritis—Sjögren syndrome (secretion inhibitor syndrome)
    P. Scleroderma (progressive systemic sclerosis)
    Q. Systemic lupus erythematosus (Kaposi–Libman–Sacks syndrome)
    R. Tuberculosis
    S. Wegener granulomatosis (Wegener syndrome)
2. Simple marginal ulcers—superficial crescentic gray-colored ulcer
    A. Infection—due to *Staphylococcus* organisms, Koch–Weeks bacillus, pseudomonas, diplobacillus of Morax–Axenfeld; usually chronic
    B. Toxic or allergic including antiinflammatory drugs
    C. Systemic disturbances, such as
        (1) Acute upper respiratory infection
        (2) Bacillary dysentery
        (3) Barre–Lieou syndrome (posterior cervical sympathetic syndrome)
        (4) Brucellosis (Bang disease)
        (5) Crohn disease (granulomatous ileocolitis)
        (6) Gout (hyperuricemia)
        (7) Influenza
        (8) Lupus erythematosus (Kaposi–Libman–Sacks syndrome)
        (9) Polyarteritis nodosa (Kussmaul disease)

* = most important

(10) Postvaccinial ocular syndrome
*(11) Rheumatoid arthritis—inferior cornea

Frueh BE, et al. Mycobacterium szulgai keratitis. *Arch Ophthalmol* 2000;118:1123–1124.

Lin JC, et al. Corneal melting associated with use of topical nonsteroidal anti-inflammatory drugs after ocular surgery. *Arch Ophthalmol* 2000;118:1129–1132.

Mondino BJ, et al. Mooren's ulcer after penetrating keratoplasty. *Am J Ophthalmol* 1987;103:53–56.

Parker AV, et al. Pseudomonas corneal ulcers after artificial fingernail injuries. *Am J Ophthalmol* 1989;107:548–560.

Roy FH. *Ocular syndromes and systemic diseases*, 3rd ed. Philadelphia: Lippincott Williams & Wilkins, 2002.

Marginal corneal ulcers

	Staphylococcus Infection	Gout	Lupus Erythematosus	Rheumatoid Arthritis	Polyarteritis Nodosa	Acute Leukemia	Mooren Ulcer
History							
1. All ages	U						
2. Associated with diabetes	S						
3. Hereditary			U	R			
4. Malignant blood disorder					U	U	
5. More in females					U		
6. More in males						S	
7. Occurs in children					U		
8. Occurs during second to third decades			U				
9. Occurs during third to fourth decades					U		
10. Occurs during fourth to fifth decades							
Physical Findings							
1. Anterior uveitis	S	R	S	S	S		S
2. Band keratopathy				S			
3. Blepharitis	U			S			
4. Cataract				S			
5. Chemosis of conjunctiva	S			S			
6. Conjunctival phlyctenules	U		S				
7. Conjunctivitis	U	U	S	U	S		U
8. Corneal epithelial keratitis	U		S	U	S		U
9. Corneal opacity				S			U
10. Corneal perforation	U						S
11. Corneal vascularization	S		S				S
12. Cotton-wool spots			U	R	S	S	
13. Dacryocystitis	S						
14. Ectropion	S						
15. Endophthalmitis	S						
16. Entropion	S						
17. Episcleritis			S	S			
18. Exophthalmos						R	
19. Hordeolum	U						
20. Hypopyon	S				S	S	
21. Keratoconjunctivitis sicca				S	U	S	
22. Lid edema	S					S	S
23. Macular edema						S	S
24. Madarosis	S						
25. Noncalcific band keratopathy			S				
26. Nystagmus				R			
27. Ocular motor disturbances			R	R	S	S	S
28. Optic nerve atrophy				S		R	S
29. Optic neuritis				S			S
30. Papilledema				U		R	S
31. Ptosis	R			R		R	
32. Retinal detachment							S
33. Retinal hemorrhage				U		U	U

* = most important

Marginal corneal ulcers (Continued)

	Staphylococcus Infection	Gout	Lupus Erythematosus	Rheumatoid Arthritis	Polyarteritis Nodosa	Acute Leukemia	Mooren Ulcer
Physical Findings							
34. Retinal vein occlusion							
35. Scleritis			S		S		
36. Scleromalacia perforans		S	S	S	S	S	S
37. Subconjunctivial nodules					S		
38. Tenonitis					S		
39. Visual field defects		S		S	S		
40. Vitreous opacities			S		R	S	
Laboratory Data							
1. Angiography—retinal							
2. Autoantibodies to nuclear and cytoplasmic constituents					U		
3. Blood tests			U				
Eosinophilia							
Sedimentation rate elevated				S			
Leukocytic count elevated				U	U		S
Neutropenia					U	U	
Normocytic hypochromic anemia				U			
Thrombocytopenia				U	U	U	
4. Conjunctival/corneal exudates for culture/gram stain				S		U	
5. Diminished serum complement levels	U						
6. Electroretinogram abnormalities			S				
7. High uric acid urine/blood		U					
8. Joint changes—roentgenogram		U					
9. Latex agglutination test—rheumatoid factor			U				
10. Lupus erythematosus cell phenomenon			U				
11. Skeletal changes—roentgenogram			S			U	

R = rarely; S = sometimes; and U = usually.

DESCEMET MEMBRANE FOLDS (USUALLY FOLLOWING HYPOTONY; SEE P. 325)

*1. Trauma, such as that due to cataract or corneal surgery
 2. Mechanical cause, such as firm, prolonged ocular bandaging or phthisis bulbi
 3. Inflammatory condition, such as that following interstitial or herpes simplex keratitis
 4. Diabetes (8%–33%)
 5. Ochronosis
 6. Toxic
   A. Quinone and hydroquinone—vertical folds
   B. Formaldehyde 26%
   C. Experimental cold injury to cornea
   D. Digitoxin
 7. Idiopathic

Angell LK, et al. Visual prognosis in patients with ruptures in Descemet's membrane due to forceps injuries. *Arch Ophthalmol* 1981;99:2137.

DESCEMET MEMBRANE TEARS (HAAB STRIAE)

*1. Acute hydrops of the cornea, such as that due to keratoconus (see p. 288)
*2. Buphthalmos (e.g., from congenital glaucoma)
 3. Conical cornea
 4. Myopia with marked anteroposterior diameter
*5. Trauma, such as birth injury or contusion

Angell LK, et al. Visual prognosis in patients with ruptures in Descemet's membrane due to forceps injuries. *Arch Ophthalmol* 1981;99:2137.

Cibis GW, Tripathi RC. The differential diagnosis of Descemet's tears (Haab's striae) and posterior polymorphous dystrophy bands. *Ophthalmology* 1982;89:614.

DESCEMET MEMBRANE THICKENING

*1. Central cornea guttata
   A. Primary
   B. Secondary cornea guttata
     *(1) Congenital luetic interstitial keratitis
      (2) Endothelial cell insult
         a. Breaks in Descemet membrane, including scrolls of Descemet membrane in healed syphilitic interstitial keratitis
         b. Chandler syndrome (iridocorneal endothelial syndrome)
         c. Cogan–Reese syndrome (iris–nevus syndrome)
        *d. Corneal dystrophy, including Fuchs syndrome
         e. Posterior keratoconus syndrome
   C. Transient cornea guttata associated with short-term episodes of iritis and corneal inflammation
 2. Peripheral Hassall Henle warts

Alvarado JA, et al. Pathogenesis of Chandler's syndrome, essential iris atrophy, and the Cogan-Reese syndrome. *Invest Ophthalmol Vis Sci* 1986;27:873–882.

* = most important

Rodrigues MM, et al. Fuchs' corneal dystrophy: a clinicopathologic study of the variation in corneal edema. *Ophthalmology* 1986;98:789–796.

Scattergood KD, et al. Scrolls of Descemet's membrane in healed syphilitic interstitial keratitis. *Ophthalmology* 1983;90:1518–1523.

RETROCORNEAL PIGMENTATION

1. Endothelial phagocytosis of free melanin pigment, such as Krukenberg spindle
2. Iris melanocytes, iris pigment epithelial cells, or pigment containing macrophages in the posterior corneal surface; can follow operative or accidental ocular trauma
3. Status post hyphema

Snip RC, et al. Posterior corneal pigmentation and fibrous proliferation by iris melanocytes. *Arch Ophthalmol* 1981; 99:1232.

LOW ENDOTHELIAL CELL COUNT (DIMINISHED NUMBER OF CORNEAL ENDOTHELIAL CELLS)

1. Acute and chronic uveitis
*2. Corneal endothelial dystrophy
3. Following cataract or other intraocular surgery
4. Cornea guttata, endothelial dystrophy, and Fuch dystrophy

Olsen T. Changes in the corneal endothelium after acute anterior uveitis as seen with the specular microscope. *Acta Ophthalmol Scand* 1980;58:250.

Murrell WJ, et al. The corneal endothelium and central corneal thickness in pigmentary dispersion syndrome. *Arch Ophthalmol* 1986;104:845–846.

SNAIL TRACKS OF CORNEA

This condition involves irregular, discontinuous grayish white streaks or patches, usually orientated horizontally and obliquely on the corneal endothelium.
1. Corneal buttons preserved in corneal storage medium
2. Following ocular surgery
3. Ocular trauma

Alfonso E, et al. Snail tracks of the corneal endothelium. *Ophthalmology* 1986;99:344–349.

KERATOCONUS (CONICAL CORNEA)

Keratoconus is characterized by noninflammatory ectasia of the cornea in its axial part, with considerable visual impairment because of development of a high degree of irregular myopic astigmatism. Keratoconus may be associated with
1. Acute hydrops of the cornea
2. Alagille syndrome
3. Anetoderma and bilateral subcapsular cataracts
4. Angelman syndrome
5. Aniridia
6. Apert syndrome (acrodysplasia)
7. Asthma, hay fever
*8. Atopic dermatitis, keratosis plantaris, and palmaris
9. Autographism
10. Avellino dystrophy

11. Blue sclerotics, including van der Hoeve syndrome (osteogenesis imperfecta) (see blue sclera, p. 231)
12. Chandler syndrome (iridocorneal endothelial syndrome)
13. Congenital hip dysplasia
14. Wearing of contact lens
15. Crouzon syndrome
16. Deep filiform corneal dystrophy
17. Ehlers–Danlos syndrome (fibrodysplasia elastica generalisata, cutis hyperelastica)
18. Essential iris atrophy
19. Facial hemiatrophy
*20. Familial
21. False chordae tendineae of left ventricle
22. Fleck corneal dystrophy
23. Focal dermal hypoplasia (Goltz syndrome)
24. Fuchs corneal endothelial dystrophy
25. Grönblad–Strandberg syndrome (pseudoxanthoma elasticum)
26. Hereditary history
27. Hyperextensible joints and mitral valve prolapse
28. Hyperornithemia
29. Infantile tapetoretinal degeneration of Leber
30. Iridocorneal dysgenesis
31. Iridoschisis
32. Joint hypermobility
33. Kurz syndrome
34. Laurence–Moon–Biedl syndrome (retinitis–polydactyly–adiposogenital syndrome)
35. Little syndrome (nail–patella syndrome)
36. Lymphogranuloma venereum
37. Marfan syndrome (arachnodactyly dystrophia mesodermalis congenita)
38. Measles retinopathy
39. Microcornea
40. Mongolism (Down syndrome)
41. Mulvihil–Smith syndrome
42. Neurocutaneous angiomatosis
43. Neurodermatitis
44. Neurofibromatosis (von Recklinghausen syndrome)
45. Noonan syndrome (male Turner syndrome)
46. Ocular hypertension
47. Pellucid marginal corneal degeneration
48. Posterior ectasia following laser in situ keratomileusis (generally if stromal bed less than 250 μ)
49. Posterior lenticonus
50. Posterior polymorphous dystrophy
51. Retinal disinsertion syndrome
52. Retinitis pigmentosa
53. Retinopathy of prematurity
54. Rieger syndrome
55. Tourette disease
56. Thalassemia syndrome
*57. Trauma, such as rubbing of eyes, birth injury, or contusion

* = most important

58. Vernal catarrh
59. Vernal conjunctivitis
60. 18q syndrome

Geggel HS, Talley AR. Delayed onset keratectasia following laser in situ keratomileusis. *J Cataract Refract Surg* 1999;25:582–586.

Krachner JH, et al. Keratoconus and related noninflammatory corneal thinning disorders. *Surv Ophthalmol* 1984; 28:293–322.

Lipman RM, et al. Keratoconus and Fuchs' corneal endothelial dystrophy in a patient and her family. *Arch Ophthalmol* 1990;108:993–994.

Rabinowitz YS. Keratoconus. *Surv Ophthalmol* 1998;42:297–319.

Roy FH. *Ocular syndromes and systemic diseases,* 3rd ed. Philadelphia: Lippincott Williams & Wilkins, 2002.

Vinokur ET, et al. The association of keratoconus, hyperextensible joints, and mitral valve prolapse. *Ophthalmology* 1986;93:95.

CORNEA PLANA (DECREASED CORNEAL CURVATURE)

1. Isolated
2. Marfan syndrome
*3. Sclerocornea

Isenberg SJ. *The eye in infancy.* Chicago: Year Book Medical, 1989.

STAPHYLOMA OF CORNEA (CORNEAL STRETCHING WITH INCARCERATION OF UVEAL TISSUE)

1. Advanced keratoconus (see p. 288)
2. Avitaminosis A with keratomalacia
3. Congenital
*4. Following corneal ulcer (see p. 281, 283), neuroparalytic keratitis, corneal leprosy, and severe corneal injury
5. Mucoviscidosis (cystic fibrosis of the pancreas)

Arffa RC. *Grayson's diseases of the cornea,* 3rd ed. St. Louis: Mosby–Year Book, 1991.

WHORL-LIKE CORNEAL LESIONS

*1. Amiodarone toxicity
2. Amodiaquine hydrochloride administration
3. Atabrine administration
*4. Chloroquine and hydroxychloroquine toxicity
5. Chlorpromazine administration
*6. Fabry disease (diffuse angiokeratosis)
7. Incontinentia pigmenti
8. Indomethacin administration
9. Meperidine hydrochloride
10. Quinacrine administration
11. Urethan administration

Arffa RC. *Grayson's diseases of the cornea*, 3rd ed. St. Louis: Mosby–Year Book, 1991.

Fraunfelder FT, Fraunfelder FW. *Drug-induced ocular side effects.* Woburn, MA: Butterworth-Heinemann, 2001.

Kaplan LJ, Cappaert WE. Amiodarone keratopathy. *Arch Ophthalmol* 1982;100:601.

Ferreira RC, et al. Corneal abnormalities associated with incontinentia pigmenti. *Am J Opthalmol* 1997;123:549–551.

CORNEAL DERMOIDS

These congenital corneal limbal lesions grow slowly. Tumors are yellowish, elevated, and variable in size; they consist of fibrofatty tissue covered by epidermal rather than by conjunctival epithelium and may contain ectodermal derivatives such as hair follicles, sebaceous glands, and sweat glands. Trauma, irritation, and puberty hasten their growth.

1. Bloch–Sulzberger syndrome (incontinentia pigmenti)
2. Cri-du-chat syndrome (cat-cry syndrome)
3. Duane retraction syndrome
4. Multiple dermoids of the cornea associated with miliary aneurysms of the retina
5. Neurocutaneous syndrome (ectomesodermal dysgenesis)
6. Nevus sebaceous of Jadassohn (linear nevus sebaceous of Jadassohn)
*7. Oculoauriculovertebral dysplasia (Goldenhar syndrome)
8. Organoid nevus syndrome
9. Ring dermoid syndrome—autosomal dominant
10. Sporadic
11. Thalidomide teratogenicities

Arffa RC. *Grayson's diseases of the cornea*, 3rd ed. St. Louis: Mosby–Year Book, 1991.

Benjamin SN, Allen HF. Classification for limbal dermoid choristomas and brachial arch anomalies. *Arch Ophthalmol* 1972;87:305–314.

Brodsky MC, et al. Oculocerebral dysgenesis in the linear nevus sebaceous syndrome. *Ophthalmology* 1997;104:497–503.

Roy FH. *Ocular syndromes and systemic diseases*, 3rd ed. Philadelphia: Lippincott Williams & Wilkins, 2002.

* = most important

Corneal dermoids

	Goldenhar Syndrome	Cri-du-chat Syndrome	Duane Retraction Syndrome	Block-Sulzberger Syndrome	Miliary Aneurysms of Retina	Thalidomide Teratogenicities	Neurocutaneous Syndrome	Nevus Sebaceous of Jadassohn Syndrome
History								
1. Drug ingestion during gestation						U		
2. Greater in females								
3. Greater left eye			U	U				
4. Hereditary			U					
5. Low birth weight	R	U	R	U	S		U	
6. Present at birth		U						
7. Unilateral	U						U	U
Physical Findings								
1. Absence/restricted adduction	S		U					
2. Antimongoloid palpebral fissures (temporal canthus lower)		U						S
3. Bulbar dermoid	U							S
4. Cataract			S					S
5. Coloboma of lids	S	R		S			S	
6. Corneal vascularization	U							U
7. Dacryocystitis								S
8. Deficiency of tears	S							
9. Epicanthal folds		U						
10. Glaucoma		U						
11. Hypertelorism						S		
12. Iris and choroid coloboma		U						
13. Microcornea	S		R				U	U
14. Microphthalmos	S							
15. Nystagmus	S	R						
16. Optic atrophy					S			S
17. Papillary conjunctivitis		R			S			
18. Papillitis							S	
19. Paralysis of extraocular muscles					S			
20. Persistent pupillary membrane	S					S		S
21. Pigmented retinopathy	S							
22. Retinal detachment					U	S	U	
23. Retinal microaneurysm					S	S		
24. Retinal vessel tortuosity					S	U		
25. Retraction of adducted globe		U						
26. Retrolenticular mass	S		U					
27. Strabismus					S	S	U	
28. Vitreous hemorrhage	S	S	R	S				
29. Widening of palpebral fissures on abduction	S		S					
Laboratory Data								
1. Chromosomal study reveals deletion of short-arm chromosome 5		U						
2. Electromyography shows disorder of paradoxic innervation			U					
3. Roentgenogram of cervical bones	U							

R = rarely; S = sometimes; and U = usually.

CORNEAL PROBLEMS ASSOCIATED WITH KERATOTIC SKIN LESIONS

1. Ectodermal dysplasia (anhidrotic)
*2. Ichthyosis
3. Keratosis follicularis
4. Keratosis follicularis spinulosa decalvans
5. Keratosis plantaris and palmaris
6. Pityriasis rubra pilaris

Arffa RC. *Grayson's diseases of the cornea*, 3rd ed. St. Louis: Mosby–Year Book, 1991.

Wilson LA. *External diseases of the eye*. New York: Harper & Row, 1979.

CORNEAL PROBLEMS ASSOCIATED WITH LID EXCRESCENCES

1. Keratosis folliculosis
2. Lipid proteinosis
*3. Molluscum contagiosum
4. Verruca vulgaris

Arffa RC. *Grayson's diseases of the cornea*, 3rd ed. St. Louis: Mosby–Year Book, 1991.

Wilson LA. *External diseases of the eye*. New York: Harper & Row, 1979.

CORNEAL DISEASE ASSOCIATED WITH LENTICULAR PROBLEMS

1. Aberfeld syndrome (ocular and facial abnormalities syndrome)—cataracts, microcornea
2. Acrodermatitis chronica atrophicans—keratomalacia, corneal opacification, cataracts
3. Addison syndrome (idiopathic hypoparathyroidism)—keratoconjunctivitis, corneal ulcers, keratitic moniliasis, cataracts
4. Amiodarone—corneal deposits, anterior subcapsular cataracts
5. Amyloidosis—amyloid deposits of cornea, corneal dystrophy, pseudopodia lentis
6. Anderson–Warburg syndrome (oligophrenia–microphthalmos syndrome)—corneal opacification and lenticular destruction with a mass visible behind the lens
7. Andosky syndrome (atopic cataract syndrome)—atopic keratoconjunctivitis, keratoconus, uveitis, subcapsular cataract
8. Aniridia—microcornea and subluxated lenses
9. Anterior chamber cleavage syndrome (Reese–Ellsworth syndrome)—corneal opacities, anterior pole cataract
10. Anterior segment ischemia syndrome—corneal edema, corneal ulceration, cataract
11. Apert syndrome (absent digits cranial defects syndrome)—exposure keratitis, cataracts, ectopia lentis
12. Arteriovenous fistula (arteriovenous aneurysm)—bullous keratopathy, cataract
13. Aspergillosis—corneal ulcer, keratitis, cataract
*14. Atopic disease (atopic eczema, Besnier prurigo)—keratoconjunctivitis, keratoconus, cataract
15. Autosomal dominant—cataracts and microcornea
16. Avitaminosis C (scurvy)—keratitis, corneal ulcer, cataract
17. Chickenpox (varicella)—corneal ulcer, corneal opacity, keratitis, cataract
18. Chlorpromazine—corneal and lens opacities
19. Cholera—keratomalacia, cataract
20. Chromosome partial deletion (short-arm) syndrome—cataracts, corneal opacities

* = most important

21. Cockayne syndrome (Mickey Mouse syndrome)—cataracts, band keratopathy, corneal dystrophy
22. Congenital spherocytic anemia (congenital hemolytic jaundice)—congenital cataract, ring-shaped pigmentary corneal deposits
23. Crouzon syndrome (Parrot-head syndrome)—exposure keratitis, cataract, corneal dystrophy
24. Cryptophthalmia syndrome (cryptophthalmos–syndactyly syndrome)—cornea differentiated from sclera, lens absence to hypoplasia, dislocation, and calcification
25. Cytomegalic inclusion disease (cytomegalovirus)—cataract, corneal opacities
26. Darier–White syndrome (keratosis follicularis)—keratosis, corneal subepithelial infiltrations, corneal ulceration, cataract
27. Dermatitis herpetiformis (Duhring–Broca disease)—corneal vascularization, cataract
28. Diphtheria—keratitis, corneal ulcer, cataract
29. Ehlers–Danlos syndrome (fibrodysplasia elastica generalisata)—microcornea, keratoconus, lens subluxation
30. Electrical injury—corneal perforation, necrosis of cornea, anterior or posterior subcapsular cataracts
31. Exfoliation syndrome (capsular exfoliation syndrome)—cataract, dislocated lens, corneal dystrophy, lens capsule exfoliation
32. Folling syndrome (phenylketonuria)—corneal opacities, cataracts
*33. Fuchs syndrome (I) (heterochromic cyclitis syndrome)—secondary cataract, edematous corneal epithelium
34. Goldscheider syndrome (epidermolysis bullosa)—bullous keratitis, corneal subepithelial blisters to corneal perforation, cataract
35. Gorlin–Goltz syndrome (multiple basal cell nevi syndrome)—cataract, corneal leukoma
36. Grönblad–Strandberg syndrome (elastorrhexis)—keratoconus, cataract, subluxation of lens
37. Hallermann–Streiff syndrome (oculomandibulofacial dyscephaly)—cataracts, microcornea
38. Hanhart syndrome (recessive keratosis palmoplantaris)—dendritic corneal lesions, keratitis, corneal haze, corneal neovascularization, cataract
39. Heerfordt syndrome (uveoparotid fever)—band keratopathy, keratoconjunctivitis, cataract
40. Hereditary ectodermal dysplasia syndrome (Siemens syndrome)—keratosis, corneal erosions, corneal dystrophy, cataract, lens luxation
*41. Herpes simplex—keratitis, corneal ulcer, cataract
*42. Herpes zoster—keratitis, corneal ulcer, cataract
43. Histiocytosis X (Hand–Schüller–Christian syndrome)—pannus, bullous keratopathy, corneal ulcer, cataract
44. Hodgkin disease—keratitis, cataract
45. Homocystinuria syndrome—dislocated lens, cataract, keratitis
46. Hutchinson–Gilford syndrome (progeria)—cataract, microcornea
47. Hydatid cyst (echinococcosis)—keratitis, corneal abscess, cataract
48. Hypervitaminosis D—band keratopathy, cataract
49. Hypoparathyroidism—keratitis, cataract
50. Hypophosphatasia (phosphoethanolaminuria)—cataract, corneal subepithelial calcifications
51. Influenza—keratitis, cataract

52. Jadassohn-type anetodermal—keratoconus, cataract
53. Jadassohn–Lewandowsky syndrome (pachyonychia congenita)—corneal dyskeratosis, cataract
*54. Juvenile rheumatoid arthritis (Still disease)—band keratopathy, cataract
55. Kussmaul disease (periarteritis nodosa)—corneal ulcer, cataract
56. Kyrle disease (hyperkeratosis penetrans)—subcapsular cataracts, subepithelial corneal opacities
57. Leri syndrome (carpal tunnel syndrome)—corneal clouding, cataract
58. Listerellosis (listeriosis)—keratitis, corneal abscess and ulcer, cataract
59. Little syndrome (nail–patella syndrome)—microcornea, keratoconus, cataract
60. Lowe syndrome (oculocerebrorenal syndrome)—cloudy cornea, cataracts, megalocornea, corneal dystrophy
61. Malaria—keratitis, cataract
62. Marchesani syndrome (brachymorphia with spherophakia)—lentic ulnar myopia, ectopia lentis, megalocornea, corneal opacity
63. Marfan syndrome (arachnodactyly–dystrophia–mesodermalis congenita)—lens dislocation, cataract, megalocornea, lenticular myopia
64. Matsoukas syndrome (oculocerebroarticuloskeletal syndromes)—cataract, corneal sclerosis
65. Meckel syndrome (dysencephalia splanchnocystica syndrome)—sclerocornea, microcornea, cataract
66. Morbilli (rubeola, measles)—corneal ulcer, cataract
67. Mucolipidosis IV (ML IV)—corneal clouding, cataract
68. Nematode ophthalmia syndrome (toxocariasis)—cataract, larvae present in the cornea
69. Neurodermatitis (lichen simplex chronicus)—keratoconjunctivitis, atopic cataracts, keratoconus
70. Ocular toxoplasmosis (toxoplasmosis)—keratitis, cataract
71. Oculodental syndrome (Peter syndrome)—macrocornea, opacities of the corneal margin, ectopic lentis, corneoscleral staphyloma
72. O'Donnell–Pappas syndrome—presenile cataract, peripheral corneal pannus
73. Paget syndrome (osteitis deformans)—corneal ring opacities, cataract
74. Passow syndrome (status dysraphicus syndrome)—neuroparalytic keratitis, zonular cataract
75. Pemphigus foliaceus (Cazenave disease)—pannus, corneal infiltration, cataract
76. Pigmentary ocular dispersion syndrome (pigmentary glaucoma)—Krukenberg spindle, equatorial pigmentation of lens capsule
77. Pseudohypoparathyroidism (Seabright–Bantan syndrome)—punctate cataracts, keratitis
78. Radiation—corneal ulcer, punctate keratitis, cataracts, exfoliation of lens capsule
79. Refsum syndrome (phytanic acid oxidase deficiency)—corneal opacities, cataracts
80. Relapsing polychondritis—corneal ulcer, cataracts, keratoconjunctivitis sicca
81. Retinal disinsertion syndrome—lens subluxation, keratoconus
82. Retinopathy of prematurity—cataracts, corneal opacification
83. Rieger syndrome (dysgenesis mesodermalis corneae et irides)—microcornea, corneal opacities in Descemet membrane, dislocated lens
84. Romberg syndrome (facial hemiatrophy)—neuroparalytic keratitis, cataracts
85. Rubella syndrome (German measles)—corneal haziness, cataracts, microcornea
86. Sabin–Feldman syndrome—posterior lenticonus, microcornea
87. Sanfilippo–Good syndrome (MPS III)—deposits in cornea and lens

* = most important

88. Schafer syndrome (keratosis palmoplantaris syndrome)—lesions in the lower portion of the cornea, cataract
89. Schaumann syndrome (sarcoidosis syndrome)—keratitis sicca, band-shaped keratitis, complicated cataract
90. Scheie syndrome (MPS IS)—diffuse haze to marked corneal clouding, cataracts
91. Stannus cerebellar syndrome—corneal vascularization, corneal opacities, cataracts
92. Stevens–Johnson syndrome (erythema multiforme exudativum)—keratitis, corneal ulcers, cataracts, pannus
93. Stickler syndrome (hereditary progressive arthroophthalmopathy)—keratopathy, cataracts
94. Thioridazine—corneal and lens opacities
95. Toxic lens syndrome—pigment precipitation on the surface of an intraocular lens, chronic uveitis
96. Trisomy syndrome—corneal and lens opacities
97. Turner syndrome (gonadal dysgenesis)—corneal nebulae, cataracts
98. Ultraviolet radiation—band keratopathy, keratitis, discoloring of lens
99. van Bogaert–Scherer–Epstein syndrome (familial hypercholesterolemia syndrome)—lipid keratopathy, cataract, juvenile corneal arcus
100. von Recklinghausen syndrome (neurofibromatosis)—nodular swelling of corneal nerves, cataracts
101. Waardenburg syndrome (interoculoiridodermatoauditive dysplasia)—microcornea, cornea plana, lenticonus
102. Wagner syndrome (hereditary hyaloideoretinal degeneration and palatoschisis)—corneal degeneration, including band-shaped keratopathy, cataracts
103. Ward syndrome (nevus jaw cyst syndrome)—congenital cataracts, congenital corneal opacities
104. Wegener syndrome (Wegener granulomatosis)—corneal ulcer, corneal abscess, cataract
105. Weil disease (leptospirosis)—keratitis, cataract
106. Werner syndrome (progeria of adults)—juvenile cataracts, bullous keratitis, trophic corneal defects
107. Yersiniosis—corneal ulcer, cataract
108. Zellweger syndrome (cerebrohepatorenal syndrome of Zellweger)—corneal opacities, cataract

Bilgami NL, et al. Marfan syndrome with microcornea, aphakia, and ventricular systolic defect. *Indian Heart J* 1981;33:78–80.

Gualtieri CT, et al. Corneal and lenticular opacities in mentally retarded young adults treated with thioridazine and chlorpromazine. *Am J Psychiatry* 1982;139:1178–1180.

Polomeno RC, Cummings C. Autosomal dominant cataracts and microcornea. *Can J Ophthalmol* 1979;14:227–229.

Roy FH. *Ocular syndromes and systemic diseases*, 3rd ed. Philadelphia: Lippincott Williams & Wilkins, 2002.

CORNEAL DISEASE ASSOCIATED WITH RETINAL PROBLEMS

1. Abdominal typhus (enteric fever)—corneal ulcer, retinal detachment, central retinal artery emboli
2. *Acanthamoeba*—keratitis, pannus, corneal ring abscess, retinal perivasculitis
3. African eyeworm disease—keratitis, central retinal artery occlusion, macular hemorrhages
4. Amyloidosis—amyloid corneal deposits, corneal dystrophy, retinal hemorrhages
5. Anderson–Warburg syndrome (oligophrenia–microphthalmos syndrome)—corneal opacification, malformed retina with retina pseudotumors

6. Angioedema (hives)—central serous retinopathy, corneal edema
7. Anterior segment ischemia syndrome—corneal edema midperiphery retinal hemorrhages
8. Apert syndrome (acrodysplasia)—exposure keratitis, retinal detachment
9. Arteriovenous fistula—bullous keratopathy, retinal hemorrhages
10. Aspergillosis—corneal ulcer, keratitis, retinal hemorrhages, retinal detachment
11. Atopic dermatitis—keratoconus and retinal detachment
12. Avitaminosis C—retinal hemorrhages, keratitis, corneal ulcer
13. *Bacillus cereus*—ring abscess of cornea, necrosis of retina
14. Bang disease (brucellosis)—keratitis, chorioretinitis, macular edema
15. Behçet syndrome (dermatostomata–ophthalmic syndrome)—keratitis, posterior corneal abscess, retinal vascular changes
16. Bietti disease (Bietti marginal crystalline dystrophy)—marginal corneal dystrophy, retinitis punctate albescens
17. Candidiasis—keratitis, corneal ulcer, retinal atrophy, retinal detachment
18. Carotid artery syndrome—corneal ulcer, loss of corneal sensation, retinal edema, engorgement of retinal veins
19. Chickenpox (varicella)—corneal ulcer, corneal opacity, retinitis, hemorrhagic retinopathy
*20. Chloroquine—corneal epithelial pigmentation, macular lesions
21. Chronic granulomatous disease of childhood—keratitis, destructive chorioretinal lesions
22. Cockayne syndrome (dwarfism with retinal atrophy and deafness)—pigmentary degeneration, band keratopathy, corneal dystrophy
23. Crohn disease (granulomatous ileocolitis)—marginal corneal ulcers, keratitis, macular edema, macular hemorrhages
24. Cryoglobulinemia—deep corneal opacities, venous stasis
25. Cystinosis (aminoaciduria)—crystals in cornea and pigment in retina
26. Dengue fever—keratitis, corneal ulcer, retinal hemorrhages
27. Diffuse keratoses syndrome—corneal nodular thickening in the stroma worse in fall, retinal phlebitis
28. Diphtheria—keratitis, corneal ulcer, central artery occlusion
29. Disseminated lupus erythematosus (Kaposi–Libman–Sacks syndrome)—keratitis, keratoconjunctivitis sicca, corneal ulcer, central retinal vein occlusion, retinal detachment
30. Ehlers–Danlos syndrome (cutis hyperelastica)—keratoconus and retinitis pigmentosa
31. Electrical injury—corneal perforation, retinal edema, retinal hemorrhages, pigmentary degeneration, retinal holes, dilatation of retinal veins
32. Fabry disease (diffuse angiokeratosis)—whorl-like changes in cornea, central retinal artery occlusion, tortuosity of retinal vessels
33. Goldscheider syndrome (epidermolysis bullosa)—bullous keratitis with opacities, retinal detachment
34. Gronblad–Strandberg syndrome (systemic elastodystrophy)—angioid streaks of the retina, macular hemorrhages, retinal detachment, keratoconus
35. Hamman–Rich syndrome (alveolar capillary block syndrome)—keratomalacia ischemic retinopathy, cystic macular changes
36. Heerfordt syndrome (uveoparotid fever)—band keratopathy, retinal vasculitis
37. Hennebert syndrome (luetic otitic nystagmus syndrome)—interstitial keratitis, disseminated syphilitic chorioretinitis
38. Histiocytosis X (Hand–Schüller–Christian syndrome)—retinal hemorrhage, retinal detachment, bullous keratopathy, corneal ulcer, pannus

* = most important

39. Hodgkin disease—keratitis, retinal hemorrhages
40. Hollenhorst syndrome (chorioretinal infarction syndrome)—hazy cornea, serous retinal detachment, pigmentary retinopathy
41. Hunter syndrome (MPS II)—splitting or absence of peripheral Bowman membrane, stromal haze, pigmentary retinal degeneration, narrowed retinal vessels
42. Hurler–Scheie syndrome (MPS IH-S)—corneal clouding, pigmentary retinopathy
43. Hurler syndrome (gargoylism)—diffuse corneal haziness, retinal pigmentary changes, megalocornea, retinal detachment
44. Hydatid cyst (echinococcosis)—keratitis, abscess of cornea, retinal detachment, retinal hemorrhages
45. Hyperlipoproteinemia—arcus juvenilis, lipemia retinalis, xanthomata of retina
46. Hyperparathyroidism—band keratopathy, vascular engorgement of retina
47. Hypovitaminosis A—keratomalacia with perforation, corneal opacity, retinal degeneration
48. Idiopathic hypercalcemia (blue-diaper syndrome)—band keratopathy, optic atrophy, papilledema
49. Indomethacin—corneal deposits, reduced retinal sensitivity
50. Influenza—keratitis, retinal hemorrhage
51. Japanese River fever (typhus)—keratitis, retinal hemorrhages
52. Juvenile rheumatoid arthritis (Still disease)—band keratopathy, macular edema
53. Kahler disease (multiple myeloma)—crystalline deposits of cornea, central retinal artery occlusion, retinal microaneurysms
54. Kussmaul disease (periarteritis nodosa)—retinal detachment, pseudoretinitis pigmentosa, corneal ulcer
55. Leber tapetoretinal dystrophy syndrome (retinal aplasia)—keratoconus, salt-and-pepper or "bone corpuscle" pigmentation, yellowish-brown or gray macular lesions
56. Lubarsch–Pick syndrome (primary amyloidosis)—amyloid corneal deposits, retinal hemorrhages
57. Lymphogranuloma venereum disease (Nicolas–Favre disease)—keratitis, pannus, corneal ulcer, keratoconus, tortuosity of retinal vessels, retinal hemorrhages
58. Marfan syndrome (arachnodactyly dystrophia mesodermalis congenita)—keratoconus, retinitis pigmentosa
59. Meckel syndrome (dysencephalia splanchnocystica syndrome)—sclerocornea, microcornea, retinal dysplasia
60. Meningococcemia—keratitis, retinal endophlebitis
61. Mikulicz–Radeski syndrome (dacryosialoadenopathy)—keratoconjunctivitis, retinal candlewax spots
62. ML IV (mucolipidosis IV)—corneal clouding, corneal opacities, retinal atrophy
63. Morbilli (measles-rubeola)—keratitis, corneal ulcer, pigmentary retinopathy, central retinal artery occlusion
64. Mucormycosis (phycomycosis)—corneal ulcer, striate keratopathy, retinitis, central retinal artery thrombosis
65. Mycosis fungoides syndrome (malignant cutaneous reticulosis syndrome)—keratoconjunctivitis, retinal edema, retinal hemorrhage
66. Myotonic dystrophy syndrome—corneal epithelial dystrophy, loss of corneal sensitivity, tapetoretinal degeneration, macular red spot, macular degeneration, chorioretinitis
67. Neurofibromatosis (von Recklinghausen syndrome)—nodular swelling nerves, hamartoma of retina
68. Norrie disease (atrophia oculi congenita)—malformation of sensory cells of retina, corneal nebulae

69. Oculodental syndrome (Peter syndrome)—corneoscleral staphyloma, megalocornea, corneal marginal opacities, macular pigmentation
70. Onchocerciasis syndrome—punctate keratitis, sclerosing keratitis, chorioretinitis, retinal degeneration
71. Paget syndrome (osteitis deformans)—corneal ring opacities, retinal hemorrhages, pigmentary retinopathy, macular changes resembling Kuhnt–Junius degeneration
72. Phenothiazine—epithelial and endothelial pigment, retinal pigmentation
73. Pierre Robin syndrome (micrognathia-glossoptosis)—retinal disinsertion, megalocornea
74. Plasma lecithin (cholesterol acyltransferase deficiency)—corneal stromal opacities, retinal hemorrhages
75. Porphyria cutanea tarda—keratitis, retinal hemorrhages, cotton-wool spots, macular edema
76. Postvaccinial ocular syndrome—corneal vesicles, and marginal ulcers, chorioretinitis, central serous retinopathy, central retinal vein thrombosis
77. Progressive systemic sclerosis—marginal corneal ulcers with cicatrization, cotton-wool spots, retinal hemorrhages
78. Radiation—corneal ulcer, punctate keratitis, keratoconjuctivitis sicca, retinal hemorrhage, macular degeneration, macular holes with vascularization
79. Refsum syndrome (phytanic acid oxidase deficiency)—band keratopathy, retinitis pigmentosa
80. Relapsing fever—interstitial keratitis, retinal hemorrhage
81. Relapsing polychondritis—corneal ulcer, retinal detachment, retinal artery thrombosis, keratoconjunctivitis sicca
82. Renal failure—cotton-wool spots, band keratopathy
83. Rendu–Osler syndrome (hereditary hemorrhagic telangiectasis)—intermittent filamentary keratitis, small retinal angiomas, retinal hemorrhages
84. Retinal disinsertion syndrome—bilateral keratoconus, retinal detachment
85. Retinoblastoma—corneal tumor, retinal neovascularization
86. Rothmund syndrome (telangiectasia–pigmentation cataract syndrome)—corneal lesions, retinal hyperpigmentation
87. Rubella syndrome (Gregg syndrome)—microcornea, pigmentary retinal changes
88. Sabin–Feldman syndrome—microcornea, chorioretinitis or atrophic degenerative chorioretinal changes
89. Sanfilippo–Good syndrome (MPS III)—slight narrowing of retinal vessels, acid mucopolysaccharide deposits in cornea
90. Schaumann syndrome (sarcoidosis syndrome)—mutton fat keratitic precipitates, keratitis sicca, band-shaped keratitis, inflammatory retinal exudates
91. Scheie syndrome (MPS IS)—diffuse to marked corneal clouding, tapetoretinal degeneration
92. Schwartz syndrome (glaucoma associated with retinal detachment)—retinal detachment, microcornea
93. Shy–Gonatas syndrome (orthostatic hypotension syndrome)—keratopathy, corneal ulcer, lattice-like white opacities in the area of Bowman membrane, retinal pigmentary degeneration
94. Smallpox—keratitis, congenital corneal clouding, chorioretinitis
95. Stannus cerebellar syndrome (riboflavin deficiency)—corneal vascularization, superficial diffuse keratitis, corneal opacities, brownish retinal patches
96. Stickler syndrome (hereditary progressive arthroophthalmopathy)—keratopathy, chorioretinal degeneration, total retinal detachment

97. Sturge–Weber syndrome (neurooculocutaneous angiomatosis)—retinal detachment, increased corneal diameter with cloudiness
98. Syphilis (acquired lues)—keratitis, retinal hemorrhages, retinal proliferation
99. Temporal arteritis syndrome (Hutchinson–Horton–Magath–Brown syndrome)—retinal detachments, narrowing of retinal vessels, central retinal artery occlusion, corneal hypesthesia
100. Trisomy 13 (Patau syndrome)—malformed cornea, retinal dysplasia
101. Tuberculosis—keratitis, pannus, corneal ulcer, retinitis
102. Ullrich syndrome (dyscraniopygophalangy)—cloudy cornea, corneal ulcers, chorioretinal coloboma
103. Ultraviolet radiation—photokeratitis, band keratopathy, herpes simplex keratitis, recurrent corneal erosions, retinal degeneration
104. Vaccinia—keratitis, pannus, corneal perforation, central serous retinopathy, pseudoretinitis pigmentosa
105. van Bogaert–Scherer–Epstein (primary hyperlipidemia)—arcus juvenilis of the cornea, lipid keratopathy, retinopathy with yellowish deposits
106. Vitreous tug syndrome—vitreous strands attached to corneal wound or scar, circumscribed retinal edema, posterior retinal detachment
107. von Gierke disease (glycogen storage disease type I)—corneal clouding, discrete nonelevated, yellow flecks in macula
108. Waardenburg syndrome (embryonic fixation syndrome)—microcornea, cornea plana, hypopigmentation and hypoplasia of retina
109. Wagner syndrome (hyaloideoretinal degeneration)—corneal degeneration, band-shaped keratopathy, hyaloideoretinal degeneration, narrowing of retinal vessels, retinal detachment, avascular preretinal membranes
110. Waldenström syndrome (macroglobulinemia syndrome)—crystalline corneal deposits, keratoconjunctivitis sicca, retinal venous thrombosis, retinal microaneurysms, cotton-wool spots
111. Weil disease (leptospirosis)—keratitis, retinitis
112. Werner syndrome (progeria of adults)—bullous keratitis, paramacular retinal degeneration
113. Wiskott–Aldrich syndrome (sex-linked draining ears, eczematoid dermatitis, bloody diarrhea)—corneal ulcers, retinal hemorrhages
114. Yersiniosis—corneal ulcer, retinal hemorrhages
115. Zellweger syndrome (cerebrohepatorenal syndrome)—corneal opacities, narrowing of retinal vessels, retinal holes without detachment, tapetoretinal degeneration
116. Zieve syndrome (hyperlipemia hemolytic anemia–icterus syndrome)—cloudy cornea, corneal ulcers, retinal lipemia

Arffa RC. *Grayson's disease of the cornea*, 3rd ed. St. Louis: Mosby–Year Book, 1991.

Roy FH. *Ocular syndromes and systemic diseases*, 3rd ed. Philadelphia: Lippincott Williams & Wilkins, 2002.

CORNEAL DISEASES ASSOCIATED WITH DEAFNESS

1. Atopic dermatitis—limbal keratitis, conjunctivitis
*2. Cogan syndrome (nonsyphilitic interstitial keratitis)—interstitial keratitis
3. Meniere disease—iritis, glaucoma
*4. Polyarteritis nodosa (Kussmaul disease)—paralimbal keratitis, corneoscleral ulceration
5. Sarcoidosis syndrome (Schaumann syndrome)—primary stromal keratitis, keratoconjunctivitis sicca

*6. Syphilis (lues)—interstitial keratitis
 7. 3-methyl-pentyn-3-yl acid phthalate (Whipcide, trichuricidal agent)—keratitis, uveitis, stromal keratitis
 8. Tuberculosis—interstitial keratitis
 9. Vogt–Koyanagi–Harada syndrome (uveitis–vitiligo–alopecia poliosis syndrome)—uveitis
10. Wegener granulomatosis—necrotizing sclerokeratitis

Heinemann MH, et al. Cogan's syndrome. *Ann Ophthalmol* 1980;12:667.

TRIGGER MECHANISMS FOR RECURRENT HERPES SIMPLEX KERATITIS

*1. Corticosteroids (topical)
*2. Emotional disturbances
*3. Exposure to sunlight (ultraviolet)
*4. Fever (most common)
 5. Gastrointestinal upsets
 6. Ingestion of food to which patient is allergic
 7. Mechanical trauma
 8. Menses

Kimura SJ. Infectious diseases of the conjunctiva and cornea. *Symposium of the New Orleans Academy of Ophthalmology*. St. Louis: CV Mosby, 1963.

PREDISPOSING FACTORS IN KERATOMYCOSIS

1. Antibiotics
2. Steroids
3. Trauma

Francois J, Ryssdlaere M. *Oculomycoses*. Springfield, IL: Charles C Thomas, 1972.

Gingrich WD. Infectious diseases of the conjunctiva and cornea. *Symposium of the New Orleans Academy of Ophthalmology*. St. Louis: CV Mosby, 1963:154.

SCLEROCORNEA

This type of developmental corneal abnormality has ill-defined limbus due to extension of opaque scleral tissue into the cornea. Vision varies with involvement. Somatic abnormalities include craniofacial, digital, skin, and testis abnormalities; deafness and mental retardation are seen.

1. Associated ocular abnormalities including:
    A. Abnormalities of Descemet membrane, endothelium, and corneal stroma
    B. Aniridia
    C. Cataract
    D. Coloboma
    E. Cornea plana—occurrence
    F. Dysgenesis of angle and iris
    G. Esotropia
    H. Glaucoma
    I. Iridocorneal synechiae
    J. Microphthalmia
    K. Nystagmus

* = most important

L. Persistent pupillary membrane
M. Posterior embryotoxon
2. Associated syndromes, including the following:
   A. Axenfeld syndrome
   B. Cross syndrome
   C. Dandy–Walker syndrome
   D. Hallermann–Streiff syndrome
   E. Hurler syndrome
   F. Hypomelanosis of Ito
   G. Lobstein syndrome
   H. Melnick-Needles syndrome
   I. Mieten syndrome
   J. Nail–patella syndrome
   K. Rieger syndrome
   L. Robert syndrome
   M. Smith–Lemli–Opitz syndrome
   N. Unbalanced 17p-10q translocation
   O. Wolf syndrome (4p-syndrome)

Isenberg SJ. *The eye in infancy.* Chicago: Year Book Medical, 1989.

Tasman W, Jaeger E, eds. *Duane's clinical ophthalmology.* Philadelphia: JB Lippincott, 1990.

POSTOPERATIVE CORNEAL MELT

This condition is characterized by central or peripheral thinning of corneal stroma after pterygium, refractive surgery, keratoplasty, glaucoma surgery, strabismus surgery, cataract surgery, or retina surgery.

1. AIDS
2. Collagen disorders
   a. Polyarteritis nodosa
   b. Rheumatoid arthritis
   c. Scleroderma
   d. Systemic lupus erythematosus
3. Delayed corneal wound healing due to drugs, including adenine arabinoside, adrenal cortex injections, aldosterones, alpha-chymotrypsin, azathioprine, betamethasone, butacaine, cocaine, cortisone, dexamethasone, fluorometholone, fluprednisolone, hydrocortisone, prednisolone, sulfacetamide, sulfamethizole, tetracaine, triamcinolone
4. Drug use
   a. Steroid therapy
   b. Stevens–Johnson syndrome
   c. Topical anesthesia abuse
   d. Topical nonsteroidal antiinflammatory agents
5. Marginal ring ulcer
   a. Acute leukemia
   b. Bacillary dysentery
   c. Brucellosis
   d. Dengue fever
   e. Gonococcal arthritis
   f. Hookworm infestation

       g. Influenza

       h. Possibly porphyria trigger mechanisms

6. Ocular predisposing factors

       a. Phlyctenular keratoconjunctivitis

       b. Superior limbic keratoconjunctivitis

       c. Trachoma

       d. Terrien disease

       e. Vernal conjunctivitis

7. Preexisting corneal dellen

8. Skin conditions

       a. Acne rosacea

       b. Benign mucosa; pemphigoid

       c. Dermatitis herpetiformis

       d. Ectodermal dysplasia

       e. Herpes zoster

       f. Ichthyosis

       g. Incontinentia pigment

       h. Leprosy

       i. Lichen planus

       j. Lyell disease

       k. Lymphopathia venereum

       l. Molluscum contagiosum

       m. Palmoplantar keratosis

       n. Pemphigus foliaceus

       o. Pityriasis rubra pilaris

       p. Psoriasis

9. Systemic diseases

       a. Brucellosis

       b. Deerfly fever

       c. Filariasis

       d. Gout

       e. *H. influenzae*

       f. Hodgkin disease

       g. Hypoparathyroidism

       h. Leprosy

       i. Lymphopathia venereum

       j. Mumps

       k. Sarcoidosis

       l. Trypanosomiasis

       m. Tuberculosis

       n. Upper respiratory infection

10. Vitamin deficiency

       a. Ariboflavinosis keratopathy

       b. Pellagra

       c. Vitamin A deficiency

       d. Vitamin B^2 deficiency

Castillo A, et al. Peripheral melt of flap after laser in situ keratomileusis. *J Refract Surg* 1998;14:61–63.

Liu SM, et al. Corneal melting after avulsion of a Molteno shunt. *J Glaucoma* 1997;6:357–358.

Wilhelmus KR. Corneal edema following argon laser iridotomy. *Ophthalmic Surg Lasers* 1992;23:533–537.

CORNEAL MUCOUS PLAQUES

These plaques are abnormal collections of a mixture of mucous, epithelial cells, and protein-aceous and lipoidal material that adhere firmly to the corneal surface.

1. Local radiation exposure
2. Herpes zoster
*3. Keratoconjunctivitis sicca
4. Other forms of keratitis
5. Vernal keratoconjuctivitis

Fraunfelder FT, et al. Corneal mucous plaques. *Am J Ophthalmol* 1977;83:31–35.

Tripathi RC, et al. Contact lens deposits and spoilage: identification and management. *Int Ophthalmol Clin* 1991; 31:91–120.

9

Intraocular Pressure

CONTENTS

GLAUCOMA SUSPECT, INFANT

  1. Amblyopia ex anopsia
*2. Corneal edema (see p. 250)
  3. Corneal enlargement
  4. Cupping and atrophy of optic disc
  5. Deep anterior chamber
*6. Epiphora, photophobia, and blepharospasm (see p. 65–66)
  7. Iridodonesis and subluxation of lens (see p. 374)
  8. Iris processes
*9. Tears in Descemet membrane (see p. 287)

Duane TD, Jaeger EA. *Clinical ophthalmology.* New York: Harper & Row, 1994.

Hoskins HD, Kass MA. *Becker-Shaffer's diagnosis and therapy of glaucoma*, 6th ed. St. Louis: CV Mosby, 1989.

Shields MB. *Textbook of glaucoma*, 3rd ed. Baltimore: Williams & Wilkins, 1992.

CONDITIONS SIMULATING CONGENITAL GLAUCOMA

  1. Blue sclera
    A. Albright hereditary osteodystrophy (pseudohypoparathyroidism)
    B. Craniofacial dysostosis (Crouzon disease)
    C. de Lange syndrome

* = most important

    D. Ehlers–Danlos syndrome

    E. Fölling syndrome

    F. Hallermann–Streiff syndrome (oculomandibulodyscephaly)

    G. Incontinentia pigmenti (Bloch–Sulzberger syndrome)

    H. Juvenile Paget disease (hyperphosphatasia, hereditary)

    I. Lowe (oculocerebrorenal) syndrome

    J. Marfan syndrome

    K. Turner (XO, gonadal dysgenesis) syndrome

    L. van der Hoeve syndrome (osteogenesis imperfecta)

    M. Werner syndrome

2. Corneal opacity

    A. Congenital malformations

        (1) Anterior corneal staphyloma

        (2) Cornea plana

        (3) Incontinentia pigmenti (Bloch–Sulzberger syndrome)

        (4) Norrie disease

     *(5) Peters anomaly

        (6) Riley–Day syndrome (congenital familial dysautonomia)

     *(7) Sclerocornea

        (8) Trisomy 13–15 syndrome (Patau syndrome)

    B. Edema

     *(1) Birth injury, such as breaks in Descemet membrane

        (2) Congenital hereditary corneal edema

        (3) Fetal uveitis

     *(4) Infectious keratitis (congenital syphilis, interstitial keratitis, rubella, variola, varicella, gonorrhea, mumps, and others)

        (5) Keratitis (chemical)

     *(6) Keratoconus

    C. Metabolic disorders/dystrophies

        (1) Congenital hereditary stromal dystrophy

        (2) Corneal amyloidosis (Lubarsch–Pick syndrome)

        (3) Corneal lipidosis

        (4) Cystinosis (Lignac–Fanconi syndrome)

        (5) Fabry disease

        (6) Hyperlipidemia

        (7) Mucopolysaccharidoses (MPS)

           a. Hunter syndrome (MPS IIB)

           b. Hurler syndrome (MPS IH)

           c. Maroteaux–Lamy syndrome (MPS VI)

           d. Morquio syndrome (MPS IV)

           e. Sanfilippo syndrome (MPS IIIC)

           f. Scheie syndrome (MPS IS)

        (8) Porphyria (congenital)

        (9) von Gierke glycogen storage disease

3. Epiphora (excessive tearing)

   *A. Lacrimal duct obstruction

   *B. Viral, chemical or allergic conjunctivitis

4. Large corneas

    A. Apert syndrome

  B. High myopia
  C. Keratoglobus
  D. Marfan syndrome
  E. Megalocornea
  F. van der Hoeve syndrome (osteogenesis imperfecta)
*5. Photophobia—anterior uveitis (many causes)

Duane TD, Jaeger EA. *Clinical ophthalmology.* New York: Harper & Row, 1994.

Roy FH. *Ocular syndromes and systemic diseases*, 3rd ed. Philadelphia: Lippincott Williams & Wilkins, 2002.

Shields MB. *Textbook of glaucoma*, 3rd ed. Baltimore: Williams & Wilkins, 1992.

Teekhasaenee C, Ritch R. Iridocorneal endothelial syndrome in Thai patients. *Arch Ophthalmol* 2000;118:187–192.

SYNDROMES AND DISEASES ASSOCIATED WITH GLAUCOMA

1. Ocular disease
    A. Corneal endothelial disorders
        (1) Fuchs endothelial dystrophy
        (2) Iridocorneal endothelial (ICE) syndrome
            a. Chandler syndrome
            b. Cogan–Reese (iris–nevus) syndrome
            c. Progressive iris atrophy
        (3) Posterior polymorphous dystrophy
    B. Developmental glaucoma with associated ocular anomalies
        (1) Aniridia
        (2) Axenfeld–Rieger syndrome
        (3) Congenital ectropion uveae
        (4) Congenital iris hypoplasia
        (5) Megalocornea
        (6) Microcornea
        (7) Peters anomaly
        (8) Sclerocornea
    C. Elevated episcleral venous pressure (see p. 235)
    D. Iris disorders
        (1) Iridoschisis
        *(2) Pigmentary glaucoma
    E. Lens disorders
        (1) Cataract
            a. Lens-particle glaucoma
            b. Phacoanaphylaxis
            c. Phacolytic (lens protein) glaucoma
            d. Phacomorphic (intumescent lens) glaucoma
        (2) Dislocation of the lens
        *(3) Exfoliation syndrome
    F. Medications or chemicals
        (1) Corticosteroids
        (2) Others
    G. Myopia
    H. Ocular hemorrhage
        (1) Degenerated ocular blood
            a. Ghost cell glaucoma

* = most important

    b. Hemolytic glaucoma
    c. Hemosideric glaucoma
*(2) Hyphema
    a. Blunt trauma
    b. Intraocular surgery
1. Intraoperative
2. Postoperative
    c. Penetrating trauma
    d. Spontaneous
1. Anterior segment neovascularization
2. Intraocular tumor
3. Pupillary vascular tufts
    (3) Orbital hemorrhage (massive)
    (4) Vitreous hemorrhage (massive)
I. Ocular inflammation
    (1) Choroiditis and retinitis
        a. Cytomegalic inclusion retinitis
        b. Sympathetic ophthalmia
        c. Toxocariasis
        d. Vogt–Koyanagi–Harada syndrome
    (2) Episcleritis
*(3) Iridocyclitis
        a. Acute anterior iridocyclitis
        b. Ankylosing spondylitis
        c. Behçet disease
        d. Fuchs heterochromic cyclitis
        e. Glaucomatocyclitic crisis (Posner–Schlossman syndrome)
        f. Infectious diseases
1. Acquired immunodeficiency syndrome (AIDS)
2. Congenital rubella
3. Disseminated meningococcemia
4. Hansen disease (leprosy)
5. Hemorrhagic fever with renal syndrome
6. Onchocerciasis (also keratitis)
7. Syphilis
        g. Juvenile rheumatoid arthritis (JRA)
        h. Pars planitis
        i. Precipitates on the trabecular meshwork (Grant syndrome)
        j. Reiter syndrome
        k. Sarcoid
        l. Trauma
    (4) Keratitis
        a. Adenovirus type 10
        b. Herpes simplex
        c. Herpes zoster
        d. Interstitial keratitis
    (5) Scleritis
*J. Ocular surgery
    (1) Aphakia or pseudophakia (see p. 405)

* = most important

(2) Corticosteroid induced

(3) Cyclodialysis cleft (sudden closure)

(4) Epithelial downgrowth

(5) Malignant (ciliary block) glaucoma

(6) Penetrating keratoplasty

    a. Distortion of angle structures

    b. Graft rejection

(7) Vitreoretinal procedures

    a. Intravitreal gas

    b. Pars plana vitrectomy

    c. Retinal photocoagulation

    d. Scleral buckling surgery

    e. Silicone oil

K. Ocular trauma

(1) Chemical burns (acid, alkali, and others)

(2) Contusion injuries

    a. Angle recession

    b. Hyphema

    c. Iritis

    d. Lens damage or dislocation

    e. Trabecular damage

(3) Penetrating injuries

    a. Epithelial downgrowth

    b. Hyphema

    c. Lens damage or dislocation

    d. Peripheral anterior synechiae

(4) Radiation damage

(5) Retained intraocular foreign body (iron, copper)

(6) Retrobulbar hemorrhage (massive)

L. Ocular tumors

(1) Benign tumors of the anterior uvea

    a. Adenomas

    b. Cysts (primary versus secondary)

    c. Iris nevi

    d. Leiomyomas

    e. Melanocytomas

    f. Melanoses

(2) Histiocytosis X

(3) Leukemias

(4) Lymphomas

(5) Metastatic tumors

    a. Carcinomas (most commonly, breast carcinoma in females and lung carcinoma in males)

    b. Melanomas

(6) Multiple myeloma

(7) Ocular tumors of childhood

    a. Juvenile xanthogranuloma

    b. Medulloepithelioma (diktyoma)

    c. Retinoblastoma

        (8) Orbital tumors
        (9) Primary uveal melanomas
        (10) Retrobulbar tumors
   M. Retinal, vitreous, and choroidal disorders
      (1) Angle closure
        a. Acute choroidal hemorrhage
        b. Central retinal vein occlusion (CRVO)
        c. Ciliochoroidal effusion

1. AIDS
2. Arteriovenous malformations
3. Inflammatory conditions
4. Nanophthalmos
5. Surgery
6. Trauma
7. Tumors
8. Uveal effusion syndrome

        d. Hemorrhagic retinal and choroidal detachment
        e. Iris retraction syndrome with retinal detachment (Campbell)
        f. Persistent hyperplastic primary vitreous (PHPV)
        g. Postoperative panretinal photocoagulation
        h. Postoperative scleral buckle
        i. Retinal dysplasia
        j. Retinopathy of prematurity (retrolental fibroplasia)
     *(2) Neovascular glaucoma (see p. 324)
      (3) Retinitis pigmentosa
      (4) Rhegmatogenous retinal detachment (Schwartz syndrome)
2. Systemic disorders
   A. AIDS
   B. Angioneurotic edema (giant urticaria)
   C. Ankylosing spondylitis (Marie–Strümpell disease)
   D. Aortic arch syndrome
   E. Behçet disease
   F. Carotid artery occlusive disease
   G. Carotid–cavernous fistula
   H. Cavernous sinus thrombosis
   I. Crouzon disease (craniofacial dysostosis)
   J. Cushing disease
   K. Developmental glaucoma as part of a syndrome
      (1) Bing–Neel [macroglobulinemia and central nervous system (CNS)] syndrome
      (2) Chondrodystrophy, joint dislocation, glaucoma, and mental retardation
      (3) Chromosomal abnormalities
        a. Chromosome partial deletion (long-arm) syndrome
        b. Pericentric inversion of chromosome II
        c. Trisomy 21 (Down syndrome)
        d. Trisomy 16–18 (Edward syndrome)
        e. Trisomy F (17–18)
        f. Trisomy 13–15 (Patau syndrome)

    g. Turner syndrome (XO, gonadal dysgenesis)

    h. 9p syndrome

(4) Cockayne syndrome

(5) Congenital rubella syndrome

(6) Cretinism (juvenile hypothyroidism)

(7) Cystinosis

(8) Dental–ocular–cutaneous syndrome

(9) Diamond–Blackfan syndrome

(10) Ehlers–Danlos syndrome

(11) Familial histiocytic dermatoarthritis syndrome

(12) Fetal alcohol syndrome

(13) Gorlin–Goltz (multiple basal cell nevi) syndrome

(14) Hallermann–Streiff syndrome (oculomandibulofacial dyscephaly)

(15) Homocystinuria

(16) Kartagener syndrome (sinusitis-bronchiectasis-situs inversus)

(17) Kimmelstiel–Wilson syndrome

(18) Klinefelter syndrome

(19) Klippel–Trenaunay–Weber syndrome

(20) Krabbe syndrome

(21) Krause syndrome (congenital encephaloophthalmic dysplasia)

(22) Lowe (oculocerebrorenal) syndrome

(23) Marfan syndrome (arachnodactyly dystrophia mesodermalis congenita)

(24) Meyer–Schwickerath–Weyers syndrome (oculodentodigital dysplasia)

(25) Miller (Wilms aniridia) syndrome

(26) MPS

    a. Hurler syndrome (MPS IH)

    b. Maroteaux–Lamy syndrome (MPS VI)

    c. Morquio syndrome (MPS IV)

(27) Nieden (telangiectasia–cataract) syndrome

(28) Pierre Robin syndrome (micrognathia-glossoptosis) syndrome

(29) Prader–Willi syndrome (hypotonia, hypogonadism, obesity, and mental retardation)

(30) Rubella syndrome

(31) Rubinstein–Taybi (broad thumb) syndrome

(32) Silverman (battered-child) syndrome

(33) Stickler syndrome (hereditary progressive arthroophthalmopathy)

(34) Treacher–Collins syndrome

(35) Ullrich syndrome (dyscraniopygophalangy)

(36) Waardenburg syndrome

(37) Wagner syndrome

(38) Weber–Christian disease

(39) Weil–Marchesani syndrome

(40) X-linked mental retardation (XLMR) syndrome

(41) Zellweger (cerebrohepatorenal) syndrome

*L. Diabetes

M. Epidemic dropsy (argemone oil poisoning)

N. Giant cell arteritis

*O. Graves disease

P. Hemorrhagic fever with renal syndrome (nephropathia epidemica)

* = most important

*Q. Herpes simplex

*R. Herpes zoster

S. Histiocytosis X

T. JRA

U. Juvenile xanthogranuloma

V. Leukemia

W. Lymphoma

X. Medications or chemicals

Y. Metastatic carcinoma

Z. Metastatic melanoma

AA. Multiple myeloma

BB. Phakomatoses

  (1) Nevus of Ota (oculodermal melanocytosis)

  (2) Sturge–Weber syndrome (encephalotrigeminal angiomatosis)

  (3) von Hippel–Lindau disease

  (4) von Recklinghausen neurofibromatosis

CC. Reiter syndrome

DD. Retinoblastoma

EE. Retrobulbar tumors

FF. Sarcoidosis

GG. Sickling disorders

HH. Superior vena cava (superior mediastinal) syndrome

II. Syphilis

JJ. Systemic corticosteroids

KK. Vogt–Koyanagi–Harada syndrome

Duane TD, Jaeger EA. *Clinical ophthalmology.* New York: Harper & Row, 1994.

Evans LS. Increased intraocular pressure in severely burned patients. *Am J Ophthalmol* 1991;111:56–58.

Grant WM. *Toxicology of the eye,* 4th ed. Springfield, IL: Charles C Thomas, 1993.

Roy FH. *Ocular syndromes and systemic diseases,* 3rd ed. Philadelphia: Lippincott Williams & Wilkins, 2002.

Shields MB. *Textbook of glaucoma,* 3rd ed. Baltimore: Williams & Wilkins, 1992.

GLAUCOMA SUSPECT, ADULT

1. Advanced age

*2. Applanation reading 21 mm Hg or greater

3. Asymmetric intraocular pressures (IOPs)

4. Black race

5. Contusion-angle deformity glaucoma in the fellow eye

*6. Diabetes mellitus

7. Diurnal fluctuation in IOP of 10 mm Hg or greater

8. Endothelial dystrophy of the cornea

*9. Exfoliative syndrome (see p. 400)

10. Family history of glaucoma

*11. Hemorrhage at optic disc margin

12. High myopia

13. IOP elevation following use of corticosteroids

14. Krukenberg spindle or dense trabecular pigment band

*15. Prominent cupping of optic disc

  A. Asymmetry of cup-to-disc ratio

      B. Cup-to-disc ratio 0.4

      C. Cupping-to-disc margin

      D. Vertical elongation of cup

16. Retinal detachment (see p. 487)

*17. Retinal vein occlusion (see p. 468–472)

18. Schiötz scale reading 4.0/5.5 or 6.25/7.5 or less

19. Thyrotropic exophthalmos

*20. Visual field changes suggestive of glaucoma

Duane TD, Jaeger EA. *Clinical ophthalmology.* New York: Harper & Row, 1994.

Shields MB. *Textbook of glaucoma,* 3rd ed. Baltimore: Williams & Wilkins, 1992.

ELEVATED INTRAOCULAR PRESSURE MEASUREMENT WITH NORMAL-APPEARING OPTIC DISC

1. Acromegaly
2. Anesthesia
    - A. Ketamine
    - B. Nitrous oxide with intravitreal gas
    - C. Succinylcholine
*3. Blepharospasm
4. Caffeine intake
5. Cardiopulmonary bypass surgery
*6. Dysthyroid ophthalmopathy
7. Elevation in hemoglobin concentration
8. Excessive water intake
9. High scleral rigidity and indentation (e.g., Schiötz) tonometry
10. Horizontal gaze position
11. Hyperthermia
12. Hyperthyroid
13. Marked emotional stress
14. Mechanical factors in checking IOP (e.g., by patient's hair interfering with applanation tonometer arm)
15. Medications or chemicals
    - *A. Corticosteroids
    - B. Cycloplegics
    - C. Others
*16. Normal variation (ocular hypertension)
*17. Preglaucoma (IOP sufficiently elevated to cause damage to the optic nerve, but damage is not yet visible ophthalmoscopically)
18. Reduced gravity
19. Tight collar, short neck, obesity
20. Tobacco smoking
*21. Tonometer in need of calibration
22. Valsalva maneuver
23. Voluntary widening of palpebral fissure

Grant WM. *Toxicology of the eye,* 4th ed. Springfield, IL: Charles C Thomas, 1993.

Munoz M, Capo H. Differential intraocular pressure in restrictive strabismus. *Am J Ophthalmol* 1991;112:352–353.

Shields MB. *Textbook of glaucoma.* Baltimore: Williams & Wilkins, 1992.

* = most important

SECONDARY OPEN-ANGLE GLAUCOMA

1. Corneal endothelial disorders
    A. Fuchs endothelial dystrophy
    B. Posterior polymorphous dystrophy
2. Elevated episcleral venous pressure (see p. 235)
3. Iris disorders
    A. Iridoschisis
    *B. Pigmentary glaucoma
4. Lens disorders
    A. Cataract
        (1) Lens particle glaucoma
        (2) Phacoanaphylaxis
        (3) Phacolytic (lens protein) glaucoma
    B. Displaced lens (see p. 317–318)
    *C. Exfoliation syndrome
5. Medications or chemicals
    *A. Corticosteroids
    B. Cycloplegic effect
    C. Others
6. Ocular hemorrhage
7. Ocular inflammation
8. Ocular surgery
    A. Alpha-chymotrypsin (enzyme glaucoma)
    *B. Corticosteroid induced
    C. Distortion of anterior chamber angle from limbal or keratoplasty sutures
    D. Early postoperative elevation of IOP following cataract surgery (especially in eyes with preexisting glaucoma)
    E. Hemorrhage
        (1) Degenerated ocular blood
            a. Ghost cell glaucoma
            b. Hemolytic glaucoma
            c. Hemosideric glaucoma
        *(2) Hyphema
        (3) Internal wound neovascularization (late postoperative hyphema)
        (4) Pseudophakia
            a. Anterior chamber intraocular lens (IOL), including uveitis, glaucoma, hyphema (UGH) syndrome
            b. Iris-fixated IOL
            c. Posterior chamber IOL (usually sulcus fixation)
        (5) Retrobulbar hemorrhage (massive)
    F. Inflammation
    G. Intravitreal gas
    H. Neodymium:yttrium-aluminum-aluminum-garnet (Nd:YAG) laser capsulotomy
    I. Pseudophakic pigmentary dispersion (e.g., with posterior chamber implant)
    J. Retained lens cortex
    *K. Retained viscoelastic
    L. Silicone oil

    M. Sudden closure of cyclodialysis cleft
    N. Vitreous filling anterior chamber

9. Ocular trauma
    A. Chemical burns (acid, alkali, other)
    B. Contusion
        (1) Angle recession
       *(2) Hyphema
        (3) Iritis
        (4) Trabecular damage
    C. Radiation damage
    D. Retained intraocular foreign body (iron, copper)
    E. Retrobulbar hemorrhage (massive)

10. Ocular tumors
11. Retinal, vitreous, and choroidal disorders
   *A. Neovascular glaucoma—open-angle stage (see p. 324)
    B. Retinitis pigmentosa
    C. Rhegmatogenous retinal detachment (Schwartz syndrome)

12. Systemic, such as ocular amyloidosis

Duane TD, Jaeger EA. *Clinical ophthalmology.* New York: Harper & Row, 1994.

Grant WM. *Toxicology of the eye*, 4th ed. Springfield, IL: Charles C Thomas, 1993.

Nelson GA, et al. Ocular amyloidosis and secondary glaucoma. *Ophthalmology* 106:1363–1366.

Roy FH. *Ocular syndromes and systemic diseases*, 3rd ed. Philadelphia: Lippincott Williams & Wilkins, 2002.

UNILATERAL GLAUCOMA

1. Corneal endothelial disorders
    A. Fuchs endothelial dystrophy with angle closure due to thickened peripheral cornea
    B. Iridocorneal endothelial (ICE) syndrome
        (1) Chandler syndrome
        (2) Iris–nevus (Cogan–Reese) syndrome
        (3) Progressive iris atrophy

2. Elevated episcleral venous pressure (see p. 235)

3. Lens disorders
    A. Cataract
        (1) Lens-particle glaucoma
        (2) Phacoanaphylaxis
        (3) Phacolytic (lens protein) glaucoma
        (4) Phacomorphic (intumescent lens) glaucoma
    B. Displacement of the lens
        (1) Buphthalmos
        (2) Cataract (mature or hypermature)
        (3) Exfoliation syndrome
        (4) Intraocular tumor
        (5) PHPV
        (6) Sturge–Weber syndrome (encephalotrigeminal angiomatosis)
        (7) Trauma
        (8) Uveitis
   *C. Exfoliation syndrome (see p. 400)

                                          * = most important

4. Medications or chemicals
    A. Alpha-chymotrypsin (enzyme glaucoma)
    B. Chemical burns
    *C. Corticosteroids (topical or periocular)
    D. Cycloplegics (angle closure or open angle)
    E. Nitrous oxide inhalation with intraocular gas
    F. Urokinase (intraocular)
    G. Others
5. Ocular hemorrhage
6. Ocular inflammation
*7. Ocular surgery
8. Ocular trauma
9. Ocular tumors
10. Retinal, vitreous, and choroidal disorders
    A. Angle closure
        (1) Acute choroidal hemorrhage
        *(2) CRVO
        (3) Ciliochoroidal effusion
            a. Arteriovenous malformations
            b. Inflammatory conditions
            c. Nanophthalmos
            d. Surgery
            e. Trauma
            f. Tumors
            g. Uveal effusion syndrome
        (4) Hemorrhagic retinal and choroidal detachment
        (5) PHPV
        *(6) Postoperative panretinal photocoagulation
        (7) Postoperative scleral buckle
        (8) Retinal dysplasia
        (9) Retinopathy of prematurity (retrolental fibroplasia)
    *B. Neovascular glaucoma (see p. 324)
        *(1) Diabetic retinopathy
        (2) Extraocular vascular disorders
            a. Carotid–cavernous fistula
            b. Carotid occlusive disease
            c. Giant cell arteritis
        (3) Ocular disorders—miscellaneous
            *a. Chronic glaucoma
            b. Endophthalmitis
            c. Intraocular malignancy
            d. Iris melanoma
            e. PHPV
            f. Photoradiation or helium ion irradiation for uveal melanoma
            g. Pseudophakia
            h. Sympathetic ophthalmia
            *i. Uveitis (chronic)
        (4) Retinal disorders—miscellaneous
            a. Coats disease

      b. Eales disease
      c. Optic-nerve glioma with venous stasis
      d. Retinal detachment (usually chronic)
      e. Retinal vascular occlusive disorders

  1. Retinal artery occlusion central or branch
 *2. Retinal vein occlusion central or branch

      f. Retinoblastoma
      g. Retinopathy of prematurity (retrolental fibroplasia)
      h. Retinoschisis
      i. Sickle cell retinopathy

  C. Open-angle glaucoma associated with rhegmatogenous retinal detachment (Schwartz syndrome)

Duane TD, Jaeger EA. *Clinical ophthalmology.* New York: Harper & Row, 1994.

Roy FH. *Ocular syndromes and systemic diseases,* 3rd ed. Philadelphia: Lippincott Williams & Wilkins, 2002.

Shields MB. *Textbook of glaucoma,* 3rd ed. Baltimore: Williams & Wilkins, 1992.

GLAUCOMA ASSOCIATED WITH DISPLACED LENS

  1. Alport syndrome
  2. Aniridia
  3. Axenfeld–Rieger syndrome
  4. Buphthalmos
 *5. Cataract (mature or hypermature)
  6. Cornea plana
  7. Crouzon disease (craniofacial dysostosis)
  8. Ectopia lentis et pupillae
  9. Ehlers–Danlos syndrome
*10. Exfoliation syndrome (see p. 400)
 11. High myopia
 12. Homocystinuria
 13. Hyperlysinemia
 14. Intraocular tumor
 15. Isolated microspherophakia
 16. Klinefelter syndrome
 17. Lowe (oculocerebrorenal) syndrome
*18. Marfan syndrome
 19. Megalocornea
 20. Oculodental syndrome
 21. Refsum syndrome
 22. Retinitis pigmentosa
 23. Scleroderma
 24. Simple ectopia lentis
 25. Stickler syndrome
 26. Sturge–Weber syndrome (encephalotrigeminal angiomatosis)
 27. Sulfite oxidase deficiency
 28. Syphilis
*29. Trauma
 30. Treacher–Collins syndrome (mandibulofacial dysostosis)
 31. Uveitis

* = most important

32. Weill–Marchesani syndrome

Duane TD, Jaeger EA. *Clinical ophthalmology*. New York: Harper & Row, 1994.

Epstein DL. *Chandler and Grant's glaucoma*, 3rd ed. Philadelphia: Lea & Febiger, 1986.

Shields MB. *Textbook of glaucoma*, 3rd ed. Baltimore: Williams & Wilkins, 1992.

GLAUCOMA AND ELEVATED EPISCLERAL VENOUS PRESSURE

1. Arteriovenous fistulas
    A. Carotid–cavernous sinus fistulas
        (1) Spontaneous
        (2) Traumatic
    B. Orbital–meningeal shunts
    C. Orbital varices
    *D. Sturge–Weber syndrome (encephalotrigeminal angiomatosis)
2. Idiopathic elevation of episcleral venous pressure
    *A. Familial
    B. Sporadic
3. Venous obstruction
    A. Cavernous sinus thrombosis
    *B. Congestive heart failure
    C. Episcleral
        (1) Chemical burns (acid, alkali, and others)
        (2) Radiation
    D. Jugular venous obstruction
    E. Ocular amyloidosis
    F. Orbital
        *(1) Dysthyroid
        (2) Orbital vein thrombosis
        (3) Phlebitis
        (4) Pseudotumor
        (5) Retrobulbar tumor
    G. Pulmonary venous obstruction
    H. Superior vena cava (superior mediastinal) syndrome

Duane TD, Jaeger EA. *Clinical ophthalmology*. New York: Harper & Row, 1994.

Shields MB. *Textbook of glaucoma*, 3rd ed. Baltimore: Williams & Wilkins, 1992.

Weinreb RN, et al. Glaucoma secondary to elevated episcleral venous pressure. In: Ritch R, et al. *The glaucomas*. St. Louis: CV Mosby, 1989.

GLAUCOMA ASSOCIATED WITH SHALLOW ANTERIOR CHAMBER

*1. Primary-angle closure
    A. Plateau iris syndrome
    *B. Relative pupillary block (most common)
2. Secondary-angle closure
    *A. CRVO (central retinal vein occlusion)
    B. Choroidal hemorrhage (acute)
    C. Ciliochoroidal effusion
        (1) AIDS
        (2) Arteriovenous malformations

      *(3) Inflammation

       (4) Nanophthalmos

       (5) Trauma

       (6) Tumor

       (7) Uveal effusion syndrome

  D. Cystinosis

  E. Drug-induced acute transitory myopia (diuretics, sulfonamides, and others)

  F. Elevated episcleral venous pressure associated with arteriovenous fistula

  G. Fuchs endothelial dystrophy—with peripheral corneal thickening

  H. Hemorrhagic retinal and choroidal detachment

   I. Hyperglycemia (acute)

   J. Inflammation

       (1) Episcleritis

       (2) Iridocyclitis with posterior synechiae and iris bombe

       (3) Posterior scleritis

  K. Intraocular tumor (posterior segment melanoma, metastatic carcinoma, retino-blastoma, medulloepithelioma, and others)

  L. Lens dislocation (see p. 401–404)

  M. Luetic interstitial keratitis

  N. Malignant (ciliary block) glaucoma

  O. Maroteaux–Lamy syndrome (MPS VI)

  P. Multiple cysts of the iris and ciliary body

  Q. Nanophthalmos

  R. Pars plana vitrectomy

  S. PHPV

 *T. Phakic or aphakic pupillary block

  U. Phakomorphic (intumescent lens) glaucoma

  V. Postoperative panretinal photocoagulation

  W. Postoperative scleral buckle

  X. Pupil dilatation, including topical dilatation and systemic decongestants, bronchodilators, gastroenterologic and genitourinary disorders.

  Y. Retinal dysplasia

  Z. Retinopathy of prematurity (retrolental fibroplasia)

Fraunfelder FT, Roy FH. *Current ocular therapy*, 5th ed. Philadelphia: WB Saunders, 2000.

Mungan N, et al. Ultrasound biomicroscopy of the eye in cystinosis. *Arch Ophthalmol* 2000;118:1329–1333.

Rho DS. Acute angle-closure glaucoma after albuterol nebulizer treatment. *Am J Ophthalmol* 2000;130:123–124.

Shields MB. *Textbook of glaucoma*, 3rd ed. Baltimore: Williams & Wilkins, 1992.

GLAUCOMA IN APHAKIA OR PSEUDOPHAKIA

  1. Alpha-chymotrypsin (enzyme glaucoma)

  2. Ciliary-block (malignant) glaucoma

 *3. Corticosteroid induced

  4. Degenerated intraocular blood

     A. Ghost cell glaucoma

     B. Hemolytic glaucoma

     C. Hemosideric glaucoma

  5. Distortion of the anterior chamber angle by limbal sutures

 *6. Early postoperative pressure elevation (especially in eyes with preexisting glaucoma)

* = most important

7. Epithelial downgrowth
8. Fibrous proliferation
*9. Following Nd:YAG capsulotomy
10. Hyphema
    A. Internal wound neovascularization (late postoperative hyphema)
    B. Pseudophakia
        (1) Anterior chamber IOL (including the UGH syndrome)
        (2) Iris-fixated IOL
        (3) Posterior-chamber IOL (usually sulcus fixation)
11. Inflammation
12. Peripheral anterior synechiae
13. Primary open-angle glaucoma
14. Pseudophakic pigmentary dispersion
*15. Pupillary block
*16. Retained lens cortex
*17. Retained viscoelastic
18. Vitreous filling the anterior chamber
19. Vitreous hemorrhage (massive)

Duane TD, Jaeger EA. *Clinical Ophthalmology.* New York: Harper & Row, 1994.

Shields MB. *Textbook of glaucoma,* 3rd ed. Baltimore: Williams & Wilkins, 1992.

Tessler DR, et al. Persistently raised intraocular pressure following extracapsular cataract extraction. *Br J Ophthalmol* 1990;74:272–274.

MEDICATIONS AND CHEMICALS THAT MAY CAUSE ELEVATED INTRAOCULAR PRESSURE

1. Anesthetic agents
    A. Ketamine
    B. Nitrous oxide (inhalation, especially in eyes with retinovitreal surgery and intra-ocular gas)
2. Anticholinergics/parasympatholytics
    A. Antidepressants
        (1) Amitriptyline (Elavil)
        (2) Imipramine (Tofranil)
        (3) Nortriptyline (Pamelor)
        (4) Protriptyline (Vivactil)
        (5) Trimipramine (Surmontil)
    B. Antihistamines
        (1) Anazolene (Vasocon-A)
        (2) Brompheniramine (Dimetane)
        (3) Cyclizine (Marezine)
        (4) Cyproheptadine (Periactin)
        (5) Diphenhydramine (Benadryl)
        (6) Orphenadrine (Norgesic)
        (7) Tripelennamine (Pyribenzamine)
    C. Antiparkinson medications
        (1) Biperiden (Akineton)
        (2) Cycrimine (Pagitane)
        (3) Trihexyphenidyl hydrochloride (Artane)

    D. Antispasmodic agents
        (1) Dicyclomine (Bentyl)
        (2) Diphemanil methylsulfate (Prantal)
        (3) Hexocyclium methylsulfate (Tral)
        (4) Hyoscyamine (Donnatal, Donnagel)
        (5) Mepenzolate (Cantil)
        (6) Methscopolamine bromide (Pamine)
        (7) Oxyphenonium bromide (Antrenyl)
        (8) Propantheline bromide (Pro-Banthine)
        (9) Tridihexethyl chloride (Pathilon)
  *E. Cycloplegics
        (1) Atropine
        (2) Cyclopentolate (Cyclogyl)
        (3) Homatropine
        (4) Tropicamide (Mydriacyl)
        (5) Scopolamine (Hyoscine)
    F. Miscellaneous
        (1) Atropine (systemic)
        (2) Glycopyrrolate (Robinul)
    G. Phenothiazine
        (1) Doxepin (Sinequan)
        (2) Haloperidol (Haldol)
        (3) Prochlorperazine (Compazine)
        (4) Promethazine (Phenergan)
        (5) Triflupromazine (Vesprin)
    H. Poisoning
        (1) Belladonna
        (2) Jimson weed
3. Argemone oil (epidemic dropsy)
4. Caffeine
5. Carbon dioxide inhalation
6. Carmustine injection
7. Chemical burns
    A. Acid
        (1) Chromic acid
        (2) Hydrochloric (muriatic) acid
        (3) Sulfuric (battery) acid
    B. Alkali
        (1) Ammonium hydroxide (ammonia)
        (2) Calcium hydroxide (lime)
        (3) Sodium hydroxide (lye)
    C. Dibent [b.f][1,4] oxazepine (CR tear gas)
    D. Formaldehyde gas (in aqueous solution formalin)
8. CNS stimulants/anorexics
    A. Dextroamphetamine
    B. Methamphetamine
    C. Phenmetrazine (Preludin)
    D. Phentermine (Ionamin)
*9. Corticosteroids

* = most important

*A. Ocular (topical)
  (1) Dexamethasone (Decadron, Maxidex)
  (2) Fluorometholone (FML, Flarex)
  (3) Prednisolone acetate (Pred Forte)
  (4) Prednisolone sodium phosphate (Inflamase)
*B. Subconjunctival depot injection
  (1) Methylprednisolone acetate
  (2) Triamcinolone
C. Systemic
  (1) Betamethasone (Celestone)
  (2) Cortisone acetate
  (3) Dexamethasone (Decadron)
  (4) Hydrocortisone (Cortef, Solu-Cortef)
  (5) Methylprednisolone (Medrol)
  (6) Paramethasone (Haldrone)
  (7) Prednisolone
  (8) Prednisone (Deltasone)
  (9) Triamcinolone (Aristocort)
10. Idiopathic lens swelling
  A. Acetylsalicylic acid (aspirin)
  B. Sulfanilamide
  C. Others
11. Intraocular injection
  A. Alpha-chymotrypsin (enzyme glaucoma)
  B. Urokinase
  *C. Viscoelastic (Healon, others)
12. Methylphenidate (Ritalin)
13. Miotics
  A. Carbachol
  B. Demecarium (Humorsol)
  C. Echothiophate (phospholine iodide)
  D. Pilocarpine
14. Succinylcholine (Anectine)
15. Sympathomimetics
  A. Ephedrine
  B. Mydriatics
    (1) Dipivalyl epinephrine (Propine)
    (2) Epinephrine (many products)
    (3) Hydroxyamphetamine (Paredrine)
    (4) Phenylephrine (Neo-Synephrine)
  C. Naphazoline (Naphcon)
  D. Pheniramine maleate (Naphcon-A)
  E. Phenylephrine (Neo-Synephrine)
  F. Tetrahydrozoline (Visine)
16. Testosterone
17. Vasodilators
  A. Elevation of IOP following subconjunctival injection
    (1) Bamethan (Bupatol)

(2) Isoxsuprine (Vasodilan)

(3) Tolazoline (Priscoline)

(4) Triaziquone (Trenimon)

B. Amyl nitrite (Vaporole)

18. Water (excessive intake)

May be potentiated by monoamine oxidase inhibitors such as phenelzine, pargyline, or tranyl-cypromine.

Duane TD, Jaeger EA. *Clinical ophthalmology.* New York: Harper & Row, 1994.

Grant WM. *Toxicology of the eye*, 4th ed. Springfield, IL: Charles C Thomas, 1993.

Shields MB. *Textbook of glaucoma*, 3rd ed. Baltimore: Williams & Wilkins, 1992.

PRIMARY LOW-TENSION GLAUCOMA

1. Nonglaucomatous optic nerve disorders resembling glaucomatous damage
    A. Developmental abnormalities
        (1) Colobomas of the optic-nerve head, including optic pits
        *(2) Large physiologic cups
        (3) Tilted discs
    B. Nonglaucomatous causes of acquired cupping
        (1) Compressive lesions
            a. Aneurysm
            b. Chiasmic arachnoiditis
            c. Cyst
            d. Tumor
        *(2) Ischemic optic neuropathy (especially arteritic)
    *C. Nonglaucomatous causes of nerve fiber bundle defects on visual field testing
        (1) Chorioretinal lesions
            a. Chorioretinitis
            b. Retinal vascular occlusions
            c. Tumors
        (2) Optic-nerve head lesions
            a. Colobomas
            b. Drusen
            c. Other
        (3) Posterior lesion of the visual pathway
            a. Meningioma
            b. Pituitary tumor
            c. Pseudotumor
            d. Other
2. Undetected high-pressure glaucoma
    A. Corneal edema giving false low measurement of IOP with applanation (e.g., Goldman or Perkins) tonometry
    B. Intermittent elevation of IOP causing damage (IOP normal at time of examination)
        (1) Glaucomatocyclitic crisis (Posner–Schlossman syndrome)
        (2) Intermittent angle closure
        (3) Others

* = most important

C. Low scleral rigidity giving false low measurement of IOP with indentation (e.g., Schiötz) tonometry

*D. Prior elevation in pressure resulting in optic nerve damage
    (1) Burned-out open-angle glaucoma
    (2) Corticosteroids
    (3) Pigmentary glaucoma
    (4) Trauma
    (5) Uveitis

E. Wide diurnal variation (multiple measurements at different times of day required to rule-out high-pressure glaucoma)

Duane TD, Jaeger EA. *Clinical ophthalmology.* New York: Harper & Row, 1994.

Shields MB. *Textbook of glaucoma*, 3rd ed. Baltimore: Williams & Wilkins, 1992.

Werner EB. Low-tension glaucoma. In: Ritch R, et al. *The glaucomas.* St. Louis: CV Mosby, 1989.

NEOVASCULAR GLAUCOMA

*1. Diabetic retinopathy

2. Extraocular vascular disorders
    A. Aortic arch syndrome
    *B. Carotid artery occlusive disease
    C. Carotid–cavernous fistula
    D. Giant cell arteritis

3. Ocular disorders—miscellaneous
    A. Chronic glaucoma
    B. Endophthalmitis
    C. Iris melanoma
    D. PHPV
    E. Pseudophakia
    F. Sympathetic ophthalmia
    *G. Uveitis

4. Retinal disorders—miscellaneous
    A. Choroidal melanoma
    B. Coats exudative retinopathy
    C. Eales disease
    D. Metastatic carcinoma
    E. Norrie disease
    F. Optic nerve glioma with subsequent venous stasis retinopathy
    G. Photoradiation or helium ion irradiation for uveal melanoma
    *H. Retinal detachment (usually chronic)
    I. Retinal vascular occlusive disorders
        (1) Branch retinal artery occlusion.
        *(2) Branch retinal vein occlusion
        *(3) Central retinal artery occlusion
        *(4) Central retinal vein occlusion
    J. Retinoblastoma
    K. Retinopathy of prematurity (retrolental fibroplasia)

    L. Retinoschisis
   M. Sickle cell retinopathy
   N. Stickler syndrome (inherited vitreoretinal degeneration)
   O. Syphilitic retinal vasculitis

Duane TD, Jaeger EA. *Clinical ophthalmology.* New York: Harper & Row, 1994.

Shields MB. *Textbook of glaucoma*, 3rd ed. Baltimore: Williams & Wilkins, 1992.

HYPOTONY

*1. Essential hypotension
 2. Secondary hypotony
     A. Cartilaginous–arthritic–ophthalmic deafness
     B. Ciliochoroidal detachment
         (1) Chorioretinal inflammation
         (2) Ocular neoplasm
       *(3) Trauma, including ocular surgery
   *C. Cyclitis
   *D. Cyclodialysis
     E. Decreased IOP from medications and chemicals
         (1) Alcuronium
         (2) Aminophylline (intravenous)
       *(3) Carbonic anhydrase inhibitors (e.g., acetazolamide, methazolamide, ethoxzolamide)
         (4) Cardiac glycosides (digitoxin, digoxin, lanatoside-C, ouabain)
         (5) Dibenamine
         (6) Dihydroergotoxine (Hydergine)
         (7) HPMPC (cidofovir)
         (8) Hyperosmotics (urea, glycerin, mannitol, ascorbic acid, glycerol, ethanol, trometamol)
         (9) Isosorbide
       (10) Pargyline (Eutonyl)
       (11) Phentolamine (Regitine)
       (12) Propranolol (Inderal)
       (13) Thiopental (Pentothal)
   *F. Deep anesthesia
     G. Deep coma and severe cerebral disease
   *H. Dehydration—severe (e.g., cholera, dysentery, diabetic coma)
   *I. Diabetic coma
   *J. Glaucoma medications (beta-blockers, sympathomimetics, miotics, carbonic anhydrase inhibitors)
     K. Hilding syndrome
     L. Horner syndrome
    M. Hyperosmolarity
     N. Intestinal perforation or obstruction
     O. Intraocular lens mal position
     P. Irradiation
     Q. Morquio–Brailsford syndrome (MPS IV)

* = most important

    R. Myotonic dystrophy
    S. Ocular ischemia
  *T. Ocular trauma with or without visible ciliary body injury
  *U. Perforating ocular trauma
  *V. Phthisis
    W. Postencephalitic syndrome
  *X. Postoperative surgical procedures especially for glaucoma
    Y. Raeder syndrome
  *Z. Retinal detachment
*AA. Systemic hypotension-severe (circulatory collapse, medications)
  BB. Uremic coma
*CC. Wound leak

Fraunfelder FT, Fraunfelder FW. *Drug-induced ocular side effects.* Woburn, MA: Butterworth-Heinemann, 2001.

Roy FH. *Ocular syndromes and systemic diseases*, 3rd ed. Philadelphia: Lippincott Williams & Wilkins, 2002.

Scott RA, Pavesio C. Ocular side-effects from systemic HPMPC (Cidofovir) for a non-ocular cytomegalovirus infection. *Am J Ophthalmol* 2000;130:126–127.

Shields MB. *Textbook of glaucoma*, 3rd ed. Baltimore: Williams & Wilkins, 1992.

GLAUCOMA ASSOCIATED WITH UVEITIS

  1. Arthritis
  2. Juvenile rheumatoid arthritis
  3. Ankylosing spondylitis, Reiter syndrome, psoriatic arthritis
  6. Fuchs heterochromic uveitis
  7. Posner–Schlossman syndrome (glaucomatocyclitic crisis)
  8. Herpes simplex
  9. Herpes zoster
10. Hansen disease
11. Rubella
12. Mumps and other viral infections
13. Gnathostomiasis
14. Traumatic uveitis
15. Phacoanaphylactic glaucoma
16. Phacolytic glaucoma
17. Pseudophakic–inflammatory glaucoma
18. Intermediate uveitis (pars planitis)
19. Posterior uveitis
        a. Ocular toxoplasmosis
        b. Acute retinal necrosis
        c. AIDS
        d. Other posterior uveitides
20. Panuveitis
        a. Sarcoidosis
        b. Behçet syndrome
        c. Sympathetic ophthalmia

* = most important

    d. Vogt–Koyanagi–Harada syndrome

    e. Congenital syphilis

    f. Acquired syphilis

    g. Tuberculosis

    h. Onchocerciasis

21. Masquerade syndromes
    a. Intraocular neoplasia (uveal malignant melanoma, intraocular lymphoma, and others)
    b. Retinal detachment

22. Open-angle glaucoma

23. Angle-closure glaucoma

24. Combined-mechanism glaucoma

Moorthy RS, et al. Glaucoma associated with uveitis. *Surv Ophthal* 1997;5:361–394.

GLAUCOMA ASSOCIATED WITH INTRAOCULAR TUMORS

1. Iris
   A. Nevus
   B. Melanocytoma
   C. Iris pigment epithelium adenoma
   D. Malignant melanoma
   E. Metastatic

2. Ciliary body
   A. Medulloepithelioma
   B. Melanocytoma
   C. Malignant melanoma
   D. Metastatic

3. Choroid
   A. Malignant melanoma
   B. Metastatic

4. Optic nerve
   A. Melanocytoma
   B. Metastatic

5. Retina—retinoblastoma

6. Metastatic
   A. Carcinoma
   B. Cutaneous melanoma
   C. Breast
   D. Lung
   E. Kidneys
   F. Testicles
   G. Prostate
   H. Pancreas
   I. Colon
   J. Gastrointestinal

7. Others
    A. Leukemia
    B. Lymphoma
    C. Phakomatoses as Sturge–Weber or neurofibromatosis
    D. Multiple myelomas
    E. Juvenile xanthogranuloma

Shields CL, et al. Prevalence and mechanisms of secondary intraocular pressure elevation in eyes with intraocular tumors. *Ophthalmolology* 1987;94:839–846.

Sullivan L, et al. The ocular manifestations of the Sturge-Weber syndrome. *J Pediatr Ophthalmol Strabismus* 1992; 29:349–356.

10

Anterior Chamber

CONTENTS

HYPOPYON (PUS IN ANTERIOR CHAMBER)

1. Hypopyon ulcer—corneal ulcer with pus in the anterior chamber
    A. Acanthamoeba
    B. Acquired immunodeficiency syndrome (AIDS)
    C. *Aspergillus* species
    D. *Candida albicans*
    E. Chemical injury
    F. *Diplococcus pneumoniae*
    G. *Escherichia coli*
    H. *Fusariam* species
    I. Herpes simplex
    J. Herpes zoster
    K. Measles
    L. Moraxella
    M. *Neisseria gonorrhoeae*
    N. *Proteus vulgaris*
    *O. *Pseudomonas aeruginosa*

　　　　　　　　　　　　　　　* = most important

    P. *Serratia* species
    Q. Smallpox
    R. Spitting-cobra venom
    S. Staphylococcus
  *T. Streptococcus

2. Severe acute iridocyclitis
3. Repeated corneal transplantation of human amniotic membrane
4. Necrosis of intraocular tumors or metastasis
5. Retained intraocular foreign bodies, including toxic lens syndrome
6. Endophthalmitis—at time of surgical treatment, accidental trauma, in drug users, or spontaneous occurrence (see p. 223)
    A. Acanthamoebae
    B. Actinomycosis
    C. Amebiasis
    D. *Aspergillosis* species
    E. Bacterial including bacillus cereus
    F. Behçet syndrome
    G. *C. albicans*
    H. Coccidioidomycosis
    I. Coenurosis
    J. Cysticercosis
    K. *Fusarium* species
    L. Hydatid cyst
    M. Influenza
    N. *Listeria monocytogenes*
    O. Lockjaw (*Clostridium tetani*)
    P. Metastatic bacterial endophthalmitis
    Q. *Moraxella* species
    R. *Mucor* species
    S. *Mycobacterium avium*
  *T. *Pseudomonas* species
    U. Relapsing fever
    V. *Serratia marcescens*
    W. Saprophytic fungi
  *X. Staphylococcus
  *Y. Streptoccus
    Z. Sterile hypopyon
        (1) Behçet syndrome (oculobuccogenital syndrome)
        (2) Endotoxin contamination of ultrasonic bath
        (3) Following cyanoacrylate sealing of a corneal perforation
        (4) Following refractive surgery
        (5) Histiocytosis X (Hand–Schüller–Christian syndrome)
        (6) Intraocular lens or instrument polishing compounds or sterilization techniques
      *(7) Juvenile rheumatoid arthritis
        (8) Laser iridotomy
        (9) Leukemia
     *(10) Reaction to lens protein

(11) Rough intraocular lens edges

(12) von Bechterev–Strumpel syndrome (rheumatoid spondylitis)

AA. Stevens–Johnson syndrome (dermatostomatitis)

BB. Tight contact lens or contact lens overwear syndrome

CC. Tuberculosis

DD. Weil disease (leptospirosis)

EE. Yersiniosis

6. Drugs, including the following:

benoxinate
butacaine
cocaine
colchicine (?)
dibucaine
dyclonine
ferrocholinate
ferrous fumarate

ferrous gluconate
ferrous succinate
ferrous sulfate
iodide and iodine solutions
    and compounds
iron dextran
iron sorbitex
phenacaine

piperocaine
polysaccharide–iron complex
proparacaine
radioactive iodides
rifabutin
tetracaine urokinase
urokinase

7. Vitreous "fluff-ball"

8. Following refractive surgery

9. Pseudohypopyon

A. Ghost cell glaucoma with khaki-colored cells

B. Accidental intraocular steroid injection

10. Acute angle-closure glaucoma

11. Non-Hodgkin lymphoma

12. Pars plana vitrectomy and silicone oil injection

Fraunfelder FT, Fraunfelder FW. *Drug-induced ocular side effects.* Woburn, MA: Butterworth-Heinemann, 2001.

Gabler B, Lohmann CP. Hypopyon after repeated transplantation of human amniotic membrane onto the corneal surface. *Ophthalmology* 2000;107:1344–1346.

Pau H. *Differential diagnosis of eye diseases*, 2nd ed. New York: Thieme Medical, 1988.

Recchia FM, et al. Endophthalmitis after pediatric strabismus surgery. *Arch Ophthalmol* 2000;118:939–944.

Roy FH. *Ocular syndromes and systemic diseases*, 3rd ed. Philadelphia: Lippincott Williams & Wilkins, 2002.

Saran BR, et al. Hypopyon uveitis in patients with acquired immunodeficiency syndrome treated for systemic *Mycobacterium avium* complex infection with rifabutin. *Arch Ophthalmol* 1994;112;1159–1161.

HYPHEMA (BLEEDING INTO THE ANTERIOR CHAMBER)

1. Trauma

A. Following laser iridectomy or strabismus surgery in aphakia

B. Honan balloon use in Fuchs heterochromic iridocyclitis

*C. Tear of ciliary body—post contusion deformity of anterior chamber

*D. To ciliary body, such as cyclodialysis

E. To iris, such as in iridodialysis or intraocular lens irritation

F. After airbag inflation

G. Metallic intraocular foreign body during magnetic resonance imaging

2. Overdistention of vessels

A. Obstruction of central retinal vein

B. Sudden lowering of high intraocular pressure

3. Fragility of vessel walls

A. Acute gonorrheal iridocyclitis

* = most important

    B. Acute herpes iridocyclitis
    C. Acute rheumatoid iridocyclitis
    D. Ankylosing spondylitis
4. Blood abnormality
    A. Anemias
    B. Association with use of aspirin
    C. Hemophilia
    D. Leukemia
    E. Purpura
    F. Sickle cell disease
5. Metabolic disease
    A. Diabetes mellitus (Willis disease)
    B. Scurvy (avitaminosis C)
6. Neovascularization of iris (see rubeosis iridis, p. 366–367)
7. Vascularized tumors of iris (see pigmented and nonpigmented iris lesions, p. 374–375)
    A. Angioma
    B. Iris vascular tufts
   *C. Juvenile xanthogranuloma (JXG)
    D. Lymphosarcoma
    E. Retinoblastoma
8. Wound vascularization following cataract extraction
9. Persistent pupillary membrane hemorrhage

Dahlmann AH, et al. Spontaneous hyphema secondary to iris vascular tufts. *Arch Ophthalmol* 2001;119:1728–1729.

Gottsch JD. Hyphema: diagnosis and management. *Retina* 1990;10:65–72.

Keszel VA, Helveston EM. Hyphema as a complication of strabismus: surgery in an aphakic eye. *Arch Ophthalmol* 1986;104:637–638.

Roy FH. *Ocular syndromes and systemic diseases*, 3rd ed. Philadelphia: Lippincott Williams & Wilkins, 2002.

Ta CN, Bowman RW. Hyphema caused by a metallic intraocular foreign body during magnetic resonance imaging. *Am J Ophthalmol* 2000;129:533–534.

SPONTANEOUS HYPHEMA

1. Delayed following glaucoma surgery
2. Diseases of blood or blood vessels
    A. Hemophilia
    B. Leukemia
    C. Malignant lymphoma
    D. Purpura
    E. Scurvy
3. Fibrovascular membranes in retrolenticular or zonular area
    A. Persistent primary vitreous
    B. Retinoschisis
    C. Retinopathy of prematurity
4. Systemic hypertension
5. Hydrophthalmos
6. Iatrogenic
7. Intraocular neoplasms
*8. JXG—yellow nodules of skin and iris
9. Malignant exophthalmos

10. Microbial keratitis, especially *Moraxella*
11. Occult trauma or trauma with late effect
*12. Rubeosis iridis
13. Severe iritis with or without
    A. Behçet disease (dermatostomatoophthalmic syndrome)
    B. Diabetes mellitus (Willis disease)
    C. Gonococcal infection
    D. Herpes zoster or herpes simplex
14. Use of warfarin, heparin, aspirin, or alcohol
15. Vascular anomalies of iris
16. Wound vascularization following cataract extraction

Koehler MP, Shelton DB. Spontaneous hyphema resulting from warfarin. *Ann Ophthalmol* 1983;15:858–859.

Mason GI, et al. Bilateral spontaneous hyphema arising from iridic microhemangiomas. *Ann Ophthalmol* 1979;11:87.

Ormerod LD, Egan KM. Spontaneous hyphaema and corneal haemorrhages as complications of microbial keratitis. *Br J Ophthalmol* 1987;71:933.

Pandolfi M. *Hemorrhages in ophthalmology*. New York: Thieme-Stratton, 1979.

SPONTANEOUS HYPHEMA IN INFANTS

1. Acute rheumatoid iridocyclitis
2. Blood dyscrasias, such as anemia, leukemia, and disseminated intravascular coagulation
3. Iritis
*4. JXG
5. Perinatal asphyxia
6. Persistent hyperplastic primary vitreous
7. Retinoblastoma
8. Retinoschisis
9. Retinopathy of prematurity
*10. Trauma without history (consider child abuse)

Appelboom T, Durso F. Retinoblastoma presenting as a total hyphema. *Ann Ophthalmol* 1985;17:508–510.

Harley RD, et al. Juvenile xanthogranuloma. *J Pediatr Ophthalmol Strabismus* 1982;19:33–39.

Ortiz JM, et al. Disseminated intravascular coagulation in infancy and in the neonate. *Arch Ophthalmol* 1982;100:1413–1415.

* = most important

Spontaneous hyphema

Key: S, R, U indicate the degree of association (as printed).

History

Finding	Systemic Hypertension	Intraocular Neoplasm Melanos	Diseases of Blood Leukemia	Severe Iritis Herpes Zoster	Rubeosis Iridis	Fibrovascular Membrane in Areas Retinopathy of Prematurity	Juvenile Xanthogranuloma
1. Acute or chronic blood disorder			S				
2. Premature Infants						U	
3. History varicella-zoster virus				U			
4. Carotid artery insufficiency					S		
5. Central retinal artery or vein occlusion					S		
6. Childhood disease							U
7. Diabetic retinopathy					S		
8. Elevated blood pressure	U						
9. Oxygen in excess in closed incubators						U	
10. Rare in children		U					
11. Rare in non-caucasians		U					

Physical Findings

Finding	Systemic Hypertension	Intraocular Neoplasm Melanos	Diseases of Blood Leukemia	Severe Iritis Herpes Zoster	Rubeosis Iridis	Fibrovascular Membrane in Areas Retinopathy of Prematurity	Juvenile Xanthogranuloma
1. Anterior chamber depth variations		S					
2. Arteriosclerosis	U						
3. Cataract							
4. Conjunctivitis				S		S	
5. Corneal, lid and epibulbar tumor							S
6. Cotton wool spots	U						
7. Chronic uveitis				U			
8. Decreased visual acuity		S		S	R		S
9. "Dragged disc" appearance		S				S	
10. Ectropion uvea						U	
11. Engorgement of conjunctival vessels				U			
12. Fatty exudates	U						
13. Fibrovascular membrane on anterior iris and chamber angle						U	
14. Freckles on iris		U					
15. Glaucoma	R	S	S	S	S	S	S
16. Heterochromia of iris		S		R	R	S	
17. Hyptony		S	S				
18. Hypopyon				S	R		
19. Iris atrophy				S			
20. Keratitis					S		
21. Macular edema				U			
22. Neuralgia		S					
23. Orbital apex syndrome				U			
24. Optic atrophy				S			
25. Optic disc edema				S		S	
26. Optic neuritis	S			S			
27. Papillary conjunctival hypertrophy				S	U		
28. Paralysis of intraocular muscles				S			
29. Pigmentary retinal changes	S			S	S		
30. Pigmented mass on iris						S	
31. Peripheral anterior synechiae				R	U		
32. Prominent episcleral vessels		U					

Spontaneous hyphema (Continued)

Physical Findings	Systemic Hypertension	Intraocular Neoplasm Melanos	Diseases of Blood Leukemia	Severe Iritis Herpes Zoster	Rubeosis Iridis	Fibrovascular Membrane in Areas Retinopathy of Prematurity	Juvenile Xanthogranuloma
33. Proptosis							R
34. Pupillary distortion		U		R			S
35. Recurrent corneal ulcer	U					U	
36. Retinal artery narrowing		S					
37. Retinal detachment	S						
38. Retinal edema	U			U		S	
39. Retinal hemorrhages						U	
40. Retinal neovascularization				U		S	
41. Retinal venous engorgement and tortuosity						U	
42. Retrolental mass					S		
43. Scleritis		S					S
44. Uveal tract tumor	S			S	S	S	
45. Vitreous hemorrhage						U	
46. Vitreous traction				S			
49. Zoster rash of eyelids							

R = rarely; S = sometimes; U = usually

Spontaneous hyphema in infants

	Juvenile Xanthogranuloma	Retinoblastoma*	Blood Dyscrasias as Anemia/Leukemia*	Acute Rheumatoid Iridocyclytis	Trauma without History*	Retrolental Fibroplasia	Persistent Hyperplastic Primary Vitreous	Retinoschisis	Iritis as Behçet Syndrome
History									
1. Bilateral									
2. Child abuse		R	S	U		U		U	S
3. Common in males					U				
4. Congenital					U			U	
5. Familial							U	U	
6. Hereditary		U	S	S					
7. Japanese/Italian extraction		U	S						S
8. Oxygen therapy						U			
9. Prematurity						U	S		
10. Virus infection									U
Physical Findings									
1. Anterior/posterior synechiae					S				S
2. Band keratopathy					U				
3. Blood stained cornea	U								
4. Cataract				U	S				
5. Cherry red spot of macula									S
6. Conjunctival/subconjunctival mass	R								S
7. Corneal abrasions					S				S
8. Corneal edema	S								
9. Corneal opacity									S
10. Cotton-wool spots			U						
11. Endophthalmitis		S							
12. Endothelial corneal damage					S				
13. Extraocular muscle paralysis			S						S
14. Eyelids, yellow/brown papules/nodules	U								
15. Galucoma	S	S		S	S	R	S		S
16. Heterchromic iris	U	U							
17. Hypopyon		U			U				
18. Hypotony									R
19. Iridodialysis					S				
20. Iris neovascularization					S				
21. Leukokoria		U							
22. Lid edema		U					U		
23. Macular edema		U			S				
24. Microphthalmia						S	S		
25. Mydriasis		U							
26. Nystagmus								S	
27. Ocular pain				U	S				
28. Optic atrophy		S		U	S				S
29. Optic neuritis									S
30. Oval/eccentric pupil	S			U					S
31. Panophthalmitis	S								
32. Papilledema		S	S						
33. Phthisis bulbi						S	S		

* = most important

Spontaneous hyphema in infants (Continued)

	Juvenile Xanthogranuloma	Retinoblastoma*	Blood Dyscrasias as Anemia/Leukemia*	Acute Rheumatoid Iridocyclytis	Trauma without History*	Retrolental Fibroplasia	Persistent Hyperplastic Primary Vitreous	Retinoschisis	Iritis as Behçet Syndrome
Physical Findings									
34. Proptosis	R				S				
35. Recessed chamber angle					S				
36. Retinal detachment			S	S	S	U	S	S	S
37. Retinal edema						S	S		
38. Retinal mass					S				
39. Retinal tractional tear	U								
40. Salmon colored iris lesion					S				
41. Scleral rupture									S
42. Scleritis					S				
43. Subluxed lens			U					S	S
44. Strabismus				S					
45. Thread-like arterioles							S		
46. Uveitis	U				U				
47. Vitreous cells					S				
48. Vitreous detachment			S	S		R		S	S
49. Vitreous hemorrhage								U	
50. Vitreous veils									
Laboratory Data									
1. Antinuclear antibody titers				U					
2. Biopsy of lid lesion	U								
3. Biopsy of tumor		S							
4. Bone marrow puncture			U						
5. Computed tomographic scan		U				S			
6. Cytology of anterior chamber	S	S	S						
7. Complete blood study (white blood cell count, hemoglobin, hematocrit)				U	S				
8. Electroretinogram abnormal								U	
9. Fluorescein angiography			S		S	S	S	S	
10. Homologous leucocytic antibody determination									U
11. Lumbosacral-spine roentgenogram									U
12. Macroglobulins negative									U
13. Orbital roentgenogram (globe calcium)			S			S			
14. Ultrasonography, ocular	U	U			U	U	S		
15. Visual fields								U	

R = rarely; S = sometimes; and U = usually.

PLASMOID AQUEOUS (AQUEOUS WITH A HIGH PROTEIN CONTENT)

1. Rheumatoid arthritis
2. Serum sickness
3. Infection with gonococcus
4. Following paracentesis or intraocular operation, such as cataract extraction
5. Severe corneal ulceration
6. Trauma

Newell FW. *Ophthalmology, principles and concepts*, 7th ed. St. Louis: CV Mosby, 1991.

CHOLESTEROLOSIS OF THE ANTERIOR CHAMBER

In this condition, cholesterol crystals develop in the anterior chamber; usually in a blind eye following trauma, but can be associated with hyphema or secondary glaucoma. It is also associated with the following:

*1. Chronic uveitis
 2. Eales disease (periphlebitis)
 3. Lens subluxation
 4. Mature or hypermature cataract
 5. Microphthalmia
*6. Phthisis bulbi
 7. Retinal detachment
 8. Traumatic cataract
 9. Vascular disorders
10. Vitreous hemorrhage

Mishra RK, et al. Cholesterol crystals in Eales disease. *Indian J Ophthalmol* 1980;28:67–68.
Wand M, Garn RA. Cholesterolosis of the anterior chamber. *Am J Ophthalmol* 1974;78:143–144.

GAS BUBBLES IN THE ANTERIOR CHAMBER

1. *Clostridium perfringens*
2. *E. coli*
3. Yttrium-aluminum-garnet (YAG) laser treatment to the anterior segment
4. Postoperative intraocular surgery

Frantz JF, et al. Acute endogenous panophthalmitis caused by clostridium perfringens. *Am J Ophthalmol* 1974;78:295–303.
Obertymski H, Dyson C. *Clostridium perfringens* panophthalmitis. *Can J Ophthalmol* 1974;9:258–259.

PIGMENTATION OF TRABECULAR MESHWORK

 1. In elderly individuals—inferior nasal or faint band circumferential
*2. Pseudoexfoliation of lens with or without glaucoma—unilateral or bilateral
*3. Pigmentary glaucoma
*4. Krukenberg spindle without glaucoma
*5. Malignant melanoma—one eye
 6. Cyst of pigment layer of iris—unilateral
 7. Previous intraocular operation, inflammation, or hyphema—scattered, mostly in lower angle
 8. Nevus—dense, isolated patch

9. Open-angle glaucoma—patchy band, whole circumference
10. Following gamma irradiation for malignancy of nasal sinus

Epstein DL. *Chandler and Grant's glaucoma*, 3rd ed. Philadelphia: Lea & Febiger, 1986.

Roth M, Simmons RJ. Glaucoma associated with precipitates on the trabecular meshwork. *Ophthalmology* 1982; 86:1614.

PIGMENT LIBERATION INTO THE ANTERIOR CHAMBER WITH DILATATION OF PUPIL

1. Diabetes mellitus (Willis disease)
2. Exercise
3. Hurler disease (mucopolysaccharidoses IH)
4. Low-tension glaucoma with pigment dispersion

Epstein DL. *Chandler and Grant's glaucoma*, 3rd ed. Philadelphia: Lea & Febiger, 1986.

Ritch R. Nonprogressive low tension glaucoma with pigmentary dispersion. *Am J Ophthalmol* 1982;94:190–196.

GRADING OF ANTERIOR CHAMBER ANGLE WIDTH (USUALLY DETERMINED BY GONIOSCOPY)

1. Grade 0: No angle structures visible—narrow angle, complete or partial closure (angle closure)
2. Grade 1: Unable to see posterior one half of trabecular meshwork—extremely narrow angle (probably capable of angle closure)
3. Grade 2: Part of Schlemm canal is visible—moderately narrow angle (may be capable of angle closure)
4. Grade 3: Posterior portion of Schlemm canal is visible—moderately open angle (incapable of angle closure)
5. Grade 4: Ciliary body is visible—open angle (incapable of angle closure)

Epstein DL. *Chandler and Grant's glaucoma*, 3rd ed. Philadelphia: Lea & Febiger, 1986.

Shields MB. *Textbook of glaucoma*, 2nd ed. Baltimore: Williams & Wilkins, 1986.

BLOOD IN SCHLEMM CANAL (REVERSAL OF NORMAL PRESSURE GRADIENT)

*1. Artifact of goniolens flange occluding the episcleral veins in one or more quadrants
2. High episcleral venous pressure
  *A. Carotid–cavernous sinus fistula (Red-eyed shunt syndrome)
  *B. Dural–cavernous fistula
  C. Mediastinal tumors
  D. Orbital arteriovenous fistula
  E. Sturge–Weber syndrome (meningocutaneous syndrome)
  F. Superior vena cava obstruction (superior vena cava syndrome)
  G. Tetralogy of Fallot
3. Low intraocular pressure
  A. Following trabeculectomy
  B. Hypotony (see p. 325)
  C. Intraocular inflammation
4. Normal eye

* = most important

Namba H. Blood reflux into anterior chamber after trabeculectomy. *Jpn J Ophthalmol* 1983;27:616–625.

Phelps CD, et al. Arterial anastomosis with Schlemm's canal. *Trans Am Ophthalmol Soc* 1985;83:304–315.

Phelps CD, et al. The diagnosis and prognosis of atypical carotid cavernous fistula. *Am J Ophthalmol* 1982;93: 423–436.

DEEP ANTERIOR CHAMBER ANGLE

1. Normal variation
2. Aphakia
3. Myopia
4. Megalocornea or conical cornea including keratoconus (see p. 288)
5. Congenital glaucoma
6. Posterior dislocation of the lens (see p. 401–404)
7. Recession of anterior chamber angle

Newell FW. *Ophthalmology, principles and concepts*, 7th ed. St. Louis: CV Mosby, 1991.

Shields MB. *Textbook of glaucoma*, 2nd ed. Baltimore: Williams & Wilkins, 1986.

NARROW ANTERIOR CHAMBER ANGLE (MAY BE CAPABLE OF ANGLE CLOSURE GLAUCOMA)

1. Normal variation
*2. Predisposition to angle closure
3. Anterior dislocation of the lens
4. Hyperopia
5. Spherophakia and microcornea
6. Postoperative intraocular operation with leaking wound (see hypotony, p. 325)
7. Choroidal detachment (see p. 532–535)
*8. Pupillary block
9. Loss of aqueous from perforating ulcer, corneal wound, or staphyloma (see hypotony, p. 325)
10. Intumescent senile cataract
11. Traumatic cataract that fluffs up
12. Primary hyperplastic primary vitreous (PHPV)
13. Peripheral anterior synechiae (see p. 341)
*14. Posterior entrapment of aqueous humor (malignant glaucoma or ciliary-block glaucoma)
15. Drugs, including the following:

acetazolamide	neostigmine	sulfamethizole
acetylcholine	physostigmine	sulfamethoxazole
alpha-chymotrypsin	pilocarpine	sulfamethoxypyridazine
demecarium	sulfacetamide	sulfanilamide
dichlorphenamide	sulfachlorpyridazine	sulfaphenazole
echothiophate	sulfadiazine	sulfapyridine
edrophonium	sulfadimethoxine	sulfasalazine
ethoxzolamide	sulfamerazine	sulfathiazole
isoflurophate	sulfameter	sulfisoxazole
methazolamide	sulfamethazine	

*16. Plateau iris

17. Diffuse ciliary body or iris tumor

Fraunfelder FT, Fraunfelder FW. *Drug-induced ocular side effects*. Woburn, MA: Butterworth-Heinemann, 2001.

Newell FW. *Ophthalmology: principles and concepts*, 7th ed. St. Louis: CV Mosby, 1991.

Taylor BC, Winslow RL. Pseudophakic flat anterior chamber following retinal detachment repair. *Ophthalmology* 1981;88:935.

IRREGULAR DEPTH OF THE ANTERIOR CHAMBER

1. Partial dislocation of lens
2. Tumor of iris or ciliary body
3. Peripheral anterior synechiae on one side of the chamber (see p. 341)
4. Iris bombe or pupillary block
5. Ruptured lens capsule with swelling on one side
6. Anatomic narrowing superiorly
7. Subacute angle-closure glaucoma
8. Cyclodialysis and traumatic recession of chamber angle

Epstein DL. *Chandler and Grant's glaucoma*, 3rd ed. Philadelphia: Lea & Febiger, 1986.

Newell FW. *Ophthalmology, principles and concepts*, 7th ed. St. Louis: CV Mosby, 1991.

PERIPHERAL ANTERIOR SYNECHIAE (ADHESION OF IRIS TISSUE ACROSS ANTERIOR CHAMBER STRUCTURES IN VARIABLE AMOUNTS NOTED WITH GONIOSCOPY)

1. Bridge corneoscleral trabecular meshwork to Schwalbe line or anterior to Schwalbe line (uncommon)
    A. Anterior chamber cleavage syndrome
        (1) Axenfeld syndrome (posterior embryotoxon)
        (2) Congenital central anterior synechiae
        (3) Following intraocular lens implantation
        (4) Reiger syndrome (dysgenesis mesostromatolysis)
    B. Essential iris atrophy (see p. 373)
    C. Iris bombe from occlusion of pupil
    D. Iris or ciliary body tumor pushing iris into contact with cornea
    E. Local adhesion with of epithelium or fibrous ingrowth
    F. Penetrating injury of the cornea
    G. Postoperative flat anterior chamber
2. Synechiae of iris limited to ciliary band, scleral spur, and trabecular meshwork (common)
    *A. Following cataract surgery, intraocular implantation, refractive surgery, or laser trabeculoplasty
    *B. Intraocular inflammation
    *C. Neovascular glaucoma from fibrovascular membrane (see p. 324)
    *D. Sequelae to angle-closure glaucoma

Epstein DL. *Chandler and Grant's glaucoma*, 3rd ed. Philadelphia: Lea & Febiger, 1986.

Kolker AE, Hetherington J. *Becker-Shaffer's diagnosis and therapy of the glaucomas*, 6th ed. St. Louis: CV Mosby, 1989.

* = most important

Newell FW. *Ophthalmology, principles and concepts*, 7th ed. St. Louis: CV Mosby, 1991.

Rouhiainen HJ, et al. Peripheral anterior synechiae formation after trabeculoplasty. *Arch Ophthalmol* 1988;106: 189–191.

NEOVASCULARIZATION OF ANTERIOR CHAMBER ANGLE (NEWLY FORMED VESSELS EXTEND INTO THE TRABECULAR MESHWORK)

1. Anterior chamber angle
   A. Congenital pupillary iris lens membrane with goniodysgenesis
   B. Traumatic chamber angle
2. Iris tumors
   A. Hemangioma
   B. Melanoma
   C. Metastatic carcinoma
3. Ocular vascular disease
   *A. Central retinal artery thrombosis
   *B. Central retinal vein thrombosis (see p. 468)
   C. Hemiretinal branch vein occlusion (HBVO)
4. Postinflammatory
   A. Anterior chamber implants
   B. Fungal endophthalmitis
   C. Radiation
   D. Retinal detachment operation
   E. Uveitis, chronic
5. Proximal vascular disease
   A. Aortic arch syndrome (Takayasu syndrome)
   B. Carotid cavernous fistula
   C. Carotid ligation
   D. Carotid occlusive disease
   E. Cranial arteritis (temporal arteritis syndrome)
6. Retinal disease
   A. Coats disease (Leber miliary aneurysms)
   *B. Diabetic retinopathy
   C. Eales disease (periphlebitis)
   D. Glaucoma, chronic
   E. Melanoma of choroid
   F. Norrie disease (fetal iritis syndrome)
   G. Persistent hyperplastic primary vitreous
   H. Retinal detachment
   I. Retinal hemangioma
   J. Retinal vessel occlusion
   K. Retinoblastoma
   L. Retrolental fibroplasia
   M. Sickle cell retinopathy (Herrick syndrome)

Cibis GW, et al. Congenital pupillary iris-lens membrane with goniodysgenesis. *Ophthalmology* 1986;93:847–852.

Kimura R. Fluorescein gonioangiography of newly formed vessels in the anterior chamber angle. *Tohoku J Exp Med* 1983;140:193–196.

Roy FH. *Ocular syndromes and systemic diseases*, 3rd ed. Philadelphia: Lippincott Williams & Wilkins, 2002.

Shihab ZM, Lee PF. The significance of normal angle vessels. *Ophthalmic Surg Lasers* 1985;16:382–385.

IRIS PROCESSES (PECTINATE LIGAMENTS IN ANTERIOR CHAMBER ANGLE)

1. Achondroplasia, diastrophic dwarfism, cartilage-hair hypoplasia, and spondyloepiphyseal dysplasia, anterior chamber cleavage syndrome, Axenfeld syndrome, Reiger syndrome, Peter anomaly.
2. Congenital glaucoma—may be associated with congenital microcoria and goniodysgenesis
3. Congenital scoliosis
4. Legg–Perthes disease (coxa plana)
5. Marfan syndrome (hypoplastic form of dystrophia mesodermalis congenita)
6. Mucopolysaccharidoses (including Hunter syndrome, Hurler syndrome, Scheie syndrome, and Sanfilippo-Good syndrome)
7. Myopic patients
*8. Normal, especially in brown-eyed persons
9. Pigmentary ocular dispersion syndrome

Dunn SP, et al. New findings in posterior amorphous corneal dystrophy. *Arch Ophthalmol* 1984;102:236–239.

Pollock A, Oliver M. Congenital glaucoma and incomplete congenital glaucoma in two siblings. *Acta Ophthalmol Scand* 1984;62:359–363.

Roy FH. *Ocular syndromes and systemic diseases*, 3rd ed. Philadelphia: Lippincott Williams & Wilkins, 2002.

WHITE MASS IN ANTERIOR CHAMBER

*1. Endophthalmitis
2. Ocular aspergillosis
3. Sterile inflammation following surgery or trauma
*4. Tumor

Katz G, et al. Ocular aspergillosis isolated in the anterior chamber. *Ophthalmology* 1993;100:1815–1818.

11

Pupil

CONTENTS

MYDRIASIS (DILATED PUPIL, USUALLY > 5 MM)

1. Physiologic
   A. Larger pupils in women than in men
   B. Larger pupils in myopes than in hypermetropes
   C. Larger pupils in blue irides than in brown irides
   D. Larger pupils in adolescents and middle-aged persons than in very young or old persons
   E. Surprise, fear, pain, strong emotion, or vestibular stimulation
   F. General anesthesia of stages I, II, and IV
   G. Autosensory pupillary reflex—stimulation of middle ear
   H. Auditory pupillary reflex—tuning fork adjacent to ear
   I. Vestibular pupillary reflex—stimulation of labyrinth by heat, cold, or rotation
   J. Vagotonic pupillary reflex—stimulation on deep inspiration
2. Drugs, including the following:

(live)
acetaminophen
acetanilid
acetophenazine
acetylcholine
adiphenine
adrenal cortex injection
albuterol

alcohol
aldosterone
alkavervir
allobarbital
alprazolam
alseroxylon
amantadine
ambutonium

amitriptyline
amobarbital
amoxapine
amphetamine
amyl nitrite
anisotropine
antazoline
antimony lithium thiomalate

antimony potassium tartrate
antimony sodium tartrate
antimony sodium
  thioglycollate
aprobarbital
aspirin
atropine
atropine methylnitrate
azatadine
baclofen
barbital
belladonna
benzathine
benzphetamine
benztropine
betamethasone
benzathine
biperiden
botulinum A
bromide
bromisovalum
brompheniramine
butabarbital
butalbital
butallylonal
butaperazine
butethal
caramiphen
carbamazepine
carbinoxamine
carbon dioxide
carbromal
carisoprodol
carphenazine
chloral hydrate
chloramphenicol
chlorcyclizine
chlordiazepoxide
chlorisondamine
chloroform
chlorpheniramine
chlorphenoxamine
chlorphentermine
chlorpromazine
chlorprothixene
cimetidine
clemastine
clidinium
clomiphene

clomipramine
clonazepam
clonidine
clorazepate
cocaine
codeine
colistimethate
colistin
contraceptives
cortisone
cryptenamine
cyclizine
cyclobarbital
cyclopentobarbital
cyclopentolate
cycrimine
cyproheptadine
deserpidine
desipramine
desoxycorticosterone
dexamethasone
dexbrompheniramine
dexchlorpheniramine
dextroamphetamine
diacetylmorphine
diazepam
dicyclomine
diethazine
diethylpropion
digitalis
digoxin
dimethindene
diphemanil
diphenhydramine
diphenylhydantoin
diphenylpyraline
diphtheria toxoid (adsorbed)
dipivefrin
disopyramide
disulfiram
doxepin
doxylamine
dipivalyl epinephrine (DPE)
droperidol
emetine
ephedrine
epinephrine
ergot
erythromycin

ether
ethopropazine
fenfluramine
fludrocortisone
fluorometholone
fluphenazine
fluprednisolone
flurazepam
fluvoxamine hydrochloride
gentamicin (?)
glutethimide
glycopyrrolate
guanethidine
halazepam
haloperidol
hashish
heptabarbital
hexachlorophene
hexamethonium
hexethal
hexobarbital
hexocyclium
homatropine
hydrabamine penicillin V
hydrabamine phenoxymethyl
  penicillin
hydrocortisone
hydromorphone
hydroxyamphetamine
imipramine
indomethacin (?)
insulin
iodide and iodine solutions
  and compounds
isocarboxazid
isoniazid
isopropamide
levallorphan
levarterenol
levodopa
lidocaine
lorazepam
loxapine
lysergic acid diethylamide
  (LSD)
lysergide
maprotiline
marijuana
measles and rubella virus
  vaccine (live)

measles virus vaccine (live)
measles, mumps, and rubella
   virus vaccine
mecamylamine
meclizine
medrysone
mepenzolate
meperidine
mephentermine
mephobarbital
meprednisone
meprobamate
mescaline
mesoridazine
metaraminol
methadone
methamphetamine
methantheline
methaqualone
metharbital
methdilazine
methitural
methixene
methohexital
methotrimeprazine
methoxamine
methscopolamine
methyl alcohol
methylatropine nitrate
methylene blue
methylpentynol
methylphenidate
methylprednisolone
methyprylon
metoclopramide
midazolam
morphine
mumps virus vaccine (live)
nalidixic acid
nalorphine
naloxone
naltrexone
naphazoline
nialamide
nitrazepam
nitroglycerin (?)
nitrous oxide
norepinephrine
nortriptyline

opium
oral contraceptives
orphenadrine
oxazepam
oxygen
oxymorphone
oxyphencyclimine
oxyphenonium
paraldehyde
paramethasone
pargyline
penicillin G
pentobarbital
pentolinium
pentylenetetrazol
perazine
pericyazine
perphenazine
phenacetin
phendimetrazine
phenelzine
pheniramine
phenmetrazine
phenobarbital
phenoxymethyl penicillin
phentermine
phenylephrine
phenylpropanolamine
phenytoin
pilocarpine
pipenzolate
piperacetazine
piperidolate
poldine
polymyxin B
potassium penicillin G
potassium penicillin V
potassium phenethicillin
potassium phenoxymethyl
   penicillin
prazepam
prednisolone
prednisone
primidone
probarbital
procaine penicillin G
prochlorperazine
procyclidine
promazine

promethazine
propantheline
propiomazine
propoxyphene
protoveratrines A and B
protriptyline
psilocybin
pyrilamine
quinidine
quinine
radioactive iodides
rauwolfia serpentina
rescinnamine
reserpine
rubella and mumps virus
   vaccine (live)
rubella virus vaccine (live)
scopolamine
secobarbital
sodium antimonylgluconate
sodium salicylate
stibocaptate
stibogluconate
stibophen
syrosingopine
talbutal
temazepam
tetraethylammonium
tetrahydrocannabinol
tetrahydrozoline
thiocarbanidin (THC) (?)
thiamylal
thiethylperazine
thiopental
thiopropazate
thioproperazine thioridazine
thiothixene
tolazoline
tranylcypromine
trazodone
triamcinolone
triazolam
tridihexethyl
trifluoperazine
trifluperidol
triflupromazine
trihexyphenidyl
trimeprazine
trimethaphan

trimethidinium
trimipramine
tripelennamine

tropicamide
urethan
veratrum viride alkaloids

vinbarbital

3. Toxins, including after-shave lotion, arsenic, *Clostridium botulinum* (gas gangrene), tetanus (lockjaw), cannabis, adrenergic agents (such as nasal sprays or asthma therapy in newborns), paraaminosalicylic acid, lead, carbon monoxide, organic phosphorus, bovine milk protein in infants with allergic malabsorption, *Datura stramonium* (Jimson weed), *Datura* wrightii (moonflower), and *Solanaceae* (nightshade), nitrocompounds and aminocompounds of benzene, carbon disulfide, and papaverine.

4. Ocular causes (mydriasis) (see fixed pupil section p. 348)
   - A. Glaucoma, usually acute
   - B. Glaucomocylitic crisis (Posner–Schlossman syndrome)
   - C. Hollenhorst syndrome (chorioretinal infarction syndrome)
   - *D. Iritis; uveitis
   - E. Intraocular foreign body (iron mydriasis)
   - F. Iris atrophy
   - G. Iris sphincter rupture
   - *H. Paralytic mydriasis following trauma
   - I. Photocoagulation complications
   - J. Retinoblastoma

5. Lesions of ciliary ganglion causing internal ophthalmoplegia (e.g., dilated pupil and absent accommodation)
   - A. Adie tonic pupil
   - B. Congenital lesion
   - C. Herpes zoster
   - D. Orbital floor fracture repair
   - E. Systemic lupus erythematosus (disseminated lupus erythematosus)
   - F. Varicella (chickenpox)
   - G. Yellow fever

6. Acute or chronic ophthalmoplegias (see p. 168–171)
7. Third-nerve lesion—also ptosis and ophthalmoplegia on affected side (see p. 168–171)
8. Coma because of alcohol ingestion, eclampsia, diabetes, uremia, epilepsy, apoplexy, or meningitis—the pupils are equally dilated and do not constrict with stimulation
9. Midbrain tumors, in which dilated pupils, paralysis of vertical gaze (especially upward gaze), and retraction nystagmus are manifested
   - A. Craniopharyngioma
   - B. Parinaud syndrome (paralysis of upgaze movements)

10. Epidural or subdural hematoma
11. Paralytic parasympathetic lesions
12. Irritative sympathetic lesion—pupillary dilatation widening of palpebral aperture and slight exophthalmos
   - A. Irritative lesion, such as tumor, encephalitis, or syringomyelia of the hypothalamus, midbrain, medulla, or cervical cord
   - B. Thoracic lesions, such as cervical rib, aneurysms of the thoracic vessels, mediastinal tumors, or tubercular pleurisy
   - *C. Cervical lesions, including nasopharyngeal tumors, thyroid swelling, or cervical nodes
   - D. Rabies (hydrophobia)
   - *E. Trauma

* = most important

   F. Visceral disease

   G. Aortic dilatation or exudative endocarditis (Roque sign)

   H. Acute abdominal conditions, such as appendicitis, cholecystitis, or colitis (Moschowitz sign)

   I. Psychiatric patients with pressure over McBurney point (Meyer phenomenon)

13. Tumors, injury, or hemorrhage of frontoparietal, parietal, temporal, or temporooccipital area—contralateral mydriasis and ipsilateral defect in the visual field
14. Fractured skull
15. Acute autonomic neuropathy
16. Acute pandysautonomia
17. Avitaminosis B_z (pellagra)
18. Chorea
19. Clivus edge syndrome
20. Craniocervical syndrome (whiplash injury)
21. Foramen lacerum syndrome (aneurysm of internal carotid artery syndrome)
22. Hemiacrosomia syndrome (hemifacial or unilateral hypertrophy)
23. Iron deficiency anemia
24. Lockjaw (tetanus)
25. Mycosis fungoides syndrome (Sézary syndrome)
26. Optic canal syndrome
27. Parkinson syndrome (shaking palsy)
28. Prematurity
29. Pulseless disease
30. Reye syndrome (acute encephalopathy syndrome)
31. Rollet syndrome (orbital apex–sphenoidal syndrome)
32. Suprarenal–sympathetic syndrome (adrenal medulla tumor syndrome)
33. Temporal arteritis
34. Weber syndrome (cerebellar peduncle syndrome)
35. Wernicke syndrome (I) (avitaminosis B_1 thiamine deficiency)
36. Zellweger syndrome (cerebrohepatorenal syndrome)

Bodker FS, et al. Postoperative mydriasis after repair of orbital floor fracture. *Am J Ophthalmol,*1993;115:372–375.

Cuppeto JR, Greco T. Mydriasis in giant cell arteritis. *J Clin Neuroophthalmol* 1985;9:267.

Fraunfelder FT, Fraunfelder FW. *Drug-induced ocular side effects.* Woburn, MA Butterworth-Heinemann, 2001.

Hendrix LE, et al. Papaverine-induced mydriasis. *AJNR Am J Neuroradiol* 1994;15:716–718.

Isenberg SJ, et al. The fixed and dilated pupils of premature neonates. *Am J Ophthalmol* 1990;110:168.

Pau H. *Differential diagnosis of eye diseases,* 2nd ed. New York: Thieme Medical, 1988.

Richardson P, Schulenburg WE. Bilateral congenital mydriasis. *Br J Ophthalmol* 1992;76:632–633.

Roy FH. *Ocular syndromes and systemic diseases,* 3rd ed. Philadelphia: Lippincott Williams & Wilkins, 2002.

RELATIVE FIXED, DILATED PUPIL

1. Midbrain damage—vascular accidents, tumors, degenerative and infectious diseases

   A. Dorsal (Edinger–Westphal nucleus and its connections)—rare, involves both pupils, pupillary near reaction often retained, and often associated with supranuclear vertical gaze palsy (upgaze)

  *B. Ventral (fascicular part of third nerve)—associated with other neurologic deficits, such as Nothnagel syndrome, Benedikt syndrome, Weber syndrome, and involves other extraocular components of the third nerve

*2. Damage to the third nerve (from interpeduncular fossa to ciliary ganglion)
    A. Basal aneurysms
    B. Supratentorial space-occupying masses, causing displacement of the brainstem or transtentorial herniation of the uncus; patient is stuporous or comatose
    C. Basal meningitis—often bilateral internal ophthalmoplegia
  *D. Ischemic oculomotor palsy
    E. Parasellar tumor (e.g., pituitary adenoma, meningioma, craniopharyngioma, naso-pharyngeal carcinoma, or distant metastases)
    F. Parasellar inflammation (e.g., Tolosa–Hunt syndrome, temporal arteritis, herpes zoster)

*3. Damage to the ciliary ganglion
    A. Viral ciliary ganglionitis or involvement of the ciliary nerves, such as from herpes zoster
    B. Orbital trauma or tumor
    C. Trauma from inferior oblique surgery
    D. Trauma from retrobulbar injections

4. Damage to short ciliary nerves
    A. Blunt trauma to the globe may injure the ciliary plexus at the iris root (traumatic iridoplegia)
    B. Choroidal trauma or tumor

*5. Damage to the iris
    A. Degenerative or inflammatory diseases of the iris
    B. Posterior synechiae
    C. Acute rise of intraocular pressure (hypoxia or sphincter damage)
    D. Blunt injury to the globe with sphincter damage (traumatic iridoplegia)
    E. Pharmacologic blockade by atropinic substances
    F. Following cataract surgery

6. Total blindness, including cortical blindness (see p. 632–636)
    A. Bilateral optic nerve
        (1) Anterior ischemic optic neuropathy
        (2) Avulsion (traumatic)
        (3) Optic neuritis
    B. Bilateral retina
        (1) Acute retinal necrosis
        (2) Central retinal artery occlusion
        (3) Central retinal vein occlusion
        (4) Retina detachment

Isenberg SJ, et al. The fixed and dilated pupils of premature neonates. *Am J Ophthalmol* 1990;110:168–171.

Lam S, et al. Atonic pupil after cataract surgery. *Ophthalmology* 1989;96:589–590.

Newell FW. *Ophthalmology: principles and concepts,* 7th ed. St. Louis: CV Mosby, 1991.

Thompson HS, et al. The fixed dilated pupil. *Arch Ophthalmol* 1971;86:21–27.

MIOSIS (SMALL PUPIL) (USUALLY <2 MM)

1. Physiologic
    A. Smaller pupil in men than in women
    B. Smaller pupil in hypermetropes than in myopes
    C. Smaller pupil in brown irides than in blue irides
    D. Smaller pupil in very young or old than in adolescents and middle-aged persons

* = most important

E. Sleep, fatigue, coma
F. Stage III anesthesia
G. Near vision (synkinesis with convergence and accommodation)
H. Vestibular stimulation
2. Drugs, including the following:

aceclidine
acetophenazine
acetylcholine
alcohol
allobarbital
alseroxylon
ambenonium
amobarbital
aprobarbital
baclofen
barbital
bethanechol
bromide
bromisovalum
bupivacaine
butabarbital
butalbital
butallylonal
butaperazine
butethal
carbachol
carbromal
carisoprodol
carphenazine
chloral hydrate
chloroform
chloroprocaine
chlorpromazine
chlorprothixene
clonidine
codeine
cyclobarbital
cyclopentobarbital
demecarium
deserpidine
diacetylmorphine
dibucaine
diethazine
digitalis(?)
diisopropyl flurophosphate
  (DFP)
dronabinol
droperidol

echothiophate
edrophonium
ephedrine (?)
ergot
ergotamine
ether
ethopropazine
fluphenazine
guanethidine
haloperidol
hashish
heptabarbital
hexachlorophene
hexethal
hexobarbital
hydromorphone
indomethacin
iodide and iodine solutions
  and compounds (?)
isocarboxazid
isoflurophate
isosorbide dinitrate (?)
levallorphan
levodopa
lidocaine
marijuana
meperidine
mephobarbital
mepivacaine
meprobamate
mesoridazine
methacholine
methadone
methaqualone (?)
metharbital
methdilazine
methitural
methohexital
methotrimeprazine
methyprylon
midazolam
morphine
nalorphine

naloxone
naltrexone
neostigmine
nialamide
nitrous oxide
opium
oxprenolol
oxymorphone
paraldehyde
pentazocine
pentobarbital
perazine
pericyazine
perphenazine
phencyclidine
phenelzine
phenobarbital
phenoxybenzamine
phenylephrine
physostigmine
pilocarpine
piperacetazine
piperazine
piperocaine
prilocaine
primidone
probarbital
procaine
prochlorperazine
promazine
promethazine
propiomazine
propoxycaine
propoxyphene
propranolol
pyridostigmine
radioactive iodides (?)
rauwolfia serpentina
rescinnamine reserpine
secobarbital
sulindac
syrosingopine
talbutal

tetracaine
tetrahydrocannabinol
thiamylal
thiethylperazine
thiopental
thiopropazate

thioproperazine
thioridazine
thiothixene
tolazoline
tranylcypromine
trifluoperazine

trifluperidol
triflupromazine
trimeprazine
vinbarbital
vitamin A

3. Ocular causes
   *A. Accommodative spasm (hysteria)
    B. Corneal irritation, such as keratitis or corneal injury
    C. Conjunctival irritation
    D. Congenital miosis (absent dilator muscle)
    E. Dislocated lenses
    F. Iritis
   *G. Posterior iris synechiae, usually irregular
    H. Retinitis pigmentosa
4. Central nervous system defects
    A. Acute pontine angle lesion, such as hemorrhage or tumor associated with disturbed conjugate gaze
    B. Arteriosclerotic and degenerative disease of the cerebrum
    C. Encephalitis
    D. Facial tetanus
    E. Giant cell (temporal arteritis)
    F. Infections or tumors of the cavernous sinus or superior orbital fissure
    G. Purulent meningitis
    H. Severe hypoxia
5. ''Cluster headache'' or histamine cephalgia–ptosis; miosis; red, watering eye on side of headache
6. Raeder paratrigeminal syndrome—ipsilateral miosis and pain—may be associated with third-nerve paralysis or corneal anesthesia
    A. Extracranial aneurysm of internal carotid
    B. Idiopathic
    C. Meningioma
    D. Migraine
    E. Posttrauma
7. Argyll Robertson pupil—small and irregular; reacts better to accommodation than to light
    A. Aberrant regeneration of the third nerve
    B. Carbon disulfide poisoning
    C. Cerebral aneurysm
    D. Chronic alcoholism
   *E. Diabetes mellitus (Willis disease)
    F. Encephalitis
    G. Friedreich ataxia
    H. Malaria
    I. Midbrain tumors, such as pinealomas and craniopharyngioma
    J. Multiple sclerosis (disseminated sclerosis)
    K. Senile and degenerative diseases of the central nervous system
    L. Syphilis (acquired lues)

* = most important

    M. Syringomyelia

    N. Trauma to skull or orbit

  8. Ataxia, spastic with congenital miosis—dominant

  9. Babinski–Nageotte syndrome (medulla tegmental paralysis)

 10. Coenurosis

 11. Craniocervical syndrome (whiplash injury)

 12. Dejerine–Klumpke syndrome (lower radicular syndrome)

 13. Devic syndrome (neuromyelitis optica)

*14. Diabetes mellitus

 15. Eaton–Lambert syndrome (myasthenic syndrome)

 16. Elevated intracranial pressure

*17. Horner syndrome (cervical sympathetic paralysis syndrome)

 18. Jugular foramen syndrome (Vernet syndrome)

 19. Lowe syndrome (oculocerebrorenal syndrome)

 20. Marfan syndrome (arachnodactyly dystrophia mesodermalis congenita)

 21. Morquio syndrome (mucopolysaccharidosis IV)

 22. Myotonic dystrophy (Curschmann–Stewart syndrome)

 23. Naffziger syndrome (scalenus anticus syndrome)

 24. Pancoast syndrome (superior pulmonary sulcus syndrome)

 25. Parkinsonism (shaking palsy)

 26. Psychogenic diseases, such as schizophrenia, dementia precox, or hysteria

 27. Refsum syndrome (phytanic acid storage disease)

 28. Retroparotid space syndrome (Villaret syndrome)

 29. Romberg syndrome (facial hemiatrophy)

 30. Spider bites

 31. Stormorken syndrome (thrombocytopathia bleeding tendency)

 32. Tetanus (lockjaw)

 33. von Herrenschwand syndrome (sympathetic heterochromia)

 34. Wallenberg syndrome (dorsolateral medullary syndrome)

 35. Wernicke syndrome (avitaminosis B_1, thiamine deficiency)

Fraunfelder FT, Fraunfelder FW. *Drug-induced ocular side effects.* Woburn, MA: Butterworth-Heinemann, 2001.

Ghanchi F, Dutton GN. Current concepts in giant cell (temporal) arteritis. *Surv Ophthalmol* 1997;42:99–123.

Roy FH. *Ocular syndromes and systemic diseases,* 3rd ed. Philadelphia: Lippincott Williams & Wilkins, 2002.

PARADOXICAL PUPILLARY REACTION (CONSTRICTS WHEN LIGHT IS WITHDRAWN)

 1. Best disease

*2. Congenital achromatopsia

*3. Congenital stationary night blindness

 4. Leber congenital amaurosis

 5. Optic nerve hypoplasia

 6. Retinitis pigmentosa

Barricks ME, et al. Paradoxical pupillary responses in congenital stationary night blindness. *Arch Ophthalmol* 1977; 95:1800–1804.

Flynn JT, et al. Paradoxical pupil in congenital achromatopsia. *Int Ophthalmol* 1981;2:91–96.

Frank JW, et al. Paradoxic pupillary phenomena. *Arch Ophthalmol* 1988;106:1564.

                                           * = most important

ABSENCE OR DECREASE OF PUPILLARY REACTION TO LIGHT

This type of absence or decreased pupillary reaction to light is caused by drugs, including the following:

acetaminophen
acetanilid
acetophenazine
alcohol
allobarbital
alprazolam
amitriptyline
amobarbital
amoxapine
amoxicillin
amphetamine
ampicillin
antazoline
antimony lithium thiomalate
antimony potassium tartrate
antimony sodium tartrate
antimony sodium
   thioglycollate
aprobarbital
aspirin
atropine
baclofen
barbital
belladonna
benztropine
biperiden
bromide
bromisovalum
brompheniramine
butabarbital
butalbital
butallylonal
butaperazine
butethal
calcifediol
calcitriol
carbenicillin (?)
carbinoxamine
carbon dioxide
carbromal
carisoprodol
carmustine
carphenazine
chloramphenicol

chlorcyclizine
chlordiazepoxide
chloroprocaine
chlorpheniramine
chlorphenoxamine
chlorpromazine
chlorprothixene
cholecalciferol
cimetidine
clemastine
clomipramine
clonazepam
clonidine
clorazepate
cloxacillin (?)
cocaine
cyclizine
cyclobarbital
cyclopentobarbital
cycrimine
desipramine
dexbrompheniramine
dexchlorpheniramine
dextroamphetamine
diacetylmorphine
diazepam
dicloxacillin (?)
diethazine
dimethindene
diphenhydramine
diphenylpyraline
diphtheria toxoid, adsorbed
doxepin
doxylamine
emetine
ergocalciferol
ergot
ethopropazine
etidocaine
fenfluramine
fluphenazine
flurazepam
glutethimide
halazepam

heptabarbital
hetacillin (?)
hexachlorophene
hexethal
hexobarbital
homatropine
imipramine
insulin
isocarboxazid
isoniazid
lidocaine
lorazepam
LSD
lysergide
meclizine
meperidine
mephobarbital
mepivacaine
meprobamate
mescaline
mesoridazine
methamphetamine
methaqualone
metharbital
methdilazine
methicillin (?)
methitural
methohexital
methotrimeprazine
methscopolamine
methyl alcohol
methyprylon
midazolam
nafcillin (?)
neomycin
nialamide
nitrazepam
nortriptyline
orphenadrine
oxacillin (?)
oxazepam
pargyline
pentobarbital
pentylenetetrazol

perazine
periciazine
perphenazine
phenacetin
phencyclidine
phenelzine
pheniramine
phenmetrazine
phenobarbital
phenylpropanolamine
phenytoin
piperacetazine
prazepam
prilocaine
primidone
probarbital
procaine
prochlorperazine
procyclidine
promazine
promethazine

propantheline
propiomazine
propoxycaine
protriptyline
psilocybin
pyrilamine
quinine
ranifidine
scopolamine
secobarbital
sodium antimonylgluconate
sodium salicylate
stibocaptate
stibogluconate
stibophen
talbutal
temazepam
tetanus immune globulin
tetanus toxoid
thiamylal
thiethylperazine

thiopental
thiopropazate
thioproperazine
thioridazine
thiothixene
tranylcypromine
triazolam
trichloroethylene
trifluoperazine
triflupromazine
trihexyphenidyl
trimeprazine
trimipramine
tripelennamine
triprolidine
urethan
vinbarbital
vitamin D
vitamin D_2
vitamin D_3

Fraunfelder FT, Fraunfelder FW. *Drug-induced ocular side effects.* Woburn, MA: Butterworth-Heinemann, 2001.

ANISOCORIA (INEQUALITY OF PUPILS OF ≥1 MM)

1. Central nervous system
   *A. Adie (tonic) pupil
   B. Aneurysm of the aorta or carotid artery
   C. Cerebrovascular accidents
   D. Cervical rib (ipsilateral constricted pupil)
   E. Encephalitis (mild cases)
   *F. Horner syndrome (cervical sympathetic paralysis syndrome)
   G. Pontine lesions
   H. Tabes dorsalis
   I. Third-nerve paresis
   J. Trigeminal neuralgia (tic douloureux)
   K. Wernicke hemianopic pupil
2. Drugs, including the following:

alcohol
antazoline
bromide
bromisovalum
brompheniramine
bupivacaine
carbinoxamine
carbromal
chloroprocaine
chlorpheniramine

clemastine
contraceptives
dexbrompheniramine
dexchlorpheniramine
diacetylmorphine
dimethindene
diphenhydramine
diphenylpyraline
disulfiram
doxylamine

dronabinol
ethchlorvynol
etidocaine
hashish
isocarboxazid
jimsonweed
lidocaine
LSD
lysergide
marijuana

mepivacaine
mescaline
methaqualone
nialamide
oral contraceptives
phenelzine
pheniramine

phenylpropanolamine
prilocaine
procaine
propoxycaine
psilocybin
pyrilamine
scopolamine

tetrahydrocannabinol
tranylcypromine
trichloroethylene
tripelennamine
triprolidine

3. Ocular conditions
   A. Artificial eye (pseudoanisocoria)
   B. Cornea, such as keratitis or abrasion
   C. Glaucoma, including pigmentary dispersion
   *D. Iris, such as iritis, synechiae, iris atrophy, or iris sphincter rupture
   E. Ocular trauma
   F. Spastic miosis
4. Physiologic
   A. Anisometropia—larger pupil with the more myopic eye
   B. Familial
   C. Lateral illumination of one eye gives more miosis in that eye than in the other
   D. Nonfamilial—normal variation (small percentage of the population)
   E. Tournay reaction—with the eyes turned sharply to the side, dilatation of the pupil of the abducting eye and miosis of pupil of the adducting eye
5. Unilateral miosis (see p. 349)
6. Unilateral mydriasis (see p. 349)

Cheng MM, Catalano RA. Fatigue-induced familial anisocoria. *Am J Ophthalmol* 1990;109:480–481.

Feibel RM, Perlmutter JC. Anisocoria in the pigmentary dispersion syndrome. *Am J Ophthalmol* 1991;111:384.

Fraunfelder FT, Fraunfelder FW. *Drug-induced ocular side effects.* Woburn, MA: Butterworth-Heinemann, 2001.

Nakagawa TA, et al. Aerosolized atropine as an unusual cause of anisocoria in a child with asthma. *Pediatr Emerg Care* 1993;9:153–154.

IRREGULARITY OF PUPIL (INCLUDING OVAL OR PEAKED PUPIL)

1. Adherent leukoma as one part of iris is pulled up to corneal scar, peripheral anterior synechiae, or corneal laceration with prolapse of iris
2. Alagille syndrome
3. Anterior chamber intraocular lens that is too long or erodes into uveal tissue
4. Argyll–Robertson pupil—small and irregular; reacts better to accommodation than to light; same type as seen in diabetic patients (pseudodiabetic pupil)
5. Congenital coloboma of the iris, usually below
6. Following laser iridectomy
7. Glaucoma—oval, dilated pupil
*8. Injury of the iris
9. Iris tuck of anterior chamber intraocular lens
*10. Iritis—usually small but pupil may be any shape with anterior or posterior synechiae
*11. Long-term intraocular inflammation
12. Medication, with faster reaction of one sector of iris than of another—miosis or mydriasis
13. Operation—as sector iridectomy or peripheral iridectomy
14. Optic atrophy due to causes such as syphilis, quinine poisoning, and internal ophthalmoplegia of vascular or traumatic origin

* = most important

15. Piece of anterior capsule into anterior chamber
16. Posterior chamber intraocular lens with loop of intraocular lens holding the midportion of iris peripherally
17. Posterior chamber lens with two haptics having the lens either behind the pupil with the haptics in front or having the lens anterior to the pupil with the haptics behind the iris
18. Segmental iris atrophy
19. Tumors of iris or ciliary body
20. Vitreous or zonules into corneal laceration
21. Vitreous strand from behind pupil to wound
22. Wound leak with or without prolapse of the iris

Fuller JR. Iris creep producing correctopia in response to Molteno implants. *Arch Ophthalmol* 2001;119:304–306.

Moster MR, et al. Laser iridectomy. *Ophthalmology* 1986;93:20–24.

Newell FW. *Ophthalmology: principles and concepts,* 7th ed. St. Louis: CV Mosby, 1991.

Reidy JJ, et al. An analysis of semiflexible, closed-loop anterior chamber intraocular lenses. *Am Intraocular Implant Soc J* 1985;11:344–352.

HIPPUS

Hippus is visible, rhythmic, but irregular pupillary oscillations that are deliberate in time. It comprises 2 mm or more excursions and has no localizing significance.

1. Normal
2. Incipient cataracts
3. Central nervous system diseases, including the presence of total third cranial nerve palsy, hemiplegia, meningitis (acute), cerebral syphilis, tabes, general paralysis, myasthenia gravis, tumors of corpora quadrigemina, epileptics, Cheyne–Strokes breathing, multiple sclerosis (disseminated sclerosis), and cerebral tumors
4. Neurasthenia (nervous exhaustion, Beard disease)
5. Drugs, including the following:

allobarbital
amobarbital
aprobarbital
barbital
butabarbital
butalbital
butallylonal
butethal
cyclobarbital

cyclopentobarbital
heptabarbital
hexethal
hexobarbital
mephobarbital
metharbital
methitural
methohexital
pentobarbital

pentylenetetrazol
phenobarbital
primidone
probarbital
secobarbital
talbutal
thiamylal
thiopental
vinbarbital

Fraunfelder FT, Fraunfelder FW. *Drug-induced ocular side effects.* Woburn, MA: Butterworth-Heinemann, 2001.

Zinn KM. *The pupil.* Springfield, IL: Charles C Thomas, 1972.

TONOHAPTIC PUPIL

Tonohaptic pupil involves a long latent period preceding both contraction to light and redilatation, followed in each instance by a short but prompt movement.

1. Catatonic state
2. Diabetes mellitus (Willis disease)

3. Diabetes insipidus
4. Dystrophia adiposogenitalis (Fröhlich syndrome) or pituitary cachexia (Simmonds disease)
5. Introverted persons of the schizophrenic group
6. Parkinsonism (shaking palsy)
7. Pigmentary retinal dystrophy
8. Postencephalitic condition
9. Schizoid state

Duke-Elder S, Scott GI. *System of ophthalmology,* Vol 12. St. Louis: CV Mosby, 1971.

LEUKOKORIA (WHITE PUPIL) (SEE LESIONS CONFUSED WITH RETINOBLASTOMA, P. 502)

  1. Angiomatosis of retina (cerebelloretinal hemangioblastomatosis)
  2. Astrocytoma
*3. Cataract (congenital)
  4. Choroidal hemangioma
*5. Coats disease (retinal telangiectasia)
  6. Coloboma of choroid and optic disc
  7. Congenital cytomegalovirus retinitis
  8. Congenital retinal detachment
  9. Exudative retinitis, chorioretinitis, or both
10. Falciform fold of retina
11. Familial exudative vitreoretinopathy
12. Herpes simplex retinitis
13. High myopia with advanced chorioretinal degeneration
*14. Medullation of nerve fiber layer
15. Metastatic endophthalmitis
16. Morning glory syndrome (hereditary central glial anomaly of the optic disc)
17. Nematode endophthalmitis (*Toxocara canis*)
18. Norrie disease (atrophia oculi congenita)
*19. Ocular toxocariasis
20. Organized vitreous hemorrhage
21. Persistent hyperplastic primary vitreous
22. Physiologic-eye photographed at 17 to 20 degrees temporal to fixation
23. Retinal dysplasia (massive retinal fibrosis)
*24. Retinoblastoma
25. Retinopathy of prematurity (ROP)
26. Retrolental membrane associated with Bloch–Sulzberger syndrome (incontinentia pigmenti)
*27. Toxoplasmosis (congenital)
28. Traumatic chorioretinitis
29. Tumors other than retinoblastoma
    A. Choroidal hemangioma
    B. Combined retinal hamartoma
    C. Diktyoma
    D. Glioneuroma
    E. Leukemia
    F. Medulloepithelioma

* = most important

G. Retinal astrocytic hamartoma

H. Retinal capillary hemangioma

30. Uveitis (peripheral)

31. Vitreous organization following unsuspected penetrating wounds

Chang-Godinich A, et al. Familial exudative vitreoretinopathy mimicking persistent hyperplastic primary vitreous. *Am J Ophthalmol* 1999;127,4:469–471.

Federman JL, et al. The surgical and nonsurgical management of persistent hyperplastic primary vitreous. *Ophthalmology* 1982;89:20.

Ing E. Personal communication. December, 2001.

Roy FH. *Ocular syndromes and systemic diseases,* 3rd ed. Philadelphia: Lippincott Williams & Wilkins, 2002.

Shapiro DR, Stone RD. Ultrasonic characteristics of retinopathy of prematurity presenting with leukokoria. *Arch Ophthalmol* 1985;103:1690–1694.

Shields JA, et al. Malignant teratoid medulloepithelioma of the ciliary body simulating persistent hyperplastic primary vitreous. *Am J Ophthalmol* 1989;107:296–300.

Leukokoria (white pupil)

	Cataract	Nematode Endophthalmitis	Coats Disease*	Persistent Hyperplastic Primary Vitreous*	Retrolental Fibroplasia	Retinal Dysplasia	Organized Vitreous Hemorrhage	Falciform Fold of Retina	Angiomatosis of Retina	Bloch-Sulzberger Syndrome	Exudative Retinitis	Diktyoma	Congenital Retinal Detachment	Norrie Disease	Juvenile Retinoschisis	Metastatic Endophthalmitis	Retinoblastoma*	Coloboma of Choroid	Medullation Nerve Layer	Traumatic Chorioretinitis	High Myopia with Retinal Degeneration
History																					
1. Bilateral	S	R	R	S	S	S	R	S	S	S		R		U	U	U	S	S	S	R	U
2. Congenital	U		S	U		U		U	R	U	U		U	U	U		U	U	U		U
3. More in females															U	U	R				
4. More in males			S																		
5. Occurs during first decade			U																		
6. Occurs from birth to 2 years of age	U	U		U	U	U		U			U		U	U	U	U	S	U	U	U	
7. Occurs during second and third decades									U												
8. Occurs during third to fifth decades																			U		U
9. Ocular trauma	S						S														
10. Oxygen therapy					S																
11. Prematurity				S	U																
Physical Findings																					
1. Angiomatosis of iris									S												
2. Chorioretinitis							S				U					U				U	
3. Ciliary body tumor												U									U
4. Dark macular spot																U					
5. Endophthalmitis		U																			U
6. Myopic crescent															U						
7. Foveal retinoschisis									S									S			
8. Glaucoma	S	S	S	S	R				S												
9. Iris tumor												U						R			
10. Lid ecchymosis																			S		
11. Microphthalmia				U	U		S	S						U					S		
12. Nystagmus	S		S			U										S	R		S		
13. Optic atrophy											S										
14. Optic neuritis											S										
15. Orbital mass																S		R			S
16. Papilledema																S					
17. Persistent hyaloid vessel				S			S	U									S				
18. Phthisis bulbi				S	S		S		S	S				U			S				
19. Pigmented retinopathy											U										
20. Retinal detachment			S	U	S	U	S	S	S	S		S		U	U	U	S		S		S
21. Retinal folds						U								S							
22. Retinal hemorrhage			S	U			S	U		S		U		U		U			U	S	
23. Retrolental mass				U	U	U		U	U	U	U		U		U		U	S			
24. Ruptures in Bruch membrane																				U	U
25. Soft retinal exudates		R	S								S										

* = most important

Leukokoria (white pupil) (Continued)

	Cataract	Nematode Endophthalmitis	Coats Disease*	Persistent Hyperplastic Primary Vitreous*	Retrolental Fibroplasia	Retinal Dysplasia	Organized Vitreous Hemorrhage	Falciform Fold of Retina	Angiomatosis of Retina	Bloch-Sulzberger Syndrome	Exudative Retinitis	Diktyoma	Congenital Retinal Detachment	Norrie Disease	Juvenile Retinoschisis	Metastatic Endophthalmitis	Retinoblastoma*	Coloboma of Choroid	Medullation Nerve Layer	Traumatic Chorioretinitis	High Myopia with Retinal Degeneration
Physical Findings																					
26. Solitary, elevated, and rounded macular lesions		U																			
27. Strabismus	U	U		S	U		U		S	S			S			S	R				
28. Telangiectatic retinal vessels			U				R		S								S	R			
29. Uveitis		U	S	S			S	S	S		S										
30. Vitreous hemorrhage		S	S	S			U									U					
31. Vitreous veils				R			U									S	U				
Laboratory Data																					
1. Blood eosinophilia		U																			
2. Electroretinogram abnormal				S	S										U						
3. Fluorescein angiography		U	U		R	S	S	U	U		U					U	R	U	U	U	U
4. Ocular ultrasonography	U	U	U	U	U		U			S	U		U	U	U		U				
5. Orbital roentgenogram							U										U				S

R = rarely; S = sometimes; and U = usually.

LONG CILIARY PROCESSES EXTENDING INTO DILATED PUPILLARY SPACE

1. Aniridia
2. Anterior rotation of ciliary processes
   A. After scleral buckling operation
   B. Angle closure
   C. Anterior choroidal separation
   D. Cyst or tumor behind iris
   E. Dislocated lens
   F. From adherence to limbal scar
   G. Plateau iris
3. Extreme mydriasis
4. Falciform detachment of the retina
5. Incontinentia pigmenti (Bloch–Sulzberger syndrome)
6. Norrie disease (atrophia oculi congenita)
7. Persistent hyperplastic primary vitreous (PHPV)
8. Retinal dysplasia of Reese
9. Retrolental fibroplasia (RLF)
10. Surgical coloboma
11. Trisomy 13 (trisomy D)

Epstein DL. *Chandler and Grant's glaucoma*, 3rd ed. Philadelphia: Lea & Febiger, 1986.

Hansen AC. Norrie's disease. *Am J Ophthalmol* 1963;66:320–332.

PERSISTENT PUPILLARY MEMBRANE

1. Fetal iritis
2. Hereditary
3. Physiologic
*4. Use of oxygen therapy in nursery for premature infants

Hornblass A. Persistent pupillary membrane and oxygen therapy in premature infants. *Ann Ophthalmol* 1971;3: 95–99.

DECENTERED PUPILLARY LIGHT REFLEX

1. Positive angle kappa—pseudoexotropia
2. Negative angle kappa—pseudoesotropia
*3. Eccentric fixation—deep unilateral amblyopia
*4. Ectopic macula—macular displacement by retinal scarring or strands, such as retrolental fibroplasia
5. Ectopic pupil

Beyer-Machule C, von Noorden GK. *Atlas of ophthalmic surgery*, Vol 1: *Lids, orbits, extraocular muscles*. New York: Thieme Medical, 1984.

PUPILLARY BLOCK FOLLOWING CATARACT EXTRACTION

1. Air pupillary block
2. Dense, impermeable anterior hyaloid membrane
3. Free vitreous block

* = most important

4. Intraocular lens effectively closing off pupil and iridectomies
5. Leaky wound
6. Nonperforating iridectomy
7. Posterior vitreous detachment associated with pooling or retrovitreal aqueous
8. Postoperative iridocyclitis
9. Subchoroidal hemorrhage
10. Swollen lens material behind the iris

Tomey KF, Traverso CE. Neodymium-YAG laser posterior capsulotomy for the treatment of aphakic and pseudopha-kic pupillary block. *Am J Ophthalmol* 1987;104:502–507.

AFFERENT PUPILLARY DEFECT

The pupil of the eye has diminished vision from disease of the retina or optic nerve and will fail to react directly to light but will constrict consensually when the healthy eye is stimulated.

1. Amblyopia (rare)
2. Branch retinal artery/vein occlusion
3. Central retinal artery/vein occlusion
4. Compressive optic neuropathy
    A. Cavernous hemangiomas
    B. Cystic tumors
        (1) Cholesterol granuloma
        (2) Conjunctival orbital cysts
        (3) Dermoid cysts
        (4) Mucoceles
    C. Inflammatory and infiltrative processes
    D. Optic nerve tumors
        (1) Optic nerve gliomas
        (2) Optic nerve meningiomas
    E. Primary malignancies
    F. Sarcoidosis
    G. Solid orbital tumors
        (1) Hemangiomas
        (2) Meningiomas
        (3) Schwannoma
    H. Thyroid ophthalmopathy
    I. Trauma
5. Diabetic retinopathy (severe)
6. Hyphema
7. Macular degeneration (rarely)
8. Neovascular glaucoma
*9. Optic neuritis
*10. Optic nerve lesion
11. Radiation
12. Reticulum cell sarcoma
13. Retinal detachment
14. *Toxoplasma* retinochoroiditis
15. Traumatic optic neuropathy and retinopathy
16. Unilateral optic nerve hypoplasia

* = most important

Browning DJ, Tiedeman JS. The test light affects quantitation of the afferent pupillary defect. *Ophthalmology* 1987; 94:53–55.

Burde RM, et al. *Clinical decisions in neuro-ophthalmology,* 2nd ed. St. Louis: CV Mosby, 1991.

Enyedi LB, et al. A comparison of the Marcus Gunn and alternating light tests for afferent pupillary defects. *Ophthalmology* 1998;105:871–873.

Girkin CA, et al. A relative afferent pupillary defect without any visual sensory deficit. *Arch Ophthalmol* 1998; 1544–1547.

12
Iris

CONTENTS

ANIRIDIA (ABSENCE OF IRIS, PARTIAL OR COMPLETE)

1. AGR triad—sporadic (bilateral or unilateral) aniridia, genitourinary abnormalities, and mental retardation
2. Associated ocular findings
    A. Cataracts
    B. Corneal dystrophy
    C. Ectopia lentis
    D. Glaucoma
   *E. Macular aplasia—autosomal dominant
    F. Microcornea and subluxated lenses
    G. Nystagmus
    H. Optic nerve hypoplasia
    I. Photophobia
    J. Poor foveal reflex
   *K. Strabismus

3. Associated with autosomal-recessive inheritance with fully developed macula
4. Associated with unilateral renal agenesis and psychomotor retardation
5. Beckwith–Wiedemann syndrome
6. Deletion of short arm of 11th chromosome
7. Gillespie syndrome (incomplete aniridia, cerebellar ataxia, and oligophrenia)
8. Homocystinuria syndrome
9. Marinesco–Sjögren syndrome (congenital spinocerebellar ataxia)
10. Miller syndrome (Wilms aniridia syndrome)
11. Partial trisomy 2q
12. Peters syndrome (oculodental syndrome)
13. Rieger syndrome (dysgenesis mesostromalis)
14. Ring chromosome 6
15. Scaphocephaly syndrome
16. Siemens syndrome (anhidrotic ectodermal dysplasia)
*17. Traumatic
18. Ullrich syndrome (dyscraniopylophalangy)

Nelson IB, et al. Aniridia: a review. *Surv Ophthalmol* 1984;28:621–642.

Pearce WG. Variability of iris defects in autosomal dominant aniridia. *Can J Ophthalmol* 1994;29:25–29.

Roy FH. *Ocular syndromes and systemic diseases,* 3rd ed. Philadelphia: Lippincott Williams & Wilkins, 2002.

COLOBOMA OF IRIS

This condition involves failure of fusions of fetal fissure in optic vesicle, usually inferior or inferonasal.

1. Acrorenoocular syndrome
2. Aicardi syndrome
3. Aniridia
4. Biemond syndrome
5. Cat eye syndrome (partial G-trisomy syndrome)
6. CHARGE association (coloboma, heart anomaly, choanal atresia, retardation, genital, and ear anomalies)
7. Chromosome partial short-arm deletion syndrome
8. Ellis–van Creveld syndrome (chondroectodermal dysplasia)
9. Epidermal nevus syndrome (ichthyosis hystrix)
10. Focal dermal hypoplasia syndrome (Goltz syndrome)
11. Hallermann–Streiff–François syndrome (dyscephalic mandibulooculofacial syndrome)
12. Hemifacial microsoma syndrome (otomandibular dysostosis)
*13. Hereditary usually dominant may be recessive
14. Hurler syndrome (mucopolysaccharidoses I)
15. Hyperchromic heterochromia
16. Jeune disease (asphyxiating thoracic dystrophy)
17. Joubert syndrome
18. Kartagener syndrome
19. Klinefelter syndrome
20. Klippel–Trenaunay–Weber syndrome (angioosteohypertrophy syndrome)
21. Langer–Giedion syndrome
22. Lanzieri syndrome

* = most important

23. Laurence–Moon–Bardet–Biedl syndrome (retinitis pigmentosapolydactyly–adiposo-genital syndrome)
*24. Marfan syndrome (dolichostenomelia–arachnodactyly–hyperchondroplasia-dystrophia mesodermalis congenita)
25. Maternal use of thalidomide
26. Maternal vitamin A deficiency
27. Meckel syndrome
28. Median facial cleft syndrome
29. Microphthalmos syndrome (Meyer–Schwickerath and Weyers syndrome)
30. Nevoid basal cell carcinoma syndrome
31. Nevus sebaceous of Jadassohn (linear sebaceous nevus syndrome of Jadassohn)
32. Obesity–cerebral–ocular–skeletal anomalies syndrome
33. Oculoauriculovertebral dysplasia syndrome
34. Organoid nevus syndrome
35. Otomandibular dysostosis (hemifacial microsomia syndrome)
36. Partial deletion of group D chromosome
37. Rieger syndrome (dysgenesis mesodermalis corneae et irides)
38. Retinal dysplasia
39. Rubinstein–Taybi syndrome (broad-thumbs syndrome)
*40. Sporadic
41. Treacher Collins syndrome (Franceschetti syndrome)
42. Trisomy 13 (D trisomy) (Patau syndrome)
43. Trisomy 17 syndrome (Edwards syndrome)
44. Turner syndrome
45. Warburg syndrome
46. White sponge nevus
47. Wolf syndrome (monosomy partial syndrome)
48. 11q syndrome
49. 13q syndrome
50. 13r syndrome
51. 18q syndrome
52. 18r syndrome
53. XYY syndrome

Isenberg SJ. *The eye in infancy.* Chicago: Year Book Medical, 1989.

Roy FH. *Ocular syndromes and systemic diseases,* 3rd ed. Philadelphia: Lippincott Williams & Wilkins, 2002.

RUBEOSIS IRIDIS (NEOVASCULARIZATION [NEWLY FORMED BLOOD VESSELS] ON THE IRIS)

1. Proximal vascular disease
    A. Aortic arch syndrome (pulseless disease; Takayasu syndrome)
    B. Carotid–cavernous fistula (carotid artery syndrome)
    C. Carotid ligation
    D. Carotid occlusive disease
    E. Cranial arteritis syndrome (giant cell arteritis)
2. Ocular vascular disease
    *A. Central retinal artery thrombosis (see p. 457)
    *B. Central retinal vein thrombosis (see p. 467)

     C. Long posterior ciliary artery occlusion

     D. Reversed flow through the ophthalmic artery

3. Retinal diseases

     A. Coats disease (retinal telangiectasia)

   *B. Diabetes mellitus

     C. Eales disease (periphlebitis)

     D. Glaucoma, chronic

     E. Melanoma of choroid

     F. Norrie disease (oligophrenia–microphthalmos syndrome)

     G. Persistent hyperplastic primary vitreous

     H. Retinal detachment

     I. Retinal hemangioma

     J. Retinoblastoma

     K. Retrolental fibroplasia

     L. Sickle cell disease (Herrick syndrome)

4. Iris tumors

     A. Hemangioma

     B. Melanoma

     C. Metastatic carcinoma

5. Postinflammatory

     A. Argon laser coreoplasty

     B. Exfoliation syndrome

     C. Fibrinoid syndrome

     D. Fungal endophthalmitis (see p. 223–225)

     E. Iris neovascularization with pseudoexfoliation

     F. Radiation

     G. Surgery for retinal detachment

     H. Uveitis, chronic

6. Vascular tufts at the pupillary margin

     A. Cataract

     B. Diabetes mellitus

     C. Myotonic dystrophy syndrome (myotonia atrophica syndrome)

     D. Ocular hypotony

     E. Respiratory failure

Roy FH. *Ocular syndromes and systemic diseases,* 3rd ed. Philadelphia: Lippincott Williams & Wilkins, 2002.

Ulbig MR, et al. Anterior hyaloidal fibrovascular proliferation after extracapsular cataract extraction in diabetic eye. *Am J Ophthalmol* 1993;115:321–326.

HYPEREMIA OF IRIS (DILATATION OF PREEXISTING VESSELS OF THE IRIS)

1. Corneal ulcer

2. Foreign body on the cornea

3. Injury, intraocular

*4. Iridocyclitis

*5. Iritis

6. Scleritis

*7. Uveitis

O'Brien CS. *Ophthalmology: notes for students.* Iowa City: Athens Press, 1930.

* = most important

HETEROCHROMIA (DIFFERENCE OF COLOR BETWEEN TWO IRIDES)

1. Hypochromic heterochromia—abnormal eye with iris of lighter color than that of the fellow eye
   - A. Anemia with unilateral iritis
   - B. Chédiak–Higashi syndrome (anomalous leukocytic inclusions with constitutional stigmata)
   - *C. Congenital, sporadic, or familial
   - D. Conradi syndrome (epiphyseal congenital dysplasia)
   - E. Fuchs syndrome (I) (heterochromic cyclitis syndrome)
   - F. Gansslen syndrome (familial hemolytic icterus)
   - G. Glaucomatocyclitic crisis (Posner–Schlossman syndrome)
   - *H. Horner syndrome (cervical sympathetic paralysis syndrome)
   - I. Hypomelanosis of Ito syndrome (incontinentia pigmenti achromiens)
   - J. Infiltration of nonpigmented tumor into iris
   - *K. Iris atrophy (diffuse and unilateral), including that caused by trauma, inflammation, or senility
   - L. Iris coloboma
   - M. Parry–Romberg syndrome (facial hemiatrophy)
   - N. Status dysraphicus syndrome (Bremer syndrome)
   - O. Tuberous sclerosis hypopigmented iris spot (Bourneville syndrome)
   - P. Waardenburg–Klein syndrome (embryonic fixation syndrome)
2. Hyperchromic heterochromia—abnormal eye with iris darker than that in the fellow eye
   - A. Anterior or posterior chamber hemorrhage, prolonged
   - B. Coloboma
   - *C. Congenital, sporadic, or familial
   - D. Embryonic fixation syndrome (Waardenburg–Klein syndrome)
   - E. Incontinentia pigmenti (Bloch–Sulzberger syndrome)
   - F. Iris abscess
   - G. Iris stromal cysts
   - H. Malignant melanoma of the iris or other pigmented tumors of the iris
   - I. Microcornea (see p. 252–253)
   - J. Monocular melanosis in which there are excess chromatophores in the stroma of the iris (melanosis bulbi)
   - *K. Neovascular, such as rubeosis iridis or hyperemia of iris, unilateral (see p. 367 or p. 366)
   - L. Neurofibromatosis (von Recklinghausen syndrome)
   - *M. Nevi of iris
   - N. Perforating injuries or contusion of the globe occurring before the subject is seven years of age
   - O. Retention of intraocular iron foreign body—siderosis
   - P. Severe contusion with hypertrophy of the superficial layers of the stroma of the iris
   - Q. Status dysraphicus (Bremer syndrome)
3. Dark central pupillary margin, pale pigment around its circumference
   - A. Hereditary osteoonychodysplasia
   - B. Normal iris

* = most important

Gutman I, et al. Hypopigmented iris spot. *Ophthalmology* 1982;89:1155.

Lois N, et al. Primary iris stromal cysts. *Ophthalmology* 1998;105:1317–1322.

Mann ES, et al. Iris coloboma with iris heterochromia. *Arch Ophthalmol* 2000;118:1590–1591.

Newell FW. *Ophthalmology: principles and concepts,* 7th ed. St. Louis: CV Mosby, 1991.

Pfeiffer N, et al. Histological effects in the iris after 3 months of Latanoprost therapy. *Arch Ophthalmol* 2001;119: 191–194.

Roy FH. *Ocular syndromes and systemic diseases*, 3rd ed. Philadelphia: Lippincott Williams & Wilkins, 2002.

Hyperchromic heterochromia (abnormal eye with iris of darker color than fellow eye)

	Siderosis	Malignant Melanoma of Iris	Neurofibromatosis	Klein-Wardenburg Syndrome	Bremer's Status Dysraphicus	Rubeosis Iridis
History						
1. Activated at puberty, during pregnancy or menopause			U			
2. Carotid artery insufficiency						S
3. Central retinal vein or artery occlusion						S
4. Diabetic retinopathy						S
5. Family or sporadic occurrence		R			U	
6. Hereditary			U	U		
7. Intraocular iron or steel foreign body	U					
8. Pigmented mass on iris		U	S			
Physical Findings						
1. Anterior chamber depth variations		U				R
2. Blepharophimosis				U		
3. Blue irides				U		
4. "Cafe au lait" spots in fundus			S			
5. Cataract	S		U		S	
6. Cells and flare	U	S				
7. Corneal edema	S					S
8. Corneal neovascularization	S					
9. Decreased visual acuity	S	S		S		S
10. Dyschromatopsia	S					
11. Ectropion uvea		S				U
12. Elephantiasis of the lids			U			
13. Enophthalmos					U	
14. Fibrovascular membrane on anterior iris and chamber angle						U
15. Fleischer's ring	U					
16. Glaucoma	R	S	R	U		U
17. Hamartoma of retina			R			
18. Hypertelorism				U		
19. Hypertrichosis				U		
20. Hyphema		S				S
21. Hypopyon	U					S
22. Hudson-Stalhi line on cornea	U					
23. Interstitial keratitis	S					
24. Iridoplegia	S					S
25. Keratitis					S	
26. Lens luxation or subluxation	S					
27. Macular edema	S					
28. Miosis					S	
29. Narrowing of palpebral fissure					S	
30. Neurofibroma of the choroid, iris, lids and ciliary body			U			
31. Night blindness	S					
32. Nodular swelling of corneal nerves			U			
33. Nystagmus						
34. Ocular hypotony					S	
35. Optic atrophy			S		S	

Hyperchromic heterochromia (abnormal eye with iris of darker color than fellow eye) (Continued)	Siderosis	Malignant Melanoma of Iris	Neurofibromatosis	Klein-Wardenburg Syndrome	Bremer's Status Dysraphicus	Rubeosis Iridis
Physical Findings						
36. Optic nerve glioma				S		
37. Papilledema					S	
38. Paresis of ocular muscles					S	
39. Phthisis bulbi	S					
40. Prominent episcleral vessels		S				
41. Proptosis			U			
42. Pulsation of the globe			U			
43. Pupillary distortion	R	S				
44. Ptosis			U		U	
45. Retinal detachment	S					
46. Rusty discoloration of conjunctiva	U					
47. Subconjunctival hemorrhage	S					
48. Synechiae	S	R				U
49. Uveitis	U	S				S
Lab Data						
1. B scan	S	U	U			
2. CT scan	S		U			
3. X ray	U					

R = Rarely; U = Usually; S = Sometimes

Hyperchromic heterochromia (abnormal eye with iris of lighter color than fellow eye)

	Horner's Syndrome	Fuch's Heterochromia	Posner-Schlossman Syndrome	Parry-Romberg's Syndrome	Chediak-Higashi Syndrome	Klein-Waardenberg's Syndrome	Bremer's Status Dysraphicus
History							
1. Familial							
2. Greater in children							U
3. Greater 20 to 50 years old		U					
4. Hereditary			U	U			
5. Lesion in the pons, cervical cord or hypothalmus				U	U	U	
6. Mild infective cyclitis							
7. Occurs in albinoid siblings born of consanguineous parents		S	S				
8. Paralysis of cervical sympathetic	S				U		
9. Photophobia					U		
Physical Findings							
1. Absence of nasal portion of eyebrows							
2. Blephanophimosis					S		
3. Blue iris						U	
4. Cataracts						U	
5. Cells and flare in anterior chamber					S		S
6. Corneal anesthesia							
7. Choroiditis							
8. Decreased pigmentation in choroid		R					
9. Elevated disc					S		
10. Enophthalmos					S		
11. Epithelial corneal edema	U			U			U
12. Glaucoma		S	U				
13. Glaucomatous cupping			U				
14. Hypertelorism			R				
15. Hypertrichosis						U	
16. Hypotony							S
17. Keratic precipitates							
18. Keratitis			U				U
19. Miosis				U		U	
20. Mydriasis							
21. Narrowness and decreased number of retinal vessels					U		
22. Nystagmus					S		S
23. Oculocutaneous albinism							
24. Optic atrophy							S
25. Outer canthus lower than inner					S		
26. Papilledema					S		
27. Paresis of ocular muscles					S		
28. Ptosis	U			U			U
29. Vitreous opacities		S					

R = rarely; S = sometimes; and U = usually.

IRIS ATROPHY

1. Anterior segment ischemia syndrome
2. Arteriovenous fistula
3. Chandler syndrome (iridocorneal endothelial syndrome)
4. Complication of light coagulation and beta radiation
5. Complication of retinal detachment operation
*6. Congenital—autosomal dominant
7. Crohn disease (granulomatous ileocolitis)
*8. Essential (progressive) atrophy
9. Glaucomatous atrophy
   A. Acute—atrophy or iridoschisis
   *B. Chronic—stromal and epithelial
10. Hallermann–Streiff–François syndrome (dyscephalic mandibulooculofacial syndrome)
11. Hilding syndrome (destructive iridocyclitis and multiple joint dislocations)
12. Homocystinuria syndrome
13. Hypothermal injury
14. Iris nevus syndrome (Cogan–Reese syndrome)
15. Ischemia
   A. Acute angle-closure glaucoma
   B. Carotid–cavernous fistula
   C. Hemoglobin sickle cell C disease
   D. Occlusive artery disease
   E. Orbital irritation
   F. Surgery angle-closure glaucoma
   *G. Trauma
16. Krause syndrome (congenital encephalo-ophthalmic dysplasia)
17. Neurogenic—tabes with stromal atrophy
18. Norrie disease (fetal iritis syndrome)
*19. Old age
20. Pierre Robin syndrome (micrognathia–glossoptosis syndrome)
21. Posterior pigment layer is swollen and degenerated
   A. Diabetes mellitus (Willis disease)
   B. Hurler syndrome (mucopolysaccharidoses I–H)
22. Postinflammatory—iritis because of diseases such as tuberculosis, syphilis (acquired lues), herpes zoster, herpes simplex, smallpox, leprosy (Hansen disease), onchocerciasis syndrome (river blindness), sporotrichosis
23. Shy–Magee–Drager syndrome (orthostatic hypotension syndrome)
24. Spontaneous progressive
   A. Congenital hypoplasia iris stroma
   B. Rieger syndrome (dysgenesis mesostromalis)
25. Takayasu syndrome (aortic arch syndrome, pulseless disease)
26. Use of quinine, chloramine, mustard gas
27. Wagner syndrome (hyaloideoretinal degeneration)
28. Xeroderma pigmentosa, including skin lesions

Rodrigues MM, et al. Clinical electron microscopic, and immunohistochemical study of the corneal endothelium and Descemet's membrane in the iridocorneal endothelial syndrome. *Am J Ophthalmol* 1986;101:16–27.

Roy FH. *Ocular syndromes and systemic diseases*, 3rd ed. Philadelphia: Lippincott Williams & Wilkins, 2002.

Shields MB, et al. The essential iris atrophies. *Am J Ophthalmol* 1978;85:749–769.

* = most important

IRIDODONESIS (TREMULOUS IRIS)

*1. Aphakia following cataract extraction
*2. Dislocation of the lens (see p. 405)
3. Hydrophthalmos or buphthalmos (see p. 222–223)
4. Hypermature senile cataract

Filatov V, et al. Dislocation of the crystalline lens in a patient with Sturge Weber syndrome. *Am J Ophthalmol* 1992;24:260–262.

Hornby SJ, et al. Visual acuity in children with coloboma. *Ophthalmology* 2000;107:511–520.

Huggon IC, et al. Contractural arachnodactyly with mitral regurgitation and iridodonesis. *Arch Dis Child* 1990;65: 317–319.

TUMORS ARISING FROM PIGMENT EPITHELIUM OF IRIS

1. Hyperplasia
    A. Primary (congenital)
        (1) At pupillary margin
        (2) At margins of colobomas
    B. Acquired
        (1) Region of sphincter—migrating epithelial cells appear in stroma as clump cells (equivocal origin)
        (2) Cells can reach anterior surface of iris and proliferate (velvety black in appearance)
    C. Secondary
        (1) Intraocular inflammation—pigmented cells proliferate around the pupillary margin onto anterior iris surface
        (2) Long-standing glaucoma
            a. Proliferation around the pupillary margin onto the anterior iris surface
            b. Migration through stroma to anterior surface at collarette
        *(3) Trauma (including operation—proliferation of pigment epithelium on anterior surface of iris, across pupil, or on posterior surface of cornea
        *(4) Drugs, including the following: demecarium, echothiophate, edrophonium, isoflurophate, neostigmine, physostigmine, pilocarpine often associated with cystic formation
2. Neoplasia
    *A. Benign—well-differentiated epithelial cells, usually pigmented, often with pseudoacinar arrangement and cysts; may have limited locally invasive properties
    B. Malignant
        (1) Carcinoma
        (2) Local invasion, intraocular metastases
        (3) Medulloepithelioma, embryonal type (diktyoma)
        (4) Papillary cystadenoma

Fraunfelder FT, Fraunfelder FW. *Drug-induced ocular side effects.* Woburn, MA: Butterworth-Heinemann, 2001.

Morris PA, Henkind P. Neoplasms of the iris pigment epithelium. *Am J Ophthalmol* 1968;66:31.

PIGMENTED LESIONS OF IRIS

1. Adenoma of iris
2. Anterior chamber intraocular lens and segmental uveal ectropion

3. Anterior staphyloma
4. Corneal or scleral perforation
*5. Cyst—congenital, spontaneous, or traumatic, including pigmentation
6. Ectopic lacrimal gland tissue
*7. Ectropion uvea
8. Epithelioma of the ciliary body
9. Exudative mass in the anterior chamber
10. Foreign body of iris, including iron with siderosis
11. Fuchs syndrome of heterochromic cyclitis with the darker normal iris considered to contain a diffuse melanoma
12. Hemangioma of the iris with pigmentation because of hemorrhage
13. Hemosiderosis because of contusions with hyphema or injuries and disease in the posterior portion of the eye with recurrent bleeding
14. Juvenile xanthogranuloma (nevoxanthoendothelioma)
15. Leiomyoma or leiomyosarcoma of the iris
16. Leukemic infiltrates and malignant lymphomas
17. Malignant melanoma of the iris
18. Metastatic carcinomas arising in the lung, breast, gastrointestinal tract, thyroid gland, prostate gland, kidney, or testicle
19. Neurofibromatosis with increased pigmentation of the iris
*20. Nevi of the iris
21. Nodular thickening and scarring of the iris
22. Pigmentary glaucoma
23. Pigment epithelial tumors of the iris
24. Segmental melanosis oculi, including congenital melanosis
25. Stromal mass in the anterior chamber
26. Uveitis, such as that because of conglomerate tuberculous lesions of the stroma or sarcoid involvement of the iris
27. Varix

Chang M, et al. Adenoma of the pigment epithelium of the ciliary body simulating a malignant melanoma. *Am J Ophthalmol* 1979;88:40–48.

Lois N, et al. Primary cysts of the iris pigment epithelium. *Ophthalmology* 1998;105:1879–1885.

Shields JA, et al. Iris varix simulating an iris melanoma. *Arch Ophthalmol* 2000;118:707–709.

Shields CL, et al. Differentiation of adenoma of the iris pigment epithelium from iris cyst and melanoma. *Am J Ophthalmol* 1986;100:678–681.

NONPIGMENTED LESIONS OF IRIS

1. Amelanotic melanoma
2. Atypical mycobacterial panophthalmitis
3. Endothelioma
4. Exudative mass in the anterior chamber
5. Fibrosarcoma
*6. Foreign body
7. Forward extension of diktyoma
8. Hemangioma of the iris
*9. Iris cyst
10. Iris lymphoma
11. Iris nodules

* = most important

    A. Ectodermal (Koeppe nodules)—pupillary margin and gray with ocular inflammation

    B. Mesodermal (Busacca nodules)—anterior surface of iris in collarette region

12. Juvenile xanthogranuloma—may be associated with diffuse infiltration of the iris
13. Lacrimal Gland Choristoma of the Iris
14. Leiomyoma or leiomyosarcoma of the iris
15. Leprosy (Hansen disease)

    A. Lepromas of the iris

    B. Leprotic pearl—minute white spots on the surface of iris

16. Metastatic carcinoma of the iris arising from the lungs, breast, gastrointestinal tract, thyroid gland, prostate gland, kidney, or testicle
17. Neurofibroma and neuroglioma
18. Sarcoid nodules—multiple, discrete, irregularly distributed over the iris
19. Seeding of tumor, such as retinoblastoma, from the posterior segment
20. Syphilis (acquired lues)

    A. Gummas—solitary, large, avascular, white lesions

    B. Papules (condylomas)—multiple, small, vascular, yellowish lesions

21. Teratoma
22. Tuberculosis

    A. Acute miliary—small grayish yellow or reddish nodules

    B. Hyalinized or fibrotic scar (Michel flecks)

    C. Tuberculoma—white-gray lesion

Chan SM, et al. Iris lymphoma in a pediatric cardiac transplant recipient. *Ophthalmology* 2000;107:1479–1482.

Imamura Y, et al. Gastric signet ring cell adenocarcinoma metastatic to the iris. *Am J Ophthalmol* 2001;131:379–381.

Kluppel M, et al. Lacrimal gland choristoma of the iris. *Arch Ophthalmol* 1999;117:110–111.

Rosenbaum PS, et al. Atypical mycobacterial panophthalmitis seen with iris nodules. *Arch Ophthalmol* 1998;116:1524–1527.

Victor V, et al. Surgical excision of iris nodules in the management of sarcoid uveitis. *Ophthalmology* 2001;108:1296–1299.

Ware GT, et al. Renal cell carcinoma with involvement of iris and conjunctiva. *Am J Ophthalmol* 1999;127,4:458–459.

CONDITIONS SIMULATING ANTERIOR UVEITIS OR IRITIS

1. Brushfield spots
2. Fuchs syndrome (II) (Stevens–Johnson syndrome)
3. Hereditary deep dystrophy of cornea
4. Hyalinized keratitic precipitate
5. Iridoschisis—splitting of iris
6. Juvenile xanthogranuloma of the iris (nevoxanthoendothelioma)
7. Malignant lymphomas or leukemia
8. Malignant melanoma
9. Metastatic tumor arising from the lungs, breast, gastrointestinal tract, thyroid gland, prostate gland, kidney, or testicle
10. Neurofibromas of the iris
11. Pigment floaters in the anterior chamber, especially after mydriasis
*12. Pseudoexfoliation of the lens capsule (glaucoma capsulare)
13. Reticulum cell sarcoma
14. Retinoblastoma

15. Scleroderma (progressive systemic sclerosis)
*16. Siderosis bulbi

Denslow GT, Kielar RA. Metastatic adenocarcinoma to the anterior uvea and increased carcinoembryonic antigen levels. *Am J Ophthalmol* 1978;85:378–382.

Schlaegel TF. *Essentials of uveitis.* Boston: Little, Brown, 1969.

SYNDROMES AND DISEASES ASSOCIATED WITH IRITIS

1. Actinomycosis
2. Amebiasis (entamoeba histolytica)
3. Amendola syndrome (Brasilian pemphigus)
4. Anderson–Warburg syndrome (congenital progressive oculoacousticocerebral dysplasia)
5. Ankylosing spondylitis (von Beckterev–Strumpell syndrome)
6. Ascariasis
7. Aspergillosis
8. Beesting of the cornea
9. Behçet syndrome (oculobuccogenital syndrome)
10. Blastomycosis
11. Brucellosis (Bang disease)
12. Candidiasis
13. Charlin syndrome (nasociliary nerve syndrome)
14. *Chlamydia* pneumoniae
15. Coccidioidomycosis
16. Cryptococcosis
17. Cysticercosis
18. Cytomegalic inclusion disease (cytomegalovirus)
19. Dengue fever
20. Endophthalmitis phacoanaphylactica
*21. Following laser iridectomy
22. Fuchs syndrome (heterochromic cyclitis syndrome)
23. Henoch–Schönlein purpura (anaphylactoid purpura)
24. Herbicide exposure—2,4-dichlorophenoxyacetic acid
*25. Herpes simplex
*26. Herpes zoster
27. Histoplasmosis
28. Histiocytosis X (xanthomatous granuloma syndrome)
29. Hypervitaminosis D
30. Leptospirosis (Weill disease)
31. Mucormycosis (phycomycosis)
32. Mustard gas injury
33. Mycoplasma pneumoniae
34. Nocardiosis
35. Onchocerciasis syndrome (*Onchocerca volvulus*)
36. Reiter syndrome (conjunctivourethrosynovial syndrome)
37. Romberg syndrome (facial hemiatrophy)
38. Rubella syndrome (Gregg syndrome)
*39. Sarcoidosis syndrome (Schaumann syndrome)
40. Sporotrichosis

* = most important

*41. Still disease (juvenile rheumatoid arthritis)
 42. Syphilis (acquired lues)
 43. Toxoplasmosis (ocular toxoplasmosis)
 44. Tuberculosis
 45. Vaccinia
 46. Vogt–Koyanagi–Harada syndrome (uveitis, vitiligo-alopecia-poliosis syndrome)

Roy FH. *Ocular syndromes and systemic diseases,* 3rd ed. Philadelphia: Lippincott Williams & Wilkins, 2002.

Solberg Y, et al. Ocular injury by mustard gas. *Surv Ophthalmol* 1997;41:461–466.

Yamada I, et al. A child with iritis due to chlamydia pneumoniae infection. *Journal of the Japanese Association for Infectious Diseases* 1994;68:1543–1547.

IRITIS (ANTERIOR UVEITIS) IN CHILDREN

 1. Anterior and posterior uveitis
     A. Retinoblastoma
    *B. Sarcoidosis syndrome (Schaumann syndrome)
     C. Sympathetic ophthalmia
     D. Vogt–Koyanagi–Harada syndrome (uveitis-vitiligo-alopecia-poliosis syndrome)
 *2. Chronic cyclitis (peripheral uveitis)
  3. Fuchs heterochromic cyclitis
  4. Iridocyclitis
     A. Acute tubulointerstitial nephritis and uveitis
     B. Ankylosing spondylitis (von Beckterev–Strumpell syndrome)
     C. Behçet syndrome (oculobuccogenital syndrome)
     D. Juvenile xanthogranuloma
     E. Kawasaki disease
     F. Leukemia
     G. Multiple sclerosis
     H. Psoriatic arthropathy
     I. Reiter syndrome
     J. Retinal capillaritis
    *K. Sarcoidosis syndrome (Schaumann syndrome)
     L. Still syndrome (juvenile rheumatoid arthritis)
    *M. Trauma
     N. Ulcerative colitis and Crohn disease
     O. Unknown
     P. Viral-associated disease
  5. Keratouveitis
    *A. Herpes simplex
    *B. Herpes zoster

Kimura SJ, Hogan MJ. Uveitis in children: analysis of cases. *Trans Am Ophthalmol Soc* 1964;62:173.

Matsuo T, Matsuo N. Bilateral iridocyclitis with retinal capillaritis in juveniles. *Ophthalmology* 1997;104:939–944.

Powell CJ, et al. Diffuse infiltrating retinoblastoma masquerading as a panuveitis. *Ophthalmology* 1986;92:119.

* = most important

Iritis (anterior uveitis) in children

Iritis (anterior uveitis) in children	Still Syndrome	Ankylosing Spondylitis	Behçet Syndrome	Sarcoidosis	Chronic Cyclitis (Para Planitis)	Fuchs Heterochromic Cyclitis	Herpes Simplex	Herpes Zoster	Vogt-Koyanagi-Harada Syndrome	Sympathetic Ophthalmia
History										
1. Before puberty	U	U								
2. Bilateral					S					
3. Familial	S									
4. Following trauma/surgery										U
5. Greater in females	S				U					
6. Greater in males		U				S				
7. Hereditary		U								
8. Occurs in young adults									U	R
9. Prominent in whites						U				
10. Prominent in blacks					U				U	
11. Seen in Japanese			S						U	
12. Virus infection			S				U	U	S	
Physical Findings										
1. Anterior and posterior synechiae	S	U	S				S			
2. Band keratopathy	S	S		R						
3. Cataract	S	S	S	R	S	S		S	S	S
4. Conjunctivitis			S	R			S	S		
5. Corneal opacity			S			S				
6. Corneal ulcer							S			
7. Corneal edema							S	S		
8. Cyclitic membrane					U					
9. Cystoid macular edema					U					
10. Choroiditis						S			S	S
11. Dacryoadenitis				U						
12. Dacryocystitis				S						
13. Decreased corneal sensitivity							U	U		
14. Dendritic corneal figure							U	S		
15. Entropion								S		
16. Exophthalmos				S						
17. Extraocular muscle paralysis				U			R	S		
18. Glaucoma	S	S	S	S		S	S	S	S	S
19. Hyphema	S									
20. Hypopyon	S	S	R				R	R		
21. Iris bombé	S									
22. Iris hypoheterchromia						U	R	R		

R = rarely; S = sometimes; and U = usually.

Iritis (anterior uveitis) in children Continued

	Still Syndrome	Ankylosing Spondylitis	Behçet Syndrome	Sarcoidosis	Chronic Cyclitis (Pars Planitis)	Fuchs Heterochromic Cyclitis	Herpes Simplex	Herpes Zoster	Vogt-Koyanagi-Harada Syndrome	Sympathetic Ophthalmia
Physical Fitness										
23. Keratitis				S			U	U		S
24. Keratitic precipitates	U	U								
25. Macular edema	S		S							
26. Macular hemorrhage				R						
27. Optic atrophy				S	S					
28. Optic neuritis	S			S	S				S	U
29. Retinal detachment						S				
30. Retinal hemorrhages				S	S				S	
31. Retinal vasculitis				S					R	
32. Scleritis			S	S						
33. Sheathing of peripheral retinal veins					U					
34. Snowballs of peripheral inferior retina					U					
35. Strabismus				S						
36. Subconjunctival nodules				U		S				
37. Vitreous hemorrhages			S		S					
38. Vitreous opacity						S				
39. White lashes						S			S	S
40. Zoster rash of lid								S	S	
Laboratory Data										
1. Antinuclear antibody test (+)	U									
2. Biopsy of inferior forniceal follicles				U						
3. Cerebrospinal fluid protein level high				S						
4. Chest roentgenogram				U						
5. Elevated sed rate		U								
6. Fluorescein angiography		U				U			U	
7. Homologous leucocytic antibody determination	U	U	S							
8. Lumbosacral spine roentgenogram		U	U							
9. Macroglobulins (−)			U							
10. Rheumatoid factor and lupus erythematosis cell test (+)	U	U								
11. Serum angiotensin-converting enzyme				U						
12. Tuberculosis skin test				U						U
13. Ultrasonography				S						
14. Viral culture serial antibody titer							U	U		

R = rarely; S = sometimes; and U = usually.

NONGRANULOMATOUS UVEITIS

1. Physical insult
   A. Endogenous
   B. Exogenous
*2. Toxic insults
   A. Autointoxication—ptomaines, protein split products, and so forth from food poisoning
   B. Bacterial endotoxins
   C. Reticulum cell sarcoma of the brain
   D. Toxins from disintegrating helminths
   *E. Viral toxins
3. Immediate hypersensitive reaction
   *A. Airborne allergens
   B. Drugs, including the following:

acetazolamide
adrenal cortex injection
aldosterone
amphotericin B
auranofin
aurothioglucose
aurothioglycanide
bacitracin
bacille Calmette–Guérin
   (BCG) vaccine
beclomethasone
benoxinate
betaxolol
brimonidine
bupivacaine
butacaine
chloramphenicol
chloroprocaine
chlortetracycline
chondroitin sulfate
chymotrypsin
cidofovir
cobalt
cocaine
colistin
contraceptives
cortisone
cytarabine
demecarium
desoxycorticosterone
dexamethasone
diisopropyl flurophosphate
   (DFP)
dibucaine

dichlorphenamide
diethylcarbamazine
diphtheria, pertussis, and
   tetanus (DPT) vaccine
disodium clodronate
disodium etidronate
disodium pamidronate
doxorubicin
dyclonine
echothiophate
edrophonium
emetine
epinephrine
erythromycin
ethoxzolamide
etidocaine
floxuridine
fludrocortisone
fluorometholone
fluorouracil
fluprednisolone
gold Au 198
gold sodium thiomalate
gold sodium thiosulfate
hyaluronate acid
hydrabamine
hydroxypropylmethylcellulose
ibuprofen
interleukin 3 and 6
iodide and iodine solutions
   and compounds
isoflurophate
latanoprost
lidocaine

measle vaccine
medrysone
meprednisone
methazolamide
methicillin
methylprednisolone
metipranolol
mitomycin
neomycin
neostigmine
paramethasone
penicillin
penicillin 0
penicillin hydrocortisone
phenacaine
phenethicillin
physostigmine
piperocaine
polymyxin B
potassium
pralidoxime
prednisolone
procaine
proparacaine
propoxycaine
quinidine
radioactive iodides
reserpine
rifampin
smallpox vaccine
sodium hyaluronate
streptokinase
streptomycin
sulfacetamide

* = most important

sulfachlorpyridazine   sulfamethoxazole   sulfisoxazole
sulfacytine   sulfamethoxypyridazine   tetracaine
sulfadiazine   sulfanilamide   tetracycline
sulfadimethoxine   sulfapyridine   thiotepa
sulfameter   sulfamerazine   triamcinolone
sulfamethazine   sulfasalazine   trifluoperazine
sulfamethizole   sulfathiazole   urokinase

       C. Foods
       D. Protein antigens (anaphylaxis)
    4. Delayed hypersensitive reaction
       A. Bacterial antigens
       B. Viral antigens
    5. Doubtful entities—nongranulomatous uveitis
       A. Amebiasis
       B. Diabetic iritis
       C. Gouty iritis
       D. Heterochromic iridocyclitis
       *E. Sarcoidosis syndrome (Schaumann syndrome)
       F. Secondary to metabolic disease, such as biliary cirrhosis and systemic xanthoma-
         tosis
       G. Uveitis associated with collagen diseases
    6. Mixed granulomatous and nongranulomatous
       A. Lens-induced uvealis
       *B. Peripheral uveitis
    7. Human leukocyte antigen (HLA)-B27 associated diseases
       A. Ankylosing spondylitis
       B. Inflammatory bowel disease
       C. Psoriasis
       D. Reiter disease
    8. Infections
       A. Herpes zoster/herpes simplex
       B. Lyme disease
       C. Syphilis

Byles DB, et al. Anterior uveitis as a side effect of topical brimonidine. *Am J Ophthalmol* 2000;130:287–291.

Chavez-de la Paz, et al. Anterior nongranulomatous uveitis after intravitreal HPMPC (Cidofovir) for the treatment of cytomegalovirus retinitis. *Ophthalmology* 1997;104:539–544.

Fraunfelder FT, Fraunfelder FW. *Drug-induced ocular side effects.* Woburn, MA: Butterworth-Heinemann, 2001.

Moorthy RS, et al. Drug-induced uveitis. *Surv Ophthalmol* 1998;42:557–570.

GRANULOMATOUS UVEITIS

   1. Proven or probable etiology
      A. Associated with nonpyogenic systemic infections
         (1) Brucellosis (*Brucella melitensis, B. abortus, B. suis*)
         (2) Leprosy (*Mycobacterium leprae*)
         (3) Leptospirosis (*Leptospira canicola, L. icterohaemorrhagiae, L. pomona*)
         *(4) Syphilis (*Treponema pallidum*)
         *(5) Tuberculosis (*Mycobacterium tuberculosis*)

B. Protozoan infections
  (1) Amebiasis (*Entamoeba coli, E. histolytica, Endolimax nana, Acanthamoeba hartmannella*)
  (2) Toxoplasmosis (*Toxoplasma gondii*)
  (3) Trypanosomiasis (*Trypanosoma cruzi, T. gambiense*)
C. Fungal infections
  (1) Actinomycosis
  (2) Aspergillosis
  (3) Blastomycosis
  (4) Candidiasis (moniliasis)
  (5) Coccidioidomycosis
  (6) Cryptococcosis (*Cryptococcus neoformans* or *Torula histolytica*)
  *(7) Histoplasmosis (*Histoplasma capsulatum*)
  (8) Mycomycosis (phycomycosis)
  (9) Nocardiosis
  (10) Sporotrichosis (*Sporotrichum schenckii*)
D. *Helminth* infestations
  (1) Ascaridiosis (*Ascaris lumbricoides*)
  (2) Cestodes
    a. Cysticercosis (*Cysticercus cellulosae*)
    b. Taeniasis (*Taenia echinococcus*)
  (3) Diptera larvae (exogenous)
  (4) Nematodes
    a. Ancylostomiasis (*Toxocara canis, Ancylostoma duodenale, Ancylostoma caninum, Necator americanus*)
    b. Onchocerciasis (*Onchocerca volvulus*)
E. Viral—herpes zoster
2. Recognized clinical and histopathologic entity, of unknown cause
  *A. Multiple sclerosis
  *B. Sarcoidosis syndrome (Schaumann syndrome)
  C. Sympathetic ophthalmia
3. Nonspecific granulomatous uveitis of unknown cause, including granulomatous ileocolitis
4. Mixed granulomatous and nongranulomatous
  A. Lens-induced uveitis
  B. Peripheral uveitis
5. Viral uveitis
  A. Proven or probable
    (1) Cytomegalic inclusion disease
    (2) Herpes simplex
    (3) Herpes zoster
    (4) Vaccinia
  B. Suspected
    (1) Behçet syndrome (oculobuccogenital syndrome)
    (2) Retinal capillaritis
    (3) Vogt–Koyanagi–Harada syndrome (uveitis–vitiligo–alopecia–poliosis syndrome)
6. Histiocytosis X (includes eosinophilic granuloma, Hand–Schüller–Christian disease and Letterer–Siwe disease)

* = most important

7. Following treatment of a choroidal melanoma with proton-beam irradiation

Cho AS, et al. Ocular involvement in patients with post-transplant lymphoproliferative disorder. *Arch Ophthalmol* 2001;119:183–185.

Matsuo T, Matsuo N. Bilateral iridocyclitis with retinal capillaritis in juveniles. *Ophthalmology* 1997;104:939–944.

Schwab IR. Herpes zoster sine herpete. *Ophthalmology* 1997;104:1421–1425.

PIGMENTED CILIARY BODY LESIONS

*1. Ciliary body cyst
2. Diffuse iris melanotic lesion
*3. Drugs including the following:

adrenal cortex injection
aldosterone
betamethasone
cortisone
demecarium
desoxycorticosterone
dexamethasone
echothiophate

edrophonium
epinephrine
fludrocortisone
fluprednisolone
hydrocortisone
isoflurophate
meprednisone
methylprednisolone

neostigmine
paramethasone
physostigmine
pilocarpine
prednisolone
prednisone
triamcinolone

4. Malignant melanoma
5. Melanocytoma of ciliary body
6. Peripheral uveal detachment
7. Posttraumatic pigmentary migration

Biswas J, et al. 7 diffuse melanotic lesion of the iris as a presenting feature of ciliary body melanocytoma: report of a case and review of the literature. *Surv Ophthalmol* 1998;42:378–383.

Fraunfelder FT, Fraunfelder FW. *Drug-induced ocular side effects.* Woburn, MA: Butterworth-Heinemann, 2001.

Lois N, et al. Cavitary melanoma of the ciliary body. *Ophthalmology* 1998;105:1091–1098.

NEUROEPITHELIAL TUMORS OF CILIARY BODY

1. Congenital
    A. Glioneuroma
    B. Medulloepithelioma
        *(1) Benign
        (2) Malignant
    C. Teratoid medulloepithelioma
        (1) Benign
        (2) Malignant
2. Acquired
    A. Adenocarcinoma
        *(1) Papillary
        (2) Pleomorphic
        (3) Solid
    B. Adenoma
        *(1) Papillary
        (2) Pleomorphic
        (3) Solid
    C. Mesectodermal leiomyoma
    D. Pseudoadenomatous hyperplasia

Shields JA, et al. Observations on seven cases of intraocular leiomyoma. *Arch Ophthalmol* 1994;112:521–528.

Shields JA, et al. Natural causes and histopathologic findings of lacrimal gland chorestoma of the iris and ciliary body. *Am J Ophthalmol* 1995;119:219–224.

INTERNAL OPHTHALMOPLEGIA

Internal ophthalmoplegia is characterized by paresis of ciliary body with loss of power of accommodation and pupil dilatation because of lesions of ciliary ganglion.

1. Acute porphyria—frequently bilateral
*2. Adie syndrome (myotonic pupil)
3. Aneurysm of the posterior communicating artery at its junction with the internal carotid—unilateral
4. Congenital—rare
*5. Cycloplegic ocular medication—most common
6. During acute illness—transient
7. During blepharoplasty—transient
8. Fisher syndrome (ophthalmoplegia–ataxia–areflexia syndrome)
9. Foramen lacerum syndrome (aneurysm of internal carotid artery)
10. Histiocytosis X (Hand–Schüller–Christian syndrome)
11. Hollenhorst syndrome (chorioretinal infarction syndrome)
*12. Increased intracranial pressure
13. Infections, including chickenpox, measles, diphtheria, syphilis, scarlet fever, pertussis, smallpox, influenza, herpes zoster, botulism, sinusitis, and viral hepatitis
14. Lubarsch–Pick syndrome (amyloidosis)
15. May be early lesion of acute or chronic ophthalmoplegia
16. Metastatic tumors of choroid
17. Nasopharyngeal carcinoma—early
18. Nothnagel syndrome (ophthalmoplegia–cerebellar ataxia syndrome)
19. Partial seizures
20. Retrobulbar injections of alcohol
21. Transscleral diathermy
22. Trauma to eye or orbit
23. Vogt–Koyanagi–Harada syndrome (uveitis–vitiligo–alopecia–poliosis syndrome)

Perlman JP, Conn H. Transient internal ophthalmoplegia during blepharoplasty: a report of three cases. *Ophthal Plast Reconstr Surg* 1991;7:141–143.

Rosenberg ML, Jabbari B. Miosis and internal ophthalmoplegia as a manifestation of partial seizures. *Neurology* 1991;41:737–739.

Roy FH. *Ocular syndromes and systemic diseases*, 3rd ed. Philadelphia: Lippincott Williams & Wilkins, 2002.

* = most important

13

Lens

CONTENTS

ANTERIOR SUBCAPSULAR CATARACT

1. Acrodermatitis chronica atrophicans
2. Addison syndrome (adrenal cortical insufficiency)
3. Albinism
4. Allopurinol therapy
5. Alport syndrome (hereditary nephritis)
6. Amiodarone usage
7. Andogsky syndrome (dermatogenous cataract)
8. Aniridia
9. Anterior chamber air
10. Atopic (eczema cataract)
11. Beesting of cornea
12. Cerebrohepatorenal syndrome (Smith–Lemli–Opitz syndrome)
13. Chlorpromazine therapy

14. Chromosomal 3; 18 translocation
15. Comedo cataract
16. Coughing
17. Cryotherapy
18. Electric cataract
*19. Diabetes mellitus (Willis disease)
20. Facial paralysis (partial)
21. Frenkel syndrome (ocular contusion syndrome)
22. Goldscheider syndrome (epidermolysis bullosa)
23. Gyrate atrophy (ornithine ketoacid aminotransferase deficiency)
24. Head-banging (chronic)
25. Hemifacial microsomia syndrome (François–Haustrate syndrome)
26. Hypermature cataract with other changes
27. Hypoparathyroidism
28. Idiopathic—10% of normal population
29. Intraocular copper and iron
30. Isotretinoin
31. Jadassohn–Lewandowsky syndrome (epidermolysis bullosa)
32. Leber congenital amaurosis
33. Marinesco–Sjögren syndrome (oligophrenia syndrome)
34. Myotonic dystrophy (Curschmann–Steinert syndrome)
35. Naphthalene ingestion
36. Neodymium:yttrium–aluminum–garnet (Nd:YAG)
37. Neurodermatitis
38. Pemphigus foliaceous (Cazenave disease)
39. Phenothiazine therapy
40. Phospholine iodide use
41. Pseudohypoparathyroidism
42. Reese–Ellsworth syndrome (anterior chamber cleavage syndrome)
43. Rothmund syndrome (telangiectasia–pigmentation–cataract syndrome)
44. Scaphocephaly
45. Schizophrenia
46. Thorazine ingestion
*47. Trauma, such as contusion
48. Tyrosinosis
49. Vitrectomy for diabetic retinopathy
50. Werner syndrome (progeria of adults)
51. Wilson disease (hepatolenticular degeneration)
52. Zinc chloride (concentrated)

McCarty CA, et al. Schizophrenia, psychotropic medication, and cataract. *Ophthalmology* 1999;106:683–687.

McKusick VA. *Mendelian inheritance in man,* 12th ed. Baltimore: Johns Hopkins University Press, 1998.

Roy FH. *Ocular syndromes and systemic disease,* 3rd ed. Philadelphia: Lippincott Williams & Wilkins, 2002.

Zadok D, Chayet A. Lens opacity after neodymium: YAG laser iridectomy for phakic intraocular lens implantation. *J Cataract Refract Surg* 1999;25:592–593.

* = most important

Anterior subcapsular cataract

	Atopic Eczema*	Electric Injury	Diabetes Mellitus*	Werner Syndrome	Myotonic Dystrophy	Intraocular Copper and Iron	Trauma (Blunt)*	Wilson Disease
History								
1. Consanguinity				S				
2. Diplopia			S		S			
3. Familial			U		U			U
4. Hereditary				U	U			
5. Intraocular foreign body history						U		
6. More than 200 volts injury		U						
7. Night blindness		S						
8. Often occurs in childhood	U							
9. Occurs in first decade								U
10. Occurs during second to third decade					S	U		
11. Onset, usually fourth decade					U			
12. Trauma history							U	
Physical Findings								
1. Absent eyelashes/eyebrows				U				
2. Angle recession							S	
3. Astigmatism					S			
4. Blepharospasm					S			
5. Blue sclera					S			
6. Bullous keratopathy					S			
7. Chemosis conjunctiva	U						S	
8. Chorioretinitis						S	S	
9. Choroidal atrophy		S						
10. Choroidal rupture		S						
11. Conjunctival giant papillary hypertrophy	S							
12. Conjunctival necrosis							S	
13. Conjunctival scarring	S						S	
14. Copper colored macular sheen						U		
15. Corneal epithelial dystrophy					S			
16. Corneal necrosis		S						
17. Corneal opacity					S		S	
18. Corneal perforation		S						
19. Corneal scarring	S	S						
20. Corneal vascularization	S							
21. Cotton-wool spots			U					
22. Dyschromatopsia						S		
23. Ectropion uvea			S					
24. Endophthalmitis						U		
25. Exophthalmos					S		S	
26. Filamentary conjunctival discharge	S							
27. Fixed and dilated pupil			S				S	
28. Hudson-Stahli line in cornea						S		
29. Hyphema						S	S	
30. Hypopyon						S		
31. Interstitial keratitis						S		

Anterior subcapsular cataract (Continued)

	Atopic Eczema*	Electric Injury	Diabetes Mellitus*	Werner Syndrome	Myotonic Dystrophy	Intraocular Copper and Iron	Trauma (Blunt)*	Wilson Disease
Physical Findings						S		
32. Iris greenish/rusty tinge			S			S		
33. Ischemic optic neuropathy						S		U
34. Kayser-Fleischer ring	S							
35. Keratoconus							S	
36. Laceration of lid	S							
37. Lid exudates/erythema							S	
38. Lid hemorrhage		U						
39. Lid necrosis/burn			U					
40. Lid telangiectasia					U			
41. Loss corneal sensitivity							S	
42. Low intraocular pressure				S	S			
43. Macular degeneration			S			S		
44. Macular edema					S			
45. Macular red spot			U					
46. Microaneurysms of retina			S		S			S
47. Nystagmus			S	S		S	S	
48. Optic nerve atrophy			S	S				
49. Optic neuritis				S				
50. Papilledema			S	U	U			S
51. Paralysis of extraocular muscles							S	U
52. Phthisis bulbi				S	S			
53. Presbyopia, early				S		S		
54. Ptosis	S							
55. Punctate keratitis			S					
56. Retinal cysts			S			S	S	
57. Retinal degeneration	S				S		S	S
58. Retinal detachment				S	U			
59. Retinal exudate/edema							S	
60. Retinal gliosis				S	U		S	S
61. Retinal hemorrhage				S				
62. Retinal holes					S			
63. Retinal neovascularization							S	
64. Retinal rusty discoloration							S	
65. Retrobulbar hemorrhage				S				
66. Rubeosis iridis	S							
67. Staphylococcal blepharitis							S	
68. Synechiae of iris	S							
69. Tranta dot			S				S	
70. Uveitis				S				S
71. Vitreous hemorrhage							S	
72. Vitreous opacity/degeneration								
Laboratory Data	U							
1. Allergy testing								
2. Blood sugar elevated			S					

* = most important

Anterior subcapsular cataract (Continued)

	Atopic Eczema*	Electric Injury	Diabetes Mellitus*	Werner Syndrome	Myotonic Dystrophy	Intraocular Copper and Iron	Trauma (Blunt)*	Wilson Disease
Laboratory Data								
3. Computed tomography scan of head								
4. Genetic studies		R						S
5. Hepatic tests				U	U			
6. Orbital roentgenogram								U
7. Serum gamma globulin concentration reduced						U	S	
8. Serum immunoglobulin E concentration elevated						U		
9. Ultrasonography	U							
10. Urine copper elevated		S				U	U	
11. Visual field defects		S	R			S		

R = rarely; S = sometimes; and U = usually.

NUCLEAR CATARACTS

1. Alcohol
2. Arteriovenous fistula
3. Associated with photocoagulation, such as argon laser use
4. Capsular exfoliation syndrome
5. Congenital dysplasia
6. Conradi syndrome (multiple epiphyseal congenital dysplasia)
7. Coppock cataract, discoid cataract, zonular cataract—autosomal dominant
8. Hyperbaric oxygen therapy
9. Maple-syrup urine disease (branched-chain ketoaciduria)
10. Matsouka syndrome (oculocerebroarticuloskeletal syndrome)
11. Micro syndrome
12. Nuclear diffuse nonprogressive cataract—autosomal dominant, rarely recessive
*13. Nuclear sclerosis
   *A. Pars plana vitrectomy for macular pucker
    B. Smoking
14. Nuclear total cataract—autosomal dominant, rarely recessive
15. Paradichlorobenzene (mothballs)
16. Perforating injuries
17. Roy syndrome II—nuclear cataract associated with smoking
*18. Rubella syndrome (German measles)
19. Siemen syndrome (hereditary ectodermal dysplasia syndrome)
20. von Gierke disease (glucose–phosphate deficiency)

Klein RE, et al. Cigarette smoking and lens opacities—the Beaver Dam Eye Study. *Am J Prev Med* 1993;9:27–30.

Leung ATS, et al. Chlorpromazine-induced refractile corneal deposits and cataract. *Arch Opthalmol* 1999;117:1662–1663.

Roy FH. *Ocular syndromes and systemic diseases,* 3rd ed. Philadelphia: Lippincott Williams & Wilkins, 2002.

Seddon J, Fong D. The association between cigarette smoking and ocular diseases. *Surv Ophthalmol* 1998;42:535–547.

LAMELLAR (STELLATE, ZONULAR, CORTICAL, CORONARY) CATARACTS

1. Alcohol
2. Aniridia
3. Argon laser
4. Autosomal-dominant congenital cataract
5. Congenital zonular cataract
6. Cortical cataract and congenital ichthyosis
7. Dermochonoral corneal dystrophy
8. Diabetes mellitus (Willis disease)
9. Females
10. Galactokinase deficiency (von Reuss syndrome)
11. Hagberg–Santavuori (neuronal ceroid–lipofuscinoses)
12. Hypertension
13. Hypoglycemia
14. Hypophosphatasia (phosphoethanolaminuria)
15. Iritis
16. Leiomyoma

* = most important

17. Mannosidosis
18. Marfan syndrome (dolichostenomelia–arachnodactyly–hyperchondroplasia–dystrophia mesodermalis congenita)
19. Marshall syndrome (atypical ectodermal dysplasia)
20. Myotonic dystrophy syndrome (Curschmann–Steinert syndrome)
21. Neurofibromatosis 2 (central neurofibromatosis)
22. Nieden syndrome (telangiectasia cataract syndrome)
23. Nonwhites
24. Obesity (abdominal)
25. Organic nitrate explosives
26. Passow syndrome (status dysraphicus syndrome)
27. Riboflavin deficiency (Stannus cerebellar syndrome)
28. Roy syndrome (cataract associated with smoking)
*29. Sunlight
30. Tetany cataract (hypoparathyroidism)
*31. Ultraviolet-B light
32. Van Bogaert–Scherer–Epstein syndrome (primary hyperlipidemia)
33. Van der Hoeve syndrome (osteogenesis imperfecta)
34. Wagner syndrome (hyaloideoretinal degeneration)
35. Zonular cataract and nystagmus—X-linked

Leske MC, et al. Diabetes, hypertension, and central obesity as cataract risk factors in a black population. *Ophthalmology* 1999;106:35–41.

McKusick VA. *Mendelian inheritance in man,* 12th ed. Baltimore: Johns Hopkins University Press, 1998.

Roy FH. *Ocular syndromes and systemic diseases,* 3rd ed. Philadelphia: Lippincott Williams & Wilkins, 2002.

Roy FH. Cigarette smoking and the risk of cataract [Letter]. *JAMA* 1993;269:748.

Younger CR, et al. Lens opacifications detected by slitlamp biomicroscopy are associated with exposure to organic nitrate explosives. *Arch Ophthalmol* 2000;118:1653–1657.

PUNCTATE CATARACTS (NUMEROUS SMALL OPACITIES)

1. Albright hereditary osteodystrophy (pseudohypoparathyroidism)
2. Argon laser
3. Autosomal dominant vitreoretinochoroidopathy (ADVIRC)
4. Cockayne syndrome (dwarfism with retinal atrophy and deafness)
5. Cretinism (hypothyroidism)
6. Galactokinase deficiency (von Reuss syndrome)
7. Hypercalcemia (adult)
8. Hyperprolactinemia
9. Incontinentia pigmenti achromians
10. Lowe syndrome (oculocerebrorenal syndrome)
11. Rothmund syndrome (telangiectasia-pigmentation-cataract syndrome)
12. Supravalvular aortic stenosis (Williams-Beuren syndrome)

Costagliola C. Hyperprolactinemia and lens opacities. *Ann Ophthal* 1992;24:418–419.

Drack AV, et al. Transient punctate lenticular opacities as a complication of Argon laser photocoagulation in an infant with retinopathy of prematurity. *Am J Ophthalmol* 1992;113:583.

McKusick VA. *Mendelian inheritance in man,* 12th ed. Baltimore: Johns Hopkins University Press, 1998.

Roy FH. *Ocular syndromes and systemic diseases,* 3rd ed. Philadelphia: Lippincott Williams & Wilkins, 2002.

POSTERIOR SUBCAPSULAR CATARACT

1. Complicated cataract
   A. Anterior segment involvement, such as that because of the following:
      (1) Acute and chronic corneal ulcer
      *(2) Iridocyclitis
      *(3) Chronic anterior uveitis
      (4) Acute or chronic glaucoma
   B. Posterior segment involvement such as that because of the following:
      *(1) Chronic posterior uveal inflammation
      (2) Long-standing retinal detachment
      (3) High myopia
      (4) Hereditary retinal lesions, including retinitis pigmentosa
      (5) Persistent hyperplastic primary vitreous
2. Congenital posterior polar lens changes
   A. Spurious posterior capsular cataract (Mittendorf dot)
   B. Posterior polar cataract—persistent fibrovascular sheath of lens with or without secondary cataract
   C. Posterior lenticonus
3. Aberfeld syndrome (ocular and facial abnormalities syndrome)
4. Acrodermatitis chronica atrophicans
5. Alcoholism
6. Aniridia
7. Anterior segment ischemia syndrome
8. Aspergillosis
9. Bassen–Kornzweig syndrome (familial hypolipoproteinemia)
10. Bloch–Sulzberger syndrome (incontinentia pigmenti)
11. Buerger disease (thromboangiitis obliterans)
12. Capsular exfoliation syndrome
13. Carotid artery syndrome
14. Chromosome partial deletion (short-arm) syndrome
15. Congenital amaurosis of Leber (Leber congenital amaurosis)
16. Cushing syndrome
*17. Diabetes mellitus (Willis disease)
18. Drugs, including dinitrophenol busulfan (Myleran), triparanol (MER-29), PUVA (psoralen plus ultraviolet light of A-wave length), allopurinol, indapamide, megestrol acetate, and phenothiazine usage
19. Electrical injury
20. Engelmann syndrome (diaphyseal dysplasia)
21. Fabry disease (glycosphingolipid lipidosis)
22. Familial hypogonadism syndrome
23. Frenkel syndrome (ocular contusion syndrome)
24. Fuchs syndrome
25. Glassblowers (heat) cataract
26. Gyrate atrophy (ornithine ketoacid aminotransferase deficiency)
27. Hagberg–Santavuori syndrome (neuronal ceroid-lipofuscinoses)
28. Hair dye
29. Hand-Schüller–Christian syndrome (xanthomatous granuloma syndrome)
30. Harada syndrome (uveitis–vitiligo–alopecia–poliosis syndrome)

* = most important

31. Heerfordt syndrome (uveoparotitis)
32. Hemochromatosis
33. Herpes simplex
34. Hodgkin disease
35. Hypertension
36. Hypoparathyroidism
37. Ionizing radiation, such as that encountered in x-ray, radium, or neutron therapy
38. Jacobsen–Brodwall syndrome
39. Kussmaul disease (necrotizing angiitis)
40. Kyrle disease (hyperkeratosis follicularis et parafollicularis in cutem penetrans)
41. Laurence–Moon–Bardet–Biedl syndrome (retinitis pigmentosa–polydactyly–adiposogenital)
42. Leprosy (Hansen disease)
43. Leri syndrome (carpal tunnel syndrome)
44. Leukemia
45. Lightning induced
46. Malaria
47. Meckel syndrome (dysencephalia splanchnocystic syndrome)
48. Myotonic dystrophy (Curschmann–Steinert syndrome)
49. Neurodermatitis (lichen simplex chronicus)
50. Neurofibromatosis 1 (von Recklinghausen syndrome)
51. Neurofibromatosis 2 (central neurofibromatosis)
52. Ocular trauma (blunt)
53. Oculootoororenoerythropoietic disease
54. O'Donnell–Pappas syndrome (foveal hypoplasia and presenile cataract—autosomal dominant)
55. Paget syndrome (osteitis deformans)
56. Pemphigus foliaceus (Cazenave disease)
57. Pernicious anemia syndrome
58. Pierre Robin syndrome (micrognathia-glossoptosis syndrome)
59. Posterior polar cataract—autosomal dominant
60. Pseudohypoparathyroidism
61. Refsum syndrome (phytanic acid storage disease)
62. Renal transplantation
63. Retinitis pigmentosa–deafness–ataxia syndrome
64. Roy syndrome I (unilateral cataract associated with smoking)
*65. Senile posterior cortical cataract
66. Sjögren syndrome (secretoinhibitor syndrome)
67. Silicone oil (intraocular)
*68. Steroid usage (topical or systemic)
69. Stickler syndrome (hereditary progressive arthro-ophthalmopathy)
70. Still disease (juvenile rheumatoid arthritis)
71. Toxocariasis (Nematode ophthalmia syndrome)
72. Trisomy (Patau syndrome)
73. Tuomaala–Haapanen syndrome (similar to pseudohypoparathyroidism)
74. Turner syndrome (gonadal dysgenesis)
75. Ultraviolet-B light
76. Uric acid (increased serum levels)
77. Vitrectomy for diabetic retinopathy

* = most important

78. Weil disease (leptospirosis)
79. Werner syndrome (progeria of adults)
80. Yersiniosis

McKusick VA. *Mendelian inheritance in man,* 12th ed. Baltimore: Johns Hopkins University Press, 1998.

Roy FH. *Ocular syndromes and systemic diseases,* 3rd ed. Philadelphia: Lippincott Williams & Wilkins, 2002.

Seddon J, Fong D. The association between cigarette smoking and ocular diseases. *Surv Ophthalmol* 1998;42: 535–547.

Tong JT, Bateman JB. Selective B-wave reduction with congenital cataract in neurofibromatosis-2. *Ophthalmology* 1999;106:1681–1683.

Posterior subcapsular cataract

	Corneal Ulcer	Glaucoma	Chronic Uveitis*	High Myopia	Retinitis Pigmentosa	Ionizing Radiation*	Diabetes Mellitus	Blunt Ocular Trauma	Steroid Use*	Fabry Disease	Kyrle Disease	Werner Syndrome	Myotonic Dystrophy
History													
1. Acute onset	U						U						
2. Associated diabetes mellitus											U		
3. Bilateral				U	U		S		U	U	S	S	U
4. Caused by microbes, parasites, or noninfectious systemic diseases			U										
5. Common during second to third decades					S							U	U
6. Common during third to fifth decades			S				U			U			
7. Common after fourth decade		U											
8. Congenital				S									
9. Consanguinity												U	
10. Exposure to roentgenograms, gamma and infrared rays, or microwaves						U							
11. Familial		S		U			U				U	U	U
12. Hereditary				U			U			U		U	U
13. Most common in blacks		S											
14. More common in males					S								
15. Preceded by mild trauma to corneal epithelium	U												
16. Prolonged topical or systemic steroids									U				
17. Trauma	S							U					
Physical Findings													
1. Absent eyelashes/scanty eyebrows						S						U	
2. Angle recession								S					
3. Anterior/posterior synechiae	S	S	U										
4. Anterior uveitis			U			S							
5. Astigmatism							S			S			
6. Blue sclera												U	
7. Bullous keratopathy												U	
8. Chorioretinitis			U					S				S	S
9. Choroidal exudative areas			U										
10. Chronic blepharitis						U							
11. Closed anterior chamber angle		U											
12. Conjunctival keratinization										S			
13. Conjunctival necrosis										S			
14. Cornea verticillata										S			
15. Corneal dystrophy										U			U
16. Corneal hypesthesia						S	S						U
17. Corneal necrosis						S							
18. Corneal opacities						S					U	U	
19. Corneal perforation	S												
20. Cystoid macular edema					S	S							
21. Dark macular spot			U										
22. Disc hamartomas/drusens					S								
23. Ectropion						U							
24. Endophthalmitis	S												
25. Enlarging myopic crescent			U										

Posterior subcapsular cataract (Continued)

	Corneal Ulcer	Glaucoma	Chronic Uveitis*	High Myopia	Retinitis Pigmentosa	Ionizing Radiation*	Diabetes Mellitus	Blunt Ocular Trauma	Steroid Use*	Fabry Disease	Kyrle Disease	Werner Syndrome	Myotonic Dystrophy
Physical Findings													
26. Entropion						U							
27. Epithelial corneal edema		U											
28. Exophthalmos								S				S	
29. Extraocular muscle palsy						S	S						
30. Folds Bowman/Descemet membranes		U											
31. Hard retinal exudates							U						
32. Hyphema								S					
33. Hypopyon	U												
34. Increased intraocular pressure		U	S			S	S		S				
35. Internuclear ophthalmoplegia										S			
36. Iridocyclitis	U												
37. Iris atrophy						S	S						
38. Keratoconus					R								
39. Lid hemorrhage								S					
40. Lid laceration								S					
41. Lid telangiectasia												S	
42. Low intraocular pressure			S					S					
43. Macular degeneration							S						S
44. Macular holes							S	S					
45. Macular red spot													U
46. Madarosis						U							
47. Microphthalmos					R								
48. Mutton fat keratic precipitates			U										
49. Myopia					U		S						
50. Nystagmus					R	S						S	
51. Optic nerve atrophy		U			S	S	R	S				S	
52. Papilledema			S					S		S			
53. Paramacular retinal degeneration												S	
54. Pigmentary changes in retina (Bone corpuscles or spiderlike figures)						U	S	S				S	
55. Pigmentary degeneration of iris		U					S						
56. Presbyopia, early							S					S	
57. Progressive external ophthalmoplegia					R							U	
58. Ptosis													R
59. Punctate keratitis						U							
60. Pupil dilated and fixed		U					S	S					
61. Retinal detachment			S	S				S					
62. Retinal exudates						S	U						
63. Retinal hemorrhage						S	U	S					
64. Retinal microaneurysms							U			U			
65. Retinal neovascularization						S	U						
66. Retinal vascular occlusion		U					S			S			
67. Retrobulbar hemorrhage								S					
68. Rupture in Bruch membrane								S					
69. Rupture of pupillary sphincter								S					
70. Strabismus					R								

* = most important

Posterior subcapsular cataract (Continued)

	Corneal Ulcer	Glaucoma	Chronic Uveitis*	High Myopia	Retinitis Pigmentosa	Ionizing Radiation*	Diabetes Mellitus	Blunt Ocular Trauma	Steroid Use*	Fabry Disease	Kyrle Disease	Werner Syndrome	Myotonic Dystrophy
Physical Findings													
71. Stromal abscess formation	U												
72. Symblepharon						S							
73. Trophic corneal defects												U	
74. Uveitis			U									S	
75. Visual field defects		U			S	U	S		U				S
76. Vitreous opacities			U										
Laboratory Data													
1. Albuminuria										S			
2. Angiotensin—converting enzyme/ lysozyme tests for sarcoid			U										
3. Blood sugar elevated							U				S		
4. Color vision abnormal					U								
5. Complement fixation test for histoplasmosis			U										
6. Chest roentgenogram			U										
7. Dark adaptation abnormal					U								
8. Electrooculogram abnormal					U								
9. Electroretinogram consistently abnormal					U								
10. Fluorescein angiograaphy			S	U	U	S	S						
11. Genetic studies											U	U	U
12. Giemsa strain smear	U												
13. Gram stain smear	U												
14. Homologous leucocytic antibody B2F testing			U										
15. Leukocyte/eosinophilic count and sedimentation rate elevated			S										S
16. Lipid storage testing										U			
17. Lumbosacral roentgenogram			U										
18. Ocular ultrasonography			S					U					
19. Purified protein derivative skin test			U										
20. Profile for immunologic abnormalities			U										
21. Venereal disease reaction level or fluorescent treponemal antibody-absorption test			U										
22. Visual field test		U			S	U	S		U				S

R = rarely; S = sometimes; and U = usually.

IRIDESCENT CRYSTALLINE DEPOSITS IN LENS

1. Idiopathic
2. Hypothyroid (cretinism)
3. Hypocalcemia
    A. Postoperative—removal of thyroid and accidental parathyroid removal
    B. Idiopathic hypoparathyroidism
    C. Pseudohypoparathyroidism (hypoparathyroid cretinism) or with hyperphosphatemia (Albright disease)
    D. Pseudopseudohypoparathyroidism (brachymetacarpal dwarfism)
4. Myotonic dystrophy (Curschmann–Steinert syndrome)
5. Drugs, including the following:

acetophenazine	gold Au 198	prochlorperazine
amiodarone	gold sodium thiomalate	promazine
auranofin	gold sodium thiosulfate	promethazine
aurothioglucose	mercuric oxide	propiomazine
aurothioglycanide	mesoridazine	silver nitrate
butaperazine	methdilazine	silver protein
carphenazine	methotrimeprazine	thiethylperazine
chlorpromazine	mild silver protein	thiopropazate
chlorprothixene	perazine	thioridazine
colloidal silver	pericyazine	thiothixene
diazepam (?)	perphenazine	trifluoperazine
diethazine	phenylmercuric acetate	triflupromazine
ethopropazine	phenylmercuric nitrate	trimeprazine
fluphenazine	piperacetazine	

6. Cataract (coralliform and aculeiform) usually autosomal dominant; sometimes recessive

Fraunfelder FT, Fraunfelder FW. *Drug-induced ocular side effects.* Woburn, MA: Butterworth-Heinemann, 2001.

McKusick VA. *Mendelian inheritance in man,* 12th ed. Baltimore: Johns Hopkins University Press, 1998.

Roy FH. *Ocular syndromes and systemic diseases,* 3rd ed. Philadelphia: Lippincott Williams & Wilkins, 2002.

OIL DROPLET IN LENS

1. Anterior displacement of lens
*2. Galactosemia–transferase deficiency (von Reuss syndrome)
3. Lenticonus

Bellows JG, Bellows RT. Displacement of the lens. In: Bellows JG, ed. *Cataract and abnormalities of the lens.* New York: Grune & Stratton, 1975:277.

Beutler E, et al. Galactokinase deficiency as cause of cataract. *N Engl J Med* 1973;288:1203–1206.

LENTICONUS (CONICAL LENS SURFACE PROTUBERANCE) AND LENTIGLOBUS (GLOBULAR LENS SURFACE PROTUBERANCE)

1. Anterior—rare and usually bilateral
    *A. Alport syndrome (hereditary nephritis)
    B. Spina bifida
    C. Waardenburg syndrome (embryonic fixation syndrome)

* = most important

2. Posterior—more common and often unilateral
    A. Associated with persistent hyperplastic primary vitreous
    B. Associated with remnants of hyaloid artery
    C. Familial posterior lenticonus and microcornea
  *D. Lowe syndrome (oculocerebrorenal syndrome)
    E. Trauma

Bleik JH, et al. Familial posterior lenticonus and microcornea. *Arch Ophthalmol* 1992;110:1208.

Junk AK, et al. Bilateral anterior lenticonus. *Arch Ophthalmol* 2000;118:895–897.

Tripathi RC, et al. Pathogenesis of cataracts in patients with Lowe's syndrome. *Ophthalmology* 1986;93:1046–1051.

LENS ABSORPTION

1. Congenital rubella syndrome (German measles)
2. Hallermann–Streiff syndrome (dyscephalic mandibulooculofacial syndrome)
3. Surgical trauma as discission
4. Trauma, blunt or penetrating

Roy FH. *Ocular syndromes and systemic diseases,* 3rd ed. Philadelphia: Lippincott Williams & Wilkins, 2002.

EXFOLIATION OF LENS CAPSULE

In this condition, superficial layers of the lens capsule split off and float in aqueous as a fine membrane.

 *1. Senile exfoliation
  2. Toxic exfoliation
    A. Atrophic eyes
    B. Prolonged iridocyclitis
    C. Lodgment of metallic foreign body, such as iron or copper
  3. Traumatic
    A. Perforating injury
    B. Contusions with suspensory ligament separated from a dislocated lens
  4. Heat exposure, such as that experienced by glassblowers

Duke-Elder S. *System of ophthalmology,* Vol XI. St. Louis: CV Mosby, 1969.

Meades K, Versace P. True exfoliation of the lens capsule. *Aust N Z J Ophthalmol* 1992;20:347–348.

MICROPHAKIA OR SPHEROPHAKIA OR MICROSPHEROPHAKIA (SMALL LENS OR HIGHLY SPHERIC LENS)

1. Achard syndrome (Marfan syndrome with dysostosis mandibulofacialis)
2. Alport syndrome (hereditary nephritis)
3. Familial anomaly
4. Homocystinuria syndrome
5. Hyperlysinemia
6. Lenticular myopia as recessive inheritance trait
7. Little syndrome (hereditary osteoorcychodysplasia)
8. Lowe syndrome (renal rickets)
*9. Marchesani syndrome (brachymorphy with spherophakia) (Weill–Marchesani syndrome)

10. Marfan syndrome (dolichostenomelia-arachnodactyly hyperchondroplasia dystrophica mesodermalis congenita)
11. Peter anomaly (anterior chamber cleavage syndrome)
12. Reticular dystrophy of the retinal pigment epithelium
13. Rubella syndrome (Gregg syndrome)
14. Waardenburg syndrome (embryonic fixation syndrome)

Roy FH. *Ocular syndromes and systemic diseases,* 3rd ed. Philadelphia: Lippincott Williams & Wilkins, 2002.

Sorsby A. *Ophthalmic genetics,* 2nd ed. New York: Appleton-Century-Crofts, 1970.

DISLOCATED LENS

1. Achard syndrome (Marfan with dysostosis)
2. Adenoma of the nonpigmented epithelium of the ciliary body
3. Apert syndrome (sphenoacrocraniosyndactyly)
4. Ascariasis
5. Associated ocular findings
   *A. Aniridia
    B. Coloboma of iris and choroid
   *C. Congenital glaucoma
    D. Ectopia lentis et pupillae
    E. Focal dermal hypoplasia (Goltz syndrome)
    F. High myopia
    G. Isolated lens dislocation (up)
    H. Megalocornea
    I. Microcornea
    J. Microspherophakia with hernia
    K. Pseudoxanthoma
    L. Retinitis pigmentosa
6. Autosomal recessive or dominant abnormality without other defects, except usually ectopic pupils
7. Capsular exfoliation syndrome
8. Crouzon disease
9. Cryptophthalmia syndrome (cryptophthalmos–syndactyly syndrome)
10. Dwarfism, genetic type
11. Ehlers–Danlos syndrome (cutis hyperelastica)
12. Gillum–Anderson syndrome (blepharoptosis, myopia, ectopia lentis)
13. Gorlin–Goltz syndrome
14. Grönblad–Strandberg syndrome (pseudoxanthoma elasticum)
15. Hereditary ectodermal dysplasia syndrome
*16. Homocystinuria—usually downward displacement of lens
17. Hyperlysinemia
18. Kniest syndrome
19. Late-onset localized junctional epidermolysis bullosa and mental retardation
20. Mandibulofacial dysostosis (Franceschetti syndrome)
21. Marchesani syndrome (brachymorphy with spherophakia)(Weill–Marchesani syndrome)
*22. Marfan syndrome (dolichostenomelia–arachnodactyly–hyperchondroplasia dystrophia mesodermalis congenita)—usually superior displacement of lens

* = most important

23. Molybdenum cofactor deficiency (combined deficiency of sulfite oxidase and xanthine dehydrogenase)
24. Oculodental syndrome (Peters syndrome)
25. Pfaundler syndrome
26. Pierre Robin syndrome
27. Pseudoexfoliation (exfoliation syndrome)
28. Recession of anterior chamber angle
29. Refsum syndrome
30. Retinal disinsertion syndrome
31. Retinoblastoma
32. Rieger syndrome (dysgenesis mesostromalis)
33. Spherophakia (see p. 400)
34. Spontaneous (degenerative)
35. Sprengel deformity
36. Sturge–Weber syndrome
37. Sulfite oxidase deficiency
38. Surgical accidents (iatrogenic)
*39. Syphilis (lues)
*40. Trauma as in Frenkel syndrome (ocular contusion syndrome), beesting, and following YAG laser
41. Treacher Collins syndrome (mandibulofacial dysostosis)
42. Uveitis
43. Wildervanck syndrome (cervicooculoacoustic syndrome)

Byrnes BA, et al. Retinoblastoma presenting with spontaneous hyphema and dislocated lens. *J Pediatr Ophthalmol Strabismus* 1993;30:334–336.

Edwards MC, et al. Isolated sulfite oxidase deficiency. *Ophthalmology* 1999;106:1957–1961.

Melamed S, et al. Neodymium:YAG laser iridotomy as a possible contribution to lens dislocation. *Ann Ophthalmol* 1986;18:281–282.

Roy FH. *Ocular syndromes and systemic diseases,* 3rd ed. Philadelphia: Lippincott Williams & Wilkins, 2002.

Dislocated lens

	Marfan Syndrome*	Weill-Marchesani Syndrome	Dwarfism as Cockayne Disease	Trauma*	Homocystinuria*	Syphilis*	Ehlers-Danlos Syndrome	Rieger Syndrome	Hyperlysinemia	Sulfite Oxidase Deficiency	Treacher-Collins Syndrome
History											
1. Autosomal dominant	U						U	U			S
2. Autosomal recessive		S	U		U						
3. Blunt ocular trauma				U							
4. Congenital	U	S				S					
5. Hereditary	U	U	U		U		U	S	S	S	U
Physical Findings											
1. Angioid streaks							U				
2. Angle recession				S							
3. Aniridia					R			S			
4. Antimongoloid obliquity (temporal canthus lower)		U									
5. Bialteral interstitial keratitis						U					
6. Blue sclera							U				
7. Cataract	U		U	S	R						
8. Central retinal artery occlusion					R						
9. Coloboma of iris	R				R						U
10. Corneal opacity		S						U			
11. Choroidal hemorrhage							S				
12. Choroiditis						U					
13. Decreased tearing			S								
14. Disciform macular degeneration							S	U			
15. Epicanthal folds							U				
16. Glaucoma		R		S	U			U			
17. Hyphema				U							
18. Iridodialysis				S							
19. Iris hypoplasia								U			
20. Iritis				U							
21. Keratoconus							U				
22. Macular edema				U							
23. Megalocornea	S	U									
24. Microcornea					R			U			
25. Microphthalmos					R			U			U
26. Myopia	U	U			U						
27. Nystagmus	U		U							U	
28. Optic atrophy		S	S		U	U		S			
29. Optic disc hypoplasia											U
30. Optic neuritis						U					
31. Papilledema					R						
32. Peripheral cystoid retinal degeneration					U						
33. Peripheral anterior synechiae				S				U			
34. Pigmented retinal appearance	S		U		U				U		
35. Retina detachment	S										
36. Spherophakia	U	U							U		
37. Strabismus	U										
38. Underdeveloped orbicularis oculi muscle											U
39. Vitreous hemorrhage							S				

* = most important

Dislocated lens (Continued)

	Marfan Syndrome*	Weill-Marchesani Syndrome	Dwarfism as Cockayne Disease	Trauma*	Homocystinuria*	Syphilis*	Ehlers-Danlos Syndrome	Rieger Syndrome	Hyperlysinemia	Sulfite Oxidase Deficiency	Treacher-Collins Syndrome
Laboratory Data											
1. Cystathionine blood/urine										U	
2. Fluorescent treponemal antibody-absorption test						U					
3. Hemocystine/methionine in blood/urine					U						
4. Lysine/homoarginine in blood/urine									U		

R = rarely; S = sometimes; and U = usually.

APHAKIA (ABSENCE OF LENS IN USUAL POSITION BEHIND THE IRIS)

1. Congenital absence of lens—rare
2. Dislocation of the lens into vitreous cavity, anterior chamber, or subconjunctival area
3. Following cataract extraction
4. Gradual absorption of the lens

Hanna C, et al. Extraocular traumatic luxation of the lens. *J Ark Med Soc* 1969;66:210.

O'Brien CS. *Ophthalmology: notes for students.* Iowa City: Athens Press, 1930.

EQUATORIAL LENS PIGMENTATION

1. Associated with myopia and retinal detachment
2. Congenital malformation
3. Pigmentary glaucoma
4. Uveitis

Delaney WV Jr. Equatorial lens pigmentation, myopia, and retinal detachment. *Am J Ophthalmol* 1975;79:194–205.

UNILATERAL CATARACTS

1. Argon laser treatment
*2. Trauma
3. Complicated cataract
    A. Anterior segment involvement, such as that because of the following:
        (1) Acute and chronic corneal ulcer
        *(2) Iridocyclitis
        (3) Chronic anterior uveitis
        (4) Acute or chronic glaucoma
    B. Posterior segment involvement, such as that because of the following:
        (1) Chronic posterior uveal inflammation
        (2) Long-standing retinal detachment
        (3) High myopia
        (4) Hereditary retinal lesions
        (5) Persistent hyperplastic primary vitreous
4. Roy syndrome I (unilateral cataract associated with smoking)
5. Congenital posterior polar lens changes
6. Glaucomatocyclitic crisis (Posner–Schlossman syndrome)
7. Conditions that give bilateral manifestations with earlier onset in one eye

Jarrett WH. Dislocation of the lens. *Arch Ophthalmol* 1967;78:289.

Roy FH. *Ocular syndromes and systemic diseases,* 3rd ed. Philadelphia: Lippincott Williams & Wilkins, 2002.

Roy FH. Cigarette smoking and the risk of cataract [Letter]. *JAMA* 1993;269:748.

LENTICULAR DISEASE ASSOCIATED WITH CORNEAL PROBLEMS

1. Aberfeld syndrome (ocular and facial abnormalities syndrome)—cataracts, microcornea
2. Acrodermatitis chronica atrophicans—keratomalacia, corneal opacification, cataracts
3. Addison syndrome (idiopathic hypoparathyroidism)—keratoconjunctivitis, corneal ulcers, keratitic moniliasis, cataracts

* = most important

4. Alport syndrome (hereditary nephritis)—anterior lenticonus, posterior polymorphous corneal dystrophy
*5. Amiodarone—corneal deposits, anterior subcapsular cataracts
6. Amyloidosis—amyloid deposits of cornea, corneal dystrophy, pseudopodia lentis
7. Anderson–Warburg syndrome (oligophrenia–microphthalmos syndrome)—corneal opacification and lenticular destruction with a mass visible behind the lens
8. Andogsky syndrome (atopic cataract syndrome)—atopic keratoconjunctivitis, keratoconus, uveitis, subcapsular cataract
9. Aniridia—microcornea and subluxated lenses
10. Anterior-chamber cleavage syndrome (Reese–Ellsworth syndrome)—corneal opacities, anterior pole cataract
11. Anterior segment ischemia syndrome—corneal edema, corneal ulceration, cataract
12. Apert syndrome (absent digits cranial defects syndrome)—exposure keratitis, cataracts, ectopia lentis
13. Arteriovenous fistula (arteriovenous aneurysm)—bullous keratopathy, cataract
14. Aspergillosis—corneal ulcer, keratitis, cataract
*15. Atopic dermatitis (atopic eczema, Besnier prurigo)—keratoconjunctivitis, keratoconus, cataract
16. Autosomal dominant—cataracts and microcornea
17. Avitaminosis C (scurvy)—keratitis, corneal ulcer, cataract
18. Chalcosis (intraocular copper containing foreign body) deposits in Descemet membrane and anterior lens capsule
19. Chickenpox (varicella)—corneal ulcer, corneal opacity, keratitis, cataract
20. Chlorpromazine—corneal and lens opacities
21. Cholera—keratomalacia, cataract
22. Chromosome partial deletion (short-arm) syndrome—cataracts, corneal opacities
23. Chrysiasis (gold)—corneal and lens deposits
24. Cockayne syndrome (Mickey Mouse syndrome)—cataracts, band keratopathy, corneal dystrophy
25. Congenital spherocytic anemia (congenital hemolytic jaundice)—congenital cataract, ring-shaped pigmentary corneal deposits
26. Crouzon syndrome (Parrot-head syndrome)—exposure keratitis, cataract, corneal dystrophy
27. Cryptophthalmia syndrome (cryptophthalmos–syndactyly syndrome)—cornea differentiated from sclera, lens absence to hypoplasia, dislocation, and calcification
28. Cytomegalic inclusion disease (cytomegalovirus)—cataract, corneal opacities
29. Darier–White syndrome (keratosis follicularis)—keratosis, corneal subepithelial infiltrations, corneal ulceration, cataract
30. Dermatitis herpetiformis (Duhring–Broca disease)—corneal vascularization, cataract
31. Dermochondral corneal dystrophy (of François)—cataract, corneal dystrophy
32. Diabetes mellitus—cataract, corneal edema secondary to rubeosis
33. Diphtheria—keratitis, corneal ulcer, cataract
34. Down syndrome (trisomy 21)—lens opacities, keratoconus
35. Ehler–Danlos syndrome (fibrodysplasia elastica generalisata)—microcornea, keratoconus, lens subluxation
36. Electrical injury—corneal perforation, necrosis of cornea, anterior or posterior subcapsular cataracts
37. Endothelial dystrophy and anterior polar cataract (Dohlman)
38. Exfoliation syndrome (capsular exfoliation syndrome)—cataract, dislocated lens, corneal dystrophy, lens capsule exfoliation

39. Fabry disease (glycosphingolipid lipidosis)—cataract, corneal dystrophy
40. Folling syndrome (phenylketonuria)—corneal opacities, cataracts
41. Fuchs syndrome (I) (heterochromic cyclitis syndrome)—secondary cataract, edematous corneal epithelium
42. Goldscheider syndrome (epidermolysis bullosa)—bullous keratitis, corneal subepithelial blisters to corneal perforation, cataract
43. Gorlin–Goltz syndrome (multiple basal cell nevi syndrome)—cataract, corneal leukoma
44. Grönblad–Strandberg syndrome (elastorrhexis)—keratoconus, cataract, subluxation of lens
45. Hallermann–Streiff syndrome (oculomandibulofacial dyscephaly)—cataracts, microcornea
46. Hanhart syndrome (recessive keratosis palmoplantaris)—dendritic corneal lesions, keratitis, corneal haze, corneal neovascularization, cataract
47. Heerfordt syndrome (uveoparotid fever)—band keratopathy, keratoconjunctivitis, cataract
48. Hereditary ectodermal dysplasia syndrome (Siemens syndrome)—keratosis, corneal erosions, corneal dystrophy, cataract, lens luxation
49. Herpes simplex—keratitis, corneal ulcer, cataracts
50. Herpes zoster—keratitis, corneal ulcer, cataract
51. Histiocytosis X (Hand–Schüller–Christian syndrome)—pannus, bullous keratopathy, corneal ulcer, cataract
52. Hodgkin disease—keratitis, cataract
53. Homocystinuria syndrome—dislocated lens, cataract, keratitis
54. Hutchinson–Gilford syndrome (progeria)—cataract, microcornea
55. Hydatid cyst (echinococcosis)—keratitis, corneal abscess, cataract
56. Hypervitaminosis D—band keratopathy, cataract
57. Hypoparathyroidism—keratitis, cataract
58. Hypophosphatasia (phosphoethanolaminuria)—cataract, corneal subepithelial calcifications
59. Influenza—keratitis, cataract
60. Jadassohn-type anetodermal—keratoconus, cataract
61. Jadassohn–Lewandowsky syndrome (pachyonychia congenita)—corneal dyskeratosis, cataract
*62. Juvenile rheumatoid arthritis (Still disease)—band keratopathy, cataract
63. Kussmaul disease (periarteritis nodosa)—corneal ulcer, cataract
64. Kyrle disease (hyperkeratosis penetrans)—subcapsular cataracts, subepithelial corneal opacities
65. Leber congenital amaurosis—cataracts, keratoconus
66. Leri syndrome (carpal tunnel syndrome)—corneal clouding, cataract
67. Listerellosis (listeriosis)—keratitis, corneal abscess and ulcer, cataract
68. Little syndrome (nail-patella syndrome)—microcornea, keratoconus, cataract
*69. Lowe syndrome (oculocerebrorenal syndrome)—cloudy cornea, cataracts, megalocornea, corneal dystrophy
70. Malaria—keratitis, cataract
71. Marchesani syndrome (brachymorphy with spherophakia)—lenticular myopia, ectopia lentis, megalocornea, corneal opacity
72. Marfan syndrome (arachnodactyly-dystrophia-mesodermalis congenita)—lens dislocation, cataract, megalocornea, lenticular myopia

* = most important

73. Matsoukas syndrome (oculocerebroarticuloskeletal syndromes)—cataract, corneal sclerosis
74. Meckel syndrome (dysencephalia splanchnocystic syndrome)—sclerocornea, microcornea, cataract
75. Micro syndrome (autosomal recessive microcephaly, microcornea, congenital cataract, mental retardation, optic atrophy, and hypogenitalism)
76. Morbilli (rubeola, measles)—corneal ulcer, cataract
77. Mucolipidosis IV (ML IV)—corneal clouding, cataract
78. Myotonic dystrophy (Curschmann–Steinert syndrome)—lens opacity, cornea–epithelial dystrophy
79. Nematode ophthalmia syndrome (toxocariasis)—cataract, larvae present in the cornea
80. Neurodermatitis (lichen simplex chronicus)—keratoconjunctivitis, atopic cataracts, keratoconus
81. Neurofibromatosis 1
82. Neurofibromatosis 2
83. Ocular toxoplasmosis (toxoplasmosis)—keratitis, cataract
84. Oculodental syndrome (Peter syndrome)—macrocornea, opacities of the corneal margin, ectopic lentis, corneoscleral staphyloma
85. O'Donnell–Pappas syndrome—presenile cataract, peripheral corneal pannus
86. Paget syndrome (osteitis deformans)—corneal ring opacities, cataract
87. Passow syndrome (status dysraphicus syndrome)—neuroparalytic keratitis, zonular cataract
88. Pemphigus foliaceus (Cazenave disease)—pannus, corneal infiltration, cataract
89. Peter anomaly (anterior chamber cleavage syndrome—lens apposition to leukoma
90. Pigmentary ocular dispersion syndrome (pigmentary glaucoma)—Krukenberg spindle, equatorial pigmentation of lens capsule
91. Pseudohypoparathyroidism (Seabright–Bantan syndrome)—punctate cataracts, keratitis
92. Radiation—corneal ulcer, punctate keratitis, cataracts, exfoliation of lens capsule
93. Refsum syndrome (phytanic acid oxidase deficiency)—corneal opacities, cataracts
94. Relapsing polychondritis—corneal ulcer, cataracts, keratoconjunctivitis sicca
95. Retinal disinsertion syndrome—lens subluxation, keratoconus
96. Retrolental fibroplasia (RLF)—cataracts, corneal opacification
97. Rieger syndrome (dysgenesis mesodermalis corneae et irides)—microcornea, corneal opacities in Descemet membrane, dislocated lens
98. Romberg syndrome (facial hemiatrophy)—neuroparalytic keratitis, cataracts
99. Rothmund syndrome (telangiectasia–pigmentation–cataract syndrome)—cataract, corneal lesions
*100. Rubella syndrome (German measles)—corneal haziness, cataracts, microcornea
101. Sabin–Feldman syndrome—posterior lenticonus, microcornea
102. Sanfilippo–Good syndrome (mucopolysaccharidosis III)—deposits in cornea and lens
103. Schafer syndrome (keratosis palmoplantaris syndrome)—lesions in the lower portion of the cornea, cataract
104. Schaumann syndrome (sarcoidosis syndrome)—keratitis sicca, band-shaped keratitis, complicated cataract
105. Scheie syndrome (mucopolysaccharidosis IS)—diffuse haze to marked corneal clouding, cataracts
106. Siderosis (intraocular iron foreign body)—iron deposition in lens and cornea
107. Stannus cerebellar syndrome—corneal vascularization, corneal opacities, cataracts

108. Steroids—cataract, may worsen certain types of corneal infections
109. Stevens–Johnson syndrome (erythema multiforme exudativum)—keratitis, corneal ulcers, cataracts, pannus
110. Stickler syndrome (hereditary progressive arthro-ophthalmopathy)—keratopathy, cataracts
111. Thioridazine—corneal and lens opacities
112. Toxic lens syndrome—pigment precipitation on the surface of an intraocular lens, chronic uveitis
113. Trisomy syndrome—corneal and lens opacities
114. Turner syndrome (gonadal dysgenesis)—corneal nebulae, cataracts
115. Ultraviolet radiation—band keratopathy, keratitis, discoloring of lens
116. van Bogaert–Scherer–Epstein syndrome (familial hypercholesterolemia syndrome)—lipid keratopathy, cataract, juvenile corneal arcus
117. von Recklinghausen syndrome (neurofibromatosis)—nodular swelling of corneal nerves, cataracts
118. Waardenburg syndrome (interoculoiridodermatoauditive dysplasia)—microcornea, cornea plana, lenticonus
119. Wagner syndrome (hereditary hyaloideoretinal degeneration and palatoschisis)—corneal degeneration, including band-shaped keratopathy, cataracts
120. Ward syndrome (nevus jaw cyst syndrome)—congenital cataracts, congenital corneal opacities
121. Wegener syndrome (Wegener granulomatosis)—corneal ulcer, corneal abscess, cataract
122. Weil disease (leptospirosis)—keratitis, cataract
123. Werner syndrome (progeria of adults)—juvenile cataracts, bullous keratitis, trophic corneal defects
*124. Wilson disease (hepatolenticular degeneration)—sunflower cataract, Kayser-Fleischer ring
125. Yersiniosis—corneal ulcer, cataract
126. Zellweger syndrome (cerebrohepatorenal syndrome of Zellweger)—corneal opacities, cataract

Dolan BJ, et al. Amiodarone keratopathy and lens opacities. *J Am Optom Assoc* 1985;56:468–470.

Roy FH. *Ocular syndromes and systemic diseases*, 3rd ed. Philadelphia: Lippincott Williams & Wilkins, 2002.

Warburg M, et al. Autosomal recessive microcephaly, microcornea, congenital cataract, mental retardation, optic atrophy, and hypogenitalism-Micro syndrome. *Am J Dis Child* 1993;147:309–312.

DRUGS ASSOCIATED WITH CATARACTS

Acetophenazine (phenothiazine)
acetohexamide
acetylcholine
adrenal cortex injection
alcohol
aldosterone
allopurinol
amiodarone (?)
amodiaquine
azathioprine (?)

bacille Calmette–Guérin (BCG) vaccine (?)
beclomethasone
benoxinate
benzodiazepine
benzphetamine (?)
betamethasone
betaxolol (?)
bleomycin
bupivacaine
busulfan

butaperazine
cactinomycin
calcitriol (?)
carbachol
carbamazepine (?)
carbromal(?)
carphenazine
chloroprocaine
chlorpropamide
chloroquine
chlorphentermine (?)

* = most important

chlorpromazine
chlorpromazine
chlorprothixene
cholecalciferol (?)
clomiphene (?)
cobalt
colchicine(?)
cortisone
danazol(?)
deferoxamine
demecarium
desoxycorticosterone
dexamethasone
dextrothyroxine (?)
diisopropyl flurophosphate (DFP)
diazoxide
dibucaine
diethazine
diethylpropion (?)
doxorubicin
droperidol (?)
dyclonine
echothiophate
ergocalciferol
ergonovine (?)
ergot (?)
ergotamine (?)
ethopropazine
ethotoin
etidocaine
etretinate
fenfluramine (?)
fludrocortisone
fluorometholone
fluphenazine
fluprednisolone
ganciclovir
glyburide
gold
haloperidol (?)
hydrocortisone
hydroxychloroquine

ibuprofen (?)
indomethacin (?)
isofluorphate
isotretinoin (?)
levobunolol (?)
lidocaine
lithium carbonate(?)
lysergic acid diethylamide (LSD)
lysergide
medrysone
megestrol acetate
mephenytoin (?)
mepivacaine
meprednisone
mescaline
mesoridazine
methdilazine
methotrimeprazine
methoxsalen (?)
methylergonovine (?)
methylprednisolone
methysergide (?)
mitomycin C (topical) (?)
mitotane
naltrexone
naproxen (?)
neostigmine
neostigmine
nifedipine (?)
oral contraceptives (?)
oxygen
paramethasone
penicillamine (?)
perazine
pericyazine
perphenazine
phenacaine
phendimetrazine (?)
phenmetrazine
phentermine (?)
phenytoin
physostigmine
pilocarpine

piperacetazine
piperazine (?)
prazosin (?)
prednisolone
prednisone (steroid)
prilocaine
procaine
prochlorperazine
promazine
promethazine
propiomazine
propoxycaine
piperocaine
psilocybin
PUVA (psoralens and ultraviolet A) (?)
quinacrine
silicone
sulfonamides (maternal ingestion)
sulindac (?)
tamoxifen
tetracaine
thiethylperazine
thiopropazate
thioproperazine
thioridazine
thiothixene
timolol (?)
tolazamide
tolbutamide
triamcinolone
trifluoperazine
trifluperidol (?)
triflupromazine
trimeprazine
trioxsalen (?)
troleandomycin (?)
urokinase (?)
verapamil (?)
vitamin D_2 (?)
vitamin D_3 (?)
warfarin

Fraunfelder FT, Fraunfelder FW. *Drug-induced ocular side effects*. Woburn, MA: Butterworth-Heinemann, 2001.

SYNDROMES AND DISEASES ASSOCIATED WITH CATARACTS

1. Aberfeld syndrome (blepharophimosis associated with generalized myopathy)
2. Acrodermatitis chronica atrophicans

   3. Addison syndrome (adrenal cortical insufficiency)
   4. Albinism
   5. Albright hereditary osteodystrophy (pseudohypoparathyroidism)
   6. Alopecia areata
  *7. Alport syndrome (hereditary nephritis)
   8. Alström disease (cataract and retinitis pigmentosa)
   9. Andogsky syndrome (atopic cataract syndrome)
  10. Anterior segment ischemia syndrome
  11. Apert syndrome (acrocephalosyndactylism syndrome)
  12. Apical malformations associated with cataracts
  13. Arteriovenous fistula
  14. Arthrogryposis multiplex congenita
  15. Aspergillosis
 *16. Atopic dermatitis syndrome
  17. Autosomal dominant foveal hypoplasia and presenile cataract syndrome (O'Don-nell–Pappas syndrome)
  18. Bassen–Kornzweig syndrome (abetalipoproteinemia)
  19. Bloch–Sulzberger syndrome (incontinentia pigmenti)
  20. Bonnevie–Ullrich syndrome (pterygolymphangiectasia)
  21. Bourneville syndrome (tuberous sclerosis)
  22. Buerger disease (thromboangiitis obliterans)
  23. Caisson syndrome (bends)
  24. Capsular exfoliation syndrome
  25. Carotid artery syndrome
  26. Cataract and hypertrophic neuropathy—autosomal recessive
  27. Cataract with microcornea and coloboma of iris—autosomal dominant
  28. Cataract, floriform—autosomal dominant
  29. Cataract and cardiomyopathy—autosomal recessive
  30. Cataract, congenital, or juvenile—autosomal recessive
  31. Cataract, congenital total, with posterior sutural opacities in heterozygotes—X-linked
  32. Cataract, congenital with absence deformity of leg—autosomal recessive
  33. Cataract, congenital, with microcornea or slight microphthalmia—X-linked
  34. Cataract, cortical, and congenital ichthyosis—autosomal recessive
  35. Cataract, mental retardation, hypogonadism (Martsolf syndrome)
  36. Cataract, microcephaly, arthrogryposis kyphosis syndrome (CAMAK syndrome)—autosomal recessive
  37. Cataract microcephaly, failure to thrive, kyphoscoliosis syndrome (CAMFAK syndrome)—autosomal recessive
  38. Cataract, nuclear and total nuclear—usually autosomal dominant rarely recessive
  39. Cataract, zonular, and nystagmus—X-linked
  40. Cat-eye syndrome (Schmid–Fraccaro syndrome)
  41. Cerebral cholesterinosis (cerebrotendinous xanthomatosis)
  42. Cerebellar ataxia, cataract, deafness, and dementia or psychosis
  43. Cerebral palsy
  44. Cerebrohepatorenal syndrome (Smith–Lemli–Opitz syndrome)
  45. Cerebrotendinous xanthomatosis
  46. Cholera
  47. Chromosome 13q partial deletion (long-arm) syndrome
  48. Chromosomal 3; 18 translocation

* = most important

49. Chromosome deletion (short-arm) syndrome
50. Cockayne syndrome (dwarfism with retinal atrophy and deafness)
51. Cerebrooculofascioskeletal syndrome (COFS syndrome)
52. Congenital cataract and hypertrophic cardiomyopathy syndrome
53. Congenital cataract with oxycephaly (tower skull)
54. Congenital hemolytic icterus
55. Congenital ichthyosiform erythroderma
56. Congenital rubella syndrome (German measles)
57. Conradi syndrome (stippled epiphyses syndrome)
58. Comedo–cataract
59. Craniofacial dysostosis (Crouzon disease)
60. Cretinism (hypothyroidism)
61. Crome syndrome (congenital cataracts, epileptic fits, mental retardation, small stature)
62. Cushing syndrome
63. Cytomegalovirus
64. Darier–White syndrome (keratosis follicularis)
65. DeBarsy syndrome
66. Dermatitis herpetiformis
*67. Diabetes mellitus (Willis disease)
68. Diarrhea
69. Diphtheria
70. Ectodermal dysplasia
71. Edward syndrome
72. Electrical injury
73. Ellis–van Creveld syndrome (chondroectodermal dysplasia)
74. Engelmann syndrome (diaphyseal dysplasia)
75. Epidermal nevus syndrome (ichthyosis hystrix)
76. Fabry disease (diffuse angiokeratosis)
77. Familial congenital cataracts, microcornea, abnormal irides, nystagmus, and glaucoma syndrome
78. Familial congenital cataract, nonprogressive neurologic disorders, and mental deficiency syndrome
79. Familial histiocytic dermatoarthritis syndrome
80. Familial hypogonadism syndrome
81. Familial t(2;16) translocation
82. Fetal alcohol syndrome
83. Folling syndrome (phenylketonuria)
84. François dyscephalic syndrome (Hallermann–Streiff syndrome)
85. Frenkel syndrome (ocular contusion syndrome)
86. Fuchs syndrome (1) (heterochromic cyclitis syndrome)
87. Galactokinase deficiency—autosomal recessive
*88. Galactosemia–transferase deficiency
89. Goldenhar syndrome (oculoauriculovertebral dysplasia)
90. Goldscheider syndrome (epidermolysis bullosa)
91. Gorlin–Goltz syndrome (multiple basal cell nevi syndrome)
92. Grönblad–Strandberg syndrome (pseudoxanthoma elasticum)
93. Gyrate atrophy (ornithine ketoacid aminotransferase deficiency)
94. Hagberg–Santavuori syndrome (neuronal ceroid–lipofuscinosis)
95. Hallermann–Streiff syndrome (oculomandibulofacial dyscephaly)

96. Hand–Schüller–Christian syndrome (histiocytosis X)
97. Harada disease (uveitis–vitiligo–alopecia-poliosis syndrome)
98. Heerfordt syndrome (uveoparotid fever)
99. Hemifacial microsomia syndrome (François–Haustrate syndrome)
100. Herpes simplex virus
101. Hilding syndrome (destructive iridocyclitis and multiple joint dislocations)
102. Hodgkin disease
103. Homocystinuria
104. Hookworm disease
105. Hruby–Irvine–Gass syndrome (cystoid maculopathy following cataract extraction with vitreous loss)
106. Hutchinson–Gilford syndrome (progeria)
107. Hydatid cyst
108. Hypercalcemia (adult)
109. Hypercalcemia (infantile) with mental retardation (supravalvular aortic stenosis syndrome)
110. Hyperprolactinemia
111. Hypertrophic cardiomyopathy
112. Hypervitaminosis A
113. Hypervitaminosis D
114. Hypocalcemia
115. Hypoglycemia
116. Hypoparathyroidism
117. Hypophosphatasia (phosphoethanolaminuria)
118. Incontinentia pigmenti achromians
119. Infantile hypoglycemia (male)
120. Influenza
121. Infrared radiation
122. Intrauterine infections
    A. herpes virus
    B. mumps
    C. rubella
    D. toxoplasmosis
    E. vaccinia
123. Jacobsen–Brodwall syndrome
124. Jadassohn–Lewandowsky syndrome (pachyonychia congenita)
125. Karsch–Neugebauer syndrome (nystagmus-split hand syndrome)
126. Klippel–Trenaunay–Weber syndrome (angioosteohypertrophy syndrome)
127. Krause syndrome (congenital encephaloophthalmic dysplasia)
128. Kussmaul disease (periarteritis nodosa)
129. Kyrle disease (hyperkeratosis penetrans)
130. Lanzieri syndrome (craniofacial malformations)
131. Laser treatment for retinopathy of prematurity
132. Laurence–Moon–Biedl syndrome (retinitis pigmentosa–polydactyly–adiposogenital)
133. Leber syndrome (optic atrophy–amaurosis–pituitary syndrome)
134. Leiomyoma
135. Leri syndrome (carpal tunnel syndrome)
136. Lightning
137. Listerellosis
*138. Lowe syndrome (oculocerebrorenal syndrome)

* = most important

139. Majewski syndrome (short-rib polydactyly syndrome)
140. Malaria
141. Male Turner syndrome (Noonan syndrome)
142. Malignant hyperpyrexia syndrome
143. Mandibulofacial dysostosis (Franceschetti syndrome)
144. Mannosidosis
145. Maple-syrup urine disease (branched-chain ketoaciduria
146. Marfan syndrome (arachnodactyly dystrophia mesodermaliscongenita)
147. Marinesco–Sjögren syndrome (congenital cataract-oligophrenia syndrome)
148. Marshall syndrome (atypical ectodermal dysplasia)
149. Martsolf syndrome
150. Matsoukas syndrome (oculocerebroarticuloskeletal syndrome)
151. Meckel syndrome (dysencephalia splanchnocystic syndrome)
152. Microcephaly, microphthalmia, cataracts, and joint contractures syndrome
153. Microphthalmia–congenital anterior polar cataract syndrome—autosomal dominant
154. Micro syndrome
155. Miller syndrome (Wilms aniridia syndrome)
156. Monilethrix
157. Morgan syndrome (intracranial exostosis)
158. Morquio–Brailsford syndrome (mucopolysaccharidoses IV)
159. Multiple sulfatase deficiency
160. Myopic (high)
161. Myotonic dystrophy (Curschmann–Steinert syndrome)
162. Nail–patella syndrome (Little syndrome)
163. Nance–Horan syndrome (cataract–dental syndrome)
164. Neurodermatitis
165. Neurofibromatosis 1 (von Recklinghausen syndrome)
166. Neurofibromatosis 2 (central neurofibromatosis)
167. Nieden syndrome (telangiectasia–cataract syndrome)
168. Norrie disease
169. Oculootoororenoerythropoietic disease
170. Optic atrophy, cataract, and neurologic disorder—autosomal dominant
171. Osteogenesis imperfecta congenita, microcephaly, and cataracts—autosomal recessive
172. Osteopetrosis (Albers–Schönberg syndrome)
173. Oxycephaly
174. Pachyonychia congenita syndrome
175. Paget syndrome (idiopathic hyperphosphatasemia)
176. Pallister–Killian syndrome
177. Partial trisomy 10q trisomy
178. Passow syndrome (syringomyelia)
179. Patau syndrome
180. Pellagra (avitaminosis B_2)
181. Pemphigus foliaceus (Cazenave disease)
182. Pernicious anemia syndrome (vitamin B_{12} deficiency)
183. Pierre Robin syndrome (micrognathia-glossoptosis syndrome)
184. Prader–Labhart–Willi syndrome (hypogenital dystrophy with diabetic tendency)
185. Pseudoexfoliation syndrome
186. Pseudohypoparathyroidism
187. Radiation

188. Reese–Ellsworth syndrome (anterior chamber cleavage syndrome)
189. Refsum syndrome (phytanic acid storage disease)
190. Renal failure (chronic)
191. Renal transplantation
192. Retinal ischemic infarction syndrome
*193. Retinitis pigmentosa–deafness–ataxia syndrome
194. Rhizomelic chondrodysplasia punctata
195. Riboflavin deficiency syndrome (oculoorogenital syndrome)
196. Ring chromosome in the D group
197. Robert syndrome
198. Robert pseudothalidomide syndrome
199. Romberg syndrome (facial hemiatrophy)
200. Rothmund syndrome (infantile poikiloderma)
*201. Roy syndrome I (unilateral cataract associated with smoking)
202. Roy syndrome II—nuclear cataract associated with smoking
203. Rubeola (measles)
204. Rubinstein–Taybi syndrome (broad-thumbs syndrome)
205. Scaphocephaly syndrome (craniofacial dysostoses)
206. Schaefer syndrome (congenital dyskeratosis)
207. Schwartz syndrome
208. Scurvy (avitaminosis C)
209. Sickle cell disease (Herrick syndrome)
210. Siemen syndrome (congenital atrophy of the skin)
211. Sjögren syndrome (secretoinhibitor syndrome)
212. Sjögren–Larsson syndrome (oligophrenia ichthyosis)
213. Smith–Lemli–Opitz syndrome
214. Split-hand with congenital nystagmus, fundal changes, cataracts—autosomal dominant
215. Spondyloepiphyseal dysplasia (SED) dwarfism
216. Stannus cerebellar syndrome (vitamin B_2 deficiency)
217. Stickler syndrome (hereditary progressive arthro-ophthalmopathy)
*218. Still disease (juvenile rheumatoid arthritis)
219. Thrombocytopenia–absent radius (TAR) syndrome
220. Toxocariasis (nematode ophthalmia syndrome)
221. Treacher Collins syndrome (mandibulofacial dysostosis)
222. Trichomegaly, spherocytosis, and cataract—autosomal dominant
223. Trichorrhexis nodosa (argininosuccinicaciduria)
224. Trisomy 13 syndrome (Patau syndrome)
225. Trisomy 16 syndrome (Edward syndrome)
226. Trisomy 20p syndrome
227. Trisomy 21 (Down syndrome)
228. Tuomaala–Haapanen syndrome
229. Turner syndrome (gonadal dysgenesis)
230. Tyrosinosis (Hanhart syndrome)
231. Usher syndrome (hereditary retinitis pigmentosa—deafness syndrome)
232. Uvea-touch syndrome
233. Van der Hoeve syndrome (brittle-bone disease)
234. Van Bogaert–Scherer–Epstein syndrome (primary hyperlipidemia)
235. Varicella infection
236. von Recklinghausen syndrome (neurofibromatosis)

* = most important

237. Wagner syndrome (hyaloideoretinal degeneration)
238. Warburg syndrome (hydrocephalus, agyria, and absent cortical laminar retinal dysplasia with or without encephalocele)
239. Ward syndrome (nevus–jaw cyst syndrome)
240. Wegener syndrome (Wegener granulomatosis)
241. Weil disease (leptospirosis)
242. Werner syndrome (scleropoililoderma)
243. Wilson disease (hepatolenticular degeneration)
244. Yersiniosis
245. Zellweger syndrome (cerebrohepatorenal syndrome)
246. 31 syndrome
247. 4p syndrome
248. 18p syndrome
249. 18q syndrome

Christiansen JP, Bradford JD. Cataract in infants treatment with argon laser photocoagulation for threshold retinopathy of prematurity. *Am J Ophthalmol* 1995;119:175–180.

Francis PJ, et al. Visual outcome in patients with isolated autosomal dominant congenital cataract. *Ophthalmology* 2001;108:1104–1108.

Ng JS, et al. Ocular complications of pediatric bone marrow transplantation. *Ophthalmology* 1999;106:160–164.

Pau H. *Differential diagnosis of eye diseases,* 2nd ed. New York: Thieme Medical, 1988.

Roy FH. *Ocular syndromes and systemic diseases,* 3rd ed. Philadelphia: Lippincott Williams & Wilkins, 2002.

LENTICULOCORNEAL ADHERENCE (LENS ADJACENT TO ENDOTHELIUM OF CORNEA)

1. Acquired anterior corneal disease as ulcer with perforation or trauma
2. Aniridia
3. Peters anomaly (oculodental syndrome)
4. Rieger anomaly (dysgenesis mesostromalis)

Kivlin JD, et al. Peters' anomaly as a consequence of genetic and nongenetic syndromes. *Arch Ophthalmol* 1986; 104:61–64.

Waring G, et al. Ultrastructure and successful keratoplasty of sclerocornea in Mieten's syndrome. *Am J Ophthalmol* 1980;90:469–475.

SPASM OF ACCOMMODATION

This condition involves increased tone of ciliary body with increased convexity of crystalline lens (see p. 619–622).

1. Alcoholism
2. Cerebrovascular accident
3. Contusion injury to the globe or head
4. Cyclic oculomotor palsy or spasm
5. Diabetes mellitus
6. Drugs, such as aceclidine, acetylcholine, carbachol, demecarium, DFP, digitalis, echothiophate, guanethidine, isoflurophate, methylene blue, morphine, neostigmine, opium, physostigmine, pilocarpine
7. Fatigue cramp of overworked ciliary muscle; most frequent with compound hyperopia and mixed astigmatism associated with anisometropia
8. Graves disease (hyperthyroidism, Basedow syndrome)

9. Infectious, such as diphtheria, helminthic infestations, or sinus disease
10. Irritative lesions of brain stem and oculomotor trunk, such as epidemic encephalitis, tabes, meningitis, influenza, scleritis, measles, or orbital inflammation
11. Middle cerebral artery occlusion
12. Ocular inflammation, such as ciliary muscle irritant
13. Pineal tumor
14. Reflex irritation, such as in trigeminal neuralgia
15. Sympathetic paralysis
16. Trauma

Fraunfelder FT, Fraunfelder FW. *Drug-induced ocular side effects.* Woburn, MA: Butterworth-Heinemann, 2001.

Pau H. *Differential diagnosis of eye diseases,* 2nd ed. New York: Thieme Medical, 1988.

Ohtsuka K, et al. Accommodation and convergence insufficiency with left middle cerebral artery occlusion. *Am J Ophthalmol* 1988;106:60–64.

Walsh FB, Hoyt WF. *Clinical neuro-ophthalmology,* 4th ed. Baltimore: Williams & Wilkins, 1988.

PARESIS OF ACCOMMODATION

This condition involves partial or total loss of physiologic ability to change the shape of the lens and thus the focus of the eye (see Mydriasis, p. 622–623); this ability is related to age (see Acquired Hyperopia, p. 344–348).

*1. Presbyopia—gradual decrease in amplitude of accommodation related to age
2. Accommodative insufficiency
   A. Asthenic individuals
   B. Illness or debilitation, including intestinal toxemia, tuberculosis, influenza, whooping cough, measles, and tonsillar and dental infections
   C. Anemia
   D. Overwork
   E. Whiplash injury
3. Ciliary body aplasia—with or without pupillary and iris abnormalities
4. Iridocyclitis—acute and chronic
5. Glaucoma with atrophy of ciliary body
6. Choroidal metastasis with suprachoroidal extension
7. Trauma, such as tears in iris sphincter, tears at root of iris, or recession of the anterior chamber angle with posterior displacement of the ciliary attachment and ocular hypotension
8. Rupture of zonular fibers and partial subluxation of lens
9. Myotonic dystrophy (Curschmann–Steinert syndrome)
10. Drugs, including the following:

acetazolamide	amphetamine	betamethasone
acetophenazine	anisindione	bethanechol
adiphenine	anisotropine	biperiden
alcohol	antazoline	bromide
alprazolam	atropine	butaperazine
ambutonium	belladonna	captopril (?)
aminosalicylate (?)	bendroflumethiazide	caramiphen
aminosalicylic acid (?)	benzathine penicillin G	carbachol
amitriptyline	benzphetamine	carbamazepine
amodiaquine	benzthiazide	carbinoxamine
amoxapine	benztropine	carbon dioxide

* = most important

carphenazine
chloramphenicol
chlordiazepoxide
chlorisondamine
chlorothiazide
chlorphenoxamine
chlorpromazine
chlorthalidone
cimetidine
clemastine
clidinium
clomipramine
clonazepam
clorazepate
cocaine
cortisone
cyclopentolate
cyclothiazide
cycrimine
desipramine
dexamethasone
dextroamphetamine
diacetylmorphine
diazepam
dibucaine
dichlorphenamide
dicyclomine
diethazine
diphemanil
diphenadione
diphenhydramine
diphenylpyraline
emetine
ergot
ethopropazine
fluorometholone
fluphenazine
glycopyrrolate
hexamethonium
hexocyclium
homatropine
hydrochlorothiazide
hydrocortisone
hydroflumethiazide
hydromorphone
hydroxyamphetamine
imipramine

indapamide
iodide and iodine solutions
   and compounds
isoniazid
isopropamide
maprotiline
marijuana
mecamylamine
medrysone
mepenzolate
meprobamate
mescaline
mesoridazine
methacholine
methamphetamine
methantheline
methaqualone
methazolamide
methdilazine
methixene
methotrimeprazine
methscopolamine
methyclothiazide
methylatropine nitrate
methylene blue
methyprylon
methysergide metolazone
mianserin
midazolam
morphine
nalidixic acid
naproxen
nitrazepam
nortriptyline
opium
orphenadrine
oxazepam
oxymorphone
oxyphencyclimine
oxyphenonium
pargyline
pentazocine
pentolinium
perazine
periciazine
perphenazine
phendimetrazine

phenindione
phenmetrazine
phentermine
pilocarpine
pimozide
pipenzolate
piperacetazine
piperazine
piperidolate
piperocaine
piroxicam (?)
poldine
polythiazide
potassium penicillin G
potassium penicillin V
potassium phenethicillin
pralidoxime
prazepam
prednisolone
primidone
procaine penicillin G
procarbazine
prochlorperazine
procyclidine
promazine
promethazine
propantheline
propiomazine
propranolol
protriptyline
psilocybin
pyrilamine
quinethazone
radioactive iodides
rubella virus vaccine (live)
scopolamine
streptomycin
temazepam
tetanus immune globulin
tetanus toxoid
tetracaine
tetraethylammonium
tetrahydrocannabinol
thiethylperazine
thiopropazate
thioproperazine
thioridazine

thiothixene

triazolam

trichlormethiazide

trichloroethylene

tridihexethyl

trifluoperazine

trifluperidol

triflupromazine

trihexyphenidyl

trimeprazine

trimethaphan

trimethidinium

trimipramine

tripelennamine

tropicamide

vinblastine

vincristine

11. Neurogenic causes
  A. Infectious conditions
      (1) Epidemic encephalitis
      (2) Anterior poliomyelitis
      (3) Exanthemas and acute infections, such as scarlet fever, mumps, measles, influenza, typhoid fever, dengue fever, viral hepatitis, amebic dysentery, and malaria
      (4) Herpes zoster
      (5) Syphilis (lues)
      (6) Tuberculosis
      (7) Leprosy (Hansen disease)
      (8) Focal infections, such as from teeth or nasal sinuses
  B. Toxic conditions
      (1) Alcohol
      (2) Lead
      (3) Arsenic
      (4) Carbon monoxide
      (5) Diphtheritic paralysis
      (6) Botulism
      (7) Extensive burn
      (8) Snake venom
  C. Degenerative conditions
      (1) Congenital hereditary ophthalmoplegia
      (2) Progressive congenital ophthalmoplegia
      (3) Hereditary ataxia
      (4) Myotonic dystrophy (Curschmann–Steinert syndrome)
      (5) Myasthenia gravis
  D. Metabolic conditions
      (1) Acute hemorrhagic anterior polioencephalitis of Wernicke
      (2) Diabetes mellitus
      (3) Lactation
      (4) Following pregnancy
  E. Isolated internal ophthalmoplegia
  F. Isolated failure of near reflex, such as with inverse Argyll–Robertson pupil
  G. Lesions of parasympathetic nuclei in midbrain
      (1) Encephalitis
      (2) Pineal tumor
      (3) Other signs of mesencephalic disease, including multiple sclerosis, infectious polyneuropathy, and vascular lesions
      (4) Syphilis—bilateral

H. Trauma to head or neck
  (1) Cerebral concussion
  (2) Craniocervical extension injuries

Pau FH. *Differential diagnosis of eye diseases,* 2nd ed. New York: Thieme Medical, 1988.

Roy FH. *Ocular syndromes and systemic diseases,* 3rd ed. Philadelphia: Lippincott Williams & Wilkins, 2002.

Walsh FB, Hoyt WF. *Clinical neuro-ophthalmology,* 4th ed. Baltimore: Williams & Wilkins, 1985.

14

Vitreous

CONTENTS

PSEUDODETACHMENT OF VITREOUS (CONDITIONS SIMULATING DETACHMENT OF VITREOUS)

1. Enormous cavity in the vitreous body with a relatively thin posterior wall
2. Membranous formations within the vitreous associated with uveitis and hemorrhage
3. Outline of the ascending portion of Cloquet canal just anterior to the disc

Tolentino FI, et al. *Vitreoretinal disorders: diagnoses and management.* Philadelphia: WB Saunders, 1976.

ANTERIOR VITREOUS DETACHMENT

In this condition, the anterior vitreous cortex may be separated from the posterior lens or posterior zonular fibers.

1. Retrolenticular—usually caused by vitreous shrinkage
   *A. Trauma (most common)
   B. Hemorrhage—usually secondary to trauma
   C. Senescence (rare)
   D. Inflammation
   E. Retinal detachment (see p. 487)
   *F. Iatrogenic after injection of vitreous substitutes (gas)
2. Retroocular
   A. Vitreous shrinkage (see p. 432)
   B. Ciliary body tumor
   C. Blood
   D. Exudate

       * = most important

3. Retrolenticular and retroocular combined occurs with rupture of the hyaloideocapsular ligament

Tolentino FI, et al. *Vitreoretinal disorders: diagnosis and management.* Philadelphia: WB Saunders, 1976.

POSTERIOR VITREOUS DETACHMENT

1. Complete posterior detachment
    A. Simple detachment—occurs in young persons
        (1) Exudate from chorioretinal focus
        (2) Hemorrhage between the vitreous and the retina
        (3) Retraction of the cortical vitreous caused by exudate within the vitreous
        (4) Vitreous hemorrhage in a young individual with vitreous shrinking due to thrombosis of central retinal vein, retinal neovascularization
    B. Complete posterior detachment with collapse
        (1) Senescent changes are primary cause
        (2) Uveitis
        (3) Trauma
        (4) Hemorrhage
        (5) Sodium hyaluronate
    C. Funnel-shaped posterior detachment
        (1) Perforating injuries of globe
        (2) Retinal neovascularization
        (3) Massive vitreous detachment
    D. Atypical complete posterior detachment—residual adherence of vitreous to a peripheral retinal area
        (1) Focus of chorioretinitis
        (2) Following cataract extraction with loss of vitreous
        (3) Following perforating wounds
        (4) Posterior uveitis with inflammatory cells
2. Partial posterior detachment (unusual)
    A. Superior detachment—primarily a senescent change; generally forerunner of posterior vitreous detachment with collapse
    B. Partial posterior detachment (not infrequent)
        (1) Preretinal hemorrhage
        (2) Retinal neovascularization
    C. Partial lateral or partial inferior detachment
        (1) Focus of choroiditis
        (2) Circumscribed retinal periphlebitis
        (3) Intraocular foreign body

Foos RY, et al. Posterior vitreous detachment in diabetic subjects. *Ophthalmology* 1980;87:122.

Jaffe NS. *The vitreous in clinical ophthalmology.* St. Louis: CV Mosby, 1969.

Nirankari VS, et al. Pseudo-vitreous hemorrhage: a new intraoperative complication of sodium hyaluronate. *Ophthalmic Surg Lasers* 1981;12:503.

Posterior vitreous detachment

	Complete, Simple Posterior Vitreous Detachment	Compete Posterior Vitreous Detachment with Collapse
Age	Young	Old or myopes of any age
Etiology	Inflammation, hemorrhage, trauma	Senescence
Refractive error	Unimportant	Myopia in younger patients
Prior vitreous degeneration	None	Fibrillary degeneration and cavities
Vitreous cells	Cells and vitreous precipitates	None
Rocking movements of vitreous	Rare	Frequent
Retinal breaks	Rare (except trauma)	10–15%
Hemorrhages	Rare in inflammatory disorders	10–15%
Vitreoretinal traction	Rare	10–15%
Prepapillary opacity	Yes	Yes
Onset	Slowly progressive	
Shape of posterior vitreous border	Spherical	Collapsed

Jaffe NS. *The vitreous in clinical ophthalmology.* St. Louis: CV Mosby, 1969.

VITREOUS HEMORRHAGE

1. Acquired lues (syphilis)
2. Arsenic toxicity
3. Ascariasis
4. Avulsed retinal vessel syndrome
5. Battered baby syndrome (Silverman syndrome)
6. Behçet syndrome (dermatostomatoophthalmic syndrome)
7. Blood disease—retinal hemorrhage breaking into vitreous
   A. Anemias
      (1) Aplastic anemia
      (2) Hemolytic anemia
      (3) Hypochromic anemia
      (4) Pernicious anemia
   B. Dysproteinemias—macroglobulins and cryoglobulins
   C. Hemophilia associated with trauma
   D. Leukemias
   E. Multiple myeloma (Kahler disease)
   F. Polycythemia vera (Vaquez disease)
   G. Thrombocytopenic purpura
8. Coats disease (retinal telangiectasia)
9. Collagen disease
   A. Dermatomyositis
   B. Disseminated lupus erythematosus (Kaposi–Libman–Sacks syndrome)
   C. Polyarteritis nodosa (Kussmaul disease)
   D. Scleroderma (progressive systemic sclerosis)
10. Complete posterior vitreous detachment with collapse (10%–15% at time of event)
11. Cysticercosis
12. Dengue fever
13. Diabetes mellitus-proliferative retinopathy
14. Dislocation of intraocular lenses
15. Disseminated intravascular coagulation
16. Drusen of optic disc
17. Eales disease
18. Exudative age-related macular degeneration
19. Familial exudative vitreoretinopathy
20. Ganciclovir Implant
21. Gronblad–Strandberg syndrome (systemic elastodystrophy)
22. Hemorrhages in the newborn
   A. Hemorrhagic disease of the newborn factor VII and prothrombin deficiency
   B. Persistent vessels of the hyaloid system
   C. Retinal hemorrhage of newborn breaking through to vitreous cavity
23. Iatrogenic globe perforation associated with strabismus surgery
24. Indomethacin reaction
25. Influenza
26. Intraocular foreign body
27. Intraocular tumor
28. Hypertension (venous occlusive disease)
29. Juvenile retinoschisis

*30. Macroaneurysm (retinal arterial)
31. Malaria
32. Malignant melanoma
33. Migration from anterior bleeding as from angle-supported, iris-supported, or posterior chamber lenses
*34. Neovascularization following vascular occlusion (primarily venous occlusive disease)
35. Neovascularization of cataract wound
36. Ocular ischemic syndrome with neovascularization of disc
37. Pars planitis
38. Persistent hyaloid artery
39. Persistent hyperplastic primary vitreous (PHPV)
*40. Posterior vitreous detachment (PVD)
41. Purtscher disease (traumatic retinal angiopathy)
42. Retinal angiomatosis (von Hippel disease)
*43. Retinal break or tear with or without retinal detachment and avulsed retinal vessels
*44. Retinal hemorrhage, including vein occlusion and sickle retinopathy, arterial macroaneurysm
45. Retinal tacks (intrusion)
46. Retinoblastoma
47. Retinopathy of prematurity-proliferative stage
48. Scleral buckle (intrusion)
49. Sleep apnea
50. Sickle cell disease (Herrick syndrome)—SA, SS, or SC
51. Surgical cataract complication with lenticular fragments dislocated into vitreous
52. Terson syndrome of associated vitreous and subarachnoid hemorrhage syndrome
53. Thalassemia (Cooley anemia)
54. Thromboangiitis obliterans (Buerger disease)
55. Tissue plasminogen activator (t-PA)
56. Tuberous sclerosis
57. von Hippel–Lindau disease (angiomatosis retinae)
58. von Willebrand syndrome
59. Trauma
60. Traumatic asphyxia
61. Tuberculosis
62. Uveitis (associated with)
63. Varicella zoster

Kokame GT. Vitreous hemorrhage after intravitreal tissue plasminogen activator (t-PA) and pneumatic displacement of submacular hemorrhage. *Am J Ophthalmol* 2000;129:546–547.

Kuhn F, et al. Terson syndrome. *Ophthalmology* 1998;105:472–477.

Potter MJ, et al. Vitrectomy for pars planitis complicated by vitreous hemorrhage: visual outcome and long-term follow-up. *Am J Ophthalmol* 2001;131:514–515.

Roy FH. *Ocular syndromes and systemic diseases,* 3rd ed. Philadelphia: Lippincott Williams & Wilkins, 2002.

Spraul CW, Grossniklaus HE. Vitreous hemorrhage. *Surv Opthalmol* 1997;42:1,3–6.

Vitreous hemorrhage

	Retinal Break	Diabetes Mellitus	Blunt Ocular Trauma	Sickle Cell Disease	Blood Disease ie Anemia	Collagen Disease ie Lupus Erythematosus	Eales Disease	Coat's Disease	Von-Hippel-Lindau Disease	Malignant Melanoma	Retinopathy of Prematurity	Retinal Vein Occlusion
History												
1. Aphakic, myopic and traumatized eyes	U											
2. Bilateral		U		U	U	S	U		U		U	
3. Congenital				U					U	R		
4. Familial	S	U		U					U	R		
5. Greater in blacks				U								
6. Greater in females						U						
7. Greater in males			U				U	U				
8. Greater in whites										U		
9. Greater over 40 years of age												U
10. History of arteriosclerosis, hypertensive disease or hyperviscosity syndromes												U
11. Occurs birth to 2 years											U	
12. Occurs 1st decade								U				
13. Occurs 2nd to 3rd decade			S			S	S		U			
14. Occurs 3rd to 4th decade				S		S	S					R
15. Oxygen therapy											U	
16. Prematurity											U	
17. Wide age range	U		U									
Physical Findings												
1. Afferent pupillary reaction abnormal	S											
2. Angioid streaks				S								
3. Angiomatosis of iris									S			
4. Anterior ischemic optic neuropathy		S										S
5. Anterior uveitis						R						
6. Arteriovenous retinal shunts		S		U								S
7. Bright choroidal plaques				U								
8. Cataract		S								R		
9. Conjunctival comma signs				U								
10. Conjunctival icterus or pallor				S								
11. Conjunctival phlyctenules						S						
12. Corneal abrasions			U									
13. Corneal epithelial keratitis						S						
14. Corneal neovascularization						S						
15. Cotton wool spots		U		U		S						U
16. Choroidal nevus										S		
17. Choroidal rupture			S							S		
18. Degenerative changes in R.P.E.	R									S		
19. Disc neovascularization		S		S								S
20. Ectropion uvea		S										S
21. Endothelial corneal damage			S									
22. Episcleritis						S						

Vitreous hemorrhage (Continued)

	Retinal Break	Diabetes Mellitus	Blunt Ocular Trauma	Sickle Cell Disease	Blood Disease ie Anemia	Collagen Disease ie Lupus Erythematosus	Eales Disease	Coat's Disease	Von-Hippel-Lindau Disease	Malignant Melanoma	Retinopathy of Prematurity	Retinal Vein Occlusion
Physical Findings												
23. Extraocular muscle paralysis		R				R				R		
24. Glaucoma		R	S						R	S	R	S
25. Hard Exudates		U					U	U	S			S
26. Hyphema			S									
27. Increased pigmentation of lids										R		
28. Iridodialysis			S									
29. Keratoconjunctivitis sicca						S						
30. Low intraocular pressure	S		S									
31. Macular edema	R	S					S			R		S
32. Macular hemorrhage		S	S	S	S							S
33. Macular holes	R		R	S								
34. Microphthalmia											R	
35. Optic atrophy		S	S	S		S				R		
36. Orbital myositis										S		
37. Panophthalmitis										R		
38. Papilledema		S			R	S						S
39. Peerivascular sheathing							U	S				S
40. Phthisis bulbi											S	
41. Pigmented or amelanotic choroidal mass										U		
42. Ptosis						R						
43. Retinal detachment	S			S			U	U	U	S	R	R
44. Retinal hemorrhages	S	U		S	S	S	U	U	S			U
45. Retinal microaneurysms		U		S	S							R
46. Retinal neovascularization		U		S	R							S
47. Retinal arterial venous anastomosis	S		U			S	R				S	S
48. Retinal vein occlusion	S			S	R		S					U
49. Retrolental mass											S	
50. Rubeosis iridis		S		S						R		S
51. Salmon patches in retina				S								
52. Scleritis						S						
53. Soft retinal exudates (cottonwool spots)		U					U	S	S			U
54. Telangiectatic retinal vessels		U						U	U			U
55. Uveitis						S						
56. Venous dilation		U	U			S	U		U		S	U
57. Visual field defects						R				R		
58. White wedge shaped infarcts in choroid				S								S
Lab Data												
1. Autoantibodies to nuclear and cytoplasmic constituents						U						
2. Biopsy										S		
3. Blood sugar elevated		U										
4. Cerebral angiography									U			

Vitreous hemorrhage (Continued)

	Retinal Break	Diabetes Mellitus	Blunt Ocular Trauma	Sickle Cell Disease	Blood Disease ie Anemia	Collagen Disease ie Lupus Erythematosus	Eales Disease	Coat's Disease	Von-Hippel-Lindau Disease	Malignant Melanoma	Retinopathy of Prematurity	Retinal Vein Occlusion
Lab Data												
5. Chest X ray abnormal							S			S		
6. CT scan:												
—Orbital mass detectable										U		
—Traumatic ocular lesion detectable			U									
7. Diminished complement levels						S						
8. Electroretinogram abnormal		S	S			R						S
9. Fluorescein angiography		U	U	U	S	U	U	U	U	U	R	U
10. Hemoglobin eletrophoresis presence of Hb-S					U							
11. L.E. cell phenomenon						S						
12. Lipid profile elevated		S										S
13. Ocular ultrasonography			U					S	U	U	U	S
14. Orbital X ray			R									
—Diffusely enlarged orbit										S		
—Erosion of optic canal										R		
15. Platelet count and Hb low					U							
16. P-32 uptake (rarely performed)										R		
17. Visual field test abnormal (rarely performed)										S		

R = rarely; S = sometimes; and U = usually.

Asteroid hyalosis versus synchysis scintillans

	Asteroid Hyalosis	*Synchysis Scintillans*
Age of patient	Elderly	Usually young
Bilaterality	Usually unilateral (75%)	Usually bilateral
Incidence	Rare	Extremely rare
Appearance	Spherical white bodies	Flat, angular crystals
Motility	Moves with vitreous structures and returns to original positions	Moves freely and falls to floor of vitreous
Chemistry	Calcium soaps	Cholesterol crystal
Associated ocular disease	None; diabetes mellitus?	Secondary to other ocular disease or trauma

Jaffe NS. *The vitreous in clinical ophthalmology.* St. Louis: CV Mosby, 1969.

VITREOUS OPACITIES

1. Opaque sheets anterior to the vitreous
    A. Elschnig pearls after extracapsular cataract extraction or needling (posterior capsule opacification)
    B. Normal posterior capsule—often following extracapsular cataract extraction or needling
    C. Soemmerring ring following extracapsular cataract extraction or needling
    D. Vitreous adhesions to iris, capsule, or intraocular lens (IOL) after cataract extraction with vitreous loss
2. Pseudoglioma–leukokoria (see p. 357)
3. Scattered opacities
    A. Amyloid disease—rare (seen in older persons)
    B. Ankylosing spondylitis
    C. Coagula of the colloid basis of the gel
    D. Crystalline deposits
        (1) Asteroid hyalosis
        (2) Synchysis scintillans
    E. Endophthalmitis
    F. Heterochromic uveitis—in persons 20 to 50 years of age; of all uveitis, iris atrophy, lens changes
    G. Myeloma, multiple—rare: in persons 50 to 70 years old, associated with bone pain, anemia
    H. Myopia, severe
    I. Pigment cells—posttraumatic (hemorrhage), senile, or melanotic, associated with rhegmatogenous retinal detachment.
    J. Protein coagulaplasmoid vitreous
        (1) Choroidal tumors (very rare—reported in metastatic breast cancer once)
        (2) Contusions
        (3) Intermediate uveitis (pars planitis)
        (4) Retinochoroiditis
    K. Red blood cells (see vitreous hemorrhage, p. 424)
    L. Snowball opacities—rare, associated with pars planitis or sarcoidosis, endophthalmitis (indolent)
    M. Tissue cells—epithelial, histiocytic, glial
    N. Toxoplasmosis—active
    O. Tumor cells—retinoblastoma in older child, reticulum cell sarcoma (older persons)
    P. Vitreous degeneration—Wagner disease, Ehlers–Danlos syndrome, and Marfan syndrome, senescent aging changes, myopia
    Q. Whipple disease
    R. White blood cells—inflammatory disease, vitreitis
    S. Retinitis pigmentosa
4. Single opacities
    A. Anterior hyaloid remnant (Mittendorf dot)—25% normal eyes, dot on posterior lens surface
    B. Hyaloid remnants (uncommon)—persistent hyperplastic primary vitreous
    C. Foreign body—history of trauma or surgery
    D. Dislocated lens (see p. 401)

E. Parasitic cysts
   (1) Hydatid disease (echinococcosis)—rare, children and young adults, tropical
   (2) Cysticercosis—rare
F. Vitreous detachment—common in older or myopic persons

Durant WJ, et al. Vitrectomy and Whipple's disease. *Arch Ophthalmol* 1984;102:851.

Hong PH, et al. Vitrectomy for large vitreous opacity in retinitis pigmentosa. *Am J Ophthalmol* 2001;131:133–134.

Recchia AE, et al. Endophthalmitis after pediatric strabismus surgery. *Arch Ophthalmol* 2000;118:939–944.

Sandgren O, et al. Vitreous amyloidosis associated with homozygosity for the transthyretin methionine gene. *Arch Ophthalmol* 1990;108:1586.

PERSISTENT HYPERPLASTIC PRIMARY VITREOUS

1. Cerebrooculodysplasia–muscular dystrophy
2. Fetal alcohol syndrome
3. Incontinentia pigmenti
4. Norrie disease
5. Septooptic pituitary
6. Sporadic unilateral and isolated finding
7. Trisomy 13
8. Warburg syndrome

Katsuya-Lauer A, et al. Persistent hyperplastic primary vitreous associated with septo-optic-pituitary dysplasia and schizencephaly. *Arch Ophthalmol* 2000;118:578–580.

BEADS IN VITREOUS (SNOWBALLS IN VITREOUS)

1. African eye-worm disease (loiasis)
2. Amyloidosis (Lubarsch–Pick syndrome)
3. Behçet syndrome (dermatostomatoophthalmic syndrome)
4. Birdshot retinochoroidopathy
5. Brucellosis (Bang disease)
6. Familial exudative vitreoretinopathy (Criswick–Schepens syndrome)
7. *Haemophilus influenzae*
8. Irvine syndrome
9. Jacobsen–Brodwall syndrome
10. Ocular toxocariasis
11. Ocular toxoplasmosis
12. Oculootoororenoerythropoietic disease
13. Pars planitis
14. Retinoblastoma
15. Sarcoidosis
16. Severe uveitis
17. Sympathetic ophthalmia
18. Toxic lens syndrome
19. Typhus (Japanese river fever)
20. Vogt–Koyanagi–Harada syndrome (uveitis–vitiligo–alopecia–poliosis syndrome)

Noda S, et al. Patients with asteroid hyalosis and visible floaters. *Jpn J Ophthalmol* 1995;37:452–455.

Schlaegel TF. The uvea. *Arch Ophthalmol* 1971;85:635.

COMPLICATIONS FOLLOWING OPERATIVE VITREOUS LOSS

1. Inflammatory complications
   A. Irritable eye (chronically)
   B. Recurrent or persistent uveitis
   C. Vitreitis with vitreous opacities
2. Wound complications
   A. Epithelial invasion or downgrowth
   B. Fibrous ingrowth
   C. Fistula or gaping of wound (with or without vitreous wick syndrome)
   *D. Infection or endophthalmitis
   E. Excessive astigmatism
3. Corneal complications
   A. Corneal edema (vitreocorneal touch)
   B. Bullous keratopathy
   C. Corneal opacification
4. Secondary glaucoma
   A. Vitreous obstruction of anterior chamber angle
   B. Pupillary block (iridohyaloid adhesions, anterior hyaloid displacement, uveitis)
   C. Iris and vitreous adherence to wound (peripheral anterior synechiae)
5. Fibroblastic and traction phenomena
   A. Pupillary membrane
   B. Pupillary distortion—"peaked" or updrawn synechiae
   C. Cystoid macular edema (CME)
   D. Retinal detachment
   E. Optic neuritis or papilledema
   F. Vitreous hemorrhage
   G. Posterior vitreous detachment

Krupin T, Kolker AG. *Atlas of complications in ophthalmic surgery.* St. Louis: CV Mosby, 1993.

Peyman GA, Shulman JA. *Intravitreal surgery: principles and practice.* New York: Appleton-Lange, 1994.

POSTOPERATIVE VITREOUS RETRACTION

Usually, this condition is manifested by circular equatorial retinal fold or star-shaped retinal fold.

1. Accidental perforation of the sclera at operation, which may be associated with hemorrhage and loss of vitreous resulting in a pathologic formation of new epiretinal membrane or proliferative vitreoretinopathy
2. Giant retinal breaks allowing a large area of direct contact between the choroid and the vitreous
3. Perforating diathermy and excessively strong or repeated applications of superficial diathermy, which may cause vitreous hemorrhage or thermal injury to the vitreous; impairment of chorioretinal blood circulation may result in exudation and hemorrhage into the vitreous
4. Venous stasis caused by the compression of vortex veins by the indentation resulting from a buckling procedure

Jaffe NS. *The vitreous in clinical ophthalmology.* St. Louis: CV Mosby, 1969.

* = most important

VITREOUS CYST (CYSTIC STRUCTURE IN VITREOUS BODY)

1. Congenital (developmental)—may be associated with hyaloid remnants
2. Acquired
   A. Infectious cyst
      (1) Coenurosis (*Coenurus cerebralis* larva of dog tapeworm)
      (2) Luetic retinochoroiditis
      (3) Toxoplasmosis
   B. Myopia
   C. Parasitic cysts
      (1) Cysticercosis—rare
      (2) Echinococcosis
      (3) Hydatid disease (echinococcosis)—rare, children and young adults, tropical
      (4) Nematode cyst (toxocariasis)
   D. Pigmentary retinopathy
   E. Retinal detachment
   F. Trauma

Cardillo JA, et al. Post-traumatic proliferative vitreoretinopathy. *Ophthalmology* 1997;104:1166–1173.

Flynn WJ, Carlson DW. Pigmented vitreous cyst. *Arch Ophthal* 1994;112:1113.

Nussenblat RB, Palestine AG. *Uveitis fundamentals and clinical practice.* Chicago: Yearbook Medical, 1989.

VITREOUS LIQUEFACTION

1. Myopia
2. Peripheral uveitis
3. Retinitis pigmentosa
4. Spontaneous
5. Trauma
6. With aging
7. With vitreous traction such as Wagner disease

Nussenblatt RB, Palestin AG. *Uveitis: fundamental and clinical practice.* Chicago: Yearbook Medical, 1989.

Takhashi M, et al. Biomicroscopic evaluation and photography of liquefied vitreous in some vitreoretinal disorders. *Arch Ophthalmol* 1981;99:1555.

15

Retina

CONTENTS

ANATOMIC CLASSIFICATION OF MACULAR DISEASES

1. Vitreoretinal surface
   A. Preretinal hemorrhage and subinternal limiting membrane hemorrhage
   B. Vitreous traction on the macula
   C. Epiretinal membrane and macular pucker
2. Nerve fiber—ganglion cell layers
   A. Hereditary cerebromacular degeneration
      (1) Sphingolipidoses
         a. Tay–Sachs disease (GM_2—gangliosidosis type I)
         b. Sandhoff disease (GM $MDSD_2$—gangliosidosis type II)
         c. Niemann–Pick disease type A (essential lipoid histiocytosis)
         d. Niemann–Pick disease type B (sea-blue histiocyte syndrome)
         e. Lactoside ceramidosis
         f. Metachromatic leukodystrophy (arylsulfatase A deficiency)
         g. Gaucher disease (glucocerebroside storage disease)
         h. Farber lipogranulomatosis
         i. Generalized gangliosidosis (GM_1—gangliosidosis type I)
         j. Mucolipidosis I (lipomucopolysaccharidosis)
      (2) Goldberg disease (unclassified syndrome with features of mucopolysaccharidoses, sphingolipidoses, and mucolipidoses)
      (3) Ceroid lipofuscinosis
         a. Hagberg–Santevuori (infantile)
         b. Jansky–Bielschowsky disease (late infantile)
         c. Spielmeyer–Vogt Batten
   B. Vitreoretinal dystrophies
      (1) Macular degeneration in congenital hereditary x-linked retinoschisis
      (2) Goldmann–Favre syndrome (vitreotapetoretinal degeneration)—recessive
3. Nerve fiber, ganglion cell, inner plexiform, inner nuclear, outer plexiform layers
   A. Ischemia secondary to inadequate perfusion of retinal vessels
      (1) Branch artery occlusion
      (2) Branch vein occlusion
      (3) Diabetes mellitus
4. Outer plexiform layer
   A. Cystoid macular degeneration (see p. 439)
      (1) With retinal vascular leakage
         a. Acute nongranulomatous iridocyclitis
         b. Acute cyclitis
         c. Hypertension
         d. Medication (epinephrine, nicotinic acid)
         e. Neoproliferative diabetic retinopathy

       f. Pars planitis

       g. Postoperative (Irvine–Gass syndrome)

       h. Radiation retinopathy

       i. Retinitis pigmentosa

       j. Sarcoidosis

       k. Vascular anomalies

  (2) Without obvious retinal vascular leakage

       a. Vitreous traction on the macula

       b. Serous detachment of sensory epithelium

       c. Serous detachment of pigment epithelium

       d. Hemorrhagic detachment of macula

       e. Choroidal tumors

B. Lipid deposits in macula secondary to vascular disease in retina

  (1) Stellate retinopathy (see p. 443)

       a. Hypertensive retinopathy

       b. Diabetic retinopathy

       c. Coats disease (retinal telangiectasia)

       d. Trauma—ocular or cerebral

       e. Retinal artery or vein occlusion (see p. 457 and 468)

       f. Retinal periphlebitis

       g. Juxtapapillary choroiditis

       h. Papilledema (see p. 593–601)

       i. Angiomatosis retinae

       j. Papillitis (see p. 578–585, 587–588)

       k. Acute, febrile illness, such as measles, influenza, meningitis, erysipelas, psittacosis, Behçet disease

       l. Chronic infections, such as tuberculosis or syphilis

       m. Coccidioidomycosis

       n. Parasitic infection, such as that due to teniae, *Giardia, Ancylostoma*

       o. Idiopathic

  (2) Circinate retinopathy

       a. Senile vascular disease

       b. Venous obstruction

       c. Diabetic retinopathy

       d. Coats disease (retinal telangiectasia)

       e. Retinal detachment

       f. Anemia

       g. Leukemia

       h. Idiopathic (primary)

       i. Retinal arterial macroaneurysm

  (3) Diabetic retinopathy

5. Outer nuclear layer or photoreceptor elements

  A. Congenital hereditary vision defects

    (1) Trichromatism (anomalous)

    (2) Dichromatism

    (3) Monochromatism

  B. Hereditary macular dystrophies

    (1) Progressive cone dystrophy

    (2) Inverse (macular) retinitis pigmentosa

C. Olivopontocerebellar degeneration

D. Light toxicity

    (1) Operating microscope burn

    (2) Solar burn

6. Pigment epithelium

  A. Hereditary macular dystrophies

    (1) Vitelliform dystrophy (Best disease)

    (2) Adult onset foveomacular vitelliform dystrophy (adult Best)

    (3) Fundus flavimaculatus

    (4) Fundus flavimaculatus with macular involvement (Stargardt disease)

    (5) Dominant drusen (Doyne honeycomb dystrophy)

    (6) Reticular pigment dystrophy (Sjögren)

    (7) Butterfly-shaped pigment dystrophy (Deutman)

    (8) Central areolar choroidal and pigment epithelial dystrophy

    (9) Sorsby fundus dystrophy

  B. Inflammatory lesions

    (1) Rubella syndrome (German measles)

    (2) Acute posterior multifocal placoid pigment epitheliopathy

  C. Toxic lesions

    (1) Chloroquine

    (2) Hydroxychloroquine

    (3) Phenothiazine

       a. Chlorpromazine

       b. Thioridazine

    (4) Sparsomycin

    (5) Ethambutol

    (6) Indomethacin

    (7) Quinine

    (8) Desferrioxamine

    (9) Penicillamine

  D. Drusen (senile, degenerative)

  E. Refsum syndrome (phytanic acid storage disease)

  F. Myotonic dystrophy syndrome

7. Bruch membrane

  A. Angioid streaks associated with

    (1) Pseudoxanthoma elasticum (Grönblad–Strandberg syndrome)

    (2) Senile elastosis of skin

    (3) Osteitis deformans (Paget disease)

    (4) Fibrodysplasia hyperelastica (Ehler–Danlos syndrome)

    (5) Sickle cell anemia

    (6) Acromegaly

    (7) Beta-thalassemia

    (8) Abetalipoproteinemia (Bassen–Kornzweig syndrome)

  B. Lacquer cracks in pathologic myopia

  C. Traumatic fracture of Bruch membrane

8. Pigment epithelium–Bruch membrane choriocapillaris

  A. Degenerative lesions

    (1) Disciform macular degeneration (senile, juvenile)

       (2) Age-related macular degeneration

       (3) Adult hereditary cerebromacular degeneration (Kufs?)

B. Serous detachment of neuroepithelium or pigment epithelium associated with the following:

       (1) Central serous chorioretinopathy

       (2) Hemangioma of choroid

       (3) Malignant melanoma

       (4) Pit of the optic disk

       (5) Hypotony (see p. 325–326)

       (6) Leukemic infiltrates of choroid

       (7) Terminal illness

       (8) Trauma

       (9) Uveitis

    (10) Optic neuritis (see p. 578–585, 587–588)

    (11) Papilledema (see p. 593–601)

    (12) Acute hypertension

    (13) Vitreous traction

    (14) Angioid streaks (see p. 526–529)

    (15) Vogt–Koyanagi–Harada syndrome

    (16) *Toxocara canis*

    (17) Myopic choroidal degeneration

    (18) Metastatic carcinoma

    (19) Choroidal nevus

    (20) Collagen vascular disease

    (21) Hemorrhagic or organized disciform detachment

9. Choroid

A. Degenerative lesions

       (1) Central areolar choroidal atrophy

       (2) Myopic choroidal atrophy

       (3) Helicoid peripapillary chorioretinal atrophy (?)

B. Inflammatory lesions

       (1) Histoplasmosis

C. Vascular occlusive lesions

10. Miscellaneous

A. Retinal inflammations (multilayer alterations that may involve the macula)

       (1) *Toxoplasma gondii*

       (2) *T. canis*

       (3) Septic emboli

       (4) Cytomegalovirus retinitis

       (5) *Candida* organisms

       (6) Bacteria

B. Congenital anomalies of the macula

       (1) Aplasia

       (2) Hypoplasia

       (3) Heterotopia

       (4) Colobomas (see p. 450)

       (5) Aberrant macular vessels

Maumenee AE, Emery JM. An anatomic classification of diseases of the macula. *Am J Ophthalmol* 1972;74:594–599.

Yannuzzi LA, et al. *The macula: a comprehensive text and atlas.* Baltimore: Williams & Wilkins, 1979.

BILATERAL MACULAR LESIONS

1. Development defects (colobomas)
2. Drugs, including the following:

allopurinol (?)
amodiaquine
broxyquinoline
chloroquine
chlorpromazine

clonidine (?)
griseofulvin (?)
hydroxychloroquine
ibuprofen (?)
indomethacin (?)

iodochlorhydroxyquin
iodoquinol
quinine
thioridazine

3. Infectious entities
    A. Herpes simplex
    *B. Cytomegalic retinitis
    C. Candidiasis and nocardiosis
    D. *T. canis* (visceral larva migrans syndrome)
    E. Congenital syphilis
    *F. Tuberculosis
    *G. Ocular histoplasmosis
    H. Congenital toxoplasmosis
4. Intrauterine inflammations
5. Noninfectious entities
    A. Best disease
    B. Stargardt disease
    *C. Exudative age-related macular degeneration
6. Presumed inflammatory origin

Bronstein MA, et al. Bilateral macular lesions. *Ann Ophthalmol* 1981;13:859–861.

Fraunfelder FT, Fraunfelder FW. *Drug-induced ocular side effects.* Woburn, MA: Butterworth-Heinemann, 2001.

PSEUDOMACULAR EDEMA

1. Exudative senile maculopathy—serous or hemorrhagic detachment of the macular retina in persons 50 years of age or older, including ''giant cyst of macula''
2. Serous detachment of retinal pigment epithelium
3. Central serous retinopathy caused by drugs, including the following:

adrenal cortex injection
aldosterone
betamethasone
cortisone
desoxycorticosterone
dexamethasone

fludrocortisone
fluprednisolone
hydrocortisone
indomethacin
methylprednisolone
oral contraceptives

paramethasone
prednisolone
prednisone
triamcinolone (?)

Fraunfelder FT, Fraunfelder FW. *Drug-induced ocular side effects.* Woburn, MA: Butterworth-Heinemann, 2001.

Gass JDM. Pathogenesis of disciform detachment of neuroepithelium. *Am J Ophthalmol* 1967;63:573–711.

MACULAR EDEMA

This condition involves the loss of foveal depression with ophthalmoscope and outline of multiple cystoid. Spaces can be retroilluminated with slit lamp; often a yellow exudate lies deep within or beneath retina in foveal area.

* = most important

1. Acquired parafoveal telangiectasis
2. Amebiasis (amebic dysentery)
3. Bang disease (brucellosis)
4. Behçet syndrome (dermatostomatoophthalmic syndrome)
*5. Carotid artery obstruction
6. Central angiospastic retinopathy
7. Coats disease
8. Choroidal tumors
9. Crohn disease
*10. Cytomegalovirus retinitis
*11. Diabetic retinopathy
12. Dominant inheritance macular dystrophy
13. Drugs, including the following:

acetazolamide
acetophenazine
adrenal cortex injection
aldosterone
allopurinol (?)
aluminum nicotinate
amithiozone
amodiaquine
aspirin
bendroflumethiazide
benoxinate
benzthiazide
betamethasone
betaxolol
broxyquinoline
bupivacaine
butacaine
butaperazine
carbromal
carphenazine
chloramphenicol
chloroquine
chlorothiazide
chlorpromazine
chymotrypsin (?)
cobalt (?)
cortisone
cyclothiazide
desoxycorticosterone
dexamethasone
dibucaine
dichlorphenamide
diethazine
diiodohydroxyquin
dipivefrin
dipivalyl epinephrine (DPE)

dyclonine
epinephrine
ergot
estradiol
ethambutol
ethopropazine
ethoxzolamide
etidocaine
fluphenazine
fluprednisolone
fludrocortisone
ganciclovir
griseofulvin
hexamethonium
hyaluronidase
hydrochlorothiazide
hydrocortisone
hydroflumethiazide
hydroxychloroquine
ibuprofen
indapamide
indomethacin (?)
iodide and iodine solutions
 and compounds
iodochlorhydroxyquin
iodoquinol
iothalamate
iothalamic acid
latanoprost
levobunolol (?)
lidocaine
meglumine and sodium
meprednisone
mesoridazine
methazolamide
methdilazine

methotrimeprazine
methyclothiazide
methylprednisolone
metisazone
naproxen
niacin
niacinamide
nicotinic acid
nicotinyl alcohol
paramethasone
perazine
periciazine
perphenazine
phenacaine
phenylephrine (?)
piperacetazine
polythiazide
prednisolone
prednisone
prilocaine
procaine
prochlorperazine
promazine
promethazine
proparacaine
propiomazine
propoxycaine
quinethazone
quinine
radioactive iodides
sodium salicylate
sulindac
tamoxifen
tetracaine
thiethylperazine
thiopropazate

thioproperazine
thioridazine
thiothalidomine
timolol

triamcinolone
trichlormethiazide
trichloroethylene
trifluoperazine

triflupromazine
trimeprazine (?)
zidovudine

14. Electrical injuries to the retina
15. Epikeratophakia complication
16. Fabry disease (ceramide trihexoside lipidosis)
17. Felty syndrome (rheumatoid arthritis with hypersplenism)
18. Following corneal-relaxing incisions
19. Goldmann–Favre disease (hyaloideoretinal degeneration)
20. Gyrate atrophy
21. Hallermann–Streiff syndrome (dyscephalic mandibulooculofacial syndrome)
22. Hemangiomas of choroid
23. Hemangioma of choroid
24. Hunter syndrome (mucopolysaccharidoses II, or MPS II)
25. Hurler syndrome (MPS I-H)
26. Hypertensive retinopathy
27. Hypotony (postoperative)
*28. Irvine–Gass syndrome
29. Large central foveal cyst
30. Leukemia
31. Meningococcemia (*Neisseria meningitidis*)
32. Macular dystrophy—dominant
33. Nematode, intraretinal
34. Nylon suture toxicity
35. Optic nerve pit
36. Pars planitis (peripheral uveitis)
37. Photocoagulation
38. Porphyria cutanea tarda
39. Posterior capsule rupture
*40. Preretinal fibrosis (macular pucker)
41. Punctata albescens retinopathy
42. Radiation retinopathy
43. Retinitis pigmentosa
44. Retinohypophysary syndrome (Lijo–Pavia–Lis syndrome)
45. Scheie syndrome
46. Scleral buckle
47. Silverman syndrome (battered baby syndrome)
48. Subacute sclerosing panencephalitis (Dawson disease)
49. Toxoplasmic chorioretinitis
50. Trauma to globe (commotio retinae)
51. Ultraviolet light from sun, operating microscope, or other bright light sources
52. Uveitis (anterior or posterior)
*53. Vein occlusion, including branch vein occlusion (see p. 468)
54. von Hippel–Lindau syndrome (retinocerebral angiomatosis)
55. Yttrium–aluminum—garnet (YAG) laser posterior capsulotomy

Axer-Siegel R, et al. Cystoid macular edema after cataract surgery with intraocular vancomycin. *Ophthalmology* 1999;106:1660–1664.

* = most important

Fraunfelder FT, Fraunfelder FW. *Drug-induced ocular side effects.* Woburn, MA: Butterworth-Heinemann, 2001.

Miyake K, et al. Latanoprost accelerates disruption of the blood–aqueous barrier and the incidence of angiographic cystoid macular edema in early postoperative pseudophakias. *Arch Ophthalmol* 1999;117:34–40.

Moroi SE, et al. Cystoid macular edema associated with latanoprost therapy in a case series for patients with glaucoma and ocular hypertension. *Ophthalmology* 1999;106:1024–1029.

Pinckers A, et al. Colour vision in retinitis pigmentosa: influence of cystoid macular edema. *Int Ophthalmol* 1993; 17:143–146.

Roy FH. *Ocular syndromes and systemic diseases,* 3rd ed. Philadelphia: Lippincott Williams & Williams, 2002.

Warwar RE. Cystoid macular edema and anterior uveitis associated with latanoprost use. *Opthalmology* 1998;105: 263–266.

ABSENCE OF FOVEAL REFLEX

The absence of foveal reflex is caused by drugs, including amodiaquine, chloroquine, diiodohydroxyquin, hydroxychloroquine, iodochlorhydroxyquin, or quinine.

Fraunfelder FT, Fraunfelder FW. *Drug-induced ocular side effects.* Woburn, MA: Butterworth-Heinemann, 2001.

MACULAR PUCKER

Macular pucker involves tiny folds that often are arranged in a stellate manner around macula and usually are associated with a preretinal membrane (preretinal macular fibrosis, preretinal vitreous membrane, surface wrinkling retinopathy, cellophane maculopathy).

1. Associated with proliferative retinopathy
   *A. Diabetes retinopathy
   B. Eales disease
   *C. Hypertension
   D. Sickle cell disease
   E. Vein occlusion
2. Central serous chorioretinopathy
   A. Psychopharmacologic medication use
   B. Corticosteroid use
   C. Hypertension
3. Congenital
4. Following photocoagulation or cryoretinopexy
5. Following traumatic posterior vitreous separation, such as blunt trauma to the eye and whiplash injury (craniocervical syndrome)
6. Loss of formed vitreous at operation
7. Idiopathic (probably related to spontaneous posterior vitreous detachment)
8. Macular detachment
9. Multiple retinal operations
10. Penetrating or blunt injuries
11. Posterior uveitis
*12. Proliferative vitreoretinopathy following vitreoretinal surgery
13. Retinal detachment
14. Trauma (blunt)
15. Vitreous hemorrhage

McDonald HR, et al. Surgical management of idiopathic epiretinal membranes. *Ophthalmology* 1986;93:978–983.

Smiddy WE, et al. Clinicopathologic study of idiopathic macular pucker in children and young adults. *Retina* 1992; 12:232–236.

Tittl MK, et al. Systemic findings associated with central serous chorioretinopathy. *Am J Ophthalmol* 1999;128: 63–68.

Uemura A, et al. Macular pucker after retinal detachment surgery. *Ophthalmic Surg Lasers* 1992;23:116–119.

MACULAR EXUDATES AND HEMORRHAGES

1. Retinal macroaneurysms
2. Hemorrhagic age-related macular degeneration (ARMD)
3. Diabetic macular edema
4. Retinal telangiectasis
5. With dense subretinal and subretinal pigment epithelium (sub-RPE [retinal pigment epithelium]) hemorrhage simulate the appearance of retinal macroaneurysms.

Yannuzzi LA, et al. *The macula: a comprehensive text and atlas.* Baltimore: Williams & Wilkins, 1979.

MACULAR STAR OR STELLATE RETINOPATHY (EXUDATES IN A STAR FORMATION RADIATING AROUND MACULA IN THE NERVE FIBER LAYER)

1. Acute febrile illness, such as measles, influenza, meningitis, erysipelas, psittacosis, Behçet disease (dermatostomatoophthalmic syndrome)
2. Cat-scratch fever
3. Chronic infections, such as tuberculosis or syphilis
4. Coccidioidomycosis
5. Gansslen syndrome (familial hemolytic icterus)
*6. Hypertension
7. Idiopathic
8. Juxtapapillary choroiditis (Jensen disease)
*9. Neuroretinitis
10. Obstruction of the artery or vein supplying the macular area (see p. 457 and 468)
11. Ocular or cerebral trauma
12. Parasitic infection, such as that due to teniae, *Giardia, Ancylostoma*
*13. Papilledema (see p. 563–601)
14. Papillitis (see p. 578–585, 587–588)
15. Retinal periphlebitis

Roy FH. *Ocular syndromes and systemic diseases,* 3rd ed. Philadelphia: Lippincott Williams & Wilkins, 2002.

Yannuzzi LA, et al. *The macula: a comprehensive text and atlas.* Baltimore: Williams & Wilkins, 1979.

* = most important

Stellate retinopathy (exudates in a star formation radiating around the macula in the nerve fiber layer)

History

	Hypertension	Ocular Trauma	Retinal Periphlebitis	Papillitis	Papilledema	Acute Febrile Illness i.e. Behçet's Disease	Chronic Infections i.e. Tuberculosis	Coccidioidomycosis
1. Communicable disease							U	
2. Elevated blood pressure	U							
3. Hereditary	S							
4. History of ocular trauma		U						
5. In young men			U					
6. Increased intracranial pressure					U			
7. Monocular loss of vision				S	U			
8. Occurs between 15 and 45 years of age						U		
9. Occurs in adults							U	
10. Occurs in people living in an endemic area								U

Physical Findings

	Hypertension	Ocular Trauma	Retinal Periphlebitis	Papillitis	Papilledema	Acute Febrile Illness i.e. Behçet's Disease	Chronic Infections i.e. Tuberculosis	Coccidioidomycosis
1. Absence of spontaneous venous pulse					S			
2. Arteriosclerosis	U							
3. Blepharitis							S	
4. Capillary nonperfusion			S					U
5. Cellulitis							S	
6. Conjunctivitis							S	
7. Corneal ulcer							S	
8. Cotton wool spots	S	S						
9. Choroidal rupture		S						
10. Choroiditis							S	
11. Dacryocystitis							S	
12. Diffuse gray-white appearance of the neurosensory retina	S							
13. Diplopia		S						
14. Disc hemorrhages						S		
15. Disc pallor (late)				U				
16. Enophthalmos		S						
17. Episcleritis	S							S
18. Fatty exudates						S		
19. Granulomatous lesion of optic nerve head								S
20. Hypopyon								S
21. Intravitreal hemorrhage			S	S				
22. Iritis		S						
23. Keratitis						S	S	
24. Keratoconjunctivitis sicca						U		
25. Lens subluxation or dislocation		S						
26. Macular edema								
27. Meibomianitis								
28. Miosis		S						
29. Mutton-fat keratic precipitates								S
30. Nystagmus							R	
31. Ocular pain		S						
32. Ocular pain on movements				U				

Stellate retinopathy (exudates in a star formation radiating around the macula in the nerve fiber layer) Continued

	Hypertension	Ocular Trauma	Retinal Periphlebitis	Papillitis	Papilledema	Acute Febrile Illness i.e. Behçet's Disease	Chronic Infections i.e. Tuberculosis	Coccidioidomycosis
Physical Findings								
33. Optic disc edema	S			U	S			
34. Optic nerve atrophy						S	S	
35. Optic nerve capillary hyperemia				U				
36. Optic neuritis						S	S	
37. Palsies of extraocular muscles								S
38. Pannus						S	S	
39. Panophthalmitis						S	S	
40. Paralysis of accommodation		S						
41. Paralysis of sixth cranial nerve								S
42. Perivascular exudates		S						
43. Perivascular sheathing		S				S		
44. Recurrent uveitis						U		
45. Relative afferent pupillary defect				U				
46. Retinal arterial narrowing	U							
47. Retinal detachment		S						
48. Retinal edema					S			
49. Retinal hemorrhages	S							
50. Retinal tears or disinsertion		S	S					
51. Retinal vasculitis		S				S		
52. Retinitis						U	S	
53. Scleral perforation							S	
54. Scleritis							S	
55. Secondary glaucoma						S		S
56. Subconjunctival nodules							S	
57. Subtle vertical striae on the temporal side of disc					S			
58. Uveitis							S	S
59. Venous dilation			S			S		
60. Venous obstruction			S					
61. Vision may be reduced		S						
62. Vitreal floaters								S
63. Vitreal opacity								S
64. Vitreous cells				S			S	S
65. Vitreous inflammation				S			S	S

R = Rarely; S = sometimes; and U = usually.

RETINOCILIARY VEIN—DISAPPEARS FROM THE RETINA AT DISC MARGIN WITHOUT CONNECTION TO CENTRAL RETINAL VEIN

1. Acquired
    A. Arachnoid cyst of the optic nerve
    B. Central retinal vein occlusion (see p. 468)
    C. Chronic atrophic papilledema from causes including craniopharyngioma (see p. 595–597)
    D. Glioma of the optic disc
2. Congenital

Wolter JJ. Retinociliary vein associated with a craniopharyngioma. *Ann Ophthalmol* 1979;11:751.

CHERRY-RED SPOT IN MACULA (RULE OUT MACULAR HEMORRHAGE)

1. Cardiac myxomas
2. Cryoglobulinemia
3. Dapsone poisoning
4. Hallervorden–Spatz disease (pigmentary degeneration of globus pallidus)
5. Hollenhorst syndrome (chorioretinal infarction syndrome)
6. Hurler syndrome (MPS I-H)
*7. Hypertension (severe)
8. Intralesional chalazion corticosteroid injection
9. Leber congenital amaurosis
10. Macular hemorrhage
*11. Macular hole with surrounding retinal detachment
12. ML I (lipomucopolysaccharidosis)
13. Myotonic dystrophy syndrome (Curschmann–Steinert syndrome)
14. Multiple sulfatase deficiency
*15. Occlusion of central retinal artery (see p. 457)
16. Quinine toxicity
17. Sphingolipidoses
    A. Cherry-red spot myoclonus
    B. Farber syndrome (Farber lipogranulomatosis)
    C. Gangliosidosis GM_1—type (juvenile gangliosidosis)
    D. Gaucher disease (glucocerebroside storage disease)
    E. Goldberg syndrome
    F. Infantile metachromatic leukodystrophy (van Bogaert–Nyssen disease)
    G. Niemann–Pick disease type A
    H. Niemann–Pick disease type B
    I. Sandhoff disease (gangliosidosis GM_2—type 2)
    *J. Tay–Sachs disease (gangliosidosis GM—type I)
18. Steroid injection intranasally
*19. Temporal arteritis (giant cell arteritis)
20. Traumatic retinal edema (commotio retinae; Berlin edema)
21. Vogt–Spielmeyer cerebral degeneration (Batten–Mayou syndrome)

Abhayambika K, et al. Peripheral neuropathy and haemolytic anaemia with cherry red spot on macula in dapsone poisoning. *J Assoc Physicians India* 1990;38:564–565.

Reed JB, et al. Bartonella henselae neuroretinitis in cat scratch disease. *Ophthalmology* 1998;105:459–466.

Roy FH. *Ocular syndromes and systemic diseases,* 3rd ed. Philadelphia: Lippincott Williams & Wilkins, 2002.

Wade NK, et al. Optic disk edema associated with peripapillary serous retinal detachment: an early sign of systemic *Bartonella henselae* infection. *Am J Ophthalmol* 2000;130:327–334.

MACULAR HEMORRHAGE

1. Choroidal neovascular membranes
   *A. Age-related macular degeneration
   B. Angioid streaks
   C. Histoplasmosis
   D. Idiopathic
   E. Pathologic myopic
   F. Posterior uveitis
2. Infectious retinitis
   *A. Cytomegalovirus retinitis
   B. Subacute bacterial endocarditis
3. Retinal vascular disease
   A. Radiation retinopathy
   B. Retinal arterial macroaneurysm
   *C. Vein occlusion
4. Systemic diseases
   A. Blood dyscrasias
      (1) Anemia
      (2) Leukemia
      (3) Polycythemia vera
      (4) Sickle cell disease
      (5) Thrombocytopenia
      (6) Waldenström macroglobulinemia
   B. Cardiovascular shock (especially gastrointestinal hemorrhage)
   *C. Diabetes mellitus
   *D. Human immunodeficiency virus (HIV)-related retinopathy
   *E. Hypertension
   F. Toxemia of pregnancy
5. Trauma
   A. Choroidal rupture
   B. Purtscher retinopathy
   C. Shaken-baby syndrome
   D. Terson syndrome
   E. Valsalva retinopathy
   F. Vitreous detachment

McCabe CM, et al. Nonsurgical management of macular hemorrhage secondary to retinal artery macroaneurysms. *Arch Ophthalmol* 2000;118:780–786.

Paris CL, et al. Neonatal macular hemorrhage. *Int Ophthalmol* 1991;15:153–155.

Stevenson A, et al. Is aspirin a factor in macular hemorrhage. *Ophthalmol Times* 1993;18:32–34

* = most important

Macular hemorrhage

	High Myopia (Fuchs Spot)*	Disciform Macular Degeneration	Inflammation as Histoplasmosis*	Angioid Streaks	Familial
History					
1. Familial					U
2. Greater in whites than blacks			U		
3. In persons 30 to 50 years	U			U	
4. In persons 50 years and older		U			
5. Mainly central visual loss		U			
6. Metamorphopsia		U			
7. More often men			U		
8. Myopia more than 12 diopters	U				
Physical Findings					
1. Circumpapillary choroiditis			U		
2. Dark spot in macula	U	S			
3. Enlarging myopic crescent	U				
4. Macular lesion in active stage, pigment ring with sensory retinal detachment			U		
5. Mottled macular appearance	U				
6. Pigment epithelial retinal detachment	U	U			
7. Ruptures in Bruch membrane	U			U	
8. Scattered atrophic chorioretinal spots in mid and far periphery			U		
9. Serous retinal separation	S	U			
Laboratory Data					
1. Fluorescein angiography	U	U	U	U	U
2. Histoplasmin skin test			U		

R = rarely; S = sometimes; and U = usually.

PARAFOVEAL TELANGIECTASIA

This condition is a retinal microvascular anomaly involving the parafoveal capillary network as well as the immediately adjacent vascular bed and is best demonstrated by fluorescein angiography.

1. Carotid artery obstruction
*2. Diabetes mellitus, usually bilateral
*3. Idiopathic
4. Localized form of Coats disease, usually unilateral
*5. Small branch vein occlusion
6. Small retinal capillary hemangioma, usually unilateral
7. Roentgenogram, irradiation

Gass JD, Oyakawa T. Idiopathic juxtafoveal telangiectasia. *Arch Ophthalmol* 1982;100:769.

Millay RH, et al. Abnormal glucose metabolism and parafoveal telangiectasia. *Am J Ophthalmol* 1986;102:363–370.

MICROHEMORRHAGIC MACULOPATHY—SMALL MONOCULAR MACULAR HEMORRHAGE THAT IS PUNCTATE, ROUND OR BILOBED

1. Increased venous stasis (Valsalva stress)
2. Impaired blood platelet aggregation
3. Medications that impair platelet function including aspirin, ibuprofen (Motrin), pentazocine, propranolol hydrochloride and oral contraceptives.

Pruett RC, Carvalho ACA, Trempe CL. Microhemorrhagic maculopathy. *Arch Ophthalmol* 1980;99:425.

MACULAR CYST

Macular cyst must be differentiated from macular hole with Hruby lens or contact lens and slit lamp.

1. Amebiasis
2. Cysticercosis—subretinal cyst
*3. Cystic degeneration—common following trauma, uveitis, and vascular disease
4. Hamman–Rich syndrome (alveolar capillary block syndrome)
5. Histoplasmosis
6. Hydatid disease (echinococcosis)
7. Parasitic and mycotic cysts

McDonnell PJ, et al. Clinical features of idiopathic macular cysts and holes. *Am J Ophthalmol* 1982;93:777–786.

Roy FH. *Ocular syndromes and systemic diseases,* 3rd ed. Philadelphia: Lippincott Williams & Wilkins, 2002.

MACULAR HOLE

Macular hole must be differentiated from macular cyst with Hruby lens or contact lens and slit lamp)

*1. Idiopathic (most common, may be bilateral)
2. From the following:
   A. Edema (see p. 439)
      (1) Inflammatory

* = most important

  (2) Toxic

  (3) Vascular

  (4) Following papilledema

B. High myopia

C. Ischemic, such as with retinal detachment or choroidal tumor—the macula is separated from choriocapillaris

D. Degenerative conditions of the retina and retinal dystrophy

E. Trauma

F. Radiation injury

G. Glaucoma

H. Posterior senile retinoschisis

 I. High tension electric shock

J. Central serous chorioretinopathy

K. Optic disc coloboma

L. Posterior retinal detachment associated with optic pits

M. Industrial laser burns

N. Lightening—induced

O. Posterior microphthalmos

P. Septic embolization

Q. Subhyaloid hemorrhage

R. Topical pilocarpine use

S. YAG laser

3. Dawson disease (subacute sclerosing panencephalitis)

4. Foveomacular retinitis—usually young males

*5. Pseudohole due to epiretinal membrane (may differentiated from true hole by fluorescein angiography)

6. Sickle cell disease

Benedict WL, Shami M. Impending macular hole associated with topical pilocarpine. *Am J Ophthalmol* 1992;114: 765–779.

Blacharski PA, Newsome DA. Bilateral macular holes after Nd:YAG laser posterior capsulotomy. *Am J Ophthalmol* 1988;105:451–459.

Gass JDM. Idiopathic senile macular hole. *Arch Ophthalmol* 1988;106:629–639.

Ho AC, et al. Unusual immunogammopathy maculopathy. *Ophthalmology* 2000;107:1099–1103.

Lansing MB, et al. The effect of pars plana vitrectomy and transforming growth factor-beta without epiretinal membrane peeling on full-thickness macular holes. *Ophthalmology* 1993;100:868–871.

Smiddy WE. Atypical presentations of macular holes. *Arch Ophthalmol* 1993;111:626–631.

MACULAR COLOBOMA

This condition involves bilaterally symmetric, circumscribed, excavated defects in choroid and retina in the region of macula associated with reduced vision

1. Autosomal dominant

2. Autosomal recessive inheritance with skeletal anomalies

3. Conditions that exhibit choroidal coloboma (see p. 555–556)

4. Down syndrome

5. Hypercalciuria, myopia, and macular coloboma

6. Isolated

7. Macular coloboma with brachydactyly
8. Sorsby syndrome I

Isenberg SJ. *The eye in infancy.* Chicago: Year Book Medical, 1989.

Yamaguchi K, Tamai M. Congenital macular coloboma in Down syndrome. *Ann Ophthalmol* 1990;22:222–223.

ELEVATED MACULAR LESION

1. Angiospastic retinopathy
2. Central serous detachment of retina
3. Chorioretinitis especially histoplasmosis and toxoplasmosis
4. Choroidal hemangioma
5. Dawson disease (subacute sclerosing panencephalitis)
6. Malignant melanoma
7. Varix of the vortex ampulla
8. Sickle cell disease

Al-Abdulla NA, et al. Sickle cell disease presenting with extensive peri-macular arteriolar occlusions in a nine-year-old boy. *Am J Ophthalmol* 2000;130:419–428.

Cunningham ET, et al. Central serous chorioretinopathy in patients with systemic lupus erythematosus. *Ophthalmology* 1996;103:2081–2090.

Newell FW. *Ophthalmology: principles and concepts,* 7th ed. St. Louis: CV Mosby, 1991.

HETEROTOPIA OF THE MACULA

This condition involves an abnormal location of the macula in relation to the optic disc; the eye with the ectopic macula tends to deviate in the same direction as macular displacement; visual fields show displacement of blind spot and cover–uncover test shows no shift of fixation.

1. Chorioretinitis
2. Congenital
*3. Retinopathy of prematurity
4. Inflammatory
*5. Proliferative diabetic retinopathy

Bresnick GH. Visual function abnormalities in macular heterotopia caused by proliferative diabetic retinopathy. *Am J Ophthalmol* 1981;92:85–102.

Stem SD, Arenberg IK. Heterotopia of the macula with associated retinal detachment. *J Pediatr Ophthalmol* 1969; 6:198–202.

WHITE OR YELLOW FLAT MACULAR LESION AND PIGMENTARY CHANGE

1. Posttraumatic—pigmentary disturbance; cysts or hole at macula
2. Postinflammatory—chorioretinal atrophy with pigment clumping at center and periphery of lesion
3. Coloboma of macula—atrophic area at macula often associated with coloboma of disc; sclera may be ectatic (see p. 450)
4. Radiation injuries—common after solar eclipse; punched-out appearance
5. Fuchs dark spot–pigmented spot associated with other signs of degenerative myopia
6. Drugs, including the following:

* = most important

adrenal cortex injection
aldosterone
allopurinol (?)
amodiaquine
betamethasone (?)
chloroquine
cortisone (?)
desoxycorticosterone (?)

dexamethasone (?)
diiodohydroxyquin
fludrocortisone
fluprednisolone (?)
griseofulvin
hydrocortisone (?)
hydroxychloroquine
indomethacin (?)

iodochlorhydroxyquin
methylprednisolone
oral contraceptives
paramethasone (?)
prednisolone (?)
prednisone (?)
quinine
triamcinolone

7. Stellate retinopathy—star-shaped exudates (see p. 443)
8. Hard exudates and circinate retinopathy (see p. 495)
9. Drusen—common, discrete yellow spots beneath the retina
10. Doyne honeycomb choroiditis—rare; honeycomb pattern of yellow patches at posterior pole; degenerative changes at macula
11. Heredomacular dystrophies
    A. Best disease (vitelliruptive macular dystrophy) up to 18 years of age; egg-yolk lesion at macula, later absorbed to leave atrophic scar
    B. Fundus flavimaculatus—yellow patches at posterior pole; degenerative changes at macula
    C. Stargardt disease (juvenile macular degeneration) to 10 years of age; variable appearance in different families; bilateral lesions showing some degree of symmetry
    D. Behr disease (optic atrophy-ataxia syndrome)—adults, similar to Stargardt type
    E. Presenile and senile—pigmentary changes followed by atrophy, bilateral and symmetric
13. Central choroidal sclerosis—rare, atrophic retina with sclerosed choroidal vessels showing clearly
14. Central areolar choroidal atrophy—rare, exudate and edema followed by sharply defined atrophic area with white strands of choroidal vessels
15. Pseudoinflammatory macular dystrophy—rare, initially edema and exudates followed by scarring with pigmentary disturbance and atrophic patches
16. Gaucher disease (glucocerebroside storage disease)—rare, ring-shaped macular lesions, lipid deposits in cornea and conjunctiva
17. Diffuse leukoencephalopathy—rare, white deposits in periphery and macular area
18. Sjögren–Larsson syndrome (oligophrenia–ichthyosis–spastic diplegia syndrome)
19. Angioid streaks (see p. 526–529)
20. Multiple evanescent white-dot syndrome (MEWDS) usually unilateral, predominantly healthy women, vitreitis
21. Acute multifocal placoid pigment epitheliopathy—rare, map-like pigmentary disturbance of posterior pole or more widespread over posterior fundus

Eagle RC, et al. Retinal pigment epithelial abnormalities in fundus flavimaculatus. *Ophthalmology* 1980;87:1189.

Fraunfelder FT, Fraunfelder FW. *Drug-induced ocular side effects and drug interactions.* Woburn, MA: Butterworth-Heinemann, 2001.

Hadden OB, Gass DM. Fundus flavimaculatus and Stargardt's disease. *Am J Ophthalmol* 1976;82:527–539.

PIGMENTARY CHANGES IN MACULA

1. Hereditary macular degeneration without cerebral or other disease
    A. Best disease (vitelliform macular dystrophy)
    B. Stargardt disease (juvenile flavimaculatus)
    C. Behr syndrome (optic atrophy-ataxia syndrome)

*2. Retinitis pigmentosa
3. Secondary pigmentary retinopathy following trauma or inflammation (see p. 497)
*4. Age-related macular degeneration
5. Metabolic disease associated with pigmentary retinopathy
    A. Abetalipoproteinemia (Bassen–Kornzweig syndrome)
    B. Alpha-lipoprotein deficiency (Tangier syndrome)
    C. Ceroid lipofuscinosis
       (1) Batten–Mayou syndrome
       (2) Dollinger–Bielschowsky syndrome, late infantile (Bielschowsky–Jansky disease)
       (3) Infantile type of neuronal ceroid lipofuscinosis
    D. Hepatic disease
    E. Refsum disease (phytanic acid storage disease)
    F. Tay–Sachs syndrome (gangliosidosis GM_2-type I)
    G. Vitamin A
    H. MPS
       (1) Hunter syndrome (MPS II)
       (2) Hurler syndrome (MPS I-H)
       (3) Sanfilippo–Good syndrome (MPS III)
       (4) Scheie syndrome (MPS I-S)
*6. Drugs, including the following:

acetophenazine	cephapirin	moxalactam
amiodarone (?)	cephradine	naproxen
amodiaquine	chloramphenicol	penicillamine
azathioprine	chloroquine	perazine
benzatropine (?)	chlorphenoxamine (?)	pericyazine
biperiden (?)	chlorpromazine	perphenazine
butaperazine	chlorprothixene	piperacetazine
carbamazepine	cisplatin	prazosin (?)
carphenazine	clofazimine	prochlorperazine
cefaclor	clonidine (?)	procyclidine (?)
cefadroxil	cobalt (?)	promazine
cefamandole	cycrimine (?)	promethazine
cefazolin	deferoxamine	propiomazine
cefonicid	diethazine	quinacrine (?)
cefoperazone	diethylcarbamazine	quinine
ceforanide	ethambutol (?)	sulindac (?)
cefotaxime	ethopropazine	tamoxifen
cefotetan	fluphenazine	thiethylperazine
cefoxitin	hydroxychloroquine	thiopropazate
cefsulodin	indomethacin (?)	thioproperazine
ceftazidime	ketoprofen (?)	thioridazine
ceftriaxone	mesoridazine	thiothixene
cefuroxime	methdilazine	trifluoperazine
cephalexin	methotrexate	triflupromazine
cephaloridine	methotrimeprazine	trihexyphenidyl (?)
cephalothin	minoxidil (?)	trimeprazine
	mitotane	

7. Inflammation
   *A. Toxoplasmosis
    B. Trauma
8. Multifocal necrotizing encephalopathy
9. Dawson disease (subacute sclerosing panencephalitis)
10. Dialinas–Amalric syndrome (deaf mutism–retinal degeneration syndrome)
11. Oculodental syndrome (Peter syndrome)
12. Sorsby syndrome (hereditary macular coloboma syndrome)

Fishman GA, et al. X-linked recessive retinitis pigmentosa. *Arch Ophthalmol* 1986;104:1329–1335.

Fraunfelder FT, Fraunfelder FW. *Drug-induced ocular side effects.* Woburn, MA: Butterworth-Heinemann, 2001.

Roy FH. *Ocular syndromes and systemic diseases,* 3rd ed. Philadelphia: Lippincott Williams & Wilkins, 2002.

BULL'S-EYE MACULAR LESION—CIRCULAR AREA OF RETINAL PIGMENT EPITHELIUM ATROPHY SURROUNDING A SPARED FOVEA

 1. Autosomal-dominant, benign, concentric annular macular dystrophy
 2. Ceroid lipofuscinosis
*3. Chloroquine or hydroxychloroquine retinopathy
 4. Cone dystrophy
 5. Hereditary ataxia
 6. NARP syndrome
 7. Spielmeyer–Vogt syndrome (Batten–Mayou syndrome)
*8. Stargardt disease (or fundus flavimaculatus)
 9. Trauma
10. Unknown

Duinkerke-Eerola, et al. Atrophic maculopathy associated with hereditary ataxia. *Am J Ophthalmol* 1980;90:846.

Isenberg SJ. *The eye in infancy.* Chicago: Year Book Medical, 1989.

Nomura R, et al. Unilateral cone dysfunction with bull's eye maculopathy. *Ophthalmology* 2001;108:49–53.

MACULAR WISPS AND FOVEOLAR SPLINTER

These are noted in focal illumination with Goldmann contact lenses but are invisible ophthalmoscopically.

1. Direct and indirect ocular concussion
2. Following absorption of small prefoveal hemorrhage
3. Foveomacular retinitis
4. Juvenile macular degeneration
5. Old, healed chorioretinitis
6. Retinitis pigmentosa
7. Spontaneous senile posterior vitreous detachment
8. Whiplash injury

Daily L. Foveolar splinter and macular wisps. *Arch Ophthalmol* 1970;83:406–411.

Daily L. Further observations on foveolar splinter and macular wisps. *Arch Ophthalmol* 1973;90:102–103.

MACULAR HYPOPLASIA (INCOMPLETE MACULAR DEVELOPMENT MANIFESTED BY DECREASED VISION)

*1. Albinism

*2. Associated with autosomal-dominant aniridia
3. Associated with microcornea and corectopia
4. Associated with myelinated nerve fibers
5. Forsius–Eriksson syndrome (Aland disease)
*6. Goldenhar–Gorlin syndrome (oculoauriculovertebral dysplasia)
7. Krause syndrome (encephaloophthalmic dysplasia)
8. Ring chromosome
9. Syndrome of foveal hypoplasia and presenile cataract (O'Donnell–Pappas syndrome)—autosomal dominant
10. Tuomaala–Haapanen syndrome
11. Waardenburg syndrome (interoculoiridodermatoauditive dysplasia)

Ghose S, Mehta U. Microcornea with corectopia and macular hypoplasia in a family. *Jpn J Ophthalmol* 1984;28: 126–130.

Margolis S, et al. Retinal and optic nerve findings in Goldenhar-Gorlin syndrome. *Ophthalmology* 1984;91: 1327–1333.

Roy FH. *Ocular syndromes and systemic diseases,* 3rd ed. Philadelphia: Lippincott Williams & Wilkins, 2002.

Szymanski KA, et al. Genetic studies of ocular albinism in a large Virginia kindred. *Ann Ophthalmol* 1984;16: 183–185.

PREMACULAR SUBHYALOID HEMORRHAGE

1. Branch retinal vein occlusion
2. Blood dyscrasia
3. Diabetic retinopathy
4. Retinal macroaneurysm
5. Terson syndrome
6. Valsalva retinopathy

Ulbig MW, et al. Long-term results after drainage of premacular subhyaloid hemorrhage into the vitreous with a pulsed Nd: YAG laser.

RETINAL VASCULAR TORTUOSITY

1. Acute malnutrition
2. Aortic coarctation
3. Bazzana syndrome (angiospastic ophthalmoauricular syndrome)
4. Choked disc (see p. 593)
5. Chronic respiratory insufficiency, such as in cystic fibrosis and familial dysautonomia (Riley–Day syndrome)
*6. Coats disease (retinal telangiectasia)
7. Congenital
8. Cri-du-chat syndrome (cat-cry syndrome)
9. Cryoglobulinemia
10. Down syndrome (trisomy 21)
11. Eales disease (periphlebitis)
12. Engelmann syndrome (diaphyseal dysplasia)
13. Fabry disease (diffuse angiokeratosis)
*14. Glaucoma, open angle
15. Granulocytic sarcoma of orbit
16. Hereditary hemorrhagic telangiectasis (Osler disease)—tortuosity and varicosity

* = most important

17. Hypertension
18. Kenny syndrome (dwarfism, thickened long bone cortex, transient hypocalcemia)
*19. Leukemia
20. Lymphogranuloma venereum (Nicolas–Favre disease)
21. Maroteaux–Lamy syndrome (mucopolysaccharidoses type VI)
22. Macroglobulinemia
23. Mosse syndrome (polycythemia–hepatic cirrhosis syndrome)
24. Myopia
25. Normal variation with fullness
26. Polycythemia with vessel fullness
27. Retinopathy of prematurity
28. Racemose hemangioma of retina, angiomatosis retinae without obvious tumor formation, or von Hippel–Lindau syndrome (retinocerebral angiomatosis)
29. Reimann syndrome (hyperviscosity syndrome)
*30. Sickle cell disease
31. Visceral larva migrans (nematode ophthalmia syndrome)

Davis JL, et al. Granulocytic sarcoma of the orbit. *Ophthalmology* 1985;92:1758–1762.

Roy FH. *Ocular syndromes and systemic diseases,* 3rd ed. Philadelphia: Lippincott Williams & Wilkins, 2002.

Wells CG, Kalina RE. Progressive inherited retinal arteriolar tortuosity with spontaneous retinal hemorrhages. *Ophthalmology* 1985;92:1015–1024.

VENOUS BEADING

*1. Diabetes mellitus
2. Loaiasis (*Loa loa*)
3. Macroglobulinemia (Waldenstrom syndrome)

Schlaegel TF. *Essentials of uveitis.* Boston: Little, Brown, 1969.

OPHTHALMODYNAMOMETRY

When blood pressure of the retinal artery is measured, a difference between the eyes of about 15% of diastolic readings is considered significant.

1. False-positive or variable readings
   A. Abnormally high or low intraocular pressure or asymmetry between the two eyes
   B. Cardiac abnormalities, such as atrial fibrillation, heart block, or extrasystoles
   C. Marked asymmetry of retinal vessels in the two eyes
   D. Measurements of ophthalmic artery pressure lower than 20 g on the instrument
   E. Poor patient cooperation
   F. Variation in systemic blood pressure between readings
2. High ophthalmodynamometry values
   A. Basilar–vertebral occlusion
   B. Bilateral distal internal carotid occlusion—unusual
   C. Progressive intracranial arterial occlusion syndrome
3. Low ophthalmodynamometry values
   A. Both sides reduced with orthostatic hypotension
   *B. Reduced on side of an occluded internal carotid artery

Walsh FB, Hoyt WF. *Clinical neuro-ophthalmology,* 4th ed. Baltimore: Williams & Wilkins, 1985.

PULSATION OF RETINAL ARTERIOLE (HIGH PULSE PRESSURE)

1. Aortic regurgitation
2. Hyperthyroidism
*3. Intraocular blood pressure higher than diastolic blood pressure but lower than systolic blood pressure

Newell FW. *Ophthalmology: principles and concepts,* 7th ed. St. Louis: CV Mosby, 1992.

RETINAL ARTERY OCCLUSION

This condition involves a sudden, painless visual loss; on ophthalmoscopic examination, a diffuse retinal pallor and a cherry-red spot in macula are noted.

1. Embolism—cardiac or pulmonary sources
    A. Air emboli following trauma or surgery
    B. Amniotic fluid embolization
    C. Cardiac myxoma
    D. Corticosteroid emboli
    E. Espildora–Luque syndrome (ophthalmic Sylvian syndrome)
    F. Fat emboli following long-bone fractures
    G. Iatrogenic trauma induced by angiography
    *H. In older patients—due to atheroma of carotid artery
    I. In young persons—due to postrheumatic vegetations (rheumatic fever), cardiac catheterization, or valvotomy
    J. Leudoemboli—vasculitis, Purtscher retinopathy, septic endocarditis
    K. Moyamoya disease (multiple progressive intracranial arterial occlusion)
    L. Nicolau syndrome (emboli of medication inadvertently introduced into artery)
    M. Synthetic material used in cardiac and vascular procedures
    N. Talc emboli—long-term intravenous drug abusers
    O. Tumors—atrial myxoma, mitral valve papillary fibroelastoma
    P. With cerebral infarction after periocular subcutaneous cosmetic silicone injection
*2. Atherosclerosis of common carotid artery (ophthalmodynamometry employed for diagnosis)
3. Ischemia
    A. Carotid occlusion or dissection
    B. Essential hypotension
    C. Following orbital floor fractures or repair
    D. Following surgery for retinal detachment
    E. Generalized shock
    F. Heart failure (rare)
    G. Kahler disease (multiple myeloma)
    H. Knee–chest position
    I. Massive hemorrhage, such as that occurring in hematemesis, gastrointestinal bleeding, or surgical procedures
    J. Migraine
    K. Mosse syndrome (polycythemia–hepatic cirrhosis syndrome)
    L. Orbital hemorrhage following retrobulbar injection
    M. After surgery for scoliosis
    N. Too rapid lowering of blood pressure in hypertensive subjects
4. Inflammation

* = most important

    A. Abdominal typhus (typhoid fever)
    B. African eye-worm disease (loiasis)
    C. Arteriole vasculitis, such as periarteritis nodosa (Kussmaul disease)
    D. Bacterial endocarditis
    E. Behçet disease (dermatostomatoophthalmic syndrome)
    F. Diphtheria
    G. Familial factor V Leiden polymorphism and positive rheumatoid factor
    H. Giant cell arteritis
    I. Herpes zoster
    J. Metastatic bacterial endophthalmitis
    K. Mucormycosis (phycomycosis)
    L. Pancreatitis
    M. Recurrent toxoplasmic retinochoroiditis
    N. Rocky Mountain spotted fever (spotted fever)
    O. Rubeola (measles)
    P. Subacute bacterial endocarditis
    Q. Systemic lupus erythematosus
    R. Takayasu disease (pulseless disease)
   *S. Temporal arteritis
    T. *Toxoplasma retinochoroiditis*
    U. Varicella (chickenpox)

5. Blood disease
    A. After platelet transfusion
    B. Following ocular trauma with secondary glaucoma in youths with sickle-trait hemoglobinopathy
    C. Polycythemia vera (Vaquez–Osler syndrome)
    D. Sickle cell disease
6. Syphilis (acquired lues)
7. Associated factors
8. Diathermy of persistent hyaloid
    A. Drusen of optic nerve (see p. 559–560)
    B. Giant cell arteritis
    C. Papilledema (see p. 593–601)
    D. Subdural cerebral hemorrhage
    E. Arteriosclerosis of central retinal artery
    F. Chronic simple glaucoma
9. After dye, yellow photocoagulation
10. Complication of retrobulbar block
11. Degos syndrome (malignant atrophic papulosis)
12. Disseminated lupus erythematosus
13. Fabry–Anderson syndrome (glycosphingolipid lipidosis)
14. Goldenhar–Gorlin syndrome (oculoauriculovertebral dysplasia)
15. Homocystinuria syndrome
16. Hyperhomocystinemia
17. Lyme disease
18. Neoplastic angioendotheliomatosis
19. Polymyalgia rheumatica
20. Protein S deficiency
21. Relapsing polychondritis

* = most important

22. Sneddon syndrome (livedo reticularis, neurologic abnormalities, and labile hypertension)
23. Use of tranexamic acid therapy

Dori D, et al. Multiple retinal arteriolar occlusions associated with coexisting primary antiphospholipid syndrome and factor V Leiden mutation. *Am J Ophthalmol* 2000;129:106–108.

Friedberg MA, Micale AJ. Monocular blindness from central retinal artery occlusion associated with chickenpox. *Am J Ophthalmol* 1994;117:117–118.

Grossman W, Ward WT. Central retinal artery occlusion after scoliosis surgery with a horseshoe headrest. *Spine* 1993;18:1226–1228.

Rao TH, et al. Central retinal artery occlusion from carotid dissection diagnosed by cervical computed tomography. *Stroke* 1994;25:1271–1272.

Roy FH. *Ocular syndromes and systemic diseases,* 3rd ed. Philadelphia: Lippincott Williams & Wilkins, 2002.

Russell SR, Folk JC. Branch retinal artery occlusion after dye yellow photocoagulation of an arterial macroaneurysm. *Am J Ophthalmol* 1987;104:186.

Retinal artery occlusion (sudden blindness with diffuse retinal pallor and cherry-red spot in macula)

	Embolism (Postrheumatic Vegetation)	Common Carotid Artery Atherosclerosis*	Ischemia (Aortic Arch Syndrome)	Inflammation (Temporal Arteritis)*	Sickle Cell Disease*	Lupus Erythematosus
History						
1. Amaurosis fugax	S	U	U			
2. Bilateral			U	S		
3. Common in blacks					U	S
4. Common in females			S			U
5. Common in young adults	U		S			U
6. Diplopia	R			S		
7. Older age			U	U		
8. Orbital and ocular pain		S				
9. Photopsias	S	S	S			
10. Subjective field loss			S			
11. Untreated group A streptococcal pharyngitis	S					
Physical Findings						
1. Acute anterior uveitis	R	R				R
2. Afferent pupillary defect				U		
3. Angioid streaks					S	
4. Arteriosclerotic retinopathy		S				
5. Arteriovenous retinal shunts			U		S	S
6. Bright choroidal plaques		U			S	
7. Cataract		S	S			
8. Conjunctival coma signs					U	
9. Conjunctival hemorrhages—petechial	U					
10. Conjunctival icterus or pallor					S	
11. Conjunctival phlyctenulae						S
12. Corneal ulcer						S
13. Cortical blindness				S		
14. Cotton-wool spots	S	S	S	U	S	S
15. Deep stromal keratitis						S
16. Dilated episcleral vessels		S				
17. Disc neovascularization					R	
18. Episcleritis						S
19. Erythema/scaling of eyelids						U
20. External ophthalmoplegia			S	S		
21. Glaucoma		S	S			
22. Hypertensive retinopathy		S				
23. Hypotony of globe		S		S		
24. Keratoconjunctivitis sicca						S
25. Lid telangiectasis						S
26. Localized yellowish deep choroidal lesions	S					
27. Macular holes					S	

Retinal artery occlusion (sudden blindness with diffuse retinal pallor and cherry-red spot in macula) Continued

	Embolism (Postrheumatic Vegetation)	Common Carotid Artery Atherosclerosis*	Ischemia (Aortic Arch Syndrome)	Inflammation (Temporal Arteritis)*	Sickle Cell Disease*	Lupus Erythematosus
Physical Findings						
28. Occluded arteries		U	S			
29. Optic atrophy		S		S	S	S
30. Optic neuritis						S
31. Papilledema	S			S		S
32. Peripapillary arteriovenous anastomosis			S			
33. Peripheral retinal holes					S	
34. Pseudo Foster-Kennedy syndrome				S		
35. Ptosis				S		R
36. Retinal detachment			S		S	S
37. Retinal hemorrhages		S		U	S	S
38. Retinal microaneurysms		S	S		S	
39. Retinal neovascularization			R		S	
40. Retinal vein occlusion						S
41. Retinal venous dilation		S	S			S
42. Retinitis proliferans			S			
43. Roth spots	U	U				
44. Rubeosis iridis/iris atrophy		S	S		R	
45. Salmon patches in retina					S	
46. Scleritis				S		S
47. Tonic pupil				S		
48. Uveitis						S
49. Vascular tortuosity					S	
50. Vitreous hemorrhage			S		S	
51. White wedge-shaped infarcts in choroid					S	
Laboratory Data						
1. Abnormal ophthalmodynamometry		S	U			
2. Biopsy of temporal artery: fragmentation of the elastic lamina, smooth muscle necrosis, cellular infiltration with lymphocytes, epithelioid cells and giant cells				U		
3. Carotid arteriography		S				
4. Depression of hemoglobin, white blood cells and platelets						U
5. Elevated antistreptolysin titer	S					
6. Elevated C reactive protein	S					
7. Elevated ESR	S			U		
8. Elevated white blood cells	U					
9. False positive STS (serologic test for syphillis)						U
10. Fluorescein angiography abnormal	U	U	U	U	U	S
11. Hemoglobin electrophoresis: presence of HbS					U	
12. L.E. cells positive						U
13. Positive antinulcear antibody trait						U
14. Positive throat culture for group A streptococcus	S					

R = rarely; S = sometimes; and U = usually.

* = most important

LOCALIZED ARTERIAL NARROWING

1. Retinal atrophy following:
   A. Degeneration
   B. Inflammation
   C. Trauma
   D. Treatment with diathermy, light, or cryopexy
2. Any vascular retinopathy

Nover A. *The ocular fundus: methods of examination and typical findings,* 4th ed. Philadelphia: Lea & Febiger, 1981.

Perkins ES, Dobree JH. *The differential diagnosis of fundus conditions.* St. Louis: CV Mosby, 1972.

GENERALIZED ARTERIAL NARROWING

1. Local causes
   A. Apparent narrowing
      (1) High hypermetropia—common, small disc, narrow vessels, sometimes pseudopapilledema (see p. 601)
      (2) Congenital microphthalmos—rare, hypermetropia, often cataract (see p. 252–253)
      (3) Aphakia—cataract operation, dislocated lens (see p. 405)
      (4) Hollenhorst syndrome (chorioretinal infarction syndrome)
      (5) Wagner syndrome (hyaloideoretinal degeneration)
   B. Trauma
      (1) Avulsion of optic nerve—rare, secondary optic atrophy
      (2) Fracture involving bony optic canal—rare, secondary optic atrophy
      (3) Following retroocular injection—rare secondary optic atrophy
      (4) Orbital hemorrhage following retroocular injection or orbital operation—rare, secondary optic atrophy
      (5) Carotid ligation for carotid—cavernous fistula, rare, secondary optic atrophy
      (6) Following angiography—rare, secondary optic atrophy
      (7) Siderosis bulbi—metallic intraocular foreign body
   C. Infection and edema
      (1) Orbital cellulitis—exophthalmos, restricted ocular movements
      (2) Following thyrotropic exophthalmos—ocular muscle paresis, lid retraction
   D. Degenerations, such as progressive cone-rod degeneration
   E. Primary tapetoretinal degenerations, such as retinitis pigmentosa; Hallgren syndrome (retinitis pigmentosa-deafness-ataxia syndrome)
2. Systemic disease
   A. Arteriosclerosis
      (1) In involutionary sclerosis—population older than 50 years of age, generalized arteriolar narrowing, diminished light reflexes
      (2) In arteriosclerotic disease
         a. Arteriosclerotic central artery occlusion—common arteriovenous crossing signs, focal arteriolar constriction
         *b. Embolus from atheromatous plaque, common, sudden onset, visible white embolus

B. Hypertensive conditions
   *(1) Essential hypertension—retinal hemorrhages, cotton-wool spots, arterio-venous crossing signs
   *(2) Malignant hypertension—retinal hemorrhages, cotton-wool spots, edema of disc
   (3) Toxemia of pregnancy—rare, sometimes hemorrhages, cotton-wool spots, edema of disc, serous detachment
   (4) Coarctation of aorta—rare, hypertensive changes vary greatly in degree
   (5) Pheochromocytoma—rare, hypertensive changes vary greatly in degree
   (6) Adrenal tumor, hyperaldosteronism (adrenal medulla tumor syndrome)—rare, hypertensive changes vary greatly in degree
   (7) Cushing tumor (adrenocortical hyperfunction)—rare, hypertensive changes vary greatly in degree
   (8) Motor-neuron disease of cervicothoracic cord hypertension; may occur after prolonged artificial pulmonary ventilation

C. Other forms of vascular disease
   (1) Retinal ischemia—hypotension following severe or recurrent bleeding, unilateral blindness in patients
   *(2) Temporal arteritis (cranial arteritis, giant-cell arteritis)—common, 50 years or older; mean age at onset, 55 years; sudden blindness at onset
   (3) Polyarteritis nodosa (Kussmaul disease)—multiple signs involving choroid, retina, cornea, episclera, and ocular muscles
   (4) Proliferative diabetic retinopathy—arterial narrowing occurs in 17% of patients with proliferative diabetic retinopathy, mainly in cicatricial stage
   (5) Cardiac arrest—thread-like arterioles, segmentation of blood column, generalized retinal pallor, pallor of disc, sometimes macular cherry-red spot
   (6) Raynaud disease (idiopathic paroxysmal digital cyanosis)—young adults, more common in women

D. Renal disease
   (1) Acute glomerulonephritis—preceding illnesses, including scarlet fever, streptococcal tonsillitis, otitis media, erysipelas (St. Anthony fire), subacute bacterial endocarditis, polyarteritis nodosa (Kussmaul disease)
   (2) Chronic glomerulonephritis—often asymptomatic and found on routine examination
   (3) Pyelonephritis and pyelitis—most common causes of renal failure

E. Diseases of the central nervous system
   (1) Migraine
   *(2) Syphilitic neuroretinitis
   (3) Viral neuroretinitis (rare complication)
   (4) Tay–Sachs disease (amaurotic familial idiocy)
   (5) Jansky–Bielschowsky disease (amaurotic familial idiocy, late form)
   (6) Myotonic dystrophy syndrome (Curschmann–Steinert syndrome)
   (7) Retinohypophysis syndrome (Lijo Pavia–Lis syndrome)
   (8) Zellweger syndrome (cerebrohepatorenal syndrome of Zellweger)

F. Toxic causes
   (1) Chloroquine, hydroxychloroquine, quinacrine, amodiaquine
   (2) Lead
   (3) Quinine—rare, may follow large dose (abortifacient) or normal dose in sensitive subjects

* = most important

G. Other causes
   (1) Caisson syndrome (bends)
   (2) Chédiak–Higashi syndrome (oculocutaneous albinism with recurrent infections; autosomal recessive)
   (3) Hunter syndrome (MPS II)
   (4) Sanfilippo–Good syndrome (MPS III)

Perkins ES, Dobree JH. *The differential diagnosis of fundus conditions.* St. Louis: CV Mosby, 1972.

Roy FH. *Ocular syndromes and systemic diseases,* 3rd ed. Philadelphia: Lippincott Williams & Wilkins, 2002.

PERIARTERITIS RETINALIS SEGMENTALIS

White or yellow plaques are arranged in segments encircling arteries like a cuff and are localized to one or more arterial branches.

  *1. Arteriosclerosis secondary to vein obstruction
   2. Herpes zoster
   3. Hypercholesterolemia
   4. Lupus erythematosus (disseminated lupus erythematosus)
   5. Metastatic uveitis
   6. Periarteritis nodosa (necrotizing angiitis)
  *7. Sarcoidosis syndrome
   8. Syphilis (acquired lues)
  *9. Temporal arteritis (giant cell arteritis)
 *10. Tuberculous retinitis
  11. Uveitis, idiopathic

Crouch ER, Goldberg MF. Retinal periarteritis secondary to syphilis. *Arch Ophthalmol* 1975;93:384–387.

Rask AJ. Peri-arteritis retinalis segmentalis. *Acta Ophthalmol* 1969;47:234–237.

FROSTED-BRANCH ANGITIS

In this condition, unusual thick sheathing surrounds all the retinal veins and less often the arteries, making them look like frosted tree branches.

   1. Herpes simplex viruses types 1 and 2
   2. Acute lymphoblastic leukemia
   3. Large cell lymphoma
   4. Crohn disease
   5. Systemic lupus erythematosus
   6. Acquired immune deficiency syndrome

Kim TS, et al. Retinal angiopathy resembling unilateral frosted branch angiitis in a patient with relapsing acute lymphoblastic leukemia. *Am J Ophthalmol* 1994;117,6:806–808.

Ridley ME, et al. Retinal manifestations of ocular lymphoma. *J Ophthalmol* 1992;99,7:1153–1161.

SHEATHING OF RETINAL VEINS

In this condition, white or gray envelopes are around veins; retinal or vitreous hemorrhage and exudates may be present.

   1. Disc only—developmental
   2. Disc and retina—papillitis or papilledema

3. Peripheral sheathing
   *A. Acute retinal necrosis
   B. Amebiasis
   C. Behçet disease (dermatostomatoophthalmic syndrome)
   D. Brucellosis—rare, tortuosity and sheathing of veins, vitreous haze, retinal hemorrhages
   E. Candidiasis
   F. Coccidioidomycosis
   G. Eales disease (periphlebitis)
   H. Diabetes mellitus
   I. Filariasis—hemorrhages and exudates
   J. Hypertension
   K. Infectious mononucleosis—peripheral or central perivascular involvement, venous engorgement and sheathing associated with retinal hemorrhages
   L. Lupus erythematosus
   M. Non-Hodgkin lymphoma
   N. Onchocerciasis syndrome (river blindness)
   O. Rickettsial infections—peripheral or central perivascular involvement, venous engorgement and sheathing associated with retinal hemorrhages
   *P. Sarcoidosis
   Q. Septicemia and bacteremia—rare, venous engorgement, usually with multiple hemorrhages and focal sheathing
   R. Sickle cell disease
   S. Syphilis (secondary) (acquired lues)
   T. Tuberculin or bacille Calmette–Guérin (BCG) vaccination—rare, sectorial, or generalized changes
   U. Viral infections, including the following:
      (1) Cytomegalovirus retinitis
      (2) Herpes simplex (likely responsible for acute retinal necrosis)
      (3) Herpes zoster ophthalmicus
      (4) Influenza
      (5) Rift Valley fever
4. Peripheral sheathing without secondary retinopathy—multiple sclerosis
5. Wide and usually dense sheathing of dilated and tortuous veins, suggestive of myelogenous leukemia

Brown S, et al. Intraocular lymphoma presenting as retinal vasculitis. *Surv Ophthalmol* 1994;39:138–140.

George RK, et al. Primary retinal vasculitis. *Opthalmology* 1996;103:384–389.

Kohno T, et al. Ocular manifestations of adult T-cell leukemia/lymphoma. *Ophthalmology* 1993;100:1794–1799.

Roy FH. *Ocular syndromes and systemic diseases,* 3rd ed. Philadelphia: Lippincott Williams & Wilkins, 2002.

ABSENT VENOUS PULSATIONS (SPONTANEOUS VENOUS PULSATIONS ABSENT AT VENULES ON THE DISC)

1. Normal individuals
*2. Impending central vein occlusion (see p. 468)
*3. Papilledema (see p. 593–601)

Ballantyne AJ, Michaelson IC. *Textbook of the fundus of the eye,* 3rd ed. Baltimore: Williams & Wilkins, 1981.

Newell FW. *Ophthalmology: principles and practice,* 7th ed. St. Louis: CV Mosby, 1991.

* = most important

DILATED RETINAL VEINS

Normally, the arteriole–venule ratio is 2:3; with an increase in this ratio, the retinal veins may be dilated.

1. Congenital
    A. Congenital tortuosity of retinal vessels—rare, sometimes associated with coarctation of aorta
    B. Fabry disease (hereditary dystrophic lipidosis)
    C. Hemangioma
    D. Longfellow–Graether syndrome
    E. Ocular fundi in newborns
    F. Racemose (arteriovenous) aneurysm—rare, arteriovenous anastomoses localized to sector of retina
    *G. Retinopathy of prematurity with plus disease
    H. von Hippel–Lindau disease (angiomatosis)—familial in 20% of cases, bilateral in 50%
2. Trauma and inflammation
    A. Anterior uveitis—dilatation of veins, often slight hyperemia of disc
    B. Carotid-cavernous fistula—fracture of base of skull, progressive exophthalmos, bruit
    C. Cavernous sinus thrombosis—rare, proptosis and orbital edema
    *D. Impending obstruction of the central retinal vein
    E. Periphlebitis—sheathing of vessels
3. Cardiovascular disease—dilatation may be present but rarely dominates the fundus picture
    A. Arteriosclerosis
    B. Involutionary sclerosis (later stages)
    C. Secondary to defective arterial flow, such as in the following:
        (1) Aortic arch syndrome (pulseless disease)
        (2) Cardiac insufficiency
        (3) Congenital heart disease
        (4) Iatrogenic (lowering of blood pressure)
        (5) Severe blood loss
        *(6) Stenosis or occlusion of common carotid
        *(7) Temporal arteritis
        (8) Venous stasis (hypotensive retinopathy of Kearns and Hollenhorst)
    D. Heritable thrombophilia and hypofibrinolysis
4. Respiratory disease—venous dilatation may occur with purplish hue of whole retina; obstruction of venous return from the head, such as in the following:
    A. Congenital septal defect (Fallot tetralogy)
    B. Emphysema
    C. Hamman–Rich syndrome (diffuse pulmonary fibrosis syndrome)
    D. Heart failure of any type
    E. Kartagener syndrome (sinusitis–bronchiectasis–situs inversus syndrome)
    F. Mechanical compression of chest
    G. Mediastinal tumor obstructing superior vena cava
5. Diseases of the central nervous system
    *A. Carotid-cavernous fistula—fractured base of skull; rupture of berry aneurysm, arteriosclerosis

B. Hemangioma of posterior fossa—rare, papilledema, often grossly dilated veins

C. Optic nerve lesion—rare, secondary to orbital space-occupying lesion

*D. Papilledema (see p. 593–601)

E. Retrolenticular syndrome (Dejerine–Roussy syndrome)

*F. Subarachnoid hemorrhage—head injury; subhyaloid hemorrhages near disc, dilated veins, sometimes papilledema

6. Blood diseases

A. Aplastic anemia—hemorrhage is the most striking sign, often spreading around the disc

B. Cryoglobulinemia—rare, may occur with multiple myeloma, veins dilated, tortuous, and sometimes beaded

C. Gansslen syndrome (familial hemolytic icterus)

D. Lymphatic leukemia

E. Macrocytic anemia of all types—common, retinopathy absent unless hemoglobin below 50%; pale fundus, superficial hemorrhages, cotton-wool spots
  (1) Pernicious anemia
  (2) Steatorrhea
  (3) Celiac disease
  (4) Carcinoma of stomach

F. Macroglobulinemia—rare; veins dilated tortuous and sometimes beaded, hemorrhages and occasionally microaneurysms

G. Monocytic leukemia

H. Myelogenous leukemia

I. Multiple myeloma (Kahler disease)

J. Polycythemia rubra vera (primary; Vaquez disease)—common in males; hemorrhages; papilledema may be marked and venous thrombosis may occur

K. Secondary polycythemia—common; hemorrhages, papilledema and venous thrombosis may occur

L. Sickle cell disease—dilatation of peripheral veins with retinal, subhyaloid, and vitreous hemorrhages

M. Thrombocytopenic purpura—retinal and subhyaloid hemorrhages near disc, moderate venous dilatation

7. Acute febrile illnesses—rare, occasional dilatation of retinal veins with a few hemorrhages and mild edema of disc

A. Infectious mononucleosis

B. Influenza

C. Rickettsial infections

D. Septicemia

8. Metabolic diseases

A. Cystic fibrosis syndrome (fibrocystic disease of pancreas)—venous congestion often swelling of disc

B. Plasma lecithin

*C. Diabetic retinopathy—larger veins affected, often beaded

9. Collagen diseases

A. Polyarteritis nodosa—among other fundus lesions, dilated veins may occur

B. Sclerosis, progressive systemic (scleroderma)

* = most important

   C. Systemic lupus erythematosus—cotton-wool spots, occasional hemorrhages, and moderate dilatation of veins
10. Toxic conditions, such as methyl alcohol ingestion

Glueck CJ, et al. Heritable thrombophilia and hypofibrinolysis—possible causes of retinal vein occlusion. *Arch Ophthalmol* 1999;117:43–49.

Newell FW. *Ophthalmology: principles and practice,* 7th ed. St. Louis: CV Mosby, 1991.

Roy FH. *Ocular syndromes and systemic diseases,* 3rd ed. Philadelphia: Lippincott Williams & Wilkins, 2002.

TORTUOSITY OF RETINAL VEINS AND HYPOPLASIA OF OPTIC NERVES

1. Endocrinopathy, especially pituitary deficiency
2. Alcohol abuse; fetal alcohol syndrome
3. Migraine disturbances
4. Agenesis of the corpus callosum associated with mutations
5. Preterm birth also associated with retinal artery/visceral tortuosity

Hellstrom A, et al. Optic nerve hypoplasia with isolated tortuosity of the retinal veins. *Arch Ophthalmol* 1999;117: 880–884.

CENTRAL RETINAL VEIN OCCLUSION

This condition is characterized by massive hemorrhage into the posterior portion of the eye and dilated retinal veins.

1. External compression of the vein
   A. Atherosclerosis of central retinal artery
   B. Connective tissue strand within the floor of the physiologic excavation
   C. Multiple crossings of the same artery and vein or congenital venous loops or twists in the retinal surface
   D. Pseudotumor cerebri
2. Degenerative or inflammatory venous disease, causing detachment, proliferation, and hydrops
   A. Acquired immunodeficiency syndrome (AIDS; HIV retinopathy)
   B. Arterial hypertension
   C. Arteriovenous malformations of retina
   D. Cardiac decompensation
   E. Closed-head trauma
   *F. Diabetes mellitus (Willis disease)
   G. Ipsilateral internal carotid artery stenosis
   H. Lyme disease
   I. Optic disc drusen
   J. Optic nerve inflammation
   K. Sarcoidosis
   L. Serpiginous choroiditis
   M. Systemic granulomatous disease, particularly tuberculosis
3. Thrombosis from venous stagnation
   A. Spasm of corresponding retinal arterioles
   B. Blood dyscrasias
      (1) Cryoglobulinemia
      (2) Emphysema with secondary erythrocytosis

(3) Deficiencies in endemic pathway (factor V R506Q mutation)

(4) Homocystinemia

(5) Increased platelet aggregation

(6) Leukemias

(7) Lymphoma

*(8) Multiple myeloma

*(9) Polycythemia vera

(10) Sickle cell disease

C. Increased viscosity of the blood

    (1) Cystic fibrosis of pancreas

    (2) Following peritoneal dialysis

    (3) Hyperproteinemia

   *(4) Macroglobulinemia

    (5) Use of tranexamic acid

D. Sudden reduction of systemic blood pressure because of cardiac decompensation, surgical or traumatic shock, or therapy for arterial hypertension

*E. Glaucoma (preexisting)

F. Increased risk of thrombosis

    (1) Hereditary

       a. Antithrombin III deficiency

       b. Protein C deficiency or protein S deficiency

       c. Rare disorders of fibrinogen and fibrinolysis

         (i) Certain dysfibrinogenemias

         (ii) Abnormal plasminogen

    (2) Acquired

       a. Carcinoma

       b. Hematologic proliferative disorders

         (i) Acute promyelocytic leukemia

         (ii) Myeloproliferative disorders (polycythemia, essential thrombo-cythemia)

       c. Behçet syndrome

       d. Lupus anticoagulant

       e. Nephrosis

       f. Complications of therapy

         (i) Oral contraceptives

         (ii) Infusion of prothrombin complex concentrates

         (iii) Heparin-induced thrombocytopenia

G. Carotid–cavernous sinus fistula

*H. Syphilis

I. With immunoglobulin G (IgG) lambda monoclonal gammopathy

J. Coil embolization of carotid–ophthalmic aneurysms

K. Oral contraceptive

Castillo B, et al. Retinal artery occlusion following coil embolization of carotid–ophthalmic aneurysms. *Arch Ophthalmol* 2000;118:851–852.

Enzenauer RW, et al. Central retinal vein occlusion in a patient with IgG lambda monoclonal gammopathy. *Arch Ophthalmol* 1999;117:134–135.

Greiner K, et al. Retinal vascular occlusion and deficiencies in the protein C pathway. *Am J Opthalmol* 1999;128: 69–74.

* = most important

Hayreh SS, et al. Systemic diseases associated with various types of retinal vein occlusion. *Am J Ophthalmol* 2001; 131:61–78.

Rath EZ, et al. Risk factors for retinal vein occlusions: a case-control study. *Ophthalmology* 1992;99:509–514.

Sagripanti A, et al. Thrombin–antithrombin III complex in acute retinal vein occlusion. *Am J Ophthalmol* 1999; 128,1:124.

Wenzler EM, et al. Hyperhomocystinemia in retinal artery and retinal vein occlusion. *Am J Ophthalmol* 1993;115: 162–167.

Central retinal vein occlusion

	External Vein Compression as Central Retinal Artery Atherosclerosis*	Inflammatory Venous Disease as Diabetes Mellitus*	Blood Dyscrasias as Leukemia	Increased Blood Viscosity as Macroglobulinemia	Glaucoma*
History					
1. Amaurosis fugax	U				
2. Common in males				U	
3. Common in persons more than 40 years		U		U	U
4. Common in persons more than 60 years	U				
5. Congenital					S
6. Familial		U	S		S
7. Orbital/ocular pain	S				
8. Photopsias	U				
Physical Findings					
1. Anterior ischemic optic neuropathy	S	S			
2. Arterial occlusions	U				
3. Arteriosclerotic retinopathy	U				
4. Bright plaques	U				
5. Cataract	S	U			S
6. Closed anterior chamber angle					U
7. Conjunctivitis, papillary			U		
8. Corneal edema	S				U
9. Corneal hypesthesia					U
10. Cotton-wool spots		U	U	S	
11. Crystalline deposits in conjunctiva/cornea				U	
12. Dilated episcleral veins	S				
13. Ectropion uvea		S			
14. Elevated intraocular pressure	S		S	U	U
15. Engorgement of conjunctival vessels			U		
16. Extraocular muscle paralysis		S	S		
17. Folds in Descemet membrane					U
18. Glaucomatous cupping					U
19. Hard exudates		U			
20. Hypopyon			S		
21. Iris atrophy	S				U
22. Iris synechiae	S				U
23. Keratoconjunctivitis sicca				U	
24. Macular edema		S	U		
25. Optic atrophy	S	S	S		U
26. Optic neuritis			S		
27. Papilledema		S	S	S	S
28. Retinal detachment			S		
29. Retinal hemorrhages	S	U	U		
30. Retinal microaneurysms	S	U		U	
31. Retinal neovascularization	S	U			
32. Retinal venous dilation	S			U	

* = most important

Central retinal vein occlusion (Continued)

	External Vein Compression as Central Retinal Artery Atherosclerosis*	Inflammatory Venous Disease as Diabetes Mellitus*	Blood Dyscrasias as Leukemia	Increased Blood Viscosity as Macroglobulinemia	Glaucoma*
Physical Findings					
33. Retinal venous thrombosis				U	
34. Rubeosis iridis	S	U			U
35. Visual field defects					U
36. Vitreous hemorrhage	S	S			
37. Vitreous opacities			S		
Laboratory Data					
1. Blood sugar elevated		U			
2. Bone marrow puncture			U	U	
3. Carotid arteriography	S				
4. Fluorescein angiography	U	U	U		
5. Lipid profile	U				
6. Peripheral blood test			U	U	
7. Serum gamma M immunoglobulin elevated				U	
8. Visual field test					U

R = rarely; S = sometimes; and U = usually.

DILATED RETINAL VEINS AND RETINAL HEMORRHAGES

  1. Carotid–cavernous fistula
 *2. Cavernous sinus fistula syndrome (carotid artery syndrome)
  3. Cavernous sinus thrombosis (hypophyseal-sphenoidal syndrome)
 *4. Central retinal vein occlusion (see p. 468)
  5. Cervical tuberculosis
  6. Choroidal melanoma remote to the neovascularization
  7. Congenital tortuosity and dilatation of the retinal vessels
  8. Cryoglobulinemia
 *9. Diabetes mellitus
 10. Intravitreal myiasis
 11. Leukemia
 12. Lymphomas
 13. Macroglobulinemia (Waldenström syndrome)
 14. Multiple myeloma (myelomatosis)
 15. Ophthalmic vein thrombosis
 16. Pappataci fever (phlebotomus fever)
 17. Paraproteinemias and dysproteinemias
 18. Polycythemia vera
 19. Retinal arteritis
*20. Sickle cell disease
*21. Syphilis (acquired lues)

Kalina RE, Kaiser M. Familial retinal hemorrhages. *Am J Ophthalmol* 1972;74:252–255.

Roy FH. *Ocular syndromes and systemic diseases,* 3rd ed. Philadelphia: Lippincott Williams & Wilkins, 2002.

RETINAL HEMORRHAGES

Retinal hemorrhages include bleeding that may be intraretinal or preretinal hemorrhages into the vitreous or subretinal hemorrhages.

  1. Congestion of the head and neck, such as in newborns, in hanging, or during choking
  2. Trauma, including electrical injury, hypothermal injury, and child abuse
  3. Vascular obstruction, such as cardiorespiratory obesity syndrome, cystic fibrosis syndrome, negative acceleration syndrome, (hydrostatic pressure syndrome), ophthalmoplegic migraine syndrome, papilledema (see p. 593–601), subarachnoid hemorrhages, superior vena cava syndrome, Symonds syndrome (benign intracranial hypertension), thrombocytopenia, thrombosis, and Wernicke syndrome (avitaminosis B_1)
  4. Inflammatory conditions, such as Criswick–Schepens syndrome (familial exudative vitreoretinopathy), Loffler syndrome (eosinophilic pneumonitis), perivasculitis, and subacute bacterial endocarditis
 *5. Acute febrile and infectious illnesses, including amebiasis ankylostomiasis, aspergillosis, bacterial endocarditis, coccidioidomycosis, cryptococcosis (torulosis), cysticercosis, dengue fever, hydatid cyst (echinococcosis), hydrophobia (rabies), infectious mononucleosis, influenza, Japanese River fever (typhus), lymphogranuloma venereum (Nicolas–Favre disease), metastatic bacterial endophthalmitis, nematode ophthalmia syndrome (toxocariasis), pertussis (whooping cough), Q fever, relapsing fever, trichinellosis, Weil disease (leptospirosis), and yersiniosis
 *6. Vascular disease, such as arteriosclerosis, atherosclerosis, arteriovenous fistula, disseminated intravascular coagulation, hypertension, Paget syndrome (hypertensive di-

* = most important

encephalic syndrome), progressive systemic sclerosis, pulmonary insufficiency, the retinopathies, particularly diabetic and hypertensive, and when the circulation through the eye is diminished in hypotensive retinopathy, such as in carotid vascular insufficiency syndrome or pulseless disease (Takayasu syndrome), suprarenal–sympathetic syndrome, temporal arteritis syndrome (cranial arteritis syndrome), and in conditions of extreme cachexia

7. Anemia that may be secondary to drugs, including the following:

acebutolol
acenocoumarin
acetaminophen
acetanilid
acetazolamide
acetohexamide
acetophenazine
actinomycin C
acyclovir
allobarbital
allopurinol
alprazolam
aminopterin
aminosalicylate (?)
aminosalicylic acid (?)
amithiozone
amitriptyline
amobarbital
amodiaquine
amoxicillin
amphotericin B
ampicillin
antazoline
anisindione
antimony lithium thiomalate
antimony potassium tartrate
antimony sodium tartrate
antimony sodium
  thioglycollate
antipyrine
aprobarbital
atenolol
auranofin
aurothioglucose
aurothioglycanide
azatadine
azathioprine
barbital
BCG vaccine
bendroflumethiazide
benzathine penicillin G

benzthiazide
bishydroxycoumarin
bleomycin
brompheniramine
busulfan
butabarbital
butalbital
butallylonal
butaperazine
butethal
cactinomycin
calcitriol
captopril
carbamazepine
carbenicillin
carbimazole
carbinoxamine
carisoprodol
carmustine
carphenazine
cefaclor
cefadroxil
cefamandole
cefazolin
cefonicid
cefoperazone
ceforanide
cefotaxime
cefotetan
cefoxitin
cefsulodin
ceftizoxime
ceftriaxone
cefuroxime
cephalexin
cephaloglycin
cephaloridine
cephalothin
cephapirin
cephradine
chlorambucil

chloramphenicol
chlordiazepoxide
chloroquine
chlorothiazide
chlorpheniramine
chlorpromazine
chlorpropamide
chlorprothixene
chlortetracycline
chlorthalidone
cholecalciferol
cimetidine
cisplatin
clemastine
clindamycin
clofibrate
clonazepam
clorazepate
cloxacillin
colchicine
cyclobarbital
cyclopentobarbital
cyclophosphamide
cycloserine
cyclosporine
cyclothiazide
cyproheptadine
cytarabine
dacarbazine
dactinomycin
dapsone
daunorubicin
deferoxamine
demeclocycline
desipramine
dexbrompheniramine
dexchlorpheniramine
diazepam
diazoxide
dichlorphenamide
dicloxacillin

dicumarol
diethazine
diltiazem
dimercaprol
dimethindene
dimethyl sulfoxide
diphenadione
diphenhydramine
diphenylhydantoin
diphenylpyraline
diphtheria and tetanus
   toxoids and pertussis
   vaccine (adsorbed)
doxorubicin
doxycycline
doxylamine
dromostanolone
droperidol
enalapril
ergocalciferol
erythromycin
ethacrynic acid
ethopropazine
ethosuximide
ethotoin
ethoxzolamide
ethyl biscoumacetate
fenfluramine
fenoprofen
flecainide
floxuridine
fluorouracil
fluoxymesterone
fluphenazine
flurazepam
furosemide
gentamicin
glutethimide
glyburide
gold Au 198
gold sodium thiomalate
gold sodium thiosulfate
griseofulvin
guanethidine
halazepam
haloperidol
heparin
heptabarbital
hetacillin

hexethal
hexobarbital
hydrabamine penicillin V
hydralazine
hydrabamine phenoxymethyl
   penicillin
hydrochlorothiazide
hydroflumethiazide
hydroxychloroquine
hydroxyurea
ibuprofen
imipramine
indapamide
indomethacin
influenza virus vaccine
interferon
isocarboxazid
isoniazid
labetalol
levodopa
lincomycin
lithium carbonate
lomustine
lorazepam
loxapine
maprotiline
measles and rubella virus
   vaccine (live)
measles, mumps and rubella
   virus vaccine (live)
measles virus vaccine (live)
mechlorethamine
mefenamic acid
melphalan
mephenytoin
mephobarbital
meprobamate
mercaptopurine
mesoridazine
methacycline
methaqualone
metharbital
methazolamide
methdilazine
methicillin
methimazole
methitural
methohexital
methotrimeprazine

methotrexate
methsuximide
methyclothiazide
methyldopa
methylene blue
methylphenidate
methylthiouracil
methyprylon
metolazone
metoprolol
metrizamide
metronidazole
mexiletine
mianserin
midazolam
minocycline
mitomycin
moxalactam
mumps virus vaccine (live)
nadolol
nafcillin
nalidixic acid
naproxen
nialamide
nifedipine
nitrazepam
nitrofurantoin
nitroglycerin
nortriptyline
oral contraceptives
orphenadrine
oxacillin
oxazepam
oxyphenbutazone
oxytetracycline
paramethadione
penicillamine
pentobarbital
perazine
periciazine
perphenazine
phenacetin
phenelzine
phenformin
phenindione
pheniramine
phenobarbital
phenprocoumon
phensuximide

phenylbutazone
phenytoin
pindolol
piperacetazine
piperazine
pipobroman
poliovirus vaccine
polythiazide
potassium penicillin G
potassium penicillin V
potassium phenethicillin
prazepam
primidone
probarbital
procaine penicillin G
procarbazine
prochlorperazine
promazine
promethazine
propiomazine
propylthiouracil
protriptyline
pyrilamine
pyrimethamine
quinacrine
quinethazone
quinidine
quinine
ranitidine

rifampin
rubella and mumps virus
  vaccine (live)
rubella virus vaccine (live)
secobarbital
semustine
sodium antimonylgluconate
stibocaptate
stibogluconate
stibophen
streptomycin
sulfonamides
suramin
talbutal
temazepam
testolactone
testosterone
tetracycline
thiabendazole
thiamylal
thiethylperazine
thioguanine
thiopental
thiopropazate
thioproperazine
thioridazine
thiotepa
thiothixene
tocainide

tolazamide
tolazoline
tolbutamide
tranylcypromine
trazodone
triazolam
trichlormethiazide
triethylenemelamine
trifluoperazine
trifluperidol
triflupromazine
trimeprazine
trimethadione
tripelennamine
triprolidine
uracil mustard
urethan
vancomycin
verapamil
vidarabine
vinbarbital
vinblastine
vincristine
vitamin A
vitamin D
vitamin D_2
vitamin D_3
warfarin

8. Vascularized neoplasms, including hereditary hemorrhagic telangiectasia (Rendu–Osler–Weber disease), and periocular and ocular metastatic tumors

9. Drugs, including the following:

acetylcholine
acid bismuth sodium tartrate
adrenal cortex injection
aldosterone
allopurinol (?)
alseroxylon
aspirin
benoxinate
betamethasone
bismuth carbonate
bismuth oxychloride
bismuth salicylate
bismuth sodium tartrate
bismuth sodium
  thioglycollate

bismuth sodium
  triglycollamate
bismuth subcarbonate
bismuth subsalicylate
butacaine
cobalt (?)
cocaine
cortisone
deserpidine
desoxycorticosterone
dexamethasone
dibucaine
dyclonine
epinephrine
ethambutol

fludrocortisone
fluorometholone
fluorouracil
fluprednisolone
glycerin
heparin
hexachlorophene
hydrocortisone
indomethacin
iodide and iodine solution
  compounds
isosorbide
ketoprofen
lincomycin
mannitol

medrysone
meprednisone
methaqualone
methylphenidate
methylprednisolone
mithramycin
mitotane
oxyphenbutazone
paramethasone
penicillamine
phenacaine
phenylbutazone
piperocaine
plicamycin
pralidoxime
prednisolone
prednisone

proparacaine
radioactive iodides
rauwolfia serpentina
rescinnamine
reserpine
sodium chloride
sodium salicylate
sulfacetamide
sulfachlorpyridazine
sulfacytine
sulfadiazine
sulfadimethoxine
sulfamerazine
sulfameter
sulfamethazine
sulfamethizole
sulfamethoxazole

sulfamethoxypyridazine
sulfanilamide
sulfaphenazole
sulfapyridine
sulfasalazine
sulfathiazole
sulfisoxazole
sulindac
syrosingopine
tamoxifen
tetracaine
triamcinolone
trichloroethylene
urea
urokinase (?)
vitamin A

10. Hematopoietic system, such as the anemias, Bing–Neel syndrome (association of macroglobulinemia and central nervous system symptoms), Fanconi syndrome (amino diabetes), Gansslen syndrome (familial hemolytic icterus), Henoch-Schönlein purpura, Herrick syndrome (sickle cell disease), Jacobsen–Brodwell syndrome, leukemias, hemophilia, polycythemia, purpuras, oculootoororenoerythropoietic disease, Plummer–Vinson syndrome (sideropenic dysphagia syndrome), Reimann syndrome (hyperviscosity syndrome), Waldenström syndrome (macroglobulinemia syndrome), Wiskott–Aldrich syndrome (purpura), also following blood transfusion with incompatibility of blood groups

11. Acosta syndrome (mountain climber syndrome)

12. Amyloidosis

13. Behçet syndrome (dermatostomatoophthalmic syndrome)

14. Bloch–Sulzberger syndrome (incontinentia pigmenti)

15. Bourneville syndrome (tuberous sclerosis)

16. Epidural steroid injection, gas myelography, or epiduroscopy

17. Following labor induced by oxytocin or dinoprostone in newborns

18. Following use of YAG laser

19. Histiocytosis X (Hand–Schüller–Christian syndrome)

20. HIV-related retinopathy

21. Hodgkin disease

22. Juvenile diabetes—dwarfism–obesity syndrome

23. Macular degeneration, age related (exudative type)

24. Morning-glory syndrome (hereditary central glial anomaly of the optic disc)

25. Mycosis fungoides syndrome (Sézary syndrome)

26. Neuroblastoma

27. Optic nerve drusen (see p. 559–560)

28. Paget syndrome (osteitis deformans)

29. Plasma lecithin (cholesterol acyltransferase deficiency)

30. Polymyalgia rheumatica

31. Polymyositis dermatomyositis (Wagner–Unverricht syndrome)

32. Porphyria cutanea tarda

33. Purtscher retinopathy
34. Radiation retinopathy
35. Sarcoidosis syndrome (Schaumann syndrome)
36. Schamberg disease (self-limiting cutaneous vasculitis)
37. Terson syndrome

Amirikia A, et al. Acute bilateral visual loss associated with retinal hemorrhages following epiduroscopy. *Arch Ophthalmol* 2000;118:287–288.

Fraunfelder FT, Fraunfelder FW. *Drug-induced ocular side effects.* Woburn, MA: Butterworth-Heinemann, 2001.

Kivlin JD, et al. Shaken baby syndrome. *Ophthalmology* 2000;107:1246–1254.

Obana A, et al. Retinal and sublyaloid hemorrhage as a complication of laser iridectomy for primary angle-closure glaucoma. *Arch Ophthalmol* 2000;118:1449–1451.

Roy FH. *Ocular syndromes and systemic diseases,* 3rd ed. Philadelphia: Lippincott Williams & Wilkins, 2002.

Yu T, et al. Epidemiology and biostatistics. *Arch Opthalmol* 1998;116:83–89.

LARGE HEMORRHAGES IN THE FUNDUS OF AN INFANT OR YOUNG CHILD (SUGGESTIVE OF INCREASED INTRACRANIAL PRESSURE AND PARALYSIS OF CRANIAL NERVES)

1. Hygroma
*2. Shaken-baby syndrome
3. Subarachnoid hemorrhage
4. Subdural hematoma

Drack AV, et al. Unilateral retinal hemorrhages in documented cases of child abuse. *Am J Ophthalmol* 1999;128,3: 340–344.

Lambert SR, et al. Optic nerve sheath and retinal hemorrhages associated with the shaken baby syndrome. *Arch Ophthalmol* 1986;104:1509–1512.

Nover A. *The ocular fundus: methods of examination and typical findings,* 4th ed. Philadelphia: Lea & Febiger, 1981.

RETINOVITREAL HEMORRHAGE IN A YOUNG ADULT

1. Incontinentia pigmenti (Bloch–Sulzberger syndrome)
2. Congenital x-linked (juvenile) retinoschisis
*3. Diabetes mellitus
*4. Sickle cell anemia
5. Trauma
6. von Hippel–Lindau syndrome

Duke-Elder S. *System of ophthalmology,* Vol. X. St. Louis: CV Mosby, 1967.

Morse PH. *Vitreoretinal disease—a manual for diagnosis and treatment,* 2nd ed. St. Louis: CV Mosby, 1989.

RETINAL HEMORRHAGE WITH CENTRAL WHITE SPOT (ROTH SPOT)

1. Collagen disease
2. Cyanosis retinae—carcinoma of the lung
*3. Diabetes mellitus
4. Following heart surgery
5. Following uncomplicated pediatric cataract extraction
*6. Hematopoietic system
    A. Anemias
    B. Leukemia
    C. Multiple myeloma (Kahler disease)
7. Intracranial hemorrhage (infants)
8. Septic retinitis
    *A. *Candida albicans* infection
    B. Kala azar
    C. Phlebitis
    D. Rheumatic mitral and aortic valvulitis
    E. Rocky mountain spotted fever
    *F. Subacute bacterial endocarditis
    G. Syphilitic aortitis
    H. Viral pneumonia
9. Vascular disease

* = most important

Retinal hemorrhage with central white spot

	Septic Retinitis—Candida Albicans	Hematopoietic System—Leukemia	Diabetes Mellitus	Vascular Disease—Arteriovenous Fistula	Collagen Disease—Polyarteritis Nodosa	Cyanosis Retinae—Carcinoma of Lung
History						
1. Acute or chronic blood disorder		U				
2. Chronic mucocutaneous candidiasis	S					
3. Congenital				S		
4. Familial			U			
5. In overweight persons			U			
6. Males between ages 20 to 50					U	
7. More in females				S		
8. More in males					U	U
9. Over age 40				U		U
10. Secondary to penetrating or blunt trauma				U		
11. Systemic dissemination in drug addicts, in debilitated patients or immunosuppressed patients	U					
Physical Findings						
1. Asteroid hyalosis				S		
2. Blepharitis	S					
3. Cataract			U	S	S	
4. Cells and flare	U			S	U	
5. Chemosis				S		
6. Conjunctival cicatrization	S					
7. Conjunctival papillary hypertrophy		S				
8. Conjunctival necrosis				S		
9. Conjunctivitis	U				S	
10. Corneal stromal infiltrate	S					
11. Corneal stromal vascularization	S			S		
12. Corneal ulcer					S	
13. Cotton wool spots		U	U		U	
14. Dacryocystitis	S					
15. Darkening of blood column in conjunctival and retinal vessels						U
16. Ectropion uvea			S	U		
17. Eczema of eyelids	S					
18. Edema of eyelids	S			S		
19. Endophthalmitis	U					
20. Engorgement of conjunctival vessels		S				
21. Exophthalmos				S		
22. Exudative detachment of retina	U				U	
23. Glaucoma			S	S	S	
24. Granuloma of eyelids						
25. Hard yellow exudates of retina			U			
26. Hyperemia of eyelids	S					
27. Hyperemia of optic nerve	S					
28. Hypopyon	U	U				
29. Iris atrophy					R	
30. Irregular sheathing of retinal veins				U		
31. Irregularity of arterial caliber						U

Retinal hemorrhage with central white spot (Continued)

	Septic Retinitis—Candida Albicans	Hematopoietic System—Leukemia	Diabetes Mellitus	Vascular Disease—Arteriovenous Fistula	Collagen Disease—Polyarteritis Nodosa	Cyanosis Retinae—Carcinoma of Lung
Physical Findings						
32. Keratitis	S					
33. Lipemia retinalis			S			
34. Macular edema		S	S			S
35. Microaneurysms of retina			U			
36. Optic atrophy		S	S	S	S	
37. Optic neuritis		S	S			
38. Papilledema		S		S		S
39. Papillitis	S					
40. Panophthalmitis	U					
41. Paralysis of extraocular muscles		S	S	S	S	
42. Perivasculitis	S					
43. Phlyctenular keratoconjunctivitis	S					
44. Pseudoretinitis pigmentosa					S	
45. Ptosis				S	S	
46. Retinal atrophy	S					
47. Retinal degeneration					S	
48. Retinal detachment		S	S			
49. Retinal embolism			U			
50. Rubeosis iridis			S			
51. Scleritis					U	
52. Segmental inflammation of retinal arteries					S	
53. Tenonitis					U	
54. Uveitis					U	
55. Vascular engorgement in retina	S	U	U			U
56. Vitreal hemorrhages			U			
57. Vitreous abscess with cellular reaction	S					
58. Vitreous opacities	S	S				
Lab Data						
1. Aqueous and/or vitreous tap for candida isolation	U					
2. Biopsy of temporal artery shows typical arteritic lesion					S	
3. Biopsy of palpable nodules in the neck						S
4. Biopsy of tender muscle positive					S	
5. Blood tests						
—Anemia		U			U	
—Eosinophilia					S	
—E.S.R. elevated					U	
—Hyperglycemia more than 140 mg/L			U			
—Immature abnormal white cells in peripheral blood and bone marrow		U				
—Leukocytosis		U			U	
—Thrombocytopenia					U	
6. Bronchosopy for visualization and biopsy	R					U
7. Carotid arteriography abnormal				U		
8. Cerebral arteriography abnormal				S		
9. Roentgenograms of the skull abnormal				S		

Retinal hemorrhage with central white spot (Continued)	Septic Retinitis—Candida Albicans	Hemopoietic System—Leukemia	Diabetes Mellitus	Vascular Disease—Arteriovenous Fistula	Collagen Disease—Polyarteritis Nodosa	Cyanosis Retinae—Carcinoma of Lung
Lab Data						
10. Roentgenograms of chest abnormal						S
11. Urinalysis						
—Cylindruria					U	
—Glycosuria			U			
—Hematuria					U	
—Ketonuria			U			
—Proteinuria					U	

R = rarely; S = sometimes; and U = usually.

Mets MB, Del Monte M. Hemorrhagic retinopathy following uncomplicated pediatric cataract extraction. *Arch Ophthalmol* 1986;104:975.

Roy FH. *Ocular syndromes and systemic diseases,* 3rd ed. Philadelphia: Lippincott Williams & Wilkins, 2002.

MICROANEURYSMS OF RETINA (PUNCTATE RED SPOTS SCATTERED OVER REGION OF POSTERIOR POLE)

1. Aging
2. Aplastic anemia—punctate hemorrhage
3. Associated with cotton-wool spots (see p. 491)
4. Bonnet–Dechaume–Blanc syndrome (cerebroretinal arteriovenous aneurysm syndrome)
5. Choroiditis
6. Chronic uveitis
7. Coats disease (retinal telangiectasia)
*8. Diabetes mellitus
9. Disseminated lupus erythematosus (Kaposi–Libman–Sacks syndrome)
10. Eales disease (periphlebitis)
11. Fabry disease (diffuse angiokeratosis)
*12. Hypertension
13. Hypotensive retinopathy, such as pulseless disease (aortic arch syndrome)
14. Kahler disease (myelomatosis)
15. Leukemias—punctate hemorrhages
16. *Loa loa* infection
17. Macroglobulinemia (Waldenström syndrome)
18. Mauriac syndrome (juvenile diabetes–dwarfism–obesity syndrome)
19. Ocular ischemic syndrome (carotid occlusive disease)
20. Osler hemorrhagic telangiectasia (hereditary hemorrhagic telangiectasis)
21. Pelizaeus–Merzbacher syndrome (aplasia axialis extracorticalis congenita)
22. Reimann syndrome (hyperviscosity syndrome)
*23. Retinoblastoma
24. Sickle cell hemoglobin C disease
25. Skin divers
26. Subacute bacterial endocarditis
27. Venous occlusion—occlusion of central retinal vein or one of its branches (see p. 468)

Polkinghorne PJ, et al. Ocular fundus lesions in divers. *Lancet* 1988;Dec:1381–1383.

Roy FH. *Ocular syndromes and systemic diseases,* 3rd ed. Philadelphia: Lippincott Williams & Wilkins, 2002.

Sanders RJ, et al. Foveal avascular zone diameter and sickle cell disease. *Arch Ophthalmol* 1991;109:812–816.

Yu T, et al. Epidemiology and biostatistics. *Arch Opthalmol* 116:83–89.

* = most important

Microaneurysms of Retina

	Diabetes Mellitus*	Hypertensive Retinopathy*	Central Retinal Vein Occlusion	Blood Disorder as Leukemia	Hypotensive Retinopathy as Pulseless Disease	Retinoblastoma*	Leber Miliary Aneurysm	Subacute Bacterial Endocarditis	Eales Disease	Fabry Disease	Osler Hemorrhagic Teleangiectasia
History											
1. Acute or chronic blood disorder				U							
2. Elevated blood pressure		U									
3. Familial	U			S		S					
4. Hereditary				S		S	U			U	U
5. Japanese extraction					U						
6. Lipoid storage disorders										U	
7. More in females					U						
8. More in males									U		
9. More than 40 years	U										
10. Occurs in children/youth					U	U	S		U		
11. Occurs in middle to older age			U			S		U			
Physical Findings											
1. Asteroid hyalosis	S										
2. Cataract	U				U					U	
3. Central retinal artery occlusion										U	
4. Choroiditis								S			
5. Corneal opacity										U	
6. Cotton-wool spots	U	U	U	U	U						
7. Endophthalmitis						U					
8. Ectropion uvea	U										
9. Exophthalmos						S					
10. Extraocular muscle paralysis	S		S	S		U			U		
11. Filamentary keratitis											U
12. Glaucoma	S		U	S		U					
13. Hard yellow exudates	U										
14. Heterochromia iridis						U					
15. Hyphema						U					
16. Hypopyon				S		U					
17. Hypotony	S										
18. Iris atrophy					S						
19. Keratoconus							S				
20. Leukokoria						U					
21. Lid edema						U		U			
22. Lipemia retinalis	U										
23. Macular edema	S			S							
24. Mydriasis						U					
25. Nystagmus							S				
26. Optic nerve atrophy	S			S		S					
27. Optic neuritis				S				S			
28. Papilledema		U	S		S		U			U	
29. Papillary hypertrophy of conjunctiva				U							

Microaneurysms of Retina (Continued)	Diabetes Mellitus*	Hypertensive Retinopathy*	Central Retinal Vein Occlusion	Blood Disorder as Leukemia	Hypotensive Retinopathy as Pulseless Disease	Retinoblastoma*	Leber Miliary Aneurysm	Subacute Bacterial Endocarditis	Eales Disease	Fabry Disease	Osler Hemorrhagic Teleangiectasia
Physical Findings											
30. Retinal detachment		S		S						U	
31. Retinal hemorrhages	U	U	U	U							R
32. Retinal neovascularization	U		U						U		
33. Roth spots				U				U			
34. Retinal pigmentation (bone corpuscle or salt and pepper-like)							U				
35. Rubeosis iridis	U		U			U					
36. Small retinal angiomas											U
37. Star-shaped angiomas of the palpebral conjunctiva											U
38. Varicosities of palpebral and bulbar conjunctiva										U	
39. Vitreal hemorrhages	S	U				U			U		
40. Vitreous opacities				U				U			
Laboratory Data											
1. Angiographic brain studies					U						
2. Biopsy of tumor						S					
3. Blood culture								U			
4. Computed tomographic scan						U					
5. Chest roentgenogram									U		
6. ELISA for tuberculosis									U		
7. Fluorescein angiography	S	U	U	S	U				U		S
8. Glucose tolerance test or random blood sugar	U										
9. Lipid profile										U	
10. Ocular ultrasonography							U				
11. Ophthalmodynamometry					U						
12. Purified protein derivative									U		
13. Ultrasound of carotids					U						
14. Venereal disease reaction level					U						
15. Visual fields			U								
16. White blood cell count, hemoglobin, hematocrit				U							

R = rarely; S = sometimes; and U = usually.

* = most important

RETINAL ARTERIOVENOUS SHUNT AT THE ARTERIOVENOUS CROSSING

1. Diabetic retinopathy
2. Leber's miliary aneurysm
3. Retinal vein occlusion
4. Takayasu disease

Tanaka T, et al. Retinal arteriovenous shunt at the arteriovenous crossing. *Ophthalmology* 1998;105:1251–1258.

Tanaka T, Shimizu K. Retinal arteriovenous shunts in Takayasu disease. *Ophthalmology* 1987;94:1380–1388.

MACROANEURYSMS OF RETINAL ARTERIES

These macroaneurysms are found within the first three orders of bifurcation of arterioles; they are frequently associated with localized hemorrhage and exudation.

  1. Congenital
*2. Generalized arteriosclerosis
*3. Hypertension
  4. Idiopathic
  5. Following open heart surgery

Kuhn F. Retinal emboli after open heart surgery. *Arch Ophthalmol* 1989;107:317.

Robertson DM. Macroaneurysm of the retinal arteries. *Trans Am Acad Ophthalmol Otolaryngol* 1973;77:55–67.

Schatz H. *Essential fluorescein angiography: a compendium of classical cases.* San Anselmo, CA: Pacific Press, 1982.

RETINAL NEOVASCULARIZATION (GROWTH OF ABNORMAL NEW BLOOD VESSELS INTO THE VITREOUS)

  1. Anemia
  2. Behçet syndrome (dermatostomatoophthalmic syndrome)
 *3. Central retinal vein occlusion (see p. 468)
 *4. Diabetes mellitus
  5. Eales disease (periphlebitis)
  6. Ehlers–Danlos syndrome (fibrodysplasia elastica generalisata)
  7. Hypertension (malignant and essential)
  8. Leukemia
  9. Lupus erythematosus
10. Macroglobulinemia (Waldenström syndrome)
11. Retinal detachment with hemorrhage
*12. Sickle cell disease
13. Syphilis (acquired lues)
14. Trauma
15. von Hippel–Lindau syndrome (retinocerebral angiomatosis)
16. Werlhof disease (hemophilia and thrombocytopenic purpura)

L'Esperance FA, James WA. *Diabetic retinopathy: clinical evaluation and management,* 2nd ed. St. Louis: CV Mosby, 1982.

Roy FH. *Ocular syndromes and systemic diseases,* 3rd ed. Philadelphia: Lippincott Williams & Wilkins, 2002.

PREDISPOSITION TO RHEGMATOGENOUS RETINAL DETACHMENT

1. Aphakia (see p. 405)

2. Branch retinal vein occlusion
3. High myopia
4. Chorioretinitis
5. Peripheral retinal degeneration
   A. Vitreous base excavation
   *B. Retinal hole
   C. Retinoschisis
   D. Cystic retinal tuft
   E. Zonular traction tuft
   F. Meridional folds
   G. Partial-thickness retinal tear
   *H. Full-thickness retinal tear
   *I. Lattice degeneration
   J. Vitreous base avulsion
6. Trauma—blunt and perforating, including operation for strabismus and block excision of epithelial implantation cysts and tumors of the anterior uvea
7. Angiomatosis retinae

Gonzales CA, et al. Bilateral rhegmatogenous retinal detachments with unilateral vitreous base avulsion as the presenting signs of child abuse. *Am J Ophthalmol* 1999;127,4:475–477.

Ikuno Y, et al. Tractional retinal detachment after branch retinal vein occlusion. *Ophthalmology* 1998;105:417–423.

Jonas JB, et al. Rhegmatogenous retinal detachment after block excision of epithelial implantation cysts and tumors of the anterior uvea. *Ophthalmology* 1999;106:1942–1946.

RETINAL DETACHMENT (LOCATION AND MORPHOLOGIC CLASSIFICATION)

1. Equator
   A. Myopic type—equatorial horseshoe tear
   B. Equatorial type associated with lattice degeneration
2. Ora serrata
   A. Aphakic, with multiple small breaks often in nasal periphery
   B. Dialysis in young, lower temporal quadrant, often bilateral
   C. Giant dialysis, often bilateral
3. Posterior pole
   A. Macular breaks, rare
   B. Other breaks at posterior pole, from cellular proliferation in inner retinal surface

Benson WE. *Retinal detachment: diagnosis and management,* 2nd ed. Philadelphia: JB Lippincott, 1988.

Bhagat N, et al. Exudative retinal detachment in relapsing polychondritis. *Ophthalmology* 2000;108:1156–1159.

Folk JC, Burton TC. Bilateral phakic retinal detachment. *Ophthalmology* 1982;89:815.

SYNDROMES AND DISEASES ASSOCIATED WITH RETINAL DETACHMENT

1. Exudative
   A. Systemic disease
      (1) Abdominal typhus
      (2) Aspergillosis
      (3) Atopic dermatitis
      (4) Blood diseases
         a. Dysproteinemias

      b. Leukemia

      c. Sickle cell disease

(5) Boutonneuse fever (rickettsia)

(6) Candidiasis

(7) Coenurosis

(8) Cryoglobulinemia

(9) Cryptococcosis

(10) Cysticercosis

(11) Disseminated intravascular coagulation

(12) Extreme venous congestion, such as occurs during choking

(13) Goldsheider syndrome (epidermolysis bullosa)

(14) Goodpasture syndrome (chronic relapsing pulmonary hemosiderosis)

(15) Grönblad–Strandberg syndrome (systemic elastodystrophy)

(16) Histiocytosis X (Hand–Schüller–Christian syndrome)

(17) Homocystinuria syndrome

(18) Hurler syndrome (MPS I-H)

(19) Hydatid cyst

(20) Hypertension—grade IV

(21) Krause syndrome (congenital encephalo-ophthalmic dysplasia)

*(22) Lupus erythematosus

(23) Lymphoma

(24) Polyarteritis nodosa (Kussmaul disease)

(25) Reese syndrome (D trisomy)

(26) Regional enteritis

(27) Relapsing polychondritis

(28) Renal disease, including chronic glomerulonephritis or uremia

(29) Rheumatoid arthritis

(30) Rheumatic fever

(31) Rift Valley fever

(32) Sturge–Weber syndrome (meningocutaneous syndrome)

(33) Syphilis

(34) Temporal arteritis syndrome (cranial arteritis syndrome)

(35) Toxemia of pregnancy

(36) Vogt–Koyanagi–Harada syndrome

B. Ocular disease

   (1) Acute retinal necrosis

   (2) Choroidal or retinal tumor

      a. Hemangioma

      b. Melanoma

      c. Metastasis—including that from breast, lung, and stomach

      d. Retinoblastoma

   (3) Colobomas of the optic nerve

   (4) Dominant myopia and retinal detachment

   (5) Familial exudative vitreoretinopathy

   (6) Harada disease and Vogt–Koyanagi syndrome

   (7) Lymphoid hyperplasia of the uveal tract

   (8) Morning-glory syndrome (hereditary central glial anomaly of the optic disk)

   (9) Nanophthalmos

(10) Norrie disease (atrophia oculi congenita)—x-linked

(11) Optic nerve pit

(12) Postinflammation of the orbit or sinuses or cyclitis

(13) Retina, congenital nonattachment and falciform folds—autosomal recessive

(14) Schwartz syndrome (glaucoma associated with retinal detachment)

(15) Scleritis (especially posterior scleritis)

(16) Sympathetic ophthalmia

(17) *Toxocara* infection

(18) Uveal effusion syndrome

C. Associated with retinal or choroidal vascular disease

   (1) Coats disease (retinal telangiectasia)

      a. In juvenile

      b. In adult

   (3) Central serous choroidopathy

   (4) Detached pigment epithelium

   (5) Eales disease (periphlebitis)

   (6) Excessive panphotocoagulation

   (7) Exudative age-related macular degeneration

   (8) Hollenhorst syndrome (chorioretinal infarction syndrome)

   (9) Incontinentia pigmenti

   (10) Osteoporosis-pseudoglioma syndrome

   (11) Post irradiation

   (12) Scleral buckling

   (13) Subpigment epithelium hemorrhage

   (14) von Hippel Lindau disease (retinocerebral angiomatosis)

D. Drugs, including the following:

aceclidine
adrenal cortex injection
aldosterone
beclomethasone
betamethasone
carbachol
chymotrypsin (?)
cortisone
demecarium (?)
dexamethasone
diisopropyl flurophosphate
   (DFP)

echothiophate
fludrocortisone
fluorometholone
fluprednisolone
ganciclovir
hydrocortisone
isoflurophate (?)
medrysone
meperidine
methyl prednisolone
methylphenidate
neostigmine (?)

oxygen
oxyphenbutazone
penicillamine
phenylbutazone
physostigmine (?)
pilocarpine
prednisone
prednisolone
sane paramethasone
triamcinolone

2. Traction

   *A. Pull of adherent and degenerated vitreous

   B. Organized vitreous band

      (1) After vitreous hemorrhage

         a. Spontaneous

         b. Traumatic

      (2) Hypertensive retinopathy

      (3) Posthemorrhagic proliferative retinopathy

      (4) Sickle cell retinopathy

   C. Postneovascularization of vitreous

* = most important

      *(1) Diabetic retinopathy, proliferative

      (2) Eales disease (periphlebitis)

      (3) Ehlers–Danlos syndrome (fibrodysplasia elastica-generalisata)

      (4) Fibrinoid syndrome

      *(5) Retinopathy of prematurity

      (6) Severe uveitis

  D. Congenital deformities, such as retinal dysplasia, coloboma, persistence of fetal vascular system, and pit of optic nerve

  E. 18Q syndrome

  F. Penetrating injury

*G. Proliferative vitreoretinopathy

  H. Puckering syndrome

  I. Retinal disinsertion syndrome

  J. Retinopathy of prematurity

  K. Warburg syndrome

3. Rhegmatogenous

  A. Accommodation spasm, including strong miotics

  B. Alport syndrome (neuropathy and deafness)

  C. Apert syndrome (acrocephalosyndactylism syndrome)

  D. Equatorial or anterior choroiditis

  E. FOAR syndrome

  F. Following YAG laser capsulotomy

  G. Hereditary ocular vitreoretinal degeneration and skeletal abnormality (cleft palate)

  H. Juxtapapillary microholes

  I. Knobloch syndrome (retinal detachment and occipital encephalocele)—autosomal recessive

  J. Marchesani syndrome

  K. Marfan syndrome (arachnodactyly dystrophia mesodermalis congenita)

  L. Marshall (D) syndrome

  M. Meckel syndrome

  N. Myopia, including staphyloma—autosomal dominant or recessive

  O. Retinal degeneration at periphery

      (1) Presenile or myopic type

      (2) Lattice and paving-stone types—autosomal dominant

  P. Retinal detachment—autosomal dominant or x-linked

  Q. Retinal vein occlusion

  R. Retinoschisis—adult or juvenile

  S. Smith–Magenis syndrome

  T. Spondyloepiphyseal dysplasia, congenital

  U. Stickler syndrome (hereditary progressive arthro-ophthalmopathy)

  V. Trauma

      (1) Direct injury—perforating wound and foreign body

      (2) Indirect injury including block excision of epithelial implantation cysts and tumors of the anterior uvea.

      (3) Post cataract operation

         a. Sunset syndrome

         b. Vitreous tug syndrome

      (4) Battered-baby syndrome (Silverman syndrome)

    *W. Viral retinitis
       (1) Acute retinal necrosis
       (2) Cytomegalovirus retinitis
    X. Vitreous degeneration
    Y. Wagner syndrome (hyaloideoretinal degeneration)

Alio JL, et al. Retinal detachment as a potential hazard in surgical correction of severe myopia with phakic anterior chamber lenses. *Am J Ophthalmol* 1993;115:145–148.

Fraunfelder FT, Fraunfelder FW. *Drug-induced ocular side effects.* Woburn, MA: Butterworth-Heinemann, 2001.

Hunyor AP, et al. Ocular-central nervous system lymphoma mimicking posterior scleritis with exudative retinal detachment. *Ophthalmology* 2000;107:1955–1959.

Ikuno Y, et al. Retinal detachment after branch retina vein occlusion. *Ophthalmology* 1997;104:27–32.

Jonas JB, et al. Rhegmatogenous retinal detachment after block excision of epithelial implantation cysts and tumors of the anterior uvea. *Ophthalmology* 1999;106:1942–1946.

Ranta P, Kivela T. Retinal detachment in pseudophakic eyes with and without Nd:YAG laser posterior capsulotomy. *Ophthalmology* 1998;105:2127–2133.

Roy FH. *Ocular syndromes and systemic diseases,* 3rd ed. Philadelphia: Lippincott Williams & Wilkins, 2002.

RETINAL FOLDS

  1. Proliferative retinal folds—inner layer outstrips outer layer
  2. Traction folds
    A. Associated with remnants of hyaloid artery
    B. Secondary to vitreous traction
    *C. Retinopathy of prematurity (cicatricial form)
  3. Falciform retinal fold (congenital retinal septum)
    A. Familial exudative vitreoretinopathy
    B. Isolated
    C. Trisomy syndrome
    D. Warburg syndrome
  4. Chronic uveitis
  5. Parasite
  6. Occult intraocular foreign body
 *7. Shaken baby syndrome
  8. Terson syndrome

Isenberg SJ. *The eye in infancy.* Chicago: Year Book Medical, 1989.

Keithahn MA, et al. Retinal folds in Terson syndrome. *Ophthalmology* 1993;100:1187–1190.

Larrison WI, et al. Posterior retinal folds following vitreoretinal surgery. *Arch Ophthalmol* 1993;111:621–625.

COTTON-WOOL SPOTS

These spots are soft exudates (fluffy, white, focal infarcts in the nerve fiber layer).

  1. Acute pancreatitis
  2. Amniotic fluid embolization
  3. Anemic conditions
    A. Cirrhosis of the liver
    B. Following cardiac surgery
    C. Gastric ulcer syndrome
    D. Hypotensive retinopathy

* = most important

   E. Ligation of the carotid artery
   F. Severe primary and secondary anemias
   G. Severe systemic blood loss
4. Blood disease
   A. Aplastic anemia
   B. Dysproteinemia
   C. Leukemia
   D. Multiple myeloma (myelomatosis)
   E. Pernicious anemia (vitamin B_{12} deficiency)
   F. Waldenström syndrome (macroglobulinemia syndrome)
5. Carbon monoxide poisoning
6. Carcinomatous cachexia
7. Collagen diseases
   A. Dermatomyositis (polymyositis dermatomyositis)
   B. Diffuse scleroderma
   C. Disseminated lupus erythematosus (systemic lupus erythematosus)
   D. Polyarteritis nodosa (necrotizing angiitis)
   E. Rheumatoid arthritis with scleromalacia perforans or polymyalgia rheumatica
*8. Diabetic retinopathy
9. Hodgkin disease
10. Infective conditions
   *A. HIV
   B. Pneumonia
   C. Rheumatic fever
   D. Rift Valley fever
   E. Rocky mountain spotted fever (spotted fever)
   F. Roth septic retinitis
   G. Subacute bacterial endocarditis
11. Microemboli following cardiac operation
12. Primary amyloidosis (idiopathic amyloidosis)
13. Primary open-angle glaucoma
14. Protein C and protein S deficiency
15. Purtscher retinopathy (fat embolism syndrome)
16. Renal disease
17. Serum disease
18. Suprarenal-sympathetic syndrome (pheochromocytoma syndrome)
19. Takayasu syndrome (aortic arch syndrome)
20. Toxemic retinopathy of pregnancy
*21. Untreated malignant hypertension

Brezin A, et al. Cotton-wool spots and AIDS-related complex. *Int Ophthalmol* 1990;14:37–41.

Mausour AM, et al. Cotton-wool spots in acquired immunodeficiency syndrome compared with diabetes mellitus, systemic hypertension, and central retinal vein occlusion. *Arch Ophthalmol* 1988;106:1074–1077.

Roy FH. *Ocular syndromes and systemic diseases,* 3rd ed. Philadelphia: Lippincott Williams & Wilkins, 2002.

* = most important

Cotton-wool spots	Malignant Hypertension	Toxemia of Pregnancy	Collagen Disease (Lupus Erythematosus)	Diabetes Mellitus	Anemic Conditions (Hypotensive Retinopathy)	Infective Conditions (Subacute Bacterial Endocarditis)	Traumatic Conditions (Purtscher Retinopathy)	Renal Disease (Renal Failure)	Blood Disease (Severe Anemia)
History									
1. Absence of renal function								U	
2. Accidents associated with sudden rise in blood pressure and congestion of head and chest							U		
3. Acute massive blood loss					U				
4. After thirty-second week of pregnancy		U							
5. Decreased blood pressure					U				S
6. Elevated blood pressure	U	U				U		U	
7. Familial	U			U					S
8. Pericarditis caused by staphylococcus epidermidis						U			
9. More in females		U	U						
10. After age 40				U					
11. Young persons	U	U	U						
Physical Findings									
1. Altered visual acuity		U		S	U				
2. Arteriosclerosis	U			S					
3. Asteroid hyalosis				S					
4. Band keratopathy								S	
5. Cataract				U					
6. Choroiditis						S			
7. Conjunctival calcium deposits								S	
8. Conjunctival petechiae						S			
9. Conjunctival phlyctenulae			S						
10. Corneal ulcer			S						
11. Cortical blindness								S	
12. Deep stromal keratitis			S						
13. Episcleritis			S						
14. Erythema or scaling of lids			S						
15. Floaters in aqueous and vitreous						S			
16. Hard yellow exudates	S			U					
17. Ischemic optic neuropathy			S	S					U
18. Keratoconjunctivitis sicca			S						
19. Lipemia retinalis				U					
20. Macular edema				S					
21. Macular star	S								
22. Microaneurysms of retina				U					
23. Optic atrophy			S	S					
24. Optic disc edema	S	S		S					
25. Optic neuritis			S			S			
26. Palpebral conjunctival pallor									U
27. Papillitis						S			
28. Posterior and macular serous detachment							U		

Cotton-wool spots (Continued)

	Malignant Hypertension	Toxemia of Pregnancy	Collagen Disease (Lupus Erythematosus)	Diabetes Mellitus	Anemic Conditions (Hypotensive Retinopathy)	Infective Conditions (Subacute Bacterial Endocarditis)	Traumatic Conditions (Purtscher Retinopathy)	Renal Disease (Renal Failure)	Blood Disease (Severe Anemia)
Physical Findings									
29. Preretinal hemorrhage						S			
30. Retinal artery occlusion			S			R			
31. Retinal arteriolar narrowing	U	U							
32. Retinal detachment			S	S					
33. Retinal edema	U						U	U	
34. Retinal hemorrhages	U	U	S		U	S	U		U
35. Retinal neovascularization				S					
36. Retinal venous dilation	S		S	U	S		U		
37. Roth spot						U	S		
38. Rubeosis iridis				U					
39. Scleritis			S						
40. Telangiectasis of lids			S						
41. Third nerve paresis				S					
42. Uveitis			S						
43. Vascular sheathing						S			U
Laboratory Data									
1. Blood culture positive for staphylococcus epidermidis						U			
2. BUN elevated								U	
3. Depression of hemoglobin, white cells and platelets			U		U				U
4. Fluorescein angiography									
Dilated capillaries at margin of lesion with aneurysm dilations	U								
Varicose looping and corkscrew coiling	U								
5. Glycosuria				U					
6. Hypercalcemia								U	
7. Hyperglycemia				U					
8. Hyponatremia								U	
9. Lupus erythematosus cell positive			U						
10. Positive immunofluorescence test (for antinuclear antibodies)			U						
11. Proteinuria		U						U	
12. Roentgenogram multiple bone fractures							U		

R = rarely; S = sometimes; and U = usually.

HARD EXUDATES (YELLOWISH WHITE DISCRETE MASSES DEEP IN THE RETINA)

1. Circinate retinopathy
2. Coats disease (retinal telangiectasia)
*3. Diabetes mellitus
*4. Exudative age-related macular degeneration
*5. Hypertensive disease
6. Radiation induced
7. Retinal arterial macroaneurysm

Berman DH, Friedman EA. Partial absorption of hard exudates in patients with diabetic end-stage renal disease and severe anemia after treatment with erythropoietin. *Retina* 1994;14:1–5.

Haik BG, et al. Radiation and chemotherapy of parameningeal rhabdomyosarcoma involving the orbit. *Ophthalmology* 1986;93:1001–1009.

Roy FH. *Ocular syndromes and systemic diseases,* 3rd ed. Philadelphia: Lippincott Williams &Wilkins, 2002.

* = most important

Hard exudates (yellowish-white discrete masses deep in retina)

	Diabetes Mellitus*	Hypertensive Disease*	Coats' Disease	Essential Hypercholesterolemic Xanthomatosis
History				
1. Bilateral	U	S		U
2. Congenital			U	
3. Elevated blood pressure		U		
4. Familial	U			U
5. More in males			S	
6. Occurs in persons up to 10 years old			U	
7. Occurs in persons 11 to 40 years old	S		R	R
8. Occurs in persons more than 40 years old		U		S
Physical Findings				
1. Anterior uveitis			U	
2. Cataract—coronary				U
3. Cataract—vesicular and posterior subcapsular cataract	U			
4. Conjunctivitis				U
5. Corneal arcus	S			U
6. Cotton-wool spots	U	U		
7. Glaucoma	S		S	
8. Lipid rings around microaneurysms				U
9. Macular edema	S	U	U	
10. Optic disc edema		S		
11. Optic nerve atrophy	S		U	
12. Retinal detachment	S	S	U	
13. Retinal hemorrhages		U	S	
14. Retinal microaneurysms	U	U	U	
15. Retinal telangiectatic vessels			S	
16. Retinal vein occlusion	S	S	U	U
17. Retinal vein sheathing	U	U		
18. Rubeosis iridis	S		U	
19. Vitreous hemorrhage	S	U	U	
Laboratory Data				
1. Elevated blood sugar	U			
2. Elevated lipid profile, including cholesterol and triglyceride	S	S		U
3. Phosphorus 32 uptake elevation			U	
4. Retinal angiography	S	U	U	U
5. Ultrasound, ocular	R		U	

R = rarely; S = sometimes; and U = usually.

RETINAL EXUDATE AND HEMORRHAGE

1. Capillary telangiectasis of retina (Reese)
2. Coats disease (retinal telangiectasia)
*3. Diabetes mellitus
4. Eales disease (periphlebitis)
5. Multiple retinal aneurysms (Leber syndrome)
6. Racemose hemangioma of the retina
7. von Hippel–Lindau, with absence of visible angioma (retinocerebral angiomatosis)

Ballantyne AJ, Michaelson IC. *Textbook of the fundus of the eye,* 3rd ed. Baltimore: Williams & Wilkins, 1981.

Michelson JB, et al. Ocular reticulum cell sarcoma. *Arch Ophthalmol* 1981;99:1409.

RETINITIS OR PSEUDORETINITIS PIGMENTOSA

Pigment may be bone corpuscular dots or heaped-up masses; salt and pepper fundus

1. Retinitis pigmentosa
    A. Abetalipoproteinemia (Bassen–Kornzweig syndrome)
    B. Alström disease (cataract and retinitis pigmentosa)
    C. Cockayne syndrome (dwarfism with retinal atrophy and deafness)
    D. Dialinas–Amalric syndrome (deaf-mutism-retinal degeneration syndrome)
    E. Hallgren syndrome (retinitis pigmentosa–deafness–ataxia syndrome)
    F. Hypotrichosis, syndactyly and retinitis pigmentosa—autosomal recessive
    G. Hunter syndrome (MPS II)
    H. Hurler syndrome (MPS I)
    I. Infantile phytanic acid storage disease
    J. Jeune syndrome
    *K. Kearns–Sayre syndrome (ophthalmoplegic retinal degeneration syndrome)
    L. Laurence–Moon–Bardet–Biedl syndrome (retinitis pigmentosa–polydac-tyly–adiposogenital syndrome)
    M. Metaphyseal chondrodysplasia with retinitis pigmentosa—autosomal recessive
    N. Microcephaly with chorioretinopathy
    O. Multiple sulfatase deficiency
    P. Muscular atrophy, ataxia, retinitis pigmentosa, diabetes mellitus—autosomal dominant
    Q. Olivopontocerebellar atrophy, type III
    R. NARP syndrome
    S. Pallidal degeneration, progressive with retinitis pigmentosa—autosomal recessive
    *T. Refsum syndrome (phytanic acid storage disease)
    U. Retinitis pigmentosa alone (usually autosomal recessive but may be autosomal dominant or sex linked)
    V. Retinitis pigmentosa associated with myopia, keratoconus, or glaucoma
    W. Retinitis pigmentosa, congenital deafness—sex linked
    X. Retinitis pigmentosa inversa (predominant—pigmentation around the disc and macula) and deafness—autosomal recessive
    Y. Retinitis pigmentosa, nerve deafness, mental retardation, and hypogonad-ism—autosomal recessive
    Z. Retinitis pigmentosa, PPRPE type (with preserved para-arteriole retinal pigment epithelium)—autosomal recessive

* = most important

AA. Retinitis pigmentosa, spastic quadriplegia, and mental retardation—autosomal recessive

BB. Rud syndrome

CC. Sanfilippo disease (MPS III)

DD. Scheie disease (MPS IS)

EE. Spielmeyer–Vogt syndrome (cerebroretinal degeneration)

FF. Usher syndrome (hereditary retinitis pigmentosa-deafness syndrome)

2. Senile changes—degenerative pigmentation

3. Vascular lesion, such as occlusion of arteriole

4. Inflammatory

    A. Behçet disease (oculobuccogenital syndrome)

    B. Chickenpox virus

    C. Cytomegalic inclusion disease

    D. Dawson disease (inclusion-body encephalitis)

    E. Fetal varicella effects

    F. Focal dermal hypoplasia (Goltz syndrome)

    G. Harada disease (Vogt–Koyanagi–Harada syndrome)

    H. Hypomelanosis of Ito

    I. Influenza virus

    J. Nematode endophthalmitis (visceral larva migrans syndrome)

    K. Onchocerciasis (river blindness)

    L. Polyarteritis nodosa (Kussmaul disease)

    M. Rubella (German measles)

    N. Rubeola (measles)

  *O. Syphilis

  *P. Toxoplasmosis

    Q. Typhoid fever (enteric fever)

    R. Vaccinia

5. Toxic

    A. Accidental intraocular injection of depot corticosteroids

    B. Chloroquine and atabrine

    C. Diaminodiphenoxyalkanes—possible drug for treatment of schistosomiasis

    D. Indomethacin

    E. Phenothiazine

        (1) Chlorpromazine

        (2) Thioridazine (Mellaril)

    F. Pregl solution (Septojod, formerly used for treatment of puerperal sepsis)

    G. Quinine

    H. Sparsomycin

6. Acute lymphocytic leukemia

7. Alagille syndrome

8. Alport syndrome

9. Bardet–Biedl syndrome

10. Battens disease

11. Cryogenic "pigmentary fallout"—following use of cryosurgery for retinal detachment

12. Cystinosis syndrome (Lignac–Fanconi syndrome)

13. External ophthalmoplegias

*14. Gardner syndrome (congenital hypertrophy of the retinal pigment epithelium and familial intestinal polyposis)

* = most important

15. Hagberg–Santavuori syndrome (neuronal ceroid lipofuscinosis)
16. Hallervorden–Spatz syndrome (pigmentary degeneration of globus pallidus)
17. Hereditary ataxias (Friedrich and Marie)
18. Leber congenital amaurosis
19. Lens dislocated into vitreous
20. MERRF syndrome
21. Mucolipidoses IV (ML IV)
22. Myotonic dystrophy syndrome (Curschmann–Steinert syndrome)
23. Neuronal ceroid lipofuscinosis
    A. Infantile form
    B. Late infantile form (Jansky–Bielschowsky)
    C. Adult form (Kufs syndrome)
24. Pelizaeus–Merzbacher syndrome (aplasia axialis extracorticalis congenita)
25. Pellagra (ariboflavinosis)
26. Progressive cone-rod degeneration
27. Renal disorders, including familial juvenile nephronophthisis (medullary cystic disease)
28. Rud syndrome (hypophyseal deficiency)
29. Sjögren–Larsson syndrome (oligophrenia–ichthyosis–spastic diplegia syndrome)
30. Tapetal-like reflex syndrome
31. Trauma, including blunt, penetrating, obstetric, and radiotherapy, Frenkel syndrome (ocular contusion syndrome)
32. Waardenburg syndrome (interoculoiridodermatoauditive dysplasia)
33. Zellweger syndrome and pseudo-Zellweger syndrome

Bateman JB, Philippart M. Ocular features of the Hagberg-Santavuori syndrome. *Am J Ophthalmol* 1986;102: 262–271.

Bloome MA, Garcia CA. *A manual of retinal and choroidal dystrophies.* East Norwalk, CT: Appleton-Century-Crofts, 1982.

Carr RE, Noble KG. Retinitis pigmentosa. *Ophthalmology* 1981;88:199.

Roy FH. *Ocular syndromes and systemic diseases,* 3rd ed. Philadelphia: Lippincott Williams & Wilkins, 2002.

Retinal bone corpuscular dots

	Retinitis Pigmentosa	Senile Degeneration	Vascular (Arterial Occlusion)	Inflammatory (Rubella)	Toxic (Chloroquine)	Cystinosis	Trauma (Blunt)	Progressive Cone-rod Degeneration	Myotonic Dystrophy
History									
1. Amaurosis fugax			S						
2. Children						U			
3. Common in males	U								
4. Glare					U				
5. Hereditary	U					U		U	U
6. Older age group		U							
7. Lacrimation							S		
8. Night blindness	U								
9. Onset, about 20 years									U
10. Photophobia						U			
11. Rubela infection, first trimester				U					
12. Trauma							U		
Physical Findings									
1. Angle recession							S		
2. Bull's eye or doughnut retinal lesion						U		U	
3. Buphthalmos				S					
4. Cataracts	S					U	S		U
5. Conjunctival hemorrhage							S		
6. Conjunctivitis				S					
7. Corneal haziness				S		U			
8. Crystals located in conjunctiva, cornea						U			
9. Cystoid macular edema	R								
10. Disc drusen	S								
11. Disc hamartoma	S								
12. Epithelial corneal edema							S		R
13. Glaucoma	S			S					
14. Hyphema							S		
15. Hypotony							S		
16. Iris atrophy				S					
17. Keratopathy				S		U			R
18. Keratoconus	R								
19. Loss of corneal sensitivity									U
20. Macular degeneration	R	U							U
21. Macular red spot									U
22. May progress to blindness	U					S			
23. Megalocornea				S					
24. Microcornea				S					
25. Microphthalmos	R			S					
26. Minute whitish corneal dots in whorl pattern					U				
27. Myopia	U								
28. Neovascular retinal proliferation			S						
29. Nystagmus	R		U				S		
30. Optic disc atrophy/pallor	U					S		U	R
31. Peripheral retinal drusen		U							

Retinal bone corpuscular dots (Continued)

	Retinitis Pigmentosa	Senile Degeneration	Vascular (Arterial Occlusion)	Inflammatory (Rubella)	Toxic (Chloroquine)	Cystinosis	Trauma (Blunt)	Progressive Cone-rod Degeneration	Myotonic Dystrophy
Physical Findings									
32. Progressive external ophthalmoplegia	R								S
33. Ptosis	R								U
34. Pupil dilated and fixed							S		
35. Retinal arteriosclerosis		U							
36. Retinal hemorrhage							S		
37. Retinal vessel attenuation	U	U	S		S			S	
38. Retrobulbar hemorrhage							S		U
39. Sheathing of retinal vessels	R		R		S				
40. Silver wire or chalky-white arterioles			U		S				
41. Spherophakia				R					
42. Strabismus	R			S					
43. Uveitis				S					
44. Vitreous opacities	U								
Laboratory Data									
1. Color vision abnormalities	U				S			U	
2. Cystine in conjunctival biopsy, cultured skin fibroblasts or polymorphonuclear leukocytes						U			
3. Dark adaptation abnormal	U								
4. Electro-oculogram	U				U			S	
5. Electroretinogram	U				U			U	
6. Fluorescein angiography							R		
Bull's eye lesion					U			U	
Diffuse hyperfluorescence scattered spicules of pigment, dye leakage from cystoid macular edema may be present	U	S		S			S		
Peripheral arteriolar occlusion			U						
7. Fluorescent rubella antibody test				U					
8. Hemoglobin electrophoresis			U						
9. Leukopenia				U				U	
10. Red blood cell count elevated			U						
11. Rubella virus hemagglutination inhibition				U					
12. Serum immunoglobulin G concentration reduced									U
13. Visual field abnormal	U	R	S		S			U	

R = rarely; S = sometimes; and U = usually.

LESIONS CONFUSED WITH RETINOBLASTOMA

1. Anomalous optic disc
2. Anteriorly dislocated lens with secondary glaucoma
*3. Coats disease (retinal telangiectasia)
4. Coloboma of choroid and optic disc (see p. 555–556)
5. Congenital corneal opacity
6. Congenital rubella syndrome (Gregg syndrome)
7. Cysts in a remnant of the hyaloid artery
8. Developmental retinal cyst
9. Glioma of the retina
10. Hematoma under retinal pigment epithelium
11. High myopia with advanced chorioretinal degeneration
12. Juvenile (x-linked) retinoschisis
13. Juvenile xanthogranuloma (nevoxanthoendothelioma)
*14. Larval granulomatosis (*T. canis*)
15. Medullation of nerve fiber layer
16. Metastatic endophthalmitis
17. Norrie disease (atrophia oculi congenita)
18. Oligodendroglioma of the retina
19. Organization of intraocular hemorrhage
*20. Persistent hyperplastic primary vitreous
21. Retinal detachment due to choroidal or vitreous hemorrhage
22. Retinal dysplasia (massive retinal fibrosis)
*23. Retinopathy of prematurity
24. Retrolental membrane associated with Bloch–Sulzberger syndrome (incontinentia pigmenti)
25. Rhegmatogenous and falciform retinal detachment
26. Secondary glaucoma
27. Sex-linked microphthalmia
28. Tapetoretinal degeneration
29. Trisomy 13 (Patau syndrome)
*30. Toxoplasmosis (ocular toxoplasmosis)
31. Traumatic chorioretinitis
*32. Tumors other than retinoblastoma
33. Uveitis in secondary retinal detachment
34. ''White-with-pressure'' sign

Howard GM. Erroneous clinical diagnoses of retinoblastoma and uveal melanoma. *Trans Am Acad Ophthalmol Otolaryngol* 1969;73:199–203.

Nicholson DH, Green WR, eds. *Pediatric ocular tumors.* New York: Masson, 1981.

* = most important

Single dark fundus lesion

	Retinal Detachment	Retinoschisis (Senile)	Macular Degeneration (Exudative)	Chorioretinitis ie Ocular Histoplasmosis	Intraocular Foreign Body	Coats' Disease	Ocular Metastatic Tumors	Choroidal Detachment	Melanocytoma of Optic Nerve	Malignant Melanoma
History										
1. Affects both sexes equally		U		U						
2. Aphakic, myopic and traumatized eyes	U									
3. Bilateral		U					S			
4. Diagnosed between two to ten years of age						U				
5. Discovery may be at birth						U				
6. Discovered in middle age									U	
7. During or immediately following an operation								U		
8. Familial blindness	S									
9. Hereditary	S		S							
10. History of ocular trauma					U			U		
11. History of scleritis or episcleritis								U		
12. More in blacks and other dark complexioned people									U	
13. Most are young adults				U	U					
14. Most common in females									U	
15. Most common in males					U	U				
16. Ocular pain							U			S
17. Onset in advanced age			U		S					
18. Onset in juvenile period			S							
19. Over 50 years of age			S							
20. Unilateral in 90%						U			U	
21. Wide age range	U			U						
Physical Findings										
1. Abnormal afferent pupillary reaction	S	S			U			S	U	
2. Anterior chamber flat					S			U		
3. Atrophic macular degeneration								U		
4. Atrophic scar around nerve head			U	U						
5. Blood vessels narrowed and yellow					U		R			U
6. Cataract	S				S	U				
7. Cholesterol crystals of retina								U		
8. Choroidal elevations of periphery										
9. Choroiditis				U						
10. Conjunctival and episcleral injection								U		
11. Corneal striae and aqueous flare								U		
12. Dark smooth multilobulated elevations								U		
13. Elevation of the retina	U	U							U	
14. Enlargement of blind spot									S	
15. Extraocular muscle paralysis							S			
16. Exudative and atrophic retinal reaction			U							
17. Glaucoma						U	S			
18. Hazy vitreous					S			U		
19. Impairment of central vision			U		S					
20. Iris discolored (green in copper, yellow in iron)					U					
21. Iritis	S									
22. Loss of vision	S		U		U			S	U	U
23. Low intraocular pressure	U							U		

Single dark fundus lesion (Continued)

	Retinal Detachment	Retinoschisis (Senile)	Macular Degeneration (Exudative)	Chorioretinitis ie Ocular Histoplasmosis	Intraocular Foreign Body	Coats' Disease	Ocular Metastatic Tumors	Choroidal Detachment	Melanocytoma of Optic Nerve	Malignant Melanoma
Physical Findings										
24. Macular edema				U						
25. Macular hemorrhages			S	S						
26. Microaneurysms in retina						U				
27. Neovascular glaucoma						S				
28. Optic nerve swelling							S			S
29. Retinal detachment	U	S				S	R	R		U
30. Retinal exudates						U				
31. Retinal folds or striae	S						U			
32. Retinal hemorrhages				U						
33. Retina is wrinkled and gray	U									
34. Retinal ischemia						U				
35. Retinal neovascularization				U						
36. Retinal tears or holes	U	S								
37. Retinal telangiectasia						U				
38. Rubeosis iridis							S			
39. Sensory retinal detachment						S				
40. Serous elevation overlying mass in retina							U			
41. Shifting subretinal fluid							U	S		
42. Splitting of the neurosensory retina		U								
43. Subretinal hemorrhages							S			
44. Tortuosity of retinal vessels	U									
45. Uveitis							U			
46. Vitreal hemorrhage						S	S			S
47. Vitreous cells	S									
48. Vitreous green or yellow and liquid					U					
49. Yellow macular deposits					U					
Laboratory Data										
1. A scan										U
2. B scan	U				U		U			U
3. 32 P test							U			U
4. Fluorescein angiography										U

R = rarely; S = sometimes; and U = usually.

SINGLE WHITE LESION OF RETINA

*1. Amelanotic melanoma
2. Astrocytoma of tuberous sclerosis
3. Degeneration of retinal pigment epithelium
4. Diktyoma
5. Glioma of optic nerve
6. Hamartomas of the optic disc of retinitis pigmentosa
7. Metastatic or direct extension of a tumor
8. Neurofibroma of von Recklinghausen syndrome
*9. Retinoblastoma
*10. *T. canis*

Nicholson DH, Green WR, eds. *Pediatric ocular tumors.* New York: Masson, 1981.

Robertson DM. Hamartomas of the optic disc with retinitis pigmentosa. *Am J Ophthalmol* 1972;74:526–531.

PALE FUNDUS LESIONS

1. Generalized pallor
   A. Albinism—photophobia; defective vision; absence of pigment in iris, retina, and choroid
   B. Chediak–Higashi syndrome (oculocutaneous albinism with recurrent infections)
   C. Waardenburg syndrome (embryonic fixation syndrome)
   D. Choroideremia—rare; night blindness; contraction of visual fields; degeneration of pigment epithelium in periphery with exposure of choroidal vessels
   E. Myopia—thinning of retina and choroidal crescent at disc
   F. Retinal ischemia
      (1) Occlusion of retinal arteries (see p. 457)
      (2) Spasm of retinal arteries—angiospasm: quinine, lead poisoning, migraine, or Raynaud disease
      (3) Anemia
   *G. Vascular retinopathies—hypertension, edema, hemorrhages, swelling of disc
   H. Leukemia
   I. The lipidoses
      (1) Congenital, rare
      (2) Infantile (Tay–Sachs disease)
      (3) Late infantile—(Jansky–Bielschowsky syndrome)—2 to 4 years of age
      (4) Juvenile—(Spielmeyer–Vogt syndrome)—5 to 8 years of age; optic atrophy
      (5) Adult—(Kufs disease)—15 to 25 years of age; eyes may be normal or show some pigmented macular changes
   J. Gaucher disease (glucocerebroside storage disease)
   K. Hereditary dystrophic lipidosis (Fabry disease)
   L. Hyperlipemia
      (1) Diabetes—rare, yellowish retinal and choroidal vessels
      (2) Essential hyperlipemic xanthomatosis—rare, yellowish retinal and choroidal vessels
   M. Oguchi disease
2. Localized pale areas
   A. Medullated nerve fibers (see p. 507)
   *B. Retinopathy of prematurity

* = most important

C. Localized retinal edema
   (1) Inflammation
   (2) Trauma
   (3) Vascular lesions
D. Retinal detachment and schisis (see p. 487)
*E. Retinoblastoma
F. Coats disease (retinal telangiectasia)
G. Coloboma (see p. 450–451)
H. Normal fundus features—pale streaks mark site of ciliary nerves
I. Atrophic areas—diathermy, light coagulation, or cryosurgery
J. Scattered retinal exudates
   (1) Preretinal—severe posterior uveitis; discrete white spots, often most marked along vessels adjacent to a patch of choroiditis
   (2) Retinal
      a. Purtscher compression syndrome—cotton-wool spots
      b. Fat emboli
      c. Hemangiomatosis—yellow exudates
      *d. Hypertensive retinopathy—cotton-wool and hard exudates
      e. Toxemia of pregnancy
      f. Hypotensive retinopathy
      g. Pulseless disease (Takayasu syndrome)
      h. Arterial occlusion
      i. Blood loss—cotton-wool spots
      j. Anemia (all types)
      k. Leukemia
      l. Purpura
      m. Macroglobulinemia (Waldenström syndrome)
      n. Hodgkin disease—soft exudates
      *o. Diabetes—cotton-wool and hard exudates
      p. Hypercholesterolemia—lipid deposits
      q. Systemic lupus erythematosus (disseminated lupus erythematosus)
      r. Dermatomyositis—cotton-wool spots
      s. Polyarteritis nodosa (Kussmaul disease)
      t. Scleroderma (progressive systemic sclerosis)
      u. Vitamin A deficiency—small white spots along course of retinal vessels
      v. Retinal capillariosis—yellowish white spots in substance of retina
      w. Leber congenital retinal aplasia—bilateral blindness, multiple white specks
      x. Female carrier of retinitis pigmentosa—brilliant silvery reflex with shining yellow spots deep to retinal vessels
3. Dystrophic conditions
   A. Gyrate atrophy—rare, irregular atrophic areas with visual defects and night blindness
   B. Choroidal sclerosis—rare, diffuse peripapillary or central choroidal atrophy with larger choroidal vessels prominent
   C. Infarction or occlusion of ciliary arteries—rare, embolism (air, fat), injury, atrophic area with prominent choroidal vessels
   D. Pseudoinflammatory macular dystrophy—rare, fourth to sixth decades, central edema, hemorrhage and exudate, bilateral and symmetric

E. Helicoid peripapillary chorioretinal atrophy—rare, congenital and adult forms, star-shaped atrophic areas radiating from disc

F. Retinitis punctata albescens—rare, onset in second and third decades, multiple discrete whitish dots which may appear crystalline, night blindness and field defects in progressive type

G. Fundus flavimaculatus—rare, onset in second and third decades, yellow flecks deep in the retina

H. Geographic choroiditis—rare, map-like pigmentary disturbance at posterior pole or more widespread over posterior fundus

I. Doyne honeycomb dystrophy—rare; middle age and older; drusen at posterior pole, with pigmentary or cystoid macular changes

J. Progressive bifocal chorioretinal atrophy—atrophy temporal to disc, extending later; night blindness in late stage

Ballantyne AJ, Michaelson IC. *Textbook of the fundus of the eye,* 3rd ed. Baltimore: Williams & Wilkins, 1981.

Bloome MA, Garcia CA. *Manual of retinal and choroidal dystrophies.* East Norwalk, CT: Appleton-Century-Crofts, 1981.

Perkins ES, Dobree JH. *The differential diagnosis of fundus conditions.* St. Louis: CV Mosby, 1972.

MEDULLATED NERVE FIBERS

In this condition, an opaque white patch is usually adjacent to and may cover the disc; it is localized to one sector of the disc and peripapillary or arcuate with a peripheral, feathered edge.

*1. Isolated finding
 2. Autosomal-recessive or -dominant inheritance
 3. Associated with the following:
     A. Aplasia of macula
     B. Coloboma of optic nerve or choroid (see p. 555–556)
     C. Conus of disc
     D. Cranial dysostosis (oxycephaly, dolichocephaly, brachycephaly, and craniofacial dysostosis)
     E. Hyaloid remnants
     F. Macular colobomas (see p. 450)
     G. Myopia
    *H. Neurofibromatosis

Ballantyne AJ, Michaelson IC. *Textbook of the fundus of the eye,* 3rd ed. Baltimore: Williams & Wilkins, 1981.

PIGMENTED FUNDUS LESIONS

1. Diffuse pigmentation
    A. Negroid fundus—accentuation of fundus pigmentation
    B. Melanosis bulbi—rare, pigmentation of external eye and fundus
    C. Nevus of Ota
    D. Waardenburg syndrome (embryonic fixation)
2. Single pigmented lesions
    A. Flat lesions
        (1) Benign melanoma—bluish, gray, or black lesion
        (2) Pigmented scar—patch of dense pigment, usually atrophic area in center

* = most important

(3) Fuchs dark spot—dark spot in macular region

*(4) Macular degeneration (exudate, age-related)

B. Raised lesions

(1) Simple detachment (see p. 487)

a. Macular, such as in central serous retinopathy

b. Associated with uveitis, such as that associated with Vogt–Koya-nagi–Harada syndrome

c. Hemorrhagic macrocyst

*(2) Malignant melanoma—raised pigmented lesion with secondary detachment, abnormal vessels

(3) Choroidal hemorrhage—trauma, spontaneous in patients with vascular disease, high myopia

*(4) Exudative macular lesion—common, old age, subretinal exudate

(5) Hemangioma of choroid—rare, raised grayish tumor near disc, secondary detachment later

*(6) Metastatic tumor—flat tumor with little pigment, primary in breast, or lung

(7) Chorioretinitis

(8) Foreign body

(9) Coats disease (retinal telangiectasia)

3. Multiple pigmented lesions

A. Scattered focal lesions

*(1) Congenital melanosis—cat's-paw patches of pigment in one sector of fundus (may be part of Gardner syndrome)

(2) Postinflammatory—flat pigment with areas of atrophy

(3) Hypertensive retinopathy—hypertensive vascular changes with scattered pigmentation

(4) Siegrist streaks—rare, chain of pigment spots along sclerosed choroidal vessel

(5) Paravenous retinochoroidal atrophy—paravenous pigmentation with chorioretinal atrophy

(6) Incontinentia pigmenti (Bloch–Sulzberger syndrome)

(7) Chorioretinal scars from cryosurgery

B. Widely disseminated pigmentary changes

(1) Genetic conditions

a. Typical retinitis pigmentosa—attenuation of retinal vessels, optic atrophy (myopia, posterior polar cataract, keratoconus)

b. Atypical retinitis pigmentosa—rare, little or no pigment, pigment in clumps

c. Retinitis pigmentosa syndromes

(i) Cockayne syndrome (dwarfism with retinal atrophy and deafness)

(ii) Hallgren syndrome (retinitis pigmentosa–deafness–ataxia syndrome)

(iii) Kearns syndrome (ophthalmoplegic retinal degeneration syndrome)

(iv) Laurence–Moon–Biedl syndrome (retinitis pigmentosa polydactyly–adiposogenital syndrome)

(v) Leber congenital retinal aplasia syndrome

        (vi) Lignac–Fanconi syndrome (cystinosis syndrome)

       (vii) Myotonic dystrophy syndrome (dystrophia myotonica syndrome)

     (viii) Pelizaeus–Merzbacher syndrome (aplasia axialis extracorticalis congenital)

   (2) Infectious conditions—secondary retinitis pigmentosa

     *a. Syphilis (congenital)—pepper-and-salt pigmentation, interstitial keratitis

      b. Syphilitic neuroretinitis—rare, retinitis pigmentosa

      c. Rubella—cataract, secondary retinitis pigmentosa (nonprogressive)

      d. Vaccinia—rare, retinitis pigmentosa, history of vaccination

   (3) Metabolic Disturbances

      a. Refsum syndrome (phytanic acid storage disease)

      b. Bassen–Kornzweig syndrome (familial hypolipoproteinemia)

   (4) Toxic conditions, such as chloroquine, phenothiazine derivatives; usually central pigmentation; cornea and lens change

4. Ciliary body and choroid

  A. Tumors

    (1) Hemangioma

    (2) Malignant melanoma

  *(3) Metastatic carcinoma, such as that from the lungs, breast, testis, kidney, prostate gland, bladder

    (4) Nevus

    (5) Neurilemmoma

    (6) Neurofibroma

  B. Detachment—serous or hemorrhagic

 *C. Lymphoma and leukemias

  D. Peripheral giant cysts

5. Vitreous body

  A. Hemorrhage

  B. Abscess

6. Staphyloma of sclera

Perkins ES, Dobree JH. *The differential diagnosis of fundus conditions.* St. Louis: CV Mosby, 1972.

Zinn K, Marmor M, eds. *The retinal pigment epithelium.* Cambridge, MA: Harvard University Press, 1979.

CHOLESTEROL EMBOLI OF RETINA (HOLLENHORST PLAQUES)

Bright-yellow plaques are often observed at bifurcation of arterioles, indicative of generalized atherosclerosis, and should signal the ophthalmologist to measure retinal artery pressures and refer the patient for general medical evaluation.

1. Abdominal aortic aneurysms

*2. Aortic stenosis

3. Arteriography showing occlusions in one or more cervical arteries

4. Atrial fibrillation

5. Bleeding duodenal or gastric ulcer

*6. Bruits in one or both carotid arteries

*7. Calcification of internal carotids (Doppler ultrasonography)

8. Congestive heart failure

* = most important

9. Coronary heart disease with myocardial infarct or angina
*10. Diabetes mellitus
11. New or old strokes or transient attacks of cerebral ischemia
12. Peripheral atherosclerosis obliterans, popliteal or femoral aneurysms
13. Renal artery occlusions
*14. Retinal arterial occlusions
15. Torsion and calcification of aorta (roentgenogram)
16. Vocal cord paralysis (aortic arch aneurysm)

Pfaffenbach DD, Hollenhorst RW. Morbidity and survivorship of patients with embolic cholesterol crystals in the ocular fundus. *Am J Ophthalmol* 1973;75:66–72.

Wylie EJ, Ehrenfeld WK. *Extracranial occlusive cerebrovascular disease: diagnosis and management.* Philadelphia: WB Saunders, 1970.

RETINAL MICROEMBOLI

1. Platelet fibrin—mural or "tail" thrombus in carotid occlusion
*2. Cholesterol–lipid-eroding atheroma in carotid bifurcation
3. Calcific or fibrinoid
   A. Calcific valvular disease dislodged spontaneously following cardiac catheterization, or angiography, or prolapse of mitral valve
   B. Rheumatic heart disease
   C. Myocardial disease
   D. Septic emboli
4. Foreign bodies
   A. Silicone or cloth particles covered cardiac valves
   B. Talc or cornstarch emboli from drug addicts
   C. Mercury
   D. Secondary to retrobulbar or intranasal methyl prednisolone acetate
5. Tumors
   A. Cardiac myxomas
   B. Metastatic tumors including malignant melanomas and breast carcinomas
6. Fat emboli from fracture of the long bones
7. Air emboli from crushing injuries of the chest

Fraunfelder FT, Roy FH. *Current ocular therapy,* 5th ed. Philadelphia: WB Saunders, 2000.

Williams IM, et al. Brain and retinal microemboli during cardiac surgery. *Ann Neurol* 1991;30:736–737.

LIPEMIA RETINALIS (ARTERIOLES AND VENULES SIMILAR IN COLOR AND APPEARING ORANGE–YELLOW TO WHITE)

1. Primary hyperlipoproteinemia
   A. Type I—familial fat-induced hyperlipoproteinemia (hyperchylomicronemia)
   B. Type III—familial hyperbetalipoproteinemia and hyperprebetalipoproteinemia (carbohydrate-induced hyperlipemia)
   C. Type IV—familial hyperprebetalipoproteinemia (carbohydrate-induced hyperlipemia)
   D. Type V—familial hyperchylomicronemia with hyperprebetalipoproteinemia (mixed hyperlipemia)
*2. Diabetes mellitus with hyperlipemia
3. Secondary hyperlipoproteinemia

A. Biliary obstruction
B. Chronic pancreatitis
C. Chronic renal failure
D. Coats disease in adults (retinal telangiectasia)
E. Glycogen storage disease
F. Hypergammaglobulinemia
G. Hypothyroidism (cretinism)
H. Idiopathic hypercalcemia
 I. Insulin-deficient diabetes mellitus (Willis disease)
*J. Malignant neoplasms
K. Nephrotic syndrome (lipoid nephrosis)
L. Progressive lipodystrophy

Martinez KR, et al. Lipemia retinalis. *Arch Ophthalmol* 1992;110:1171.

Spaeth GL. Ocular manifestations of the lipidoses. In: Tasman W, ed. *Retinal diseases in children*. New York: Harper & Row, 1971.

HEMORRHAGIC OR SEROUS EXUDATES BENEATH PIGMENT EPITHELIUM

1. Angioid streaks (see p. 526–529)
2. Best macular degeneration (vitelliruptive macular dystrophy)
3. Coats disease (retinal telangiectasia)
4. Doyne honeycomb macular degeneration
*5. Histoplasmosis (histoplasmosis choroiditis)
*6. Macular drusen in age-related macular degeneration
7. Myopia
8. Solid neoplasms
9. Trauma

Gitter KA, et al. Traumatic hemorrhagic detachment of retinal pigment epithelium. *Arch Ophthalmol* 1968;79:729–732.

Pager CK, et al. Malattia leventinese presenting with subretinal neovascular membrane and hemorrhage. *Am J Ophthalmol* 2001;131:517–518.

RETINAL VASCULAR TUMORS AND ANGIOMATOSIS RETINAE SYNDROMES

1. Associated with pheochromocytoma
2. Blue rubber bleb nevus syndrome (Bean syndrome)
3. Bonnet–Dechaune–Blanc syndrome (neuroretinal angiomatosis syndrome)
4. Cavernous retinal hemangioma—intraretinal angiomas
*5. Coats disease (retinal telangiectasia)
6. Gorlin syndrome
7. Racemose angioma—with arteriovenous anomalies of central nervous system (Wyburn–Mason syndrome)
8. Retinal telangiectasis (Leber military aneurysms)—telangiectasia retinae of Reese
9. Sturge–Weber syndrome (meningocutaneous syndrome)
*10. von Hippel–Lindau syndrome (retinocerebral angiomatosis retinae)

Crompton JL, Taylor D. Ocular lesion in the blue rubber nevus syndrome. *Ophthalmology* 1981;65:133–137.

De Potter P, et al. Combined hamartoma of the retina and retinal pigment epithelium in Gorlin syndrome. *Arch Ophthalmol* 2000;118:1004–1006.

Geeraets WJ. *Ocular syndromes*, 3rd ed. Philadelphia: Lea & Febiger, 1976.

* = most important

Retinal vascular tumors

	Retinal Telangiectasia	Cavernous Retinal Hemangioma	Wynburn Mason Syndrome	Coats' Disease	Von Hippel-Lindau Syndrome	Sturge-Weber Syndrome	Pheochromocytoma
History							
1. Bilateral	S		S	S	S		
2. Congenital	U	U	R	U	R	U	
3. Greater in males	S	S		S			
4. Occurs during second to third decades					U		
5. Occurs before fourth decade				U			
6. Occurs during fourth to sixth decades							U
7. Onset during first decade of life	U	U		U			
Physical Findings							
1. Third, fourth, and sixth nerve palsies				S			
2. Angiomatosis of iris					S		
3. Choroidal hemangioma						U	
4. Conjunctival telangiectasia						S	
5. Glaucoma	R			S	S	S	
6. Optic atrophy							
7. Papilledema				S			U
8. Port-wine lid stain						S	
9. Ptosis				R			
10. Pulsatile exophthalmos				S			
11. Retinal hemorrhage	U		S	U	S		S
12. Soft exudates of retina	S		S	S	S		S
13. Telangiectatic retinal vessels	U	U		U	S	U	S
14. Total retinal detachment	R				U	S	S
15. Uveitis	R				S		
Laboratory Data							
1. Computed tomographic scan of head			U				
2. Cerebral angiography			U		S	R	
3. Fluorescein angiography	S	S	U	S	U	S	S
4. Ocular ultrasound	R	S	R	U	U	U	U
5. Urinary catecholamine and vanillylmandelic acid							U
6. Visual field test	S	S	U	S	U	S	S

R = rarely; S = sometimes; and U = usually.

Traumatic retinopathies

	Purtscher Retinopathy	Commotio Retinae	Traumatic Asphyxia	Fat Emoblism
Type of trauma	Chest compression	Local	Chest	Fractures
Accompanying signs	None	None	Cyanosis	Chest, cerebral, and cutaneous signs
Onset of systemic picture	None	None	Immediate	Symptom-free, 48-hour interval
Initial vision	Variable	20/200	Variable	Occasionally reduced
Duration of loss of vision	Several weeks	Days	Several weeks	Several weeks
Ultimate vision	Normal	Normal	Variable	Normal
External eye	Normal	Contused	Hemorrhage	Normal or petechiae
Fundus picture	Exudates and hemorrhage	Retinal edema	Normal or hemorrhage	Exudate, edema, and hemorrhages
Onset of fundus abnormalities	Within 1 to 2 days	A few hours	Immediate or a few hours	After 1 to 2 days

Ballantyne AJ, Michaelson IC. *Textbook of the fundus of the eye*, 3rd ed. Baltimore: Williams & Wilkins, 1981.

RETINAL "SEA-FANS"

These are vasoproliferative lesions with a characteristic fan-shaped appearance, also called a "parachute" lesion.

   1. Aortic arch syndrome (pulseless disease)
   2. Carotid–cavernous fistula (carotid artery syndrome)
 *3. Central and branch retinal vein occlusion (see p. 468)
   4. Chronic myelocytic leukemia
 *5. Diabetes mellitus
   6. Eales disease (periphlebitis)
   7. Facioscapulohumeral muscular dystrophy (FSH [facio scapulo numeral] syndrome)
   8. Incontinentia pigmenti I (Block–Sulzberger syndrome)
   9. Familial exudative vitreoretinopathy (Criswick–Schepens syndrome)
 10. Hemoglobin C trait
 11. Leukemia
 12. Long-standing retinal detachment
 13. Lupus erythematosus
 14. Macroglobulinemia
 15. Multiple sclerosis
 16. Polycythemia vera (erythremia)
*17. Retinopathy of prematurity
 18. Sarcoidosis syndrome
*19. Sickle cell disease
 20. Talc and cornstarch emboli
 21. Uveitis, including pars planitis

Gurwin EB, et al. Retinal telangiectasis in facioscapulohumeral muscular dystrophy with deafness. *Arch Ophthalmol* 1985;103:1695–1707.

Jampol LM, Goldberg MH. Peripheral proliferative retinopathies. *Surv Ophthalmol* 1980;25:1–14.

Rodgers R, et al. Ocular involvement in congenital leukemia. *Am J Ophthalmol* 1986;101:730–732.

Roy FH. *Ocular syndromes and systemic diseases,* 3rd ed. Philadelphia: Lippincott Williams & Wilkins, 2002.

RETINAL VESSELS DISPLACED TEMPORALLY

  1. Familial vitreoretinopathy
  2. Hamartomas
  3. Inflammation
  4. Myopia with lattice-like retinal degeneration
*5. Retinopathy of prematurity
*6. Sickle cell disease (drepanocytic anemia)
  7. Trauma

Ballantyne AJ, Michaelson IC. *Textbook of the fundus of the eye,* 3rd ed. Baltimore: Williams & Wilkins, 1981.

Nover A. *The ocular fundus: methods of examination and typical findings,* 4th ed. Philadelphia: Lea & Febiger, 1981.

RETINAL VESSELS DISPLACED NASALLY

  1. Axial myopia
*2. Glaucoma

3. Inflammation
4. Trauma

Ballantyne AJ, Michelson IC. *Textbook of the fundus of the eye,* 3rd ed. Baltimore: Williams & Wilkins, 1981.

Nover A. *The ocular fundus: methods of examination and typical findings,* 4th ed. Philadelphia: Lea & Febiger, 1981.

PERIPHERAL FUNDUS LESIONS

1. Pale raised lesions
    A. Vitreous opacities—white fluffy or discrete opacities, associated with pars planitis or sarcoid uveitis
    B. Retinopathy of prematurity—retinal edema and dense white lesions with neovascularization
    C. Toxocariasis (nematode ophthalmia syndrome)—vitreous opacities with peripheral granuloma
    D. Leprosy (Hansen disease)—peripheral exudates with anterior uveal involvement
    E. Vitreoretinal dystrophies—bands in vitreous with retinoschisis or retinal detachment
    F. Angiomatosis—retinal tumor with enlarged, feeding vessels
    *G. Retinoblastoma—raised, creamy-white, fluffy lesion without inflammatory signs
2. Flat lesions
    A. Coloboma—pale area with pigmented edge in region of fetal cleft
    B. Chorioretinitis
        (1) Disseminated, congenital syphilis—pepper-and-salt or larger confluent lesions
        (2) Toxoplasmosis—pigmented scars of old lesions
        (3) Cytomegalic inclusion disease—localized chorioretinitis or general peripheral infiltration
        *(4) Histoplasmosis—peripheral punched-out lesions with or without pigmentation
    C. Peripheral degenerations
        (1) Senile changes—of eyes older than years of age, depigmented areas with pigmented margins (cobblestone degeneration)
        (2) Secondary pigmentary degeneration—peripheral pigmentary changes similar to senile type or to retinitis pigmentosa
        (3) Cystoid degeneration—multiple cystic spaces and thin areas in peripheral retina
        *(4) Lattice degeneration—lace work of white lines with depigmented and pigmented patches
        (5) Cystinosis (cystine storage aminoaciduria dwarfism syndrome)—granular rings of pigment in periphery of fundus, similar to cobblestone degeneration
    D. Equatorial linear pigment disturbance
        (1) Ophthalmomyiasis internal
        (2) Histoplasmosis syndrome
    E. Retinitis
        *(1) Acute retinal necrosis
        *(2) Cytomegalovirus retinitis

* = most important

3. Dark raised lesions
  A. Choroidal detachment (see p. 532–535)
      (1) Spontaneous—slowly progressive detachment, no inflammatory signs
     *(2) Postoperative—intraocular operation; particularly for cataract and glaucoma; shallow anterior chamber; leaking wound
      (3) Exudative
          a. Inflammatory—shallow anterior chamber, myopia, and peripheral detachment
          b. Vascular—nephritis, hypertension, toxemia of pregnancy, polyarteritis nodosa, leukemia
         *c. Tumors—intraocular tumors; tumors of orbit and lacrimal gland
          d. Traumatic—contusion injuries, perforating wounds, hypotony, anterior chamber may be shallow or deep if perforation occurs posteriorly
  B. Exudative retinal detachment (see p. 487)
     *(1) Secondary to general disease with retinopathy—hypertension, toxemia of pregnancy, leukemia, dysproteinemia, polyarteritis nodosa, rickettsial arteritis, venous congestion, talc and cornstarch emboli
      (2) Secondary to local disease of the eye—inflammatory signs with exudative detachment, Harada disease, sympathetic ophthalmitis, scleritis, tenonitis, choroidal tumor, and ophthalmomyiasis
  C. Simple detachment—myopia in two thirds of patients, trauma, may follow cataract extraction or discission for congenital cataract
  D. Cysts
      (1) Ciliary body—larger cysts usually push iris forward; rarely, cyst extends backward to be seen ophthalmoscopically
      (2) Pars plana—may enlarge and appear as a multilocular reddish-brown cyst
  E. Scleral indentation—retinal detachment operation
  F. Neoplasms of ciliary body
      (1) Benign epithelioma—brown spot to 2 mm in diameter on surface of ciliary body
     *(2) Other tumors—diktyoma, leiomyoma, reticuloses, neurofibroma, malignant melanoma, rare, usually present as a mass protruding through the root of iris; may cause glaucoma; dark bulge seen ophthalmoscopically; lens changes adjacent to tumor
  G. Neoplasms of choroid
      (1) Congenital melanosis—cat's-paw patches of pigment in one sector of fundus
      (2) Choroidal nevus—flat, bluish gray or black lesion
     *(3) Malignant melanoma—raised, pigmented lesion with secondary detachment
      (4) Secondary metastatic—rare, primary lesion in breast, lung, and so on
4. Vascular lesions
  A. Periphlebitis (Eales disease) common; young adults; sheathing of peripheral veins; hemorrhages in new vessels and later retinal detachment (see p. 487)
 *B. Perivasculitis secondary to uveitis—perivascular infiltration, particularly in pars planitis, sarcoidosis, Behçet disease, and toxoplasmosis
  C. Systemic diseases
      (1) Rickettsia—engorgement of veins, retinal edema, hemorrhages, and exudates

(2) Multiple sclerosis (disseminated sclerosis)—sheathing of veins (see p. 468)

(3) Polyarteritis nodosa (necrotizing angiitis)—hemorrhages, exudates, and serous detachment of retina (see p. 488)

(4) Tuberculin or BCG inoculation—rare, sheathing of peripheral veins with hemorrhages

*(5) Sickle cell retinopathy (Herrick syndrome)—dilatation of peripheral veins, hemorrhages, and connective tissue sheets in periphery; new vessel formation

Mason GI. Bilateral ophthalmomyiasis interna. *Am J Ophthalmol* 1981;91:65–70.

Perkins ES, Dobree JH. *The differential diagnosis of fundus conditions.* St. Louis: CV Mosby, 1972.

Tasman W, Shields JA. *Disorders of the peripheral fundus.* New York: Harper & Row, 1980.

RETINAL DISEASE ASSOCIATED WITH CORNEAL PROBLEMS

1. Abdominal typhus (enteric fever)—corneal ulcer, retinal detachment, central retinal artery emboli

2. Acanthamoeba—keratitis, pannus, corneal ring abscess, retinal perivasculitis

3. African eyeworm disease—keratitis, central retinal artery occlusion, macular hemorrhages

4. Amyloidosis—amyloid corneal deposits, corneal dystrophy, retinal hemorrhages

5. Anderson–Warburg syndrome (oligophrenia-microphthalmos syndrome)—corneal opacification, malformed retina with retina pseudotumors

6. Angioedema (hives)—central serous retinopathy, corneal edema

*7. Anterior segment ischemia syndrome—corneal edema midperiphery retinal hemorrhages

8. Apert syndrome (acrodysplasia)—exposure keratitis, retinal detachment

9. Arteriovenous fistula—bullous keratopathy, retinal hemorrhages

10. Aspergillosis—corneal ulcer, keratitis, retinal hemorrhages, retinal detachment

11. Atopic dermatitis—keratoconus and retinal detachment

12. Avitaminosis C—retinal hemorrhages, keratitis, corneal ulcer

13. Bacillus cereus—ring abscess of cornea, necrosis of retina

14. Bang disease (brucellosis)—keratitis, chorioretinitis, macular edema

15. Behçet syndrome (dermatostomata-ophthalmic syndrome)—keratitis, posterior corneal abscess, retinal vascular changes

16. Bietti disease (Bietti marginal crystalline dystrophy)—marginal corneal dystrophy, retinitis punctate albescens

17. Candidiasis—keratitis, corneal ulcer, retinal atrophy, retinal detachment

*18. Carotid artery syndrome—corneal ulcer, loss of corneal sensation, retinal edema, engorgement of retinal veins

19. Chickenpox (varicella)—corneal ulcer, corneal opacity, retinitis, hemorrhagic retinopathy

20. Chloroquine—corneal epithelial pigmentation, macular lesions

21. Chronic granulomatous disease of childhood—keratitis, destructive chorioretinal lesions

22. Cockayne syndrome (dwarfism with retinal atrophy and deafness)—pigmentary degeneration, band keratopathy, corneal dystrophy

* = most important

23. Crohn disease (granulomatous ileocolitis)—marginal corneal ulcers, keratitis, macular edema, macular hemorrhages
24. Cryoglobulinemia—deep corneal opacities, venous stasis
25. Cystinosis (aminoaciduria)—crystals in cornea and pigment in retina
26. Dengue fever—keratitis, corneal ulcer, retinal hemorrhages
27. Diffuse keratoses syndrome—corneal nodular thickening in the stroma worse in fall, retinal phlebitis
28. Diphtheria—keratitis, corneal ulcer, central artery occlusion
29. Disseminated lupus erythematosus (Kaposi–Libman–Sacks syndrome)—keratitis, keratoconjunctivitis sicca, corneal ulcer, central retinal vein occlusion, retinal detachment
30. Ehlers–Danlos syndrome (cutis hyperelastica)—keratoconus, and retinitis pigmentosa
31. Electrical injury—corneal perforation, retinal edema, retinal hemorrhages, pigmentary degeneration, retinal holes, dilatation of retinal veins
32. Fabry disease (diffuse angiokeratosis)—whorl-like changes in cornea, central retinal artery occlusion, tortuosity of retinal vessels
33. Goldscheider syndrome (epidermolysis bullosa)—bullous keratitis with opacities, retinal detachment
34. Gronblad–Strandberg syndrome (systemic elastodystrophy)—angioid streaks of the retina, macular hemorrhages, retinal detachment, keratoconus
35. Hamman–Rich syndrome (alveolar capillary block syndrome)—keratomalacia ischemic retinopathy, cystic macular changes
36. Heerfordt syndrome (uveoparotid fever)—band keratopathy, retinal vasculitis
37. Hennebert syndrome (luetic otitic nystagmus syndrome)—interstitial keratitis, disseminated syphilitic chorioretinitis
38. Histiocytosis X (Hand–Schüller–Christian syndrome)—retinal hemorrhage, retinal detachment, bullous keratopathy, corneal ulcer, pannus
39. Hodgkin disease—keratitis, retinal hemorrhages
40. Hollenhorst syndrome (chorioretinal infarction syndrome)—hazy cornea, serous retinal detachment, pigmentary retinopathy
41. Hunter syndrome (MPS II)—splitting or absence of peripheral Bowman membrane, stromal haze, pigmentary retinal degeneration, narrowed retinal vessels
42. Hurler–Scheie syndrome (MPS IH-S)—corneal clouding, pigmentary retinopathy
43. Hurler syndrome (gargoylism)—diffuse corneal haziness, retinal pigmentary changes, megalocornea, retinal detachment
44. Hydatid cyst (echinococcosis)—keratitis, abscess of cornea, retinal detachment, retinal hemorrhages
45. Hyperlipoproteinemia—arcus juvenilis, lipemia retinalis, xanthomata of retina
46. Hyperparathyroidism—band keratopathy, vascular engorgement of retina
47. Hypovitaminosis A—keratomalacia with perforation, corneal opacity, retinal degeneration
48. Idiopathic hypercalcemia (blue-diaper syndrome)—band keratopathy, optic atrophy, papilledema
49. Indomethacin—corneal deposits, reduced retinal sensitivity
50. Influenza—keratitis, retinal hemorrhage
51. Japanese River fever (typhus)—keratitis, retinal hemorrhages
52. Juvenile rheumatoid arthritis (Still disease)—band keratopathy, macular edema
53. Kahler disease (multiple myeloma)—crystalline deposits of cornea, central retinal artery occlusion, retinal microaneurysms

54. Kussmaul disease (periarteritis nodosa)—retinal detachment, pseudoretinitis pigmentosa, corneal ulcer

55. Leber tapetoretinal dystrophy syndrome (retinal aplasia)—keratoconus, salt-and-pepper or "bone corpuscle" pigmentation, yellowish brown or gray macular lesions

56. Lubarsch–Pick syndrome (primary amyloidosis)—amyloid corneal deposits, retinal hemorrhages

*57. Lymphogranuloma venereum disease (Nicolas–Favre disease)—keratitis, pannus, corneal ulcer, keratoconus, tortuosity of retinal vessels, retinal hemorrhages

58. Marfan syndrome (arachnodactyly dystrophia mesodermalis congenita)—keratoconus, retinitis pigmentosa

59. Meckel syndrome (dysencephalia splanchnocystic syndrome)—sclerocornea, microcornea, retinal dysplasia

60. Meningococcemia—keratitis, retinal endophlebitis

61. Mikulicz–Radeski syndrome (dacryosialoadenopathy)—keratoconjunctivitis, retinal candlewax spots

62. ML IV (mucolipidosis IV)—corneal clouding, corneal opacities, retinal atrophy

63. Morbilli (measles-rubeola)—keratitis, corneal ulcer, pigmentary retinopathy, central retinal artery occlusion

64. Mucormycosis (phycomycosis)—corneal ulcer, striate keratopathy, retinitis, central retinal artery thrombosis

65. Mycosis fungoides syndrome (malignant cutaneous reticulosis syndrome)—keratoconjunctivitis, retinal edema, retinal hemorrhage

66. Myotonic dystrophy syndrome—corneal epithelial dystrophy, loss of corneal sensitivity, tapetoretinal degeneration, macular red spot, macular degeneration, chorioretinitis

*67. Neurofibromatosis (von Recklinghausen syndrome)—nodular swelling nerves, hamartoma of retina

68. Norrie disease (atrophia oculi congenita)—malformation of sensory cells of retina, corneal nebulae

69. Oculodental syndrome (Peters syndrome)—corneoscleral staphyloma, megalocornea, corneal marginal opacities, macular pigmentation

70. Onchocerciasis syndrome—punctate keratitis, sclerosing keratitis, chorioretinitis, retinal degeneration

71. Paget syndrome (osteitis deformans)—corneal ring opacities, retinal hemorrhages, pigmentary retinopathy, macular changes resembling Kuhnt–Junius degeneration

72. Phenothiazine—epithelial and endothelial pigment, retinal pigmentation

73. Pierre Robin syndrome (micrognathia–glossoptosis)—retinal disinsertion, megalocornea

74. Plasma lecithin (cholesterol acyltransferase deficiency)—corneal stromal opacities, retinal hemorrhages

75. Porphyria cutanea tarda—keratitis, retinal hemorrhages, cotton-wool spots, macular edema

76. Postvaccinial ocular syndrome—corneal vesicles, and marginal ulcers, chorioretinitis, central serous retinopathy, central retinal vein thrombosis

77. Progressive systemic sclerosis—marginal corneal ulcers with cicatrization, cotton-wool spots, retinal hemorrhages

78. Radiation—corneal ulcer, punctate keratitis, keratoconjuctivitis sicca, retinal hemorrhage, macular degeneration, macular holes with vascularization

*79. Refsum syndrome (phytanic acid oxidase deficiency)—band keratopathy, retinitis pigmentosa

* = most important

80. Relapsing fever—interstitial keratitis, retinal hemorrhage
81. Relapsing polychondritis—corneal ulcer, retinal detachment, retinal artery thrombosis, keratoconjunctivitis sicca
82. Renal failure—cotton-wool spots, band keratopathy
83. Rendu–Osler syndrome (hereditary hemorrhagic telangiectasis)—intermittent filamentary keratitis, small retinal angiomas, retinal hemorrhages
84. Retinal disinsertion syndrome—bilateral keratoconus, retinal detachment
*85. Retinoblastoma—corneal neovascularization, retinal tumor
86. Rothmund syndrome (telangiectasia-pigmentation cataract syndrome)—corneal lesions, retinal hyperpigmentation
87. Rubella syndrome (Gregg syndrome)—microcornea, pigmentary retinal changes
88. Sabin–Feldman syndrome—microcornea, chorioretinitis or atrophic degenerative chorioretinal changes
89. Sanfillipo–Good syndrome (mucopolysaccharidosis III)—slight narrowing of retinal vessels, acid mucopolysaccharide deposits in cornea.
*90. Schaumann syndrome (sarcoidosis syndrome)—mutton fat keratitic precipitates, keratitis sicca, band-shaped keratitis, inflammatory retinal exudates
91. Scheie syndrome (MPS I-S)—diffuse to marked corneal clouding, tapetoretinal degeneration
92. Schwartz syndrome (glaucoma associated with retinal detachment)—retinal detachment, microcornea
93. Shy–Gonatas syndrome (orthostatic hypotension syndrome)—keratopathy, corneal ulcer, lattice-like white opacities in the area of Bowman membrane, retinal pigmentary degeneration
94. Smallpox—keratitis, congenital corneal clouding, chorioretinitis
95. Stannus cerebellar syndrome (riboflavin deficiency)—corneal vascularization, superficial diffuse keratitis, corneal opacities, brownish retinal patches
96. Stickler syndrome (hereditary progressive arthroophthalmopathy)—keratopathy, chorioretinal degeneration, total retinal detachment
97. Sturge-Weber syndrome (neurooculocutaneous angiomatosis)—retinal detachment, increased corneal diameter with cloudiness
*98. Syphilis (acquired lues)—keratitis, retinal hemorrhages, retinal proliferation
*99. Temporal arteritis syndrome (Hutchinson–Horton–Magath–Brown syndrome)—retinal detachments, narrowing of retinal vessels, central retinal artery occlusion, corneal hypesthesia
100. Trisomy 13 (Patau syndrome)—malformed cornea, retinal dysplasia
*101. Tuberculosis—keratitis, pannus, corneal ulcer, retinitis
102. Ullrich syndrome (dyscraniopygophalangy)—cloudy cornea, corneal ulcers, chorioretinal coloboma
103. Ultraviolet radiation—photokeratitis, band keratopathy, herpes simplex keratitis, recurrent corneal erosions, retinal degeneration
104. Vaccinia—keratitis, pannus, corneal perforation, central serous retinopathy, pseudo-retinitis pigmentosa
105. van Bogaert–Scherer–Epstein (primary hyperlipidemia)—arcus juvenilis of the cornea, lipid keratopathy, retinopathy with yellowish deposits
106. Vitreous tug syndrome—vitreous strands attached to corneal wound or scar, circumscribed retinal edema, posterior retinal detachment
107. von Gierke disease (glycogen storage disease type I)—corneal clouding, discrete nonelevated, yellow flecks in macula

108. Waardenburg syndrome (embryonic fixation syndrome)—microcornea, cornea plana, hypopigmentation and hypoplasia of retina
109. Wagner syndrome (hyaloideoretinal degeneration)—corneal degeneration, band-shaped keratopathy, hyaloideoretinal degeneration, narrowing of retinal vessels, retinal detachment, avascular preretinal membranes
110. Waldenström syndrome (macroglobulinemia syndrome)—crystalline corneal deposits, keratoconjunctivitis sicca, retinal venous thrombosis, retinal microaneurysms, cotton-wool spots
111. Weil disease (leptospirosis)—keratitis, retinitis
112. Werner syndrome (progeria of adults)—bullous keratitis, paramacular retinal degeneration
113. Wiskott–Aldrich syndrome (sex-linked draining ears, eczematoid dermatitis, bloody diarrhea)—corneal ulcers, retinal hemorrhages
114. Yersiniosis—corneal ulcer, retinal hemorrhages
115. Zellweger syndrome (cerebrohepatorenal syndrome)—corneal opacities, narrowing of retinal vessels, retinal holes without detachment, tapetoretinal degeneration
116. Zieve syndrome (hyperlipemia hemolytic anemia-icterus syndrome)—cloudy cornea, corneal ulcers, retinal lipemia

Arffa RC. *Grayson's disease of the cornea,* 3rd ed. St. Louis: Mosby-Yearbook, 1991.

Roy FH. *Ocular syndromes and systemic diseases,* 3rd ed. Philadelphia: Lippincott Williams & Wilkins, 2002.

RETINAL LESIONS ASSOCIATED WITH DEAFNESS

1. Alport syndrome (hereditary familial congenital hemorrhagic nephritis)
2. Alström disease—retinitis pigmentosa
3. Choroideremia, obesity, and congenital deafness
4. Cockayne syndrome (dwarfism with retinal atrophy and deafness)
5. Dialinas–Amalric syndrome (deaf-mutism-retinal degeneration syndrome)
*6. Harada syndrome (Vogt–Koyanagi–Harada syndrome)
7. Hallgren syndrome (retinitis pigmentosa–deafness–ataxia syndrome)
8. Hunter syndrome (MPS II)
9. Laurence–Moon–Bardet–Biedl syndrome (retinitis pigmentosa–polydactyly adiposogenital syndrome)
10. Norrie disease—mental retardation, X-linked retinal malformation, and hearing loss
*11. Refsum syndrome (phytanic acid storage disease)
12. Retinal vessel changes, muscular dystrophy, mental retardation, and hearing loss
13. Rubella (German measles)—cardiac disorders, cataract, salt-and-pepper pigmentation
14. Sanfilippo syndrome (MPS III, autosomal recessive)
*15. Syphilis—acquired or congenital
16. Usher syndrome (hereditary retinitis pigmentosa—deafness syndrome)
17. Waardenburg syndrome (embryonic fixation syndrome)

Ayazi S. Choroideremia obesity, and congenital deafness. *Am J Ophthalmol* 1981;92:63–69.

Millay RH, et al. Ophthalmologic and systemic manifestations of Alström's disease. *Am J Ophthalmol* 1986;102: 482–490.

SUBRETINAL FIBROSIS

1. Central serous chorioretinopathy
2. Long-standing rhegmatogenous retinal detachment

* = most important

3. Proliferative vitreoretinopathy
4. Vogt–Koyanagi–Harada disease

Kuo IC, et al. Subretinal fibrosis in patients with Vogt–Koyanagi–Harada disease. *Ophthalmology* 2000;107: 1721–1728.

Rathinam SR, et al. Vogt–Koyanagi–Harada syndrome after cutaneous injury. *Ophthalmology* 1999;106:635–638.

EPIRETINAL MEMBRANES—MEMBRANES THAT GROW ON THE INNER SURFACE OF THE RETINA

*1. After retinal photocoagulation, cryotherapy, or reattachment of retina
 2. Following blunt or penetrating injuries
*3. Idiopathic
 4. Nonproliferative retinal vascular disorders
*5. Proliferative retinopathies
 6. Rhegmatogenous retinal detachment (see p. 468)
 7. Sickle cell disease, including sickle cell C, sickle cell S, and sickle cell B with thalassemia
 8. Vitreous hemorrhage (see p. 424)

Carney MD, Jampol LM. Epiretinal membranes in sickle cell retinopathy. *Arch Ophthalmol* 1987;105:214–217.

Cherfan GM, et al. Nuclear sclerotic cataract after vitrectomy for idiopathic epiretinal membranes causing macular pucker. *Am J Ophthalmol* 1991;111:434–438.

Lansing MB, et al. The effect of pars plana vitrectomy and transforming growth factor-beta without epiretinal membrane peeling on full-thickness macular holes. *Ophthalmology* 1993;100:871–872.

LINEAR STREAKS PATTERN IN FUNDUS

*1. Angioid streaks (see p. 526–529)
 2. Bird-shot retinochoroidopathy
 3. Choroidal rupture
 4. Demarcation lines
*5. Presumed ocular histoplasmosis syndrome—peripheral, parallel to equator
 6. Migrating parasites
    A. Botfly larvae
    B. Trematodes
*7. Retinal and choroidal detachment
*8. Snail-track configuration of lattice degeneration

Fountain JA, Schloegel TF. Linear streaks of the equator in the presumed ocular histoplasmosis syndrome. *Arch Ophthalmol* 1981;99:246.

YELLOW–ORANGE LESIONS OF SUBRETINAL FUNDUS

 1. Acute inflammatory lesions of pigment epithelium, choriocapillaris, and choroid
*2. Detachment of retinal pigment epithelium
 3. Isolated pocket of subretinal fluid
 4. Subretinal fluid following scleral buckling procedure

Avirs LR, Hilton GF. Lesions simulating serous detachments of the pigment epithelium. *Arch Ophthalmol* 1980; 98:1427–1429.

Lobes LR, Grand MG. Subretinal lesions following scleral buckling procedure. *Arch Ophthalmol* 1980;98:680–683.

TALC RETINOPATHY—DRUG ADDICTS WHO INJECT DRUGS INTRAVENOUSLY

1. Optic disc neovascularization (see p. 562–563)
2. Peripheral retinal neovascularization (see p. 514)
3. Vitreous hemorrhage (see p. 424)

O'Brien RJ, Schroedl BL. Talc retinopathy. *Optom Vis Sci* 1991;68:54–57.

Tse DT, Ober RR. Talc retinopathy. *Am J Ophthalmol* 1980;90:624–640.

CRYSTALLINE RETINOPATHY

1. Bietti crystalline dystrophy (Bietti disease)
2. Chronic retinal detachment
3. Cystinosis (cystine storage–aminoaciduria–dwarfism syndrome)
4. Gyrate atrophy with hyperornithemia (ornithine ketoacid aminotransferase deficiency)
5. Hyperoxaluria (oxalosis)
6. Nitrofurantoin therapy
7. Retinal pathology
8. Sjögren–Larson syndrome (oligophrenia-ichthyosis-spastic diplegia syndrome)
*9. Talc emboli
*10. Tamoxifen retinopathy

Ahmed I, et al. Crystalline retinopathy associated with chronic retinal detachment. *Arch Ophthalmol* 1998;116: 1449–1454.

Ibanez HE, et al. Crystalline retinopathy associated with long-term nitrofurantoin therapy. *Arch Ophthalmol* 1994; 112:304–305.

Willemsen MA, et al. Juvenile macular dystrophy associated with deficient activity of fatty aldehyde dehydrogenase in Sjögren-Larsson syndrome. *Am J Ophthalmol* 2000;130:782–789.

PULFRICH STEREO-ILLUSION PHENOMENON

This condition involves central serous elevation of the macula with abnormal latency of the visual-evoked potential.

*1. Optic nerve disease—demyelinating optic neuropathy
2. Media opacity
3. Anisocoria
4. Macular disease

Greenberg HS. Visual-evoked responses. *J Clin Neuro Ophthalmol* 1981;1:273.

Hofeldt AJ, et al. Pulfrich stereo-illusion phenomenon in serous sensory retinal detachment of the macula. *Am J Ophthalmol* 1985;100:576–580.

PARAFOVEAL TELANGIECTASIA

This type of retinal microvascular anomaly involves the parafoveal capillary network as well as immediately adjacent vascular bed and is best demonstrated by fluorescein angiography.

*1. Carotid artery obstruction
*2. Diabetes mellitus usually bilateral
*3. Idiopathic
4. Localized form of Coats disease, usually unilateral
5. Small-branch venular occlusion

* = most important

6. Small retinal capillary hemangioma, usually unilateral
7. Roentgenogram, irradiation

Gass JD, Oyakawa T. Idiopathic juxtafoveal telangiectasia. *Arch Ophthalmol* 1982;100:769.

Millay RH, et al. Abnormal glucose metabolism and parafoveal telangiectasia. *Am J Ophthalmol* 1986;102:363–370.

HEREDITARY PEDIATRIC RETINAL DEGENERATIONS

1. Acquired
   A. Juvenile retinitis pigmentosa
   B. Early onset retinitis pigmentosa
      (1) Autosomal dominant
      (2) Autosomal recessive
      (3) X-linked recessive
2. Congenital
   A. Complicated Leber congenital amaurosis
      (1) Multiple neurologic abnormalities
      (2) Others
      (3) Saldino–Mainzer syndrome
      (4) Senior–Loken syndrome (tubulointerstitial nephropathy syndrome)
      (5) Zellweger syndrome (cerebrohepatorenal syndrome of Zellweger)
   B. Uncomplicated Leber congenital amaurosis

Foxman SG, et al. Classification of congenital and early onset retinitis pigmentosa. *Arch Ophthalmol* 1985;103:1502–1506.

Nickel B, Hoyt CS. Leber's congenital amaurosis. *Arch Ophthalmol* 1982;100:1089–1092.

RETICULAR PATTERN OF DARK LINES IN FUNDUS

1. Granular pigmentary pattern of the peripheral fundus
2. Multiple drusen of peripheral fundus
3. Reticular degeneration of the pigment epithelium (peripheral)
4. Reticular pattern dystrophy of posterior fundus (Sjögren reticular dystrophy, Mesker macroreticular dystrophy, pattern dystrophy of the retinal pigment epithelium, Doyne honeycomb reticular degeneration)
5. Tapetochoroidal hypopigmentation

Gass JDM, et al. Drusen and disciform macular detachment and degeneration. *Arch Ophthalmol* 1973;90:206–217.

Lewis H, et al. Reticular degeneration of the pigment epithelium. *Ophthalmology* 1985;92:1485–1495.

RETINAL PIGMENT EPITHELIAL TEARS

This condition involves a flat, uniform, crescent-shaped area of exposed choroid of pigment epithelial elevation.

1. Acute retinal necrosis
*2. After laser photocoagulation
3. Along margin of retinal detachment
*4. Associated with pigment epithelial detachments
5. Spontaneous
6. Trauma

Fox GM, Blumenkranz M. Giant retinal pigment epithelial tears in acute retinal necrosis. *Am J Ophthalmol* 1993;
116:302–306.

Levin LA, et al. Retinal pigment epithelial tears associated with trauma. *Am J Ophthalmol* 1991;112:396–400.

Schoeppner G, et al. The risk of fellow eye visual loss with unilateral retinal pigment epithelial tears. *Am J Ophthalmol* 1989;108:683–685.

RETINAL PIGMENT EPITHELIAL FOLDS

1. Choroidal folds (see p. 530)
2. Pigment epithelial detachment
3. Retinal pigment epithelial tears (rips)
4. Retinal striae
*5. Subretinal neovascularization

Schatz H, et al. Retinal pigment epithelial folds associated with retinal pigment epithelial detachment in macular degeneration. *Ophthalmology* 1990;97:658–665.

Schoeppner G, et al. The risk of fellow eye visual loss with unilateral retinal pigment epithelial tears. *Am J Ophthalmol* 1989;108:683–685.

MIZUO PHENOMENON

This condition involves a change of color of the fundus from red in the dark-adapted state to golden immediately or shortly after the onset of light.

1. Oguchi disease
2. X-liked juvenile retinoschisis
3. X-linked recessive cone dystrophy

de Jong PTV, et al. Mizuo phenomenon in X-linked retinoschisis. *Arch Ophthalmol* 1991;109:1104–1108.

Mizuo GA. A new discovery in dark adaptation in Oguchi's disease. *Acta Soc Ophthalmol Jpn* 1913;17:1148–1150.

Usui T, et al. Mizuo phenomenon observed by scanning laser ophthalmoscopy in a patient with Oguchi disease. *Am J Ophthalmol* 2000;130:359–361.

WHITE-DOT FOVEA

This is a ring-like lesion in the macula with numerous confluent white dots arranged in a ring around the foveal margin.

1. Crystalline retinopathies
2. Epiretinal membrane with pseudohole
3. Gunn dots
4. Macular halo syndrome
5. Macular hole
6. Niemann–Pick disease
7. Vitreomacular fraction syndrome

* = most important

16 =

Choroid

CONTENTS

ANGIOID STREAKS

Angioid streaks are ruptures of Bruch membrane characterized ophthalmoscopically by brownish lines surrounding the disc and radiating toward the periphery.

1. AC hemoglobinopathy
2. Acanthocytosis (abetalipoproteinemia, Bassen–Kornzweig syndrome)
3. Acromegaly
4. Acquired hemolytic anemia
5. Beta thalassemia minor
6. Calcinosis
7. Chronic congenital idiopathic hyperphosphatasemia
8. Chronic familial hyperphosphatemia
9. Cardiovascular disease with hypertension
10. Cooley anemia
11. Diffuse lipomatosis

12. Dwarfism
13. Epilepsy
14. Facial angiomatosis
15. Fibrodysplasia hyperelastica (Ehlers–Danlos syndrome)
16. François dyscephalic syndrome (Hallermann–Streiff syndrome)
17. Hemochromatosis
18. Hereditary spherocytosis
19. Hypercalcinosis
20. Idiopathic thrombocytic purpura
21. Lead poisoning
22. Myopia
23. Neurofibromatosis
24. Ocular melanocytosis
25. Optic disc drusen
26. Osteitis deformans (Paget disease)
27. Pituitary tumor
28. Previous choroidal detachment
*29. Pseudoxanthoma elasticum (Grönblad–Strandberg syndrome)
30. Senile (actinic) elastosis of the skin
31. Sickle cell disease (Herrick syndrome)
32. Sturge–Weber syndrome
33. Trauma
34. Tuberous sclerosis
35. Thrombocytopenic purpura

Aessopos A, et al. Angioid streaks in sickle-thalassemia. *Am J Ophthalmol* 1994;117:589–592.

Mansour AM. Is there an association between optic disc drusen and angioid streaks? *Graefes Arch Clin Exp Ophthalmol* 1992;230:595–596.

Roy FH. *Ocular syndromes and systemic diseases*, 3rd ed. Philadelphia: Lippincott Williams & Wilkins, 2002.

* = most important

Angioid streaks (rupture of bruch membrane with brownish lines around disc and radiating toward periphery)

	Senile (Actinic) Elastosis	Pseudoxanthoma Elasticum (Gronblad-Strandberg Syndrome)	Fibrodysplasia Hyperplastica (Ehlers-Danlos Syndrome)	Osteitis Deformans (Paget Disease)	Cardiovascular Disease with Hypertension	Sickle Cell Disease	Dwarfism	Acromegaly	Pituitary Tumor	Epilepsy	Lead Poisoning	Thrombocytopenic Purpura	Facial Angiomatosis	Previous Choroidal Detachment	François Dycephalic Syndrome	Ocular Melanocytosis
History																
1. Autosomal dominant			U	U												
2. Autosomal recessive		U				U										
3. Congenital																U
4. Develop with age/ exposure to sun	U															
5. Elevated blood pressure					U											
6. Familial	U														U	
7. Hereditary		U	U	U	U								U			
8. Metamorphopsia									U							
9. Micropsia									U							
10. More in blacks						U										
11. More in children												S				
12. More in males					U											
13. More in whites																U
14. Ocular/periocular trauma														U		
15. Onset after 40 years				U				U								
16. "Pica" in children											U					
17. Severer in females				U												
18. Unilateral														U		U
Physical Findings																
1. Anterior synechiae														U		
2. Bilateral microphthalmos															U	
3. Black sunbursts, retina						U										
4. Blue sclera			U												S	
5. Buphthalmos													U			
6. Cataract		S					U								U	
7. Chalk-white vessels of retina						U										
8. Chorioretinal hyperpigmentation								S							U	
9. Choroidal coloboma														S		
10. Choroidal detachment		U												U		
11. Choroidal hemangioma													U			
12. Cotton-wool spots					U											
13. Decreased intraocular pressure									S					U		
14. Descemet wrinkles		S		S												
15. Exophthalmos		S							S						S	
16. Extraocular muscle paralysis				U									U			
17. Gaze paresis										U						
18. Hemianopia									U						U	
19. High myopia			S						S							
20. Holes in periphery/macula						U	U									
21. Hyloid/vitreous anterior displacement														U		
22. Increased intraocular pressure					U									U	S	
23. Increased pigment episclera/ sclera/uvea																U
24. Keratoconus		U	S													

Angioid streaks (rupture of bruch membrane with brownish lines around disc and radiating toward periphery) (Continued)

	Senile (Actinic) Elastosis	Pseudoxanthoma Elasticum (Gronblad-Strandberg Syndrome)	Fibrodysplasia Hyperplastica (Ehlers-Danlos Syndrome)	Osteitis Deformans (Paget Disease)	Cardiovascular Disease with Hypertension	Sickle Cell Disease	Dwarfism	Acromegaly	Pituitary Tumor	Epilepsy	Lead Poisoning	Thrombocytopenic Purpura	Facial Angiomatosis	Previous Choroidal Detachment	François Dycephalic Syndrome	Ocular Melanocytosis
Physical Findings																
25. Macular hemorrhages		U			S							U				
26. Malignant melanoma																S
27. Microcornea			U												U	
28. Nevus of ota																U
29. Nystagmus									U						U	
30. Optic atrophy		S		S			U		U				S		S	
31. Optic neuritis											U	U				
32. Optic nerve cupping					S								S			
33. Papilledema					U				U		U	U				
34. Peripheral artery occlusion						U										
35. Port-wine stain of face													U			
36. Ptosis									U	S						
37. Retinal atrophy						U										
38. Retinal degeneration									S							
39. Retinal detachment		U	U													
40. Retinal edema					U											
41. Retinal hemorrhage					U	U					U	U				
42. Shiny dots in macula											U					
43. Skin papules	U	S	S													
44. Strabismus			U						U						S	
45. Vascular sheathing											U					
46. Visual field defects		U		U					U							
47. Vitreous hemorrhage		U			S	U										
Laboratory Data																
1. Bones, roentgenogram		S		U			U	U								
2. Computed tomographic scan							U	S	U	S			U		S	
3. Cerebral angiography									S				U			
4. Electroencephalogram										U						
5. Fluorescein angiography		S	S											U	U	U
6. Hemoglobin electrophoresis						U										
7. Lipid profile tests					U											
8. Peripheral blood test (hemoglobin, hematocrit, red blood cell, and platelet counts)					U							U				
9. Pituitary panel, including prolactin, growth hormone, adrenocorticotropic hormone, follicle-stimulating hormone, luteinizing hormone, thyroid-stimulating hormone									U							
10. Pneumoencephalogram									S							
11. Serum alkaline phosphatase				U												
12. Skin biopsy	U	U	U													
13. Skull roentgenogram						S	U	U	U							
14. Ultrasonography, ocular														U	S	R
15. Urinary calcium levels			S	U												

R = rarely; S = sometimes; and U = usually.

CHOROIDAL FOLDS

Choroidal folds are folds of the posterior pole, at the level of the choroid, with Hruby lens and pattern of alternating light lines on fluorescein angiography.

1. Choroidal tumor, such as a melanoma
2. Disciform degeneration
3. Exophthalmos
4. Graves disease (Basedow syndrome)
5. High hyperopia
6. Idiopathic—no underlying pathologic state
7. Infection of paranasal sinuses
8. Long-standing orbital inflammation
9. Massive cranioorbital hemangiopericytoma
*10. Ocular hypotony (see p. 325)
11. Orbital mass
12. Papilledema (see p. 593)
13. Posteriorly located choroidal detachment
14. Postoperative condition, such as scleral buckle
15. Primary retinal detachment
16. Subretinal neovascularization
17. Uveitis

Griebel SR, Kosmorsky GS. Choroidal folds associated with increased intracranial pressure. *Am J Ophthalmol* 2000; 129:513–516.

Leventer DB. Frontoethmoidal mucoceles causing bilateral chorioretinal folds. *Arch Ophthalmol* 2001;119:922.

Shields JA, et al. Clinicopathologic correlation of choroidal folds: secondary to massive cranioorbital hemangiopericytoma. *Ophthal Plast Reconstr Surg* 1992;8:62–68.

LESIONS CONFUSED WITH MALIGNANT MELANOMA

1. Ciliary body and choroid
    A. Angioid streaks (see p. 526)
    B. Choroiditis
    C. Coats disease
    D. Detachment
    E. Leukemia and lymphoma
    F. Limited choroidal hemorrhage
    G. Lymphoid hyperplasia
    H. Nodular hyperplasia
    I. Sclerouveitis
    J. Tumors
        (1) Hemangioma
        (2) Melanocytoma
        (3) Meningioma
        (4) Metastatic carcinoma, including lung
        (5) Neurilemmoma
        (6) Neurofibroma
        (7) Neuroendocrine tumor
        (8) Nevus
        (9) Retinal oligodendroglioma
    K. Uveal effusion

2. Optic-nerve head
    A. Congenital crater
    B. Melanocytoma
3. Retina
    A. Chorioretinitis
    B. Ciliary body and choroid'
    C. Disciform macular degeneration
    D. Foreign body
    E. Hemorrhagic macrocyst of retina
    F. Lesions of pigment epithelium
    G. Retinal detachment
        (1) Macular
        (2) More extensive
    H. Retinoschisis
4. Scleral thickening as amyloidosis
5. Vitreous body
    A. Abscess
    B. Hemorrhages

Brannan SO, et al. A choroidal amyloid-rich neuroendocrine tumor. *Arch Ophthalmol* 1999;117:1081–1083.

Eagle RC, et al. Choroidal metastasis as the initial manifestation of a pigmented neuroendocrine tumor. *Arch Ophthalmol* 2000;118:841–845.

Marek J, et al. Retinal oligodendroglioma. *Am J Ophthalmol* 1999;128:389–391.

Shields JA, Shields CL. *Intraocular tumors: a text and atlas*. Philadelphia: WB Saunders, 1992.

Simon CK, et al. Bilateral uveal effusion associated with scleral thickening due to amyloidosis. *Arch Ophthalmol* 2000;118:1293–1295.

CHOROIDAL HEMORRHAGE

1. Acute choroiditis
*2. After glaucoma filtering procedure (especially with Sturge–Weber syndrome)
3. Choroidal vascular aneurysm
4. Choroidal vascular sclerosis, such as senile macular degeneration with hemorrhage (disciform degeneration of the macula)
5. General diseases
    A. Arteriosclerosis
    B. Blood dyscrasias
        (1) Leukemia
        (2) Pernicious anemia
        (3) Purpura
        (4) Thrombocytopenia
    C. Diabetes mellitus (Willis disease)
    D. Ehlers–Danlos syndrome (fibrodysplasia elastica generalisata)
    E. Paget disease (osteitis deformans)
    F. Valsalva maneuver
6. Myopia—accompanied by choroidal atrophy
7. Papilledema—rare

Boker T, Steinmetz R. Hyperopia and choroidal neovascularization. *Ophthalmology* 1994;101:972.

Madreperla SA, et al. Choroidal hemangiomas. *Ophthalmology* 1997;104:1773–1779.

* = most important

Roy FH. *Ocular syndromes and systemic diseases*, 3rd ed. Philadelphia: Lippincott Williams & Wilkins, 2002.

VanMeurs JC, van der Bosch WA. Suprachoroidal hemorrhage following a Valsalva maneuver. *Arch Ophthalmol* 1993;111:1025–1026.

CHOROIDAL DETACHMENT

Choroidal detachment can be differentiated from retinal detachment and tumor by its solid appearance, smooth surface, and appearance of normal retinal vessels with color unchanged and good transillumination.

*1. Acute ocular hypotony (see p. 325)
     A. Myopia
     B. Operative or perforating wounds, including those required for surgical treatment of cataract, glaucoma, grafting of cornea, and retinal detachment
     C. Severe uveitis with severe visual loss, intense ocular pain, unusually low tension, and extremely deep anterior chamber in women
     D. Yttrium–aluminum–garnet (YAG) laser cyclophotocoagulation
 2. Inflammatory disease
     A. Acute sinusitis
     B. Chronic cyclitis
     C. Harada disease (Vogt–Koyanagi–Harada syndrome)
     D. Orbital abscess
     E. Orbital pseudotumor
     F. Scleritis and tenonitis
     G. Sympathetic ophthalmia
 3. Neoplastic disease
     A. Intraocular tumor, such as metastatic or malignant melanoma
     B. Leukemia
     C. Orbital tumor
 4. Spontaneous detachment associated with uveal effusion, such as nonrhegmatogenous retinal detachment, shifting subretinal fluid, and peripheral annular choroidal detachment affecting males almost exclusively
 5. Trauma
     A. Complication of scleral buckling retinal detachment surgery
     B. Contusion of globe without perforation
     C. Following perforation injury, including that because of perforating corneal ulcer
     D. Phthisical eye with traction of organized inflammatory tissue
 6. Vascular disease
     A. Diabetes mellitus (Willis disease)
     B. Disseminated intravascular coagulation
     C. Hypertension
     D. Leukemia
     E. Multiple myeloma (Kahler disease)
     F. Nephritis
     G. Oral acetazolamide
     H. Periarteritis nodosa (Kussmaul disease)
     I. Syphilitic vascular disease
     J. Toxemia of pregnancy

* = most important

Kurtz S, et al. Orbital pseudotumor presenting as acute glaucoma with choroidal and retinal detachment. *German J Ophthalmol* 1993;2:61–62.

Lakhanpal V. Experimental and clinical observations on massive suprachoroidal hemorrhage. *Trans Am Ophthalmol Soc* 1993;91:545–652.

Roy FH. *Ocular syndromes and systemic diseases*, 3rd ed. Philadelphia: Lippincott Williams & Wilkins, 2002.

Choroidal detachment (solid appearance, smooth surface and normal retinal vessels with unchanged color)

	Inflammatory Disease as Harada Disease	Vascular Disease as Diabetes Mellitus	Neoplastic Disorder as Malignant Melanoma	Ocular Trauma as Blunt Trauma	Acute Ocular Hypotony	Spontaneous Detachment with Uveal Effusion as Nonrhegmatogenous Retinal Detachment
History						
1. Bilateral	U	U				
2. Common in males				U		U
3. Familial		U				
4. Japanese/Italian extraction	U					
5. Occurs in persons 11 to 40 years		S				
6. Occurs in young adults	U	U				
7. Ocular pain					S	
8. Surgery					U	
9. Virus infection	U					
10. Visual distortion			S			S
Physical Findings						
1. Acute diffuse exudative choroiditis	U					U
2. Cataracts	S		U		S	
3. Cyclodialysis cleft					S	
4. Corneal abrasions				S		
5. Corneal arcus		S				
6. Cotton-wool spots		U				
7. Choroidal folds					S	
8. Choroidal nevus			S			
9. Choroidal rupture				U	S	S
10. Decreased intraocular pressure				S	U	U
11. Endothelial corneal damage				S		
12. Extraocular muscle paralysis			S			
13. Exudative iridocyclitis	U					S
14. Glaucoma	U	S	S	S		
15. Hyphema				S		
16. Hypermetropia			U			
17. Increased lid pigmentation			S			
18. Iridodialysis				S		
19. Macular edema					S	
20. Macular hemorrhage	S					
21. Optic nerve atrophy		S	S	S		
22. Oribital mass			S			
23. Papilledema	U		S			
24. Phthisis bulbi	S					
25. Pigmentary retinopathy	U		S			
26. Pigmentary iris degeneration					S	
27. Pigmented/amelanotic choroidal mass			U			
28. Poliosis	U					
29. Recessed chamber angle				S		
30. Retinal detachment	U	S	U	S		U
31. Retinal edema	U					S
32. Retinal folds					U	

Choroidal detachment (solid appearance, smooth surface and normal retinal vessels with unchanged color) (Continued)

	Inflammatory Disease as Harada Disease	Vascular Disease as Diabetes Mellitus	Neoplastic Disorder as Malignant Melanoma	Ocular Trauma as Blunt Trauma	Acute Ocular Hypotony	Spontaneous Detachment with Uveal Effusion as Nonrhegmatogenous Retinal Detachment
Physical Findings						
33. Retinal hemorrhage			S	S′		
34. Retinal microaneurysms		U				
35. Retinal vein occlusion		S				
36. Scleral rupture				S	S	
37. Shallow anterior chamber					S	
38. Subluxed lens				S		
39. Sympathetic ophthalmitis	U					
40. Uveitis	U					
41. Vitreous detachment				S		S
42. Vitreous hemorrhage			S	S		
43. Vitreous opacities	U					
44. White lashes	U					
Laboratory Data						
1. Abnormal blood sugar		U				
2. Computed tomographic scan of globe			S	S		
3. Fluorescein angiography	U	U	U	U		S
4. Phosphorus 32 uptake elevated			U			
5. Ultrasonography, globe	S		S	U	U	U

R = rarely; S = sometimes; and U = usually.

CONDITIONS SIMULATING POSTERIOR UVEITIS OR CHOROIDITIS

1. Angioid streaks (see p. 526)
2. Central serous retinopathy
   A. Central serous retinopathy and exudative chorioretinopathy associated with systemic vasculitis
   B. Central serous retinopathy associated with crater-like holes in the optic disc
   C. Choroidal
   D. Chorioretinal
   E. Retinal
3. Chorioretinopathy with hereditary microcephaly
4. Circinate retinopathy
5. Congenital macular dysplasia
6. Doyne homogeneous retinal degeneration
7. Drug-induced macular disease
   A. Chloroquine (Aralen)
   B. Indomethacin (Indocin)
   C. Thioridazine (Mellaril)
8. Drusen because of the following:
   A. Disease (vascular, inflammatory, or neoplastic)
   B. Heredity (primary degeneration)
   C. Senility
9. Fundus flavimaculatus
10. Helicoid peripapillary chorioretinal degeneration
11. Hemangioma of the choroid
12. Idiopathic hyperlipemia
13. Ischemic ocular inflammation
14. Ischemic optic neuropathy (vascular pseudopapillitis)
15. Jensen disease (juxtapapillary retinopathy)
16. Macular degeneration
17. Malignant melanoma
18. Metastatic carcinoma
19. Night-blinding retinochoroidopathies
    A. Predominantly choroidal heredodegenerations
       (1) Choroidal sclerosis
       (2) Choroideremia
       (3) Fuchs spot
       (4) Gyrate atrophy of choroid
       (5) Myopic retinopathy and choroidopathy
    B. Predominantly tapetoretinal heredodegenerations
       (1) Retinitis pigmentosa group
       (2) Retinitis punctata albescens
20. Opacities of the macular retina
    A. Cotton-wool patches (see p. 491–494)
    B. Glial scars
    C. Hemorrhage
    D. Hemosiderin
    E. Inspissated exudates
    F. Lipoid deposits

    G. Pigment epithelium
        (1) Pigment epithelium migration
        (2) Pigment epithelium secretion
        (3) Pigment epithelium seeds
        (4) Proliferation in response to demand for phagocytes
        (5) Proliferation with formation of cuticular masses
        (6) Proliferation with metaplasia
        (7) Simple proliferation
21. Peripheral chorioretinal atrophy
22. Pigmentary perivenous—chorioretinal degeneration
23. Primary familial amyloidosis
24. Relapsing polychondritis
25. Retinal perforation during surgical treatment for strabismus
26. Retinal vasculitis
    A. Involvement of central retinal vein (papillophlebitis)
    B. Retinal periarteritis
    C. Retinal periphlebitis
27. Retinoblastoma
28. Sickle cell retinopathy
29. Solar burns
30. Sorsby pseudoinflammatory (hemorrhagic) macular degeneration
31. Vitreous hemorrhage (see p. 421–422)

Schlaegel TF. *Essentials of uveitis.* Boston: Little, Brown, 1969.

Suran A, et al. *Immunology of the eye, workshop III. Immunologic aspects of ocular disease: infection, inflammation, and allergy.* Oxford: IRL Press, 1981.

CHOROIDITIS (POSTERIOR UVEITIS)

1. Anterior and posterior uveitis
    A. Herpes viruses
    B. Peripheral uveitis (cyclitis)
    C. Sarcoidosis syndrome (Schaumann syndrome)
    D. Syphilis (acquired lues)
    E. Toxoplasmosis
    F. Tuberculosis
    G. Unknown
    H. Vogt–Koyanagi–Harada syndrome (uveitis–vitiligo–alopecia–poliosis syndrome)
2. Acquired immunodeficiency syndrome (AIDS)
3. Acute posterior multifocal placoid pigment epitheliopathy
4. Behçet syndrome
5. Bird-shot choroidopathy
6. Candidiasis
7. Cat-scratch disease
8. Cryptococcosis
9. Cytomegalovirus inclusion disease
10. Coccidioidomycosis
11. Epstein–Barr virus
12. Lyme disease

13. Histoplasmosis
14. Multiple evanescent white dot syndrome
15. Multiple sclerosis
16. *Pneumocystis carinii*
17. Punctate inner choroidopathy
18. Sarcoidosis syndrome (Schaumann syndrome)
19. Serpiginous choroidopathy
20. Syphilis (acquired lues)
21. Systemic lupus erythematosus
22. Toxocariasis
*23. Toxoplasmosis
24. Unknown
25. Varicella zoster

Demiroglu H, et al. Risk factor assessment and prognosis of eye involvement in Behçet's disease in Turkey. *Ophthalmology* 1997;104:701–705.

Kerrison JR, et al. Retinal pathologic changes in multiple sclerosis. *Retina* 1994;14:445–451.

Ormerod LD, et al. Retinal and choroidal manifestations of cat-scratch disease. *Ophthalmology* 1998;105:1024–1031.

Schubert HD, et al. Cytologically proven seronegative Lyme choroiditis and vitreitis. *Retina* 1994;14:39–41.

CONDITIONS SIMULATING POSTERIOR UVEITIS IN CHILDREN

1. Coats syndrome (retinal telangiectasia)
2. Cockayne disease (dwarfism with retinal atrophy and deafness)
3. Cystinosis syndrome (Lignac–Fanconi syndrome)
4. Hypogammaglobulinemia
5. Idiopathic hyperlipemia
6. Leukemia
7. Massive retinal fibrosis
*8. Retinoblastoma

Freidman AH, et al. *An atlas of uveitis: diagnosis and management.* Baltimore: Williams & Wilkins, 1982.

Kraus M, et al. *Uveitis—pathophysiology and therapy,* 2nd ed. New York: Thieme, 1986.

CHOROIDITIS (POSTERIOR UVEITIS) IN CHILDREN

1. Ankylosing spondylitis
2. Anterior and posterior uveitis
    A. Sarcoidosis syndrome (Schaumann syndrome)
    B. Sympathetic ophthalmia
    C. Vogt–Koyanagi–Harada syndrome
3. Arteritis
4. Behçet disease (dermatostomatoophthalmic syndrome)
5. Chorioretinitis of unknown cause
    A. Disseminated chorioretinitis
    B. Juxtapapillary chorioretinitis
6. Cytomegalovirus inclusion disease (cytomegalovirus)
7. Diffuse unilateral subacute neuroretinitis
8. Herpes simplex chorioretinitis
9. Human immunodeficiency virus retinopathy
10. Inability of leukocytes to kill microorganisms

11. Intermediate uveitis
12. Juvenile psoriatic arthritis
13. Juvenile rheumatoid arthritis
14. *Nematode* (*Toxocara*) retinochoroiditis
15. Reiter disease (idiopathic blennorrheal arthritis syndrome)
16. Reticulum cell sarcoma of brain
17. Rubella
18. Subacute sclerosing panencephalitis
19. Syphilitic retinochoroiditis
*20. Toxoplasmic retinochoroiditis
21. Tuberculosis

Kanski JJ, Shun-Shin A. Systemic uveitis syndrome in childhood: an analysis of cases. *Ophthalmology* 1984;91: 1247–1251.

Kraus M, et al. *Uveitis—pathophysiology and therapy*, 2nd ed. New York: Thieme, 1986.

Okada AA, Foster CS. Posterior uveitis in the pediatric population. *Int Ophthalmol Clin* 1992;32:121–152.

SYNDROMES AND DISEASES ASSOCIATED WITH UVEITIS

1. Arthralgia
    A. Hilding syndrome (destructive iridocyclitis and multiple joint dislocations)
    B. Histoplasmosis
    C. Whipple disease (intestinal lipodystrophy)
2. Arthritis
    A. Ankylosing spondylitis
    B. Behçet syndrome (dermatostomatoophthalmic syndrome)
    C. Bleu syndrome
    D. Familial histiocytic dermatoarthritis syndrome
    E. Felty syndrome (rheumatoid arthritis with hypersplenism)
    F. Gonorrhea
    G. Juvenile rheumatoid arthritis (Still disease)
    H. Leprosy (Hansen disease)
    I. Mucocutaneous lymph node syndrome
    J. Progressive systemic sclerosis
    K. Psoriatic arthritis
    L. Reiter syndrome (polyarthritis enterica)
    M. Rheumatoid arthritis (adult)
    N. Sarcoidosis syndrome (Schaumann syndrome)
    O. Sporotrichosis
    P. Ulcerative colitis
    Q. Van Metre peripheral polyarthritis or monoarthritis
    R. Whipple disease (intestinal lipodystrophy)
    S. Yersiniosis
3. Cataract
    A. Acrodermatitis chronica atrophicans
    B. Andogsky syndrome (dermatogenous cataract)
    C. Anterior segment ischemia syndrome
    D. Arteriovenous fistula
    E. Atopic dermatitis
    F. Carotid artery syndrome (carotid vascular insufficiency syndrome)

* = most important

    G. Cerebral palsy

    H. Chickenpox

    I. Cockayne syndrome (dwarfism with retinal atrophy and deafness)

    J. Cytomegalic inclusion disease

    K. Electrical injury

    L. Familial histiocytic dermatoarthritis syndrome

    M. Hallermann–Streiff–François syndrome (dyscephalic mandibulooculofacial syndrome)

    N. Herpes simplex

    O. Herpes zoster

    P. Hilding syndrome (destructive iridocyclitis and multiple joint dislocations)

    Q. Histiocytosis X (Hand–Schüller–Christian syndrome)

    R. Hodgkin disease (lymph node disease)

    S. Homocystinuria syndrome

    T. Hypervitaminosis D

    U. Influenza

    V. Juvenile rheumatoid arthritis (Still disease)

    W. Kussmaul disease (periarteritis nodosa)

    X. Leptospirosis (Weil disease)

    Y. Listerellosis

    Z. Malaria

  AA. Measles (rubeola)

  BB. Moniliasis (idiopathic hypoparathyroidism)

  CC. Myotonic dystrophy syndrome

  DD. Oculootoororenoerythropoietic disease

  EE. Passow syndrome (syringomyelia)

  FF. Radiation

  GG. Relapsing polychondritis

  HH. Rubella syndrome

  II. Sarcoidosis syndrome (Schaumann syndrome)

  JJ. Stevens–Johnson syndrome (erythema multiforme exudativum)

  KK. Stickler syndrome (hereditary progressive arthroophthalmyopathy)

  LL. Toxocariasis (visceral larva migrans syndrome)

  MM. Toxoplasmosis

  NN. Werner syndrome (progeria of adults)

  OO. Yersiniosis

4. Conjunctivitis

    A. Acanthamoeba

    B. Actinomycosis

    C. African eyeworm disease

    D. Amebiasis

    E. Andogsky syndrome (dermatogenous cataract)

    F. Angular conjunctivitis

    G. Ascariasis

    H. Atopic dermatitis

    I. Bacillary dysentery (shigellosis)

    J. Bacterial endocarditis

    K. Behçet syndrome (dermatostomato-ophthalmic syndrome)

    L. Boutonneuse fever (rickettsia, Marseilles fever)

    M. Brucellosis

    N. Candidiasis

    O. Charlin syndrome (nasal nerve syndrome)

    P. Chlamydia

    Q. Coccidioidomycosis

    R. Coenurosis

    S. Cogan syndrome (nonsyphilitic interstitial keratitis)

    T. Crohn disease (granulomatous ileocolitis)

    U. Cytomegalic inclusion disease

    V. Disseminated lupus erythematosus (Kaposi–Libman–Sacks syndrome)

    W. Epidermic keratoconjunctivitis

    X. *Escherichia coli*

    Y. Felty syndrome (rheumatoid arthritis with hypersplenism)

    Z. *Haemophilus aegyptius*

  AA. Herpes simplex

  BB. Herpes zoster

  CC. Hodgkin disease

  DD. Infectious mononucleosis

  EE. Influenza

  FF. Kussmaul disease (periarteritis nodosa)

  GG. Leptospirosis (Weil disease)

  HH. Listerellosis

   II. Lymphogranuloma venereum

  JJ. Measles (rubeola)

  KK. Meningococcemia

  LL. Metastatic bacterial endophthalmitis

 MM. Mikulicz–Radecki syndrome (dacryosialoadenopathy)

  NN. Moniliasis (idiopathic hypoparathyroidism)

  OO. Moraxella lacunata

  PP. Mucocutaneous lymph node syndrome

  QQ. Mumps

  RR. Mycosis fungoides syndrome (Sézary syndrome)

  SS. Nocardiosis

  TT. Ocular vaccinia

  UU. Pneumococcus

  VV. Polymyositis dermatomyositis

 WW. Progressive systemic sclerosis (scleroderma)

  XX. Psoriatic arthritis

  YY. Q fever

  ZZ. Radiation

 AAA. Reiter syndrome (polyarthritis enterica)

 BBB. Relapsing fever

 CCC. Rocky Mountain spotted fever

 DDD. Rubella syndrome

 EEE. St. Anthony fire (erysipelas)

 FFF. Seborrheic dermatitis

 GGG. Sporotrichosis

 HHH. Staphylococcus

  III. Stevens–Johnson syndrome (erythema multiforme exudativum)

JJJ. Streptococcus
KKK. Syphilis (acquired lues)
LLL. Trichinellosis
MMM. Tuberculosis
NNN. Vaccinia
OOO. Xeroderma pigmentosum
PPP. Yersiniosis

5. Cornea

A. Acanthamoeba
B. Acrodermatitis chronic atrophicans
C. Actinomycosis
D. African eyeworm disease
E. Andogsky syndrome (dermatogenous cataract)
F. Angioedema (Quincke disease)
G. Angular conjunctivitis (Morax–Axenfeld bacillus)
H. Ankylosing spondylitis
I. Anterior segment ischemia syndrome
J. Arteriovenous fistula
K. Atopic dermatitis
L. Bee sting of the cornea
M. Behçet syndrome (dermatostomatoophthalmic syndrome)
N. Brucellosis (Bang disease)
O. Candidiasis
P. Charlin syndrome (nasal nerve syndrome)
Q. Chickenpox
R. Chlamydia
S. Cockayne syndrome (dwarfism with retinal atrophy and deafness)
T. Cogan syndrome (I) (nonsyphilitic interstitial keratitis)
U. Crohn disease (granulomatous ileocolitis)
V. Cystinosis syndrome
W. Cytomegalic inclusion disease
X. Disseminated lupus erythematous (Kaposi–Libman–Sacks syndrome)
Y. Electrical injury
Z. Epidemic keratoconjunctivitis
AA. *E. coli*
BB. Felty syndrome (rheumatoid arthritis with hypersplenism)
CC. Gonorrhea
DD. *H. aegyptius*
EE. Herpes simplex
FF. Herpes zoster
GG. Hilding syndrome (destructive iridocyclitis and multiple joint dislocations)
HH. Histiocytosis X (Hand–Schüller–Christian syndrome)
II. Hodgkin disease (lymph node disease)
JJ. Homocystinuria syndrome
KK. Hypervitaminosis D
LL. Hypothermal injury
MM. Influenza
NN. Japanese River fever (mite borne typhus)
OO. Juvenile rheumatoid arthritis (Still disease)

PP. Juvenile xanthogranuloma (nevoxanthoendothelioma)
QQ. Kussmaul disease (periarteritis nodosa)
RR. Leprosy (Hansen disease)
SS. Leptospirosis (Weil disease)
TT. Lewis syndrome (tuberoserpiginous syphilid of Lewis)
UU. Listerellosis
VV. Lockjaw
WW. Lymphogranuloma venereum
XX. Malaria
YY. Measles (rubeola)
ZZ. Meningococcemia
AAA. Mikulicz–Radecki syndrome (dacryosialoadenopathy)
BBB. Moniliasis–idiopathic hypoparathyroidism (Addison syndrome)
CCC. *Moraxella lacunata*
DDD. Mumps
EEE. Mycosis fungoides syndrome (Sézary syndrome)
FFF. Myotonic dystrophy syndrome
GGG. Nocardiosis
HHH. Ocular vaccinia
III. Onchocerciasis syndrome
JJJ. Passow syndrome (status dysraphicus)
KKK. Plague
LLL. *Pneumococcus*
MMM. Postvaccinial ocular syndrome
NNN. Progressive systemic sclerosis (scleroderma)
OOO. Psoriasis
PPP. Psoriatic arthritis
QQQ. Radiation
RRR. Reiter syndrome (polyarthritis enterica)
SSS. Relapsing fever
TTT. Relapsing polychondritis
UUU. Rheumatoid arthritis (adult)
VVV. Rubella syndrome
WWW. St. Anthony fire (erysipelas)
XXX. Sarcoidosis syndrome (Schaumann syndrome)
YYY. Seborrheic dermatitis
ZZZ. Sporotrichosis
AAAA. *Staphylococcus*
BBBB. Stevens–Johnson syndrome (erythema multiforme exudativum)
CCCC. Stickler syndrome (hereditary progressive arthroophthalmopathy)
DDDD. *Streptococcus*
EEEE. Syphilis
FFFF. Thelaziasis
GGGG. Toxoplasmosis
HHHH. Tuberculosis
IIII. Vaccinia
JJJJ. Werner syndrome (progeria of adults)

      KKKK. Xeroderma pigmentosum
      LLLL. Yersiniosis
  6. Diarrhea
        A. Amebiasis
        B. Bacillary dysentery
        C. *Chlamydia*
        D. Crohn disease (granulomatous ileocolitis)
        E. *E. coli*
        F. Listerellosis
        G. Psoriatic arthritis
        H. Regional enteritis (ulcerative colitis)
        I. Rubella syndrome
        J. *Staphylococcus*
        K. Ulcerative colitis (regional enteritis)
        L. Whipple disease (intestinal lipodystrophy)
        M. Yersiniosis
  7. Disc neovascularization
        A. Ischemic uveitis of Knox
        B. Papillophlebitis
  8. Exophthalmus (proptosis)
        A. Actinomycosis
        B. Angioedema
        C. Arteriovenous fistula
        D. Coenurosis
        E. Cryptococcosis
        F. Disseminated lupus erythematosus (Kaposi–Libman–Sacks syndrome)
        G. Hallermann–Streiff–François syndrome (dyscephalic mandibulooculofacial syndrome)
        H. Herpes zoster
        I. Histiocytosis X (Hand–Schüller–Christian syndrome)
        J. Juvenile xanthogranuloma (nevoxanthoendothelioma)
        K. Kussmaul disease (periarteritis nodosa)
        L. Mumps
        M. Polymyositis dermatomyositis
        N. Relapsing polychondritis
        O. Streptococcus
        P. Trichinellosis
        Q. Werner syndrome (progeria of adults)
  9. Exudative detachment
        A. Acute retinal necrosis syndrome
        B. Bacterial endocarditis
        C. Boutonneuse fever (rickettsia, Marseilles fever)
        D. Cryptococcosis
        E. Histiocytosis X (Hand–Schüller–Christian syndrome)
        F. Japanese River fever (typhus)
        G. Kussmaul disease (periarteritis nodosa)
        H. Mycosis fungoides syndrome
        I. Oculootororenoerythropoietic disease
        J. Pappataci fever (sandfly fever)

K. Periocular and ocular metastatic tumors
L. Progressive systemic sclerosis (scleroderma)
M. Rheumatic fever
N. Rocky Mountain spotted fever
O. Sarcoidosis syndrome (Schaumann syndrome)
P. Schwartz syndrome (glaucoma associated with retinal detachment)
Q. Stickler syndrome (hereditary progressive arthroophthalmopathy)
R. Toxocariasis (visceral larva migrans syndrome)
S. Toxoplasmosis
T. Weber–Christian syndrome (subcutaneous inflammatory lesions)

10. Glaucoma
A. Acanthamoeba
B. Angioedema
C. Arteriovenous fistula
D. Acariasis
E. Atopic dermatitis
F. Behçet syndrome (dermatostomatoophthalmic syndrome)
G. Brucellosis (late manifestation) (Bang disease)
H. Carotid artery syndrome
I. Coats disease (retinal telangiectasia)
J. Coccidioidomycosis
K. Coenurosis
L. Electrical injury
M. *E. coli*
N. Familial histiocytic dermatoarthritis syndrome
O. Hallermann–Streiff–François syndrome (dyscephalic mandibulooculofacial syndrome)
P. Homocystinuria syndrome
Q. Juvenile rheumatoid arthritis (Still disease)
R. Juvenile xanthogranuloma (nevoxanthoendothelioma)
S. Leprosy (Hansen disease)
T. Listerellosis
U. Measles (rubeola)
V. Oculootoororenoerythropoietic disease
W. Onchocerciasis syndrome
X. Periocular and ocular metastatic tumors
Y. Pneumococcus
Z. Posner–Schlossman syndrome (glaucomatocyclitic crisis)
AA. Pseudouveitis, glaucoma, hyphema syndrome (PUGH syndrome)
BB. Radiation
CC. Relapsing polychondritis
DD. Rubella syndrome
EE. Sarcoidosis syndrome (Schaumann syndrome)
FF. Schwartz syndrome (glaucoma associated with retinal detachment)
GG. *Staphylococcus*
HH. Stickler syndrome (hereditary progressive arthro-ophthalmopathy)
II. *Streptococcus*
JJ. Trichinellosis
KK. Uveitis, glaucoma, hyphema syndrome (UGH syndrome)

        LL. Weber-Christian syndrome (subcutaneous inflammatory lesions)

11. Hepatomegaly
    A. Cytomegalic inclusions disease
    B. Toxocariasis (visceral larva migrans syndrome)
    C. Toxoplasmosis

12. Influenza-like disease
    A. Acanthamoeba
    B. Amebiasis
    C. Bacillary dysentery
    D. Boutonneuse fever (rickettsia, Marseilles fever)
    E. Brucellosis (Bang disease)
    F. Chickenpox
    G. *Chlamydia*
    H. *E. coli*
    I. Gonorrhea
    J. *H. aegyptius*
    K. Histoplasmosis
    L. Influenza
    M. Japanese River fever (mite-borne typhus)
    N. Leptospirosis (Weil disease)
    O. Malaria
    P. Measles (rubeola)
    Q. Meningococcemia
    R. Mumps
    S. Pappataci fever (sandfly fever)
    T. Plague (bubonic plague)
    U. Pneumococcus
    V. Q fever
    W. Relapsing fever
    X. Rocky Mountain spotted fever
    Y. Staphylococcus
    Z. Streptococcus
    AA. Toxoplasmosis
    BB. Tuberculosis

13. Iris neovascularization, such as Knox ischemic ocular inflammation (rubeosis iridis)

14. Jaundice
    A. Leptospirosis

15. Meningism (meningitis)
    A. Acanthamoeba
    B. Behçet syndrome (dermatostomato-ophthalmic syndrome)
    C. Cryptococcosis
    D. Gonorrhea
    E. Herpes simplex
    F. Histoplasmosis
    G. Leptospirosis (Weil disease)
    H. Listerellosis
    I. Meningococcemia
    J. Sympathetic ophthalmia

       K. Toxoplasmosis

       L. Tuberculosis

16. Microphthalmia

       A. Cytomegalic inclusion disease

       B. Hallermann–Streiff–François syndrome (dyscephalic mandibulooculofacial syndrome)

       C. Mumps

       D. Rubella syndrome

       E. Toxoplasmosis

17. Nodules in the leg

       A. Histoplasmosis

       B. Sarcoidosis syndrome (Schaumann syndrome)

       C. Ulcerative colitis

18. Optic neuritis (papillitis)

       A. Angioedema

       B. Behçet syndrome (dermatostomatoophthalmic syndrome)

       C. Boutonneuse fever (rickettsia, Marseilles fever)

       D. Brucellosis (Bang disease)

       E. Candidiasis

       F. Chickenpox

       G. Cytomegalic inclusion disease

       H. Disseminated lupus erythematosus (Kaposi–Libman–Sacks syndrome)

       I. Electrical injury

       J. Felty syndrome (rheumatoid arthritis with hypersplenism)

       K. Herpes zoster

       L. Hodgkin disease (lymph node disease)

       M. Infectious mononucleosis

       N. Influenza

       O. Juvenile rheumatoid arthritis (Still disease)

       P. Leptospirosis

       Q. Malaria

       R. Measles

       S. Meningococcemia

       T. Mikulicz–Radecki syndrome (dacryosialoadenopathy)

       U. Mumps

       V. Ocular vaccinia

       W. Onchocerciasis syndrome

       X. Pappataci fever (sandfly fever)

       Y. Postvaccinial ocular syndrome

       Z. Q fever

      AA. Reiter syndrome (polyarthritis enterica)

      BB. Regional enteritis (ulcerative colitis)

      CC. Rocky Mountain spotted fever

      DD. Sarcoidosis syndrome (Schaumann syndrome)

      EE. Stevens–Johnson syndrome (erythema multiforme exudativum)

      FF. *Streptococcus*

      GG. Sympathetic ophthalmia

      HH. Syphilis (acquired lues)

       II. Toxocariasis (visceral larva migrans syndrome)

JJ. Toxoplasmosis
KK. Trichinellosis
LL. Tuberculosis
MM. Vaccinia

19. Papilledema
    A. Angioedema
    B. Arteriovenous fistula
    C. Acariasis
    D. Bacterial endocarditis
    E. Behçet syndrome (dermatostomatoophthalmic syndrome)
    F. Brucellosis (Bang disease)
    G. Chickenpox
    H. Coccidioidomycosis
    I. Cryptococcosis
    J. Cysticercosis
    K. Disseminated lupus erythematosus (Kaposi–Libman–Sacks syndrome)
    L. Histiocytosis X (Hand–Schüller–Christian syndrome)
    M. Hodgkin disease (lymph node disease)
    N. Hypervitaminosis D
    O. Malaria
    P. Moniliasis—idiopathic hypoparathyroidism (Addison disease)
    Q. Mycosis fungoides syndrome (Sézary syndrome)
    R. Papillophlebitis
    S. Pappataci fever (sandfly fever)
    T. Passow syndrome (status dysraphicus)
    U. Periocular and ocular metastatic tumors
    V. Progressive systemic sclerosis
    W. Sarcoidosis syndrome (Schaumann syndrome)
    X. Syphilis
    Y. Trichinellosis
    Z. Whipple disease (intestinal lipodystrophy)

20. Paralysis of extraocular muscle
    A. African eyeworm disease
    B. Arteriovenous fistula
    C. Bacterial endocarditis
    D. Brucellosis
    E. Cerebral palsy
    F. Chickenpox
    G. Coccidioidomycosis
    H. Cysticercosis
    I. Disseminated lupus erythematosus
    J. Electrical injury
    K. Herpes simplex
    L. Herpes zoster
    M. Hodgkin disease (lymph node disease)
    N. Hypothermal injury
    O. Infectious mononucleosis
    P. Influenza

   Q. Kussmaul disease (periarteritis nodosa)

   R. Lockjaw (tetanus)

   S. Malaria

   T. Measles (rubeola)

   U. Meningococcemia

   V. Multiple sclerosis

   W. Mumps

   X. Ocular vaccinia

   Y. Passow syndrome (status dysraphicus)

   Z. Periocular and ocular metastatic tumors

  AA. Reiter syndrome (polyarthritis enterica)

  BB. Relapsing fever

  CC. Relapsing polychondritis

  DD. Rocky Mountain spotted fever

  EE. Streptococcus

  FF. Syphilis (acquired lues)

  GG. Trichinellosis

21. Perivenous sheathing

   A. *Acanthamoeba*

   B. Amebiasis

   C. Boutonneuse fever (rickettsia, Marseilles fever)

   D. Brucellosis (Bang disease)

   E. Candidiasis

   F. Coccidioidomycosis

   G. Metastatic bacterial endophthalmitis

   H. Metastatic fungal endophthalmitis

   I. Multiple sclerosis

   J. Myotonic dystrophy syndrome

   K. Ocular vaccinia

   L. Onchocerciasis syndrome

   M. Plague

   N. Postvaccinial ocular syndrome

   O. Q fever

   P. Sarcoidosis syndrome (Schaumann syndrome)

   Q. Syphilis (acquired lues)

   R. Toxocariasis (visceral larva migrans syndrome)

   S. Toxoplasmosis

   T. Tuberculosis

   U. Vaccinia

   V. Weber–Christian syndrome (subcutaneous inflammatory lesions)

22. Pneumonitis

   A. *Chlamydia*

   B. Cytomegalic inclusion disease

   C. Plague (Bubonic plague)

   D. Pneumococcus

   E. Rubella syndrome

   F. Toxocariasis

   G. Whipple disease (intestinal lipodystrophy)

23. Prostatitis
    A. Gonococcosis
    B. Whipple disease (intestinal lipodystrophy)
24. Salt-and-pepper fundus
    A. Choroideremia in males
    B. Cockayne disease (dwarfism with retinal atrophy and deafness)
    C. Cystinosis
    D. Prenatal influenza
    E. Prenatal syphilis
25. Skin lesions
    A. Acrodermatitis chronica atrophicans
    B. African eyeworm disease
    C. Andogsky syndrome (dermatogenous cataract)
    D. Angioedema
    E. Atopic dermatitis
    F. Behçet syndrome (dermatostomato-ophthalmic syndrome)
    G. Chickenpox
    H. Disseminated lupus erythematosus (Kaposi–Libman—Sacks syndrome)
    I. Familial histiocytic dermatoarthritis syndrome
    J. Herpes simplex
    K. Herpes zoster
    L. Histiocytosis X (Hand–Schüller–Christian syndrome)
    M. Juvenile xanthogranuloma (nevoxanthoendothelioma)
    N. Leprosy (Hansen disease)
    O. Lewis syndrome (tuberoserphiginous syphilid of Lewis)
    P. Listerellosis
    Q. Measles (rubeola)
    R. *Moraxella lacunata*
    S. Mucocutaneous lymph node syndrome
    T. Mycosis fungoides syndrome (Sézary syndrome)
    U. Polymyositis dermatomyositis
    V. Postvaccinial ocular syndrome
    W. Psoriasis
    X. Psoriatic arthritis
    Y. St. Anthony fire (erysipelas)
    Z. Schistosomiasis (bilharziasis)
    AA. Seborrheic dermatitis
    BB. Sporotrichosis
    CC. *Staphylococcus*
26. Stomatitis
    A. Behçet syndrome (dermatostomatoophthalmic syndrome)
    B. Disseminated systemic histoplasmosis—not the ocular form
    C. Herpes simplex
    D. Lewis syndrome (tuberoserpiginous syphilid of Lewis)
    E. Reiter syndrome (polyarthritis enterica)
    F. Regional enteritis
    G. Ulcerative colitis

27. Tonsillitis
    A. Whipple disease (intestinal lipodystrophy)
28. Trauma (nonpenetrating)

Friedman AH, et al. *An atlas of uveitis: diagnosis and management.* Baltimore: Williams & Wilkins, 1982.

Kraus M, et al. *Uveitis—pathophysiology and therapy*, 2nd ed. New York: Thieme, 1986.

Roy FH. *Ocular syndromes and systemic diseases*, 3rd ed. Philadelphia: Lippincott Williams & Wilkins, 2002.

Characteristics of granulomatous and nongranulomatous inflammation in posterior uvea

Symptomatology	Granulomatous Uveitis	Nongranulomatous Uveitis	
		Acute, Self-limited Insult	Chronic or Often Repeated Insult
Anterior ocular changes	Sometimes epithelioid or "mutton-fat" keratotic deposits; often Koeppe nodules	Usually none	None in early irreversible in stage; terminal stages
Vitreous changes	Usually heavy vitreous blurring; heavy veil-like opacities	Slight to intense general blurring; fine muscae or string-like fibrinous opacities	Slowly increasing blue with heavy opacities in terminal stages
Retinal and subretinal edema	Usually slight or moderate and localized around exudates; intense only when there is a secondary allergic reaction	Marked and generalized, with blurring of neuro-retinal vascular bed	Low grade at onset; may become intense in later stages
Choroidal exudates	Heavy massive exudates— edges may be blurred by surrounding retinal and subretinal edema	No heavy massive exudates; occasionally localized areas of deeper infiltration	Great tendency to localized deep ill-defined infiltrates (lymphocyte, etc.)
Secondary retinal involvement	Almost invariable with retinal destruction	None or limited to pigment and neuroepithelium	None in early stage; irreversible in later stages with involvement of neuro-epithelium
Residual organic damage in retina and choroid	Heavy glial scars with massive pigment heaping which often surrounds the lesion	No fine granular changes in pigment epithelium but damage to neuroepithelium and occasionally superficial gliosis	Fine granular change in early stages; superficial gliosis in terminal stages

Schlaegel TF. *Essentials of uveitis*. Boston: Little, Brown, 1983.

CHORIORETINITIS JUXTAPAPILLARIS

This large, irregular opaque mass that protrudes three to four diopters and obscures the retinal vessels is seen near the disc and may be confused with acute optic neuritis or a tumor.

1. Acanthamoeba keratitis of fellow eye
2. Bird-shot retinochoroidopathy
3. *Coccidioides immitis*
4. Histoplasmosis
5. Sarcoidosis syndrome (Schaumann syndrome)
6. Syphilis (acquired lues)
7. Toxoplasmosis
8. Tuberculosis

Eide N, Skjeldal O. Juxtapapillary chorioretinitis in neurosyphilis. *Acta Ophthalmol* 1984;62:351–358.

Haessler FH. *Eye signs in general disease*. Springfield, IL: Charles C Thomas, 1960:98.

John KJ, et al. Chorioretinitis in the contralateral eye of a patient with acanthamoeba keratitis. *Ophthalmology* 1988; 95:635–639.

Woods AC. *Endogenous inflammations of the uveal tract*. Baltimore: Williams & Wilkins, 1961.

CHOROIDAL NEOVASCULARIZATION

Choroidal neovascularization comprises new vessel formation from choriocapillaris through a defect in the Bruch membrane as suggested by fluorescein angiography.

1. Choroidal neovascular ingrowth at the margin of the optic nerve head
    A. Angioid streaks (see p. 526)
    B. Hyaline bodies of optic nerve head
    C. Idiopathic choroidal neovascularization
    D. Macular drusen
    E. Multiple evanescent white-dot and acute idiopathic blind spot enlargement syndrome
    F. Optic-nerve coloboma
    G. Peripapillary choroiditis
    H. Presumed ocular histoplasmosis syndrome
    I. Pseudotumor cerebri (Symond syndrome)
    J. Serpiginous choroiditis
2. Choroidal neovascular ingrowth through breaks in Bruch membrane in the macular area
3. Acute posterior multifocal placoid pigment epitheliopathy
    A. Angioid streaks (see p. 526)
    B. Behçet syndrome (dermatostomatoophthalmic syndrome) or Best disease
    C. Bird-shot retinochoroidopathy
    D. Choroidal rupture
    E. Choroidal tumors
    F. Chronic uveitis
    G. Foveomacular dystrophy
    H. Fundus flavimaculatus
    I. Idiopathic choroidal neovascularization
    *J. Macular drusen
    K. Morning glory syndrome
    L. Myopic degeneration

* = most important

M. Parafoveal telangiectasis
N. Photocoagulation of macular lesions with argon laser
O. Presumed ocular histoplasmosis syndrome
P. Osteogenesis imperfecta (van der Hoeve syndrome)
Q. Retinitis pigmentosa
R. Rubella syndrome (Gregg syndrome)
S. Sarcoidosis syndrome (Schaumann syndrome)
T. Scars from previous deep macular hemorrhage
U. Senile disciform macular degeneration (Kuhnt–Junius disease)
V. Serpiginous choroiditis
W. Sorsby fundus dystrophy
X. Tilted disc syndrome
Y. Toxocariasis
Z. Toxoplasma retinochoroiditis
AA. Trauma
BB. Vein occlusion
CC. Vogt–Koyanagi–Harada syndrome (uveitis–vitiligo–alopecia–poliosis syndrome)

Callanan D, Gass JD. Multifocal choroiditis and choroidal neovascularization associated with the multiple evanescent white dot and acute idiopathic blind spot enlargement syndrome. *Ophthalmology* 1992;99:1678–1685.

Dailey JR, et al. Peripapillary choroidal neovascular membrane associated with an optic nerve coloboma. *Arch Ophthalmol* 1993;111:441–442.

Feist RM, et al. Choroidal neovascularization in a patient with adult foveomacular dystrophy and a mutation in the retinal degeneration slow gene. *Am J Ophthalmol* 1994;118:259–260.

Lewis H, et al. Macular translocation for subfoveal choroidal neovascularization in age-related macular degeneration: a prospective study. *Am J Ophthalmol* 1999;128:135–146.

Roy FH. *Ocular syndromes and systemic diseases*, 3rd ed. Philadelphia: Lippincott Williams & Wilkins, 2002.

Shields JA, et al. Adenoma of the retinal pigment epithelium simulating a juxtapapillary choroidal neovascular membrane. *Arch Ophthalmol* 2001;119:289–292.

ISCHEMIC INFARCTS OF CHOROID (ELSCHNIG SPOTS)

When healed, these may show small, disseminated yellowish scars with central pigment deposits and may be associated with retinal separation when acute.

1. Chronic glomerulonephritis
2. Collagen disease, such as scleroderma
*3. Malignant hypertension
4. Toxemia of pregnancy

Klein BA. Ischemic infarcts of choroid (Elschnig spots). *Am J Ophthalmol* 1968;66:1069–1074.

Venecia G, et al. The eye in accelerated hypertension—Elschnig's spots in nonhuman primates. *Arch Ophthalmol* 1980;98:913.

CHORIORETINAL AND CHORIOVITREAL NEOVASCULARIZATION

This type of new vessel formation from choroid into the retina or vitreous usually occurs after photocoagulation or after any of the following:

1. Atrophic scars in the presumed ocular histoplasmosis syndrome
2. Central serous chorioretinopathy
*3. Diabetes mellitus (Willis disease)

4. Diseases of the retinal pigment epithelium
5. Eales disease (periphlebitis)
6. Leber syndrome (optic atrophy—amaurosis pituitary syndrome)
7. Sarcoidosis syndrome (Schaumann syndrome)
8. Sickle cell disease (Herrick syndrome)

Chandra SR, et al. Choroidovitreal neovascular ingrowth after photocoagulation for proliferative diabetic retinopathy. *Arch Ophthalmol* 1980;98:1593.

Dizon-Moore RV, et al. Chorioretinal and choriovitreal neovascularization. *Arch Ophthalmol* 1981;99:842.

UVEAL EFFUSION

Uveal effusion involves leaking of fluid from the choriocapillaris into the choroid or subretinal space or both.

1. Hydrostatic
  A. Dural arteriovenous fistula
  *B. Hypotony, wound leak
  C. Nanophthalmos
2. Idiopathic
3. Inflammatory
  A. After panretinal photocoagulation
  B. HIV
  C. Scleritis, infected scleral buckle
  D. Systemic lupus erythematosus
  E. Trauma, intraocular surgery
  F. Uveitis, sympathetic ophthalmia, Harada disease

Uyama M, et al. Uveal effusion syndrome. *Ophthalmology* 2000;107:441–449.

Wisotsky BJ, et al. Angle closure glaucoma as an initial presentation of systemic lupus erythematosus. *Ophthalmology* 1998;105:1170–1172.

CHOROID COLOBOMA

1. Aicardi syndrome
2. Basal cell nevus syndrome (Gorlin syndrome)
3. Cat-eye syndrome (partial G-trisomy)
4. CHARGE association among coloboma, heart anomaly, choanal atresia, retardation, genital and ear anomalies
5. Doubtful association
  A. Crouzon syndrome (dysostosis craniofacialis)
  B. Ellis–Van Crevald syndrome (chondroectodermal dysplasia)
  C. Hallerman–Streiff syndrome (dyscephalic mandibulooculofacial)
  D. Incontinentia pigmenti I (Block–Sulzberger syndrome)
  E. Kartagener syndrome (bronchiectasis-dextrocardia-sinusitis)
  F. Laurence–Moon–Bardet–Biedl syndrome (retinitis pigmentosa–polydactyl–adiposogenital syndrome)
  G. Pierre Robin syndrome (micrognathia–glossoptosis syndrome)
  H. Stickler syndrome (hereditary progressive arthro-ophthalmopathy)
  I. Tuberous sclerosis (Bourneville syndrome)

* = most important

6. Goldenhar syndrome (oculoauriculovertebral dysplasia)
7. Goltz syndrome (focal dermal hypoplasia syndrome)
8. Isolated, sporadic
9. Joubert syndrome with bilateral chorioretinal coloboma (coloboma, chorioretinal with cerebellar vermis aplasia)
10. Klinefelter syndrome (gynecomastia-aspermatogenesis syndrome)
11. Lenz microphthalmia syndrome
12. Linear sebaceous nevus syndrome
13. Median facial cleft syndrome
14. Meckel syndrome (dysencephalia splanchnocystic syndrome)
15. Retinal astrocytoma
16. Retinal dysplasia
17. Retinoblastoma
18. Rubinstein–Taybi syndrome (broad-thumbs syndrome)
19. Triploidy
*20. Trisomy (Edward syndrome)
21. Trisomy (Patau syndrome)
22. Turner syndrome
23. Warburg syndrome
24. 13q syndrome

Daufenbach DR, et al. Chorioretinal colobomas in a pediatric population. *Ophthalmology* 1998;105:1455–1458.

Isenberg SJ. *The eye in infancy.* Chicago: Year Book Medical, 1989.

Ward JR, et al. Upper-limb defect associated with developmental delay, unilateral poorly developed antihelix, hearing deficit, and bilateral choroid coloboma: a new syndrome. *J Med Genet* 1992;29:589–591.

CHOROIDAL ISCHEMIA

This condition involves decreased choroidal perfusion demonstrated by fluorescein angiography.

1. Arteritic anterior ischemic optic neuropathy
2. Disseminated intravascular coagulation
*3. Hypertension, severe
4. Renal failure
5. Systemic lupus erythematosus
6. Toxemia of pregnancy
7. Thrombotic thrombocytopenic purpura

Kinyoun JL, Kalina RE. Visual loss from choroidal ischemia. *Am J Ophthalmol* 1986;101:650–656.

Slavin ML, Barondes MJ. Visual loss caused by choroidal ischemia preceding anterior ischemic optic neuropathy in giant cell arteritis. *Am J Ophthalmol* 1994;117:81–86.

PARS PLANITIS (PERIPHERAL UVEITIS)

In pars planitis, inferior exudates in the peripheral retina, ora, pars plana, and peripheral vitreous, vitreous ray and cells, posterior cortical cataract, perivasculitis, partial thrombosis of central retinal vein, glaucoma, peripheral retinal hemorrhages, and retinal detachment may be present.

1. Dental infection
2. Hereditary

*3. Idiopathic

4. Multiple sclerosis (disseminated sclerosis)

5. Nematodiases

6. Rheumatic disease

7. Sarcoidosis syndrome (Schaumann syndrome)

8. Sinus infection

9. Streptococcal hypersensitivity

10. Syphilis (acquired lues)

11. Toxoplasmosis

12. Ulcerative colitis (inflammatory bowel disease)

Josephberg RG, et al. A fluorescein angiographic study of patients with pars planitis and peripheral exudation (snowbanking) before and after cryopexy. *Ophthalmology* 1994;101:262–266.

Phillips WB, et al. Pars planitis presenting with vitreous hemorrhage. *Ophthalmic Surg Lasers* 1993;24:630–631.

Differential diagnosis of pars planitis

	Chronicity	Vitreous Opacities	Retinal Edema	Fluorescein Leakage	Organized Vitreous	Distinguishing Features
Acute nongranulo-matous iritis	−	±	±	±	−	Acute red eye
Acute recurrent cyclitis	+	+	+	+	+	Localized area of inflammation in ciliary body
Nematode	+	+	+	+(?)	+	Nodular focus and dragged retina, one eye
Irvine-Gass syndrome	+	+	+	+	±	Usually postoperative
Behçet syndrome	+	+	+	+(?)	+	Retinal vasculitis
Peripheral toxo-plasmosis	±	+	±	±	±	Localized area of inflammation
Sarcoidosis	+	+	+	+	+	Other ocular signs of sarcoidosis

* = most important

17

Optic Nerve

CONTENTS

BLURRED OPTIC-NERVE HEADS

CILIOOPTIC VEIN

This vein appears at the disc edge and dips into the optic nerve to anastomose with branches of the central retinal vein

1. Congenital
2. Neurofibromatosis (von Recklinghausen syndrome)
3. Sturge–Weber syndrome (meningocutaneous syndrome)

Zaret CR, et al. Cilio-optic vein associated with phakomatosis. *Ophthalmology* 1980;87:330–334.

DRUSEN OF OPTIC NERVE

These white or yellow conglomerate, translucent bodies in the optic nerve may cause field defects.

1. Alagille syndrome
2. Alport syndrome (hereditary nephritis)
3. Angioid streaks (pseudoxanthoma elasticum; Grönblad–Strandberg syndrome)
4. Associated with corneal dystrophy
5. Diabetes mellitus (Willis disease)
6. Friedreich ataxia
7. Glaucoma
8. Hereditary—autosomal dominant
9. High myopia
10. Idiopathic
11. Meningioma (unusual)
12. Pituitary tumor (unusual)
13. Retinal vein occlusion
14. Retinitis pigmentosa
15. Systemic lupus erythematosus (SLE)
16. Status dysraphicus syndrome (Passow syndrome)
17. Syphilis (acquired lues)
19. Tuberous sclerosis (Bourneville syndrome)
20. Wilson disease (hepatolenticular degeneration)

Chern S, et al. Central retinal vein occlusion associated with drusen of the optic disc. *Ann Ophthalmol* 1991;23: 66–69.

Newell FW. *Ophthalmology: principles and concepts*, 7th ed. St. Louis: CV Mosby, 1991.

Nischal KK, et al. Ocular ultrasound in Alagille syndrome. *Ophthalmology* 1997;104:79–85.

Roy FH. *Ocular syndromes and systemic diseases*, 3rd ed. Philadelphia: Lippincott Williams & Wilkins, 2002.

FLUID ENLARGEMENT OF RETROBULBAR OPTIC NERVE OR SHEATH (DEMONSTRATED BY COMPUTED TOMOGRAPHIC SCANNING AND ECHOGRAPHY)

1. Arachnoiditis
2. Basilar artery aneurysm
3. Bilateral temporal lobe cysts
4. Central retinal vein occlusion (see p. 468–472)
5. Facial trauma
6. Iliojejunal bypass
7. Occipital intradural arteriovenous malformation
8. Optic-nerve meningioma
9. Optic-nerve sheath cyst
10. Pseudotumor cerebri
11. Subdural hematoma
12. Trauma (intrasheath hemorrhage of optic nerve)
13. Uveal meningeal syndrome

Hupp SL, Glaser JS. Optic nerve sheath decompression. *Arch Ophthalmol* 1987;105:386–389.

HYPEREMIA OF OPTIC DISC

1. Central retinal vein thrombosis (see p. 468–472)
2. Hemangioma
3. Hypermetropia

4. Hypertensive retinopathy
5. Ischemic optic neuropathy
6. Neovascularization
7. Optic neuritis (see p. 578)
8. Papilledema (see p. 593)
9. Polycythemia vera (Vaquez disease)
10. von Hippel–Lindau disease (retinocerebral angiomatosis)

Duke-Elder S, Scott GI. *System of ophthalmology*, vol 12. St. Louis: CV Mosby, 1971.

ISCHEMIC OPTIC NEUROPATHY

The anterior form is occlusive disease of the optic-nerve head and retrolaminar region of the optic nerve; the posterior form is occlusion of one or more nutrient arteries to the rest of the optic nerve. Onset is usually sudden, with painless unilateral visual loss and visual-field defect.

1. Compression
   A. Orbital hemorrhage (trauma)
   B. Thyroid disease (Graves disease)
2. Drugs
   A. Sumatriptan
   B. Vigabatrin
3. Systemic diseases (often in combination)
   A. Arteriosclerosis
   B. Arrhythmia
   C. Atherosclerosis
   D. Cerebrovascular disease
   E. Diabetes mellitus
   F. Gastrointestinal ulcer
   G. Hypercholesterolemia
   H. Hyperhomocystinemia
   I. Hyperparathyroidism
   J. Hypertension, nocturnal hypotension
   K. Ischemic heart disease
   L. Sickle cell disease
   M. Takayasu disease
4. Vasculitis
   A. Allergic vasculitis
   B. Buerger disease
   C. Churg–Strauss syndrome (allergic granulomatosis and angiitis)
   D. Collagen diseases, including polyarteritis nodosum and systemic lupus
   E. Giant cell (temporal) arteritis
   F. Postimmunization
   G. Postviral vasculitis
   H. Syphilis
5. Miscellaneous
   A. Acute anemia

B. Anemia combined with hypotension
C. Carotid artery disease
D. Fabry disease (angiokeratoma corporis diffusum)
E. Hypertensive with peritoneal dialysis
F. Low tension glaucoma
G. Glucose-6-phosphate dehydrogenase deficiency
H. Migraine
I. Polycythemia vera
J. Radiation
K. Retinal artery occlusion
L. Tobacco
M. Various vascular disorders (e.g., cavernous sinus thrombosis)

Feldon SE. Anterior ischemic optic neuropathy: trouble waiting to happen. *Ophthalmology* 1999;106:651–653.

Jackson TL, et al. Hypotensive ischemic optic neuropathy and peritoneal dialysis. *Am J Ophthalmol* 1999;128: 109–110.

Moster ML. Visual loss after coronary artery bypass surgery. *Surv Ophthalmol* 1998;42:453–455.

Pianka P, et al. Hyperhomocystinemia in patients with nonarteritic anterior ischemic optic neuropathy, central retinal artery occlusion and central retinal vein occlusion. *Ophthalmology* 2000;107:1588–1592.

Salomon O, et al. Analysis of prothrombotic and vascular risk factors in patients with nonarteritic anterior ischemic optic neuropathy. *Ophthalmology* 1999;106:739–742.

LINEAR HEMORRHAGE ON OPTIC DISC

1. Diabetes mellitus
2. Drusen of optic nerve
3. Glaucoma
4. Ischemic optic neuropathy
   A. Altitudinal field loss
   B. Dense arcuate field loss
   C. Sector-shaped field loss
5. Isolated finding
6. Leukemia
7. Systemic hypertension

Jonas JB, Xu L. Optic disk hemorrhages in glaucoma. *Am J Ophthalmol* 1994;118:1–8.

Shihab ZM, et al. The significance of disc hemorrhage in open-angle glaucoma. *Ophthalmology* 1982;89:211.

NEOVASCULARIZATION OF OPTIC DISC (GROWTH OF BLOOD VESSELS ONTO OPTIC DISC)

1. Anemia
2. Age-related macular degeneration (AMD)
3. Arterial insufficiency
4. Behçet disease (oculobuccogenital syndrome)
5. Buerger disease (thromboangiitis obliterans)
6. Coats disease (retinal telangiectasia)
7. Choroidal rupture
8. Diabetes mellitus
9. Drusen of optic nerve head

10. Eales disease (periphlebitis)
11. Geographic helicoid peripapillary choroidopathy
12. Glaucoma, chronic uncontrolled
13. Hereditary drusen of Bruch membrane
14. von Hippel–Lindau disease (retinocerebral angiomatosis)
15. Hypertensive retinopathy, advanced
16. Incontinentia pigmenti achromians (hypomelanosis of Ito syndrome)
17. Infection
    A. Endophthalmitis
    B. Congenital rubella syndrome (Gregg syndrome)
    C. Histoplasmosis
    D. Toxoplasmosis
18. Intraocular inflammation
    A. Rheumatoid arthritis
    B. Sarcoidosis syndrome (Schaumann syndrome)
    C. Uveitis (unspecified)
19. Myopia, severe
20. Norrie disease (fetal iritis syndrome)
21. Pseudotumor cerebri (Symond syndrome)
22. Retinal vein occlusion (see p. 468–472)
23. Retinitis pigmentosa
24. Retinopathy of prematurity (ROP)
25. Sickle cell disease (Herrick syndrome)
26. Takayasu disease (aortic arch syndrome)
27. Trauma
28. Tumors
    A. Benign
        (1) von Hippel–Lindau disease
        (2) Juxtapapillary capillary hemangioma
        (3) Nevus
    B. Malignant
        (1) Choroidal melanoma
        (2) Leukemia
        (3) Lymphoma
        (4) Metastatic tumors
29. Vogt-Koyangi-Harada syndrome (uveitis-vitiligo-alopecia-poliosis)

Roy FH. *Ocular syndromes and systemic diseases*, 3rd ed. Philadelphia: Lippincott Williams & Wilkins, 2002.

Sanislo SR, et al. Corticosteroid therapy for optic disc neovascularization secondary to chronic uveitis. *Am J Ophthalmol* 2000;130:724–731.

To KW, et al. Bilateral optic disc neovascularization in association with retinitis pigmentosa. *Can J Ophthalmol* 1991;26:152–155.

NEURORETINITIS (INFLAMMATION OF OPTIC NERVE AND ADJACENT RETINA)

1. *Bartonella henselae* infection
2. Cat-scratch disease

3. Herpes simplex
4. Idiopathic
5. Mumps (epidemic parotitis)
6. *Nematode*
7. *Salmonella*
8. Syphilis
9. *Toxocara canis*
10. Toxoplasmosis

Fish RH, et al. Toxoplasmosis neuroretinitis. *Ophthalmology* 1993;100:1177–1182.

Gray AV, et al. Bartonella henselae inflection associated with peripapillary angioma, branch retinal artery occlusion, and severe vision loss. *Am J Ophthalmol* 1999;127,2:223–224.

OPTIC-NERVE ATROPHY

1. Chromosome disorders
   A. Angelman syndrome (happy puppet syndrome; microdeletion of chromosome 15q11–13)
   B. Chromosome deletion (long arm) syndrome (de Grouchy syndrome)
   C. Cri-du-chat syndrome (cat-cry syndrome; deletion of short arm of chromosome 5)
   D. Patau syndrome (trisomy syndrome)
   E. Subacute sclerosing panencephalitis (Dawson disease)
2. Demyelinating and degenerative diseases
   A. Arylsulfatase A deficiency syndrome (ADL, metachromatic leukodystrophy)
   B. Devic syndrome (optical myelitis)
   C. Hereditary motor sensory neuropathy (HMSN I; Charcot–Marie–Tooth syndrome)
   D. Hereditary optic atrophy (Behr syndrome)
   E. Multiple sclerosis
3. Dermatologic disorders
   A. Keratodermia palmaris et plantaris
   B. McCune–Albright syndrome (fibrosus dysplasia)
   C. Naegeli syndrome (reticular pigmented dermatosis)
   D. Porphyria cutanea tarda
   E. Pseudoxanthoma elasticum (Grönblad–Strandberg syndrome)
   F. Wrinkly-skin syndrome
4. Drugs, poisons, and vaccines, including the following:

acetophenazine	auranofin (?)	calcifediol
acetylsalicylic acid	aurothioglucose (?)	calcitriol
adrenal cortex injection	aurothioglycanide (?)	carbamazepine
aldosterone	barbital	carbon dioxide
allobarbital	beclomethasone	carbromal
amobarbital	benzathine penicillin G	carphenazine
antimony lithium thiomalate	betamethasone	cephaloridine (?)
antimony potassium tartrate	bromide (?)	chloramphenicol (?)
antimony sodium tartrate	bupivacaine (?)	chloroprocaine (?)
antimony sodium thioglycollate	butabarbital	chloroquine
antipyrine	butalbital	chlorpromazine
aprobarbital	butallylonal	cholecalciferol
aspirin	butaperazine	cisplatin
	butethal	clindamycin

cocaine
colchicine compounds
cortisone
cyclobarbital
cyclopentobarbital
danazol
dapsone
desoxycorticosterone
dexamethasone
diatrizoate meglumine or
    sodium
diethazine
ergocalciferol
ethambutol
ethopropazine
etidocaine (?)
fludrocortisone
fluorometholone
fluphenazine
fluprednisolone
gentamicin
glutethimide
gold Au 198
gold sodium thiomalate (?)
gold sodium thiosulfate (?)
heptabarbital
hexachlorophene
hexamethonium
hexethal
hexobarbital
hydrabamine phenoxymethyl
    penicillin
hydrocortisone
hydroxychloroquine
ibuprofen
interferon
iodine and iodine solutions
    and
iodochlorhydroxyquin
iodoquinol
isocarboxazid (?)
isoniazid
lidocaine (?)
medrysone
mephobarbital
mepivacaine (?)
meprednisone

mesoridazine
methaqualone(?)
metharbital
methdilazine
methitural
methohexital
methotrimeprazine
methyl alcohol
methylene blue
methylprednisolone
methyprylon
mitotane
nadolol(?)
nalidixic acid
naproxen (?)
oxyphenbutazone
penicillamine
pentobarbital
perazine
pericyazine
perphenazine
phenelzine (?)
phenobarbital
phenoxymethyl penicillin
phenylbutazone
piperacetazine
potassium penicillin G
potassium penicillin V
potassium phenethicillin
prednisolone
prilocaine (?)
primidone
probarbital
procaine penicillin G
procaine (?)
procarbazine
prochlorperazine
promazine
promethazine
propiomazine
propoxycaine (?)
quinine
radioactive iodides
silicone
streptomycin
secobarbital
sodium antimonylgluconate

sodium salicylate
stibocaptate
stibogluconate
stibophen
sulfacetamide
sulfachlorpyridazine
sulfacytine
sulfadimethoxine
sulfamerazine
sulfameter
sulfamethazine
sulfamethizole
sulfamethoxazole
sulfamethoxypyridazine
sulfanilamide
sulfaphenazole
sulfapyridine
sulfasalazine
sulfathiazole
sulfisoxazole
sulthiame
talbutal
tamoxifen
thiamylal
thiethylperazine
thiopental
thiopropazate
thioproperazine
thioridazine
tobramycin
tranylcypromine (?)
triamcinolone
trichloroethylene
trifluoperazine
triflupromazine
trimeprazine
tryparsamide
vaccines—influenza
vinbarbital
vinblastine
vincristine
vitamin A
vitamin D (retinol)
vitamin D_2 (ergocalciferol)
vitamin D_3 (cholecalciferol)
warfarin

5. Endocrine
   A. Cretinism (hypothyroidism)
   B. Cushing syndrome (adrenocortical syndrome)
   C. Diabetes mellitus
   D. DIDMOAD (diabetes mellitus and insipidus with optic atrophy and deafness) syndrome; Wolfram syndrome, Marquardt–Loriaux syndrome)
   E. Fröhlich syndrome (dystrophia adiposogenitalis)
   F. Hyperparathyroidism
   G. Hypophosphatasia (phosphoethanolaminuria)
   H. Juvenile diabetes mellitus (Mauriac syndrome)
   I. Pituitary gigantism syndrome (Launois syndrome)
   J. Simmonds syndrome (hypopituitarism syndrome)
   K. Retinohypophysis syndrome (Lijo Pavia–Lis syndrome)
   L. Zollinger–Ellison syndrome (polyglandular adenomatosis syndrome)
6. Granulomatoses
   A. Sarcoidosis
   B. Tuberculosis
   C. Wegener syndrome (Wegener granulomatosis)
7. Infectious
   A. African eye-worm disease (loiasis)
   B. Anthrax
   C. Congenital cytomegalic inclusion disease
   D. Congenital rubella syndrome (Gregg syndrome)
   E. Cysticercosis
   F. Deerfly fever (tularemia)
   G. Encephalitis
   H. Encephalomeningitis
   I. Echinococcosis (hydatid cyst)
   J. Lyme disease (borreliosis, relapsing fever)
   K. Malaria
   L. Meningitis
   M. Measles (morbilli)
   N. von Mikulicz–Radecki syndrome (dacryosialoadenopathy)
   O. Mumps (epidemic parotitis)
   P. Mycoplasma pneumoniae
   Q. Onchocerciasis syndrome (river blindness)
   R. Rocky Mountain spotted fever
   S. Syphilis (congenital or acquired)
   T. Toxoplasmosis
   U. Yellow fever
8. Inherited
   A. Congenital optic atrophy (autosomal dominant or recessive)
   B. Jensen syndrome (opticoacoustic nerve atrophy with dementia; X-linked)
   C. Juvenile optic atrophy (autosomal dominant)
   D. Metaphyseal dysplasia, anetoderma and optic atrophy (autosomal recessive)
   E. Myotonic dystrophy
   F. Optic atrophy, cataract and neurologic disorder (dominant)
   G. Optic atrophy, non-Leber type, early onset (X-linked)

H. Optic atrophy, polyneuropathy, and deafness (X-linked)
I. Optic atrophy, spastic paraplegia syndrome (X-linked)
J. Optic atrophy, spastic paraplegia, dementia (autosomal dominant)
K. Optic atrophy, nerve deafness, and distal neurogenic amyotrophy (recessive)
L. Optic atrophy with demyelinating of central nervous system (autosomal dominant)
M. Optic atrophy hypoplasia, familial, bilateral (autosomal dominant)
9. Inherited metabolic disorders
A. Leukodystrophies
(1) Adrenoleukodystrophy (ALD)
(2) Canavan disease (spongy degeneration of the nervous system)
(3) Cockayne syndrome
(4) Homocystinuria syndrome
(5) Krabbe disease
(6) Maple syrup urine disease
(7) Menkes disease (kinky-hair syndrome)
B. Peroxisome abnormalities
(1) Defective biogenesis:
a. Infantile Refsum syndrome (heredopathia atactica polyneuritiformis)
b. Neonatal ALD (adrenal cortical atrophy, patchy brain demyelination)
c. Zellweger syndrome (cerebrohepatorenal syndrome)
(2) Refsum syndrome (heredopathia atactica polyneuritiformis
(3) Rhizomeric chondrodysplasia punctata
(4) Single enzyme deficiency
a. Primary hyperoxaluria type I
b. X-linked ALD
C. Storage disorders
(1) Lipoidoses
a. Generalized gangliosidosis
(i) Gangliosidosis GM2, type
(ii) Generalized gangliosidosis GM type
(iii) Juvenile gangliosidosis GM type
b. Sphingolipidoses (arylsulfatase A deficiency syndrome
(i) Arylsulfatase A deficiency syndrome (metachromatic leukodystrophy)
(a) Late infant form: Greenfield disease
(b) Adult form: Bogaert–Nijssen–Peiffer syndrome
(c) Austin disease (multiple sulfatase deficiency
(d) Fabry disease (angiokeratoma corporis diffusum)
(e) Krabbe disease (globoid cell leukodystrophy)
(f) Niemann–Pick syndrome (essential lipoid histiocytosis)
(g) Tay–Sachs syndrome (hexosaminidase deficiency)
(2) Glucose-phosphate dehydrogenase deficiency (von Gierke disease)
(3) Mucolipidoses IV (ML IV)
(4) Mucopolysaccharidoses (MPS) or lysosomal storage diseases
a. MPS I-H (Hurler syndrome; chondroosteodystrophy or lipochondrodystrophy)
b. MPS I-S (Scheie syndrome)

      c. MPS II (Hunter syndrome)

      d. MPS III (Sanfilippo syndrome)

      e. MPS IV (Morquio syndrome)

      f. MPS VI (Maroteaux–Lamy syndrome)

    (5) Neural ceroid lipofuscinosis

      a. Infantile type: Haltia–Santavuori disease

      b. Late infantile type: Jansky–Bielschowsky disease (internuclear ophthalmoplegia)

      c. Juvenile type: Batten disease (Spielmeyer–Vogt–Sjögren syndrome; cerebroretinal degeneration)

    (6) Other disorders involving lipids

      a. Bassen–Kornzweig syndrome (familial hypolipoproteinemia)

      b. Refsum syndrome (heredopathia atactica polyneuritiformis)

10. Local

    A. Aphakic cystoid macula edema (ACME; Irvine–Gass syndrome)

    B. Bird-shot chorioretinopathy

    C. Coats disease

    D. Drusen of optic nerve

    E. Glaucoma

    F. Vascular occlusion

11. Mental and psychomotor deficiency, retardation

    A. Drummond syndrome (idiopathic hypercalcemia)

    B. Familial dysautonomia (Riley–Day syndrome)

    C. Hallervorden–Spatz syndrome

    D. Hallgren syndrome (retinitis pigmentosa–deafness–ataxia syndrome)

    E. Kloepfer disease

    F. Rubinstein–Taybi syndrome

12. Miscellaneous

    A. Albinism

    B. Anemia

    C. Arachnoidal adhesion (e.g., caused by tabes)

    D. Bloch–Sulzberger disease (incontinentia pigmenti)

    E. Bobble-head doll syndrome (massive dilatation of third ventricle)

    F. Bonnet–Dechaume–Blanc syndrome (neuroretinoangiomatosis)

    G. Brown–Sequard syndrome

    H. Cerebellar ataxia (Louis–Bar syndrome)

    I. Cerebral palsy

    J. Cystic fibrosis syndrome

    K. Foster–Kennedy syndrome (basal–frontal syndrome)

    L. Histiocytosis X eosinophil granuloma (Hand–Schuller–Christian syndrome)

    M. Incipient prechiasmal optic nerve compression syndrome

    N. Laurence–Moon–Bardet–Biedl syndrome (retinitis pigmentosa–polydactyly–adiposogenital syndrome)

    O. Leber syndrome

    P. Oculodental syndrome (Peter syndrome)

    Q. Optic cochleodental degeneration syndrome

    R. Peliazeus–Merzbacher disease (aplasia axialis extracorticalis congenita)

    S. Posthypoxic syndrome

    T. Pseudotumor cerebri

    U. Rieger syndrome
    V. Russell syndrome
    W. Status dysraphicus syndrome (Passow syndrome)
    X. Sphenomaxillary fossa syndrome (pterygopalatine fossa syndrome)
    Y. Wagner disease (hereditary vitreoretinal degeneration)

13. Nutritional deficiency
    A. Avitaminosis B (Wernicke syndrome, beriberi)
    B. Avitaminosis B (pellagra)
    C. Garland syndrome (central nervous system deficiency)
    D. (?) Infantile neuroaxonal dystrophy (possible vitamin E deficiency, Seitelberger disease II)
    E. Kwashiorkor syndrome (hypoproteinemia syndrome)
    F. (?) Oculoorogenital syndrome (avitaminosis B with possible avitaminosis A)

14. Orbital
    A. Hutchinson–Pepper syndrome (metastatic infraorbital neuroblastoma)
    B. Rollet syndrome (orbital apex syndrome)
    C. Superior orbital fissure syndrome (Rochon–Duvigneaud syndrome)

15. Rheumatoid
    A. von Bechterew–Stumpelld syndrome (ankylosing spondylitis)
    B. Behçet disease (oculobuccogenital syndrome)
    C. Polymyalgia rheumatica
    D. SLE

16. Skeletal disorders
    A. Achondroplasia
    B. Albers–Schonberg syndrome (osteopetrosis)
    C. Anencephaly
    D. Apert syndrome (acrocephalosyndactylism syndrome)
    E. Brachmann–de Lange syndrome
    F. Camurati–Engelmann syndrome (progressive diaphyseal dysplasia)
    G. Chondrodystrophia calcificans congenita (Conradi syndrome)
    H. Cloverleaf skull syndrome (Kleeblattschädel deformity)
    I. Craniometaphyseal dysplasia (Pyle syndrome)
    J. Craniostenosis
        (1) Oxycephaly
        (2) Plagiocephaly
        (3) Scaphocephaly
        (4) Trigonocephaly
    K. Crouzon syndrome (craniofacial dysotosis)
    L. Enchondromatosis syndrome (Ollier syndrome)
    M. Generalized gangliosidosis GM type
    N. Greig syndrome (hypertelorism ocularis)
    O. Hallermann–Streiff–François syndrome (oculomandibulofacial dyscephaly)
    P. Hutchinson–Gilford progeria syndrome (progeria)
    Q. Marchesani syndrome
    R. McCune–Albright syndrome (fibrosus dysplasia)
    S. Metaphyseal dysplasia, anetoderma, and optic atrophy
    T. Microcephaly
    U. Osteogenesis imperfecta (van der Hoeve syndrome)
    V. Paget syndrome (osteitis deformans)

    W. Primary hyperoxaluria type (osteodystrophy hydrocephalus)

    X. Zellweger syndrome (cerebrohepatorenal syndrome)

17. Trauma

    A. Direct and indirect optic nerve trauma

    B. Electrical injury

    C. Mechanical injury/surgical trauma (orbital floor fracture, malar fractures, Krönlein lateral orbitotomy)

    D. Ocular contusion

    E. Optic-nerve evulsion

    F. Radiation

18. Tumors

    A. Craniopharyngiomas

    B. Ectopic pinealomas

    C. Gliomas

    D. Hemangiomas

    E. Meningiomas

    F. Nasopharyngeal carcinomas

    G. Neuroblastomas

    H. Pituitary adenomas

    I. Pseudo–Foster Kennedy syndrome

    J. Pseudo–pseudo–Foster Kennedy syndrome

    K. von Recklinghausen syndrome (neurofibromatosis)

    L. Tumors extending into fourth ventricle and cerebellum causing papilledema

19. Vascular

    A. Aneurysm of internal carotid artery (foramen lacerum syndrome)

    B. Arteriosclerosis

    C. Cavernosus sinus thrombosis (Foix syndrome)

    D. Giant cell (temporal arteritis)

    E. Hollenhorst syndrome (chorioretinal infarction syndrome)

    F. Kussmaul disease (necrotizing angiitis)

    G. Occlusion of the carotid artery

    H. Sickle cell disease (Herrick syndrome)

    I. Takayasu syndrome (aortic arch syndrome)

Fraunfelder FT, Fraunfelder FW. *Drug-induced ocular side effects and drug interactions.* Woburn, MA: Butterworth-Heinemann, 2001.

Gamez J, et al. Bilateral optic nerve atrophy in myotonic dystrophy. *Am J Ophthalmol* 2001;131:398–400.

Girkin CA, et al. Radiation optic neuropathy after stereotactic radiosurgery. *Ophthalmology* 1997;104:1634–1643.

Roy FH. *Ocular syndromes and systemic diseases*, 3rd ed. Philadelphia: Lippincott Williams & Wilkins, 2002.

Swartz N, Savino PJ. Is all nondefinable optic atrophy Leber's hereditary optic neuropathy? *Surv Ophthalmol* 1994; 39:146–150.

Optic-Nerve Atrophy and Deafness

1. Adult form of arylsulfatase A deficiency (Bogaert–Nijssen–Peiffer syndrome; optico-cochleodental degeneration)

2. Camuati–Engelmann syndrome (progressive diaphyseal dysplasia)

3. HMSN I (Charcot–Marie–Tooth syndrome)

4. Congenital rubella syndrome (German measles, Gregg syndrome)

5. Cockayne syndrome (dwarfism with retinal atrophy and deafness)
6. Craniometaphyseal dysplasia (Pyle syndrome)
7. DIDMOAD syndrome (optic atrophy, sensorineural deafness, diabetes mellitus and diabetes insipidus)
8. Dominant inheritance—congenital deafness and progressive optic nerve atrophy
9. Friedreich ataxia (optic atrophy, ataxia, and progressive hearing loss)
10. Generalized gangliosidosis GM type
11. Hallgren syndrome (retinitis pigmentosa–deafness–ataxia syndrome)
12. Juvenile diabetes mellitus
13. Krabbe syndrome (infantile globoid [II] cell leukodystrophy)
14. ML IV
15. MPS I-H (Hurler syndrome)
16. MPS II (Hunter syndrome)
17. MPS IV (Morquio syndrome)
18. (?) MPS (Maroteaux–Lamy syndrome)
19. (?) Niemann–Pick syndrome (essential lipoid histiocytosis)
20. Osteogenesis imperfecta
21. Recessive: nerve deafness, optic atrophy, and distal neurogenic amyotrophy
22. Refsum syndrome (phytanic acid oxidase deficiency)
23. Rosenberg–Chutorian syndrome
24. Sylvester disease
25. Treft syndrome

Emery JM, et al. Krabbe's disease. *Am J Ophthalmol* 1972;74:400–406.

Roy FH. *Ocular syndromes and systemic diseases*, 3rd ed. Philadelphia: Lippincott Williams & Wilkins, 2002.

Shields JA, et al. Pigmented adenoma of the optic nerve head simulating a melanocytoma. *Ophthalmology* 1992; 99:1705–1709.

Syndromes and Diseases Associated with Optic Atrophy

1. Achondroplasia
2. Acquired lues (syphilis)
3. African eye worm disease (loiasis)
4. Albers–Schonberg syndrome (osteopetrosis)
5. Albinism
6. Albright syndrome (fibrous dysplasia)
7. Anemia
8. Anencephaly
9. Aneurysm of internal carotid artery syndrome (foramen lacerum syndrome)
10. Anthrax
11. Apert syndrome (acrocephalosyndactylism syndrome)
12. Arachnoidal adhesion, including tabes
13. Arteriosclerosis
14. Arylsulfatase A deficiency syndrome (metachromatic leukodystrophy)
15. Avitaminosis B_2 (pellagra)
16. Bassen–Kornzweig syndrome (familial hypolipoproteinemia)
17. Batten–Mayou syndrome (cerebroretinal degeneration)
18. Behçet syndrome (oculobuccogenital syndrome)
19. Behr syndrome (optic atrophy-ataxia)
20. Bielschowsky–Jansky disease (internuclear ophthalmoplegia)

21. Bloch–Sulzberger disease (incontinentia pigmenti)
22. Bobble-head doll syndrome
23. Bonnet–Dechaume–Blanc syndrome (neuroretinoangiomatosis)
24. Brown–Marie syndrome (hereditary ataxia syndrome)
25. Brown–Séquard syndrome (lesion of spinal cord)
26. Carbon monoxide
27. Central nervous system deficiency—bitemporal pallor because of deficient diet (Garland syndrome)
28. Cerebral palsy
29. Cerebellar ataxia
30. Charcot–Marie–Tooth syndrome (progressive neuritic muscular syndrome)
31. Chondrodystrophia calcificans congenita (Conradi syndrome)
32. Chromosome deletion (long-arm) syndrome (de Grouchy syndrome)
33. Coats disease (retinal telangiectasia)
34. Cockayne syndrome (dwarfism with retinal atrophy and deafness)
35. Congenital cytomegalic inclusion disease
36. Congenital optic atrophy—autosomal dominant or recessive
37. Congenital syphilis
38. Craniometaphyseal dysplasia (Pyle syndrome)
39. Craniostenosis (including oxycephaly, scaphocephaly, trigonocephaly, and plagiocephaly)
40. Cretinism (hypothyroidism)
41. Cri-du-chat syndrome (cat-cry syndrome)
42. Crouzon syndrome (craniofacial dysostosis)
43. Cushing syndrome (adrenocortical syndrome)
44. Cystic fibrosis syndrome (fibrocystic disease of pancreas)
45. Cysticercosis
46. Dawson disease (subacute sclerosing panencephalitis)
47. Deerfly fever (tularemia)
48. de Lange syndrome (congenital muscular hypertrophy-cerebral syndrome)
49. Devic syndrome (optical myelitis)
50. Diabetes mellitus
51. Didmoad–Wolfram syndrome (diabetes mellitus and insipidus with optic atrophy and deafness)—autosomal recessive
52. Diencephalic syndrome (Penfield syndrome)
53. Disseminated lupus erythematosus (Kaposi–Libman–Sacks syndrome)
54. Dollinger–Bielschowsky syndrome (lipidosis)
55. Drugs, including the following:

acetophenazine	antimony sodium	bupivacaine (?)
allobarbital	thioglycollate	butabarbital
alseroxylon (?)	antipyrine	butalbital
aminosalicylate (?)	aprobarbital	butallylonal
aminosalicylic acid (?)	aspirin	butaperazine
amobarbital	barbital	butethal
amodiaquine	betamethasone	calcitriol
antimony lithium thiomalate	bromide (?)	carbromal
antimony potassium tartrate	bromisovalum	carphenazine
antimony sodium tartrate	broxyquinoline	chloramphenicol

chloroprocaine (?)
chloroquine
chlorpromazine
cholecalciferol
clindamycin
cobalt (?)
cocaine
cortisone
cyclobarbital
cyclopentobarbital
cycloserine (?)
dapsone
deferoxamine
deserpidine(?)
dexamethasone
dextrothyroxine (?)
diethazine
digitalis (?)
diiodohydroxyquin
ergocalciferol
ergonovine (?)
ergot (?)
ergotamine (?)
ethambutol
ethopropazine
etidocaine (?)
ferrocholinate (?)
ferrous fumarate (?)
ferrous gluconate (?)
ferrous succinate (?)
ferrous sulfate (?)
fluorometholone
fluphenazine
gentamicin
heptabarbital
hexachlorophene
hexamethonium
hexethal
hexobarbital
hydrocortisone
hydroxychloroquine
iodide and iodine solutions
   and compounds
iodochlorhydroxyquin
iodoquinol
iron dextran (?)
iron sorbitex
isoniazid

levothyroxine (?)
lidocaine (?)
liothyronine
liotrix (?)
medrysone
mephobarbital
mepivacaine (?)
mesoridazine
metharbital
methdilazine
methitural
methohexital
methotrexate (?)
methotrimeprazine
methyl alcohol
methylene blue
methylergonovine (?)
methylprednisolone
methysergide (?)
nitroglycerin (?)
oral contraceptives
oxyphenbutazone
pentobarbital
perazine
pericyazine
perphenazine
phenobarbital
phenylbutazone
piperacetazine
polysaccharide iron complex
   (?)
prednisolone
prilocaine (?)
primidone
probarbital
procaine (?)
prochlorperazine
promazine
promethazine
propiomazine
propoxycaine (?)
propoxyphene
quinine
radioactive iodides
rauwolfia serpentina (?)
rescinnamine (?)
reserpine (?)
secobarbital

sodium antimonylgluconate
sodium salicylate
stibocaptate
stibogluconate
stibophen
streptomycin
sulfacetamide (?)
sulfachlorpyridazine (?)
sulfacytine (?)
sulfadiazine (?)
sulfadimethoxine (?)
sulfamerazine (?)
sulfameter (?)
sulfamethazine
sulfamethizole (?)
sulfamethoxazole (?)
sulfamethoxypyridazine
sulfanilamide (?)
sulfaphenazole
sulfapyridine (?)
sulfasalazine (?)
sulfathiazole (?)
sulfisoxazole (?)
suramin
syrosingopine (?)
talbutal
thiamylal
thiethylperazine
thiopental
thiopropazate
thioproperazine
thioridazine
thyroglobulin (?)
thyroid (?)
tobramycin
trichloroethylene
trifluoperazine
triflupromazine
trimeprazine
tryparsamide
vinbarbital
vinblastine
vincristine
vitamin A
vitamin D
vitamin D_2
vitamin D_3

56. Drummond syndrome (idiopathic hypercalcemia)
57. Drusen of optic nerve
58. Dyschondroplasia syndrome (Ollier syndrome)
59. Electrical injury
60. Encephalitis, acute
61. Engelmann syndrome (diaphyseal dysplasia)
62. Exfoliation syndrome
63. Foix syndrome (cavernous sinus thrombosis)
64. Foster–Kennedy syndrome (basal–frontal syndrome)
65. Friedreich ataxia (optic atrophy and sensorineural deafness)—recessive
66. Fröhlich syndrome (dystrophia adiposogenitalis)
67. Galactosyl ceramide lipidosis (globoid cell leukodystrophy)
68. Gangliosidosis GM 1, type
69. Generalized gangliosidosis (infantile)
70. Greig syndrome (hypertelorism ocularis)
71. Glaucoma
72. Glucose-phosphate dehydrogenase deficiency (von Gierke disease)
73. Grönblad-Strandberg syndrome (systemic elastodystrophy)
74. Hallermann–Streiff–François syndrome (oculomandibulofacial dyscephaly)
75. Hallervorden–Spatz syndrome (pigmentary degeneration of globus pallidus)
76. Hallgren syndrome (retinitis-pigmentosa deafness-ataxia syndrome)
77. Happy-puppet syndrome (puppet children)
78. Herrick syndrome (sickle cell disease)
79. Histiocytosis X (Hand–Schüller–Christian syndrome)
80. Hollenhorst syndrome (chorioretinal infarction syndrome)
81. Homocystinuria syndrome
82. Hutchinson syndrome (progeria)
83. Hydatid cyst
84. Hydrocephalus chondrodystrophicus congenita (Kleeblattschädel syndrome)
85. Hyperparathyroidism
86. Hypophosphatasia (phosphoethanolaminuria)
87. Incipient prechiasmal optic nerve compression syndrome
88. Infantile neuroaxonal dystrophy (Seitelberger disease II)
89. Infantile type of neuronal ceroid lipofuscinosis
90. Infections such as basal meningitis, infectious encephalomeningitis (especially measles epidemic parotitis), congenital neurosyphilis (rare before 2 years of age), and toxoplasmosis
91. Irvine syndrome (spontaneous rupture of vitreous face with vitreous adhesions to the wound followed by macular edema)
92. Jensen syndrome (opticoacoustic nerve atrophy with dementia)—X-linked
93. Juvenile diabetes—rare
94. Juvenile optic atrophy—autosomal dominant
95. Keratodermia palmaris et plantaris
96. Kloepfer disease
97. Krabbe disease (meningocutaneous syndrome)
98. Kussmaul disease (necrotizing angiitis)
99. Kwashiorkor (hypoproteinemia syndrome)
100. Laurence–Moon–Bardet–Biedl syndrome (retinitis pigmentosa–polydactyly–adiposogenital syndrome)

101. Leber syndrome (optic atrophy-amaurosis-pituitary syndrome)
102. Leigh disease (subacute necrotizing encephalomyelopathy)
103. Leukemia
104. Malaria
105. Maple syrup urine disease (branched-chain ketoaciduria)
106. Marchesani syndrome (brachymorphy with spherophakia)
107. Maroteaux–Lamy disease (MPS VI)
108. Marquardt–Loriaux syndrome
109. Measles (morbilli)
110. Menkes disease (kinky-hair disease)
111. MERRF syndrome
112. Metachromatic leukodystrophy (Greenfield disease)
113. Metaphyseal dysplasia, anetoderma, and optic atrophy—autosomal recessive
114. Microcephaly
115. Micro syndrome
116. Mikulicz–Radecki syndrome (dacryosialoadenopathy)
117. ML IV
118. MPS IH (Hurler syndrome)
119. MPS IS (Scheie syndrome)
120. MPS II (Hunter syndrome)
121. MPS IV (Morquio syndrome)
122. Multiple sclerosis (disseminated sclerosis)
123. Mumps
124. Naegeli syndrome (reticular pigmented dermatosis)
125. Niemann–Pick syndrome (essential lipoid histiocytosis)
126. Occlusion of carotid artery
127. Oculodental syndrome (Peter syndrome)
128. Oculoorogenital syndrome (riboflavin deficiency syndrome)
129. Onchocerciasis syndrome (river blindness)
130. Optic atrophy, cataract and neurologic disorder—dominant
131. Optic atrophy, nerve deafness, and distal neurogenic amyotrophy—recessive
132. Optic atrophy, non-Leber type, with early onset—x-linked
133. Optic atrophy, polyneuropathy and deafness—x-linked
134. Optic atrophy, spastic paraplegia syndrome—x-linked
135. Optic atrophy with demyelinating of central nervous system—autosomal dominant
136. Optic nerve hypoplasia, familial, bilateral—autosomal dominant
137. Opticocochleodental degeneration syndrome
138. Orbital operation, such as following orbital floor fracture, reduction of malar fractures and Krönlein lateral orbitotomy
137. Osteogenesis imperfecta (van der Hoeve syndrome)
139. Paget syndrome (osteitis deformans)
140. Passow syndrome (syringomyelia)
141. Pelizaeus–Merzbacher disease (aplasia axialis extracorticalis congenita)
142. Pituitary gigantism syndrome (Launois syndrome)
143. Polymyalgia rheumatica
144. Porphyria cutanea tarda
145. Posthypoxic encephalopathy syndrome
146. Radiation
147. Refsum syndrome (phytanic acid oxidase deficiency)

148. Relapsing fever
149. Retinohypophysary syndrome (Lijo Pavia–Lis syndrome)
150. Rieger syndrome (hypodontia and iris dysgenesis)
151. Riley–Day syndrome (congenital familial dysautonomia)
152. Rochon–Duvigneaud syndrome (superior orbital fissure syndrome)
153. Rocky Mountain spotted fever
154. Rollet syndrome (orbital apex-sphenoidal syndrome)
155. Rosenberg–Chutorian syndrome
156. Rubella syndrome (German measles)
157. Rubinstein–Taybi syndrome (broad thumb syndrome)
158. Russell syndrome
159. Sabin–Feldman syndrome
160. Sanfilippo disease (MPS III)
161. Scaphocephaly syndrome
162. Schaumann syndrome (sarcoidosis syndrome)
163. Schilder syndrome (encephalitis periaxialis diffusa)
164. Simmonds syndrome (hypopituitarism syndrome)
165. Spastic paraplegia, optic atrophy, dementia—autosomal dominant
166. Sphenomaxillary fossa syndrome (pterygopalatine fossa syndrome)
167. Spielmeyer–Vogt syndrome (cerebroretinal degeneration)
168. Spongy degeneration of the white matter
169. Suprarenal—sympathetic syndrome (adrenal medulla tumor syndrome)
170. Sylvester disease
171. Simmond syndrome (benign intracranial hypertension)
172. Takayasu syndrome (aortic arch syndrome)
173. Tay–Sachs syndrome (hexosaminidase deficiency)
174. Temporal arteritis syndrome (Hutchinson–Horton–Magath-Brown syndrome)
175. Toxins, including lead, chronic cyanide intoxication such as from eating cassava, thallium (used for treatment of scalp fungi)
176. Trauma, evulsion of optic nerve, and ocular contusion
177. Treft syndrome
178. Trisomy D syndrome (Patau syndrome)
179. Tuberculosis
180. Tumors, including craniopharyngiomas, ectopic pinealomas, gliomas, hemangiomas, meningiomas, nasopharyngeal carcinomas, neuroblastomas, pituitary adenomas, and tumors extending into fourth ventricle and cerebellum causing papilledema
181. Tunbridge–Paley disease
182. Vaccinia
183. Vascular accident
184. von Bekterev–Strumpell syndrome (ankylosing spondylitis)
185. von Recklinghausen syndrome (neurofibromatosis)
186. Wagner syndrome (hyaloideoretinal degeneration)
187. Wegener syndrome (Wegener granulomatosis)
188. Wernicke syndrome (thiamine deficiency)
189. Wrinkly-skin syndrome
190. Yellow fever
191. Zellweger syndrome (cerebrohepatorenal syndrome)
192. Zollinger–Ellison syndrome (polyglandular adenomatosis syndrome)

Fraunfelder FT, Fraunfelder FW. *Drug-induced ocular side effects and drug interactions.* Woburn, MA: Butterworth-Heinemann, 2001.

McKusick VA. *Mendelian inheritance in man*, 12th ed. Baltimore: Johns Hopkins University Press, 1998.

Rizzo JF, et al. Optic atrophy in familial dysautonomia. *Am J Ophthalmol* 1986;102:463–467.

Roy FH. *Ocular syndromes and systemic diseases*, 3rd ed. Philadelphia: Lippincott Williams & Wilkins, 2002.

OPTIC-NERVE HYPOPLASIA

1. Chromosome disorders
   A. Down syndrome (trisomy 21)
   B. Deletion of long chromosome (13)
   C. Edward syndrome (trisomy 18)
   D. Patau syndrome (trisomy 13)
   E. Ring chromosome mosaicism
   F. 13 q deletion syndrome
2. Idiopathic
3. Neurologic conditions
   A. Agenesis of the corpus callosum
   B. Anencephaly
   C. Basal encephalocele
   D. Behavioral problems
   E. Cerebellar atrophy
   F. Cerebral atrophy
   G. Cerebral infarcts
   H. Cerebral palsy
   I. Colpocephaly
   J. Congenital suprasellar tumors
   K. Congenital third, fourth, and sixth nerve palsies and up-gaze palsies
   L. Encephaloceles
   M. Hydranencephaly
   N. Hydrocephaly
   O. Mental retardation
   P. Migration disturbances
   Q. Perinatal encephalopathy
   R. Porencephaly
   S. Posterior pituitary ectopia
4. Ocular conditions
   A. Albinism
   B. Aniridia
   C. Astigmatism
   D. Blepharophimosis
   E. Colobomas (optic disc and chorioretinal)
   F. High myopia
   G. Microphthalmos
   H. Retinal vascular tortuosity
5. Systemic conditions
   A. Aicardi syndrome
   B. Albinism
   C. Chondrodysplasia punctata
   D. Cleft lip and palate

   E. Diabetes mellitus (maternal)—segmental optic nerve hypoplasia in infant
   F. Duane retraction syndrome
   G. Fetal alcohol syndrome, especially pituitary abnormalities with isolated tortuosity
      of retinal veins
   H. Goldenhar–Gorlin syndrome
   I. Hemifacial atrophy
   J. Hypertelorism
   K. Intrauterine infections—including cytomegalovirus and hepatitis
       (1) Cytomegalovirus
       (2) Hepatitis
   L. Inherited (autosomal dominant or recessive)
   M. Klippel–Trenaunay–Weber syndrome
   N. Meckel syndrome
   O. Median cleft face syndrome
   P. de Morsier syndrome (septooptic dysplasia and mutations in the homeobox gene
      HESX1/hesx1)
   Q. Osteogenesis imperfecta
   R. Potter syndrome
   S. Syndrome of nevus sebaceus of Jadassohn
   T. Topless optic disk syndrome
6. Toxins (maternal use of)
   A. Alcohol
   B. Lysergic acid diethylamide (LSD)
   C. Phencyclidine (PCP)
   D. Phenytoin
   E. Quinine
   F. Tobacco

Brodsky MC, et al. Congenital optic disc anomalies [review]. *Surv Ophthalmol* 1994;32:89–112.

Brodsky MC. Optic nerve hypoplasia with posterior pituary ectopia: male predominance and nonassociation with breech delivery. *Am J Ophthalmol* 1999;127,2:238–239.

Helstrom A, et al. Optic nerve hypoplasia with isolated tortuosity of the retinal veins. *Arc Ophthalmol* 1999;117: 880–884.

Chismire KJ, Witkop GS. Angle dysgenesis in a patient with blepharophimosis syndrome. *Am J Ophthalmol* 1994; 117:676–677.

Siatkowski RM, et al. The clinical, neuroradiographic, and endocrinologic profile of patients with bilateral optic nerve hypoplasia. *Ophthalmology* 1997;104:493–496.

OPTIC NEURITIS (PAPILLITIS AND RETROBULBAR NEURITIS

This condition is characterized by progressive loss of vision and possibly complete amaurosis; pain in or behind the eye, especially on lateral movement; Marcus Gunn pupillary phenomenon; and central or paracentral scotoma.

1. Demyelinating and degenerative diseases
   A. Adrenoleukodystrophy
   B. Hereditary ataxia (Brown–Marie syndrome)
   C. Multiple sclerosis
   D. Opticomyelitis (Devic disease)
2. Drugs, poisons, vaccines
   A. Drugs, including the following:

acetohexamide
acetyldigitoxin
alcohol
allobarbital
aminosalicylate
aminosalicylic acid (?)
amiodarone (?)
amitriptyline
amobarbital
aprobarbital
barbital
bromisovalum
broxyquinoline
bupivacaine (?)
butabarbital
butalbital
butallylonal
butethal
calcitriol (?)
caramiphen
carbromal
carmustine
chloral hydrate (?)
chloramphenicol
chloroprocaine (?)
chlorpropamide (?)
cholecalciferol
cisplatin
clindamycin
clophene (?)
cyclobarbital
cyclopentobarbital
cycloserine (?)
deferoxamine
desipramine
deslanoside
dextrothyroxine (?)
didanosine
diethylpropion (?)
digitalis
digitoxin
digoxin
diiodohydroxyquin
diphtheria and tetanus
   toxoids (adsorbed)
diphtheria and tetanus
   toxoids and pertussis
diphtheria toxoid (adsorbed)
disulfiram

ergocalciferol (?)
ergonovine
ergotamine
ethambutol
ethchlorvynol
ethionamide
etidocaine (?)
etoposide
etretinate
fenoprofen
ferrocholinate (?)
ferrous fumarate (?)
ferrous gluconate (?)
ferrous succinate
ferrous sulfate (?)
fluorouracil (?)
gitalin
glyburide
heptabarbital
hexethal
hexobarbital
ibuprofen
imipramine
indomethacin (?)
influenza virus vaccine
interferon alpha, beta, or
   gamma
iodide and iodine solutions
   and compounds
iodochlorhydroxyquin
iodoquinol
iron dextran (?)
iron sorbitex (?)
isocarboxazid (?)
isoniazid
isotretinoin
kanamycin (?)
lanatoside C
levothyroxine (?)
lidocaine
liothyronine (?)
liotrix (?)
measles and rubella virus
   vaccine (live)
measles, mumps, and rubella
   virus vaccine
mephobarbital
mepivacaine (?)
metharbital

methitural
methohexital
methyl alcohol
methylergonovine
methysergide
metronidazole(?)
minoxidil(?)
mumps virus vaccine (live)
naproxen
nialamide (?)
nitrofurantoin (?)
nortriptyline
nystatin
oral contraceptives
ouabain
oxyphenbutazone
penicillamine
pentobarbital
phenobarbital
phenylbutazone
piroxicam (?)
poliovirus vaccine (?)
polysaccharide–iron complex
   (?)
prilocaine (?)
primidone
probarbital
procaine (?)
procarbazine
propoxycaine (?)
protriptyline
quinacrine
quinidine
rabies immune globulin
rabies vaccine
radioactive iodides
rifampin (?)
rubella and mumps virus
   vaccine (live)
rubella virus vaccine (live)
secobarbital
smallpox vaccine
streptomycin
sulfacetamide
sulfachlorpyridazine
sulfacytine
sulfadiazine
sulfadimethoxine
sulfamerazine

sulfameter
sulfamethizole
sulfamethoxazole
sulfamethoxypyridazine
sulfanilamide
sulfaphenazole
sulfapyridine
sulfasalazine
sulfathiazole
sulfisoxazole

sulindac (?)
talbutal
tamoxifen (?)
tetanus immune globulin (?)
tetanus toxoid (?)
thiamylal
thiopental
thyroglobulin (?)
thyroid (?)
tolazamide

tolbutamide
trichloroethylene
tryparsamide
vaccine (adsorbed)
vinbarbital
vinblastine
vincristine
vitamin D
vitamin D_2 (?)
vitamin D_3 (?)

   B. Poisons (inhalation, skin absorption, or ingestion): alcohol, arsenicals (inorganic, gaseous, or organic), carbon disulfide, carbon tetrachloride, chlorodinitrobenzene and dinitrobenzene, copper, dinitrotoluene, Lysol solution, mercury, methyl bromide, methyl alcohol, siderosis (exogenous: intraocular foreign body or endogenous: iron metabolism disorders), tobacco, toluene (methyl benzene), trichlorethylene, tricresil phosphate, venoms (e.g., bee sting), vinyl benzene (styrene)

   C. Vaccines and toxoids: Bacille Calmette-Guérin (bCG) vaccination, diphtheria toxoid (absorbed), diphtheria and tetanus toxoids (absorbed), influenza virus vaccine, measles or mumps or rubella live vaccine, poliovirus vaccine, rabies immune globulin, rabies vaccine, smallpox vaccine, tetanus immune globulin (?), tetanus toxoid (?), bee and wasp sting.

  3. Infection and inflammation

   A. Bacterial

    (1) Anthrax

    (2) Botulism (toxin from clostridium botulinum)

    (3) Brucellosis (undulant fever)

    (4) Diphtheria

    (5) Endocarditis

    (6) Leptospirosis (Weil syndrome)

    (7) Lyme disease (borreliosis, relapsing fever)

    (8) Mycoplasma pneumoniae

    (9) Pertussis (whooping cough)

    (10) Streptococcus (scarlet fever)

    (11) Syphilis (acquired lues)

    (12) Tuberculosis

    (13) Typhoid fever (abdominal typhus)

   B. Fungal

    (1) Candidiasis

    (2) Coccidioidomycosis

    (3) Mucormycosis

    (4) Torulosis (cryptococcus)

   C. Viral

    (1) Acquired immune deficiency syndrome (AIDS)

    (2) Bornholm disease (epidemic pleurodynia)

    (3) Chickenpox (varicella)

    (4) Epidemic keratoconjunctivitis

    (5) Equine encephalitis

    (6) Hepatitis A, B, C

       (7) Infectious mononucleosis

       (8) Influenza

       (9) Measles (rubeola)

      (10) Mumps

      (11) Pappataci fever (sandfly fever)

      (12) Poliomyelitis

      (13) Smallpox

      (14) Yellow fever

   D. Protozoan

       (1) Malaria

       (2) Toxoplasmosis

       (3) Trypanosomiasis

   E. Rickettsia

       (1) Boutonneuse fever rickettsia (Marseilles fever)

       (2) Japanese river fever (typhus)

       (3) Q fever

       (4) Rocky Mountain spotted fever

   F. Orbit

       (1) Herpes zoster

       (2) Infections of the gasserian ganglion

       (3) von Mikulicz–Radecki syndrome (dacryosialoadenopathy)

       (4) Rollet syndrome (orbital apex syndrome)

       (5) Tolosa–Hunt syndrome (painful ophthalmoplegia)

   G. *Helminth* infestations

       (1) Acanthamoeba

       (2) Echinococcosis (hydatid cyst)

       (3) Onchocerciasis (river blindness)

       (4) Toxocariasis (nematode ophthalmia syndrome)

       (5) Trichinellosis

   H. Spread from sphenoid and posterior ethmoidal sinuses

    I. Postinfectious

       (1) Guillain–Barré syndrome (acute infectious neuritis)

       (2) Reye syndrome (acute encephalopathy syndrome)

       (3) Subacute sclerosing panencephalitis (Dawson disease)

       (4) Vogt–Koyanagi–Harada syndrome (uveitis–vitiligo–alopecia–poliosis syndrome)

4. Noninfectious arteritis, hypersensitivity vasculitis

   A. Involving small vessels

       (1) Drugs

       (2) Henoch–Schönlein

   B. Involving small and medium-sized vessels

       (1) Polyarteritis nodosa (Kussmaul disease)

       (2) Necrotizing granulomatous arthritis

          a. Sarcoidosis

          b. Wegener granulomatosis (Wegener syndrome)

       (3) Buerger disease (thromboangiitis obliterans)

       (4) Localized arteritis

          a. Idiopathic

          b. Polyarteritis nodosa

    C. Involving large, medium and small vessels
       (1) Arteritis in collagen vascular disease
          a. Behçet disease (oculobuccogenital syndrome)
          b. Progressive systemic sclerosis (PSS; scleroderma)
          c. Rheumatoid arthritis
          d. SLE
       (2) Giant cell (temporal) arteritis
       (3) Takayasu syndrome (aortic arch syndrome)
    D. Idiopathic paroxysmal digital cyanosis (Raynaud disease)
    E. Multiple myeloma (Kahler disease)
  5. Others
    A. Chorioretinitis
    B. Cystic fibrosis syndrome
    C. Hutchinson–Gilfor (progeria) syndrome
    D. Hysteria
    E. McCune–Albright syndrome (fibrous dysplasia)
    F. Naegeli syndrome (melanophoric nevus)
    G. Paget disease (osteitis deformans)
    H. Parkinson syndrome (paralysis agitans)
    I. Relapsing polychondritis
    J. Stevens–Johnson syndrome (erythema multiforme exudativum)
    K. Uveitis, including sympathetic ophthalmia
  6. Systemic diseases
    A. Endocrine
       (1) Diabetes mellitus
       (2) Hypoparathyroidism
       (3) Hyperthyroidism (Basedow syndrome)
       (4) Hyperthyroidism
       (5) Juvenile diabetes–dwarfism–obesity syndrome (Mauriac syndrome)
       (6) Lactation
       (7) Pregnancy
       (8) Puberty
       (9) Retinohypophysary syndrome (Lijo Pavia–Lis syndrome)
    B. Nutritional diseases
       (1) Beriberi (vitamin B deficiency)
       (2) Carcinomatosis
       (3) Hyperemesis gravidarum
       (4) Pellagra (vitamin B deficiency)
    C. Rheumatic disease, arthritis
       (1) Felty syndrome
       (2) Juvenile rheumatoid arthritis (Still disease)
       (3) Polymyalgia rheumatica
       (4) Reiter syndrome (polyarthritis enterica)
       (5) Rheumatoid arthritis
    D. Miscellaneous
       (1) Amyloidosis (Lubarsch–Pick syndrome)
       (2) Chronic glomerulonephritis with secondary renal hypertension or pyelone-
          phritis
       (3) Emphysema

       (4) Hepatic failure
       (5) Hypertension
       (6) Porphyria
       (7) Trauma
  A. Mechanical
  B. Radiation
       (1) Electromagnetic
            a. High voltage/lighting
            b. Microwave
            c. Laser burn
            d. X-ray
       (2) Radioactive source
            a. a-ruthenium
            b. b-betatron
            c. g-cobalt
            d. pisotope
8. Tumors
  A. Craniopharyngioma
  B. Hemangiopericytoma of optic nerve
  C. Myeloproliferative diseases
       (1) Hodgkin disease
       (2) Leukemia
       (3) Lymphoma
  D. Neuroblastoma

Beck RW, et al. Fellow eye abnormalities in acute unilateral optic neuritis. *Ophthalmology* 1993;100:691–698.

Fraunfelder FT, Fraunfelder FW. *Drug-induced ocular side effects and drug interactions.* Woburn, MA: Butterworth-Heinemann, 2001.

Maltzman JS, et al. Optic neuropathy occurring after bee and wasp sting. *Ophthalmology* 2000;107:193–195.

Straussberg R, et al. Epstein-Barr virus infection associated with encephalitis and optic neuritis. *J Pediatr Ophthalmol Strabismus* 1993;30:262–263.

Blurred optic nerve heads

	Vision	Visual Fields	Retinal Veins	Color of Nerve Head	Retinal Hemorrhages	Peripapillary Retinal Edema	Vitreous Cells	Symmetry of Nerve Heads	Comments
1. Early papilledema	Normal	Normal (except blind spot enlargement)	Slightly distended; early loss of spontaneous pulsations	Pink	±	±	–	Often asymmetric	Headaches
2. Advanced papilledema	Normal or, at times, somewhat reduced	Normal (except blind spot enlargement)	Distended without spontaneous pulsations	Very pink to pale	+	+	–	Often symmetric	Sixth nerve palsies are additional clue to increased pressure
3. Hyperopia and physiologic variants	Normal	Normal	Normal	Normal	–	–	–	Often symmetric	Fundus seen with + lens; central disc cupping usually present
4. Optic neuritis	Impaired	Central scotoma ± peripheral loss	Distended ± spontaneous pulsations	Pink	±	±	±	Usually unilateral	Precipitous onset; may have pain with ocular motility
5. Optic nerve tumor	Normal or markedly reduced	Normal or markedly reduced	Normal or distended	May be pigmented if disc tumor contains melanin; very pink to pale	±	±	–	Usually unilateral	May involve only the orbital or intracranial optic nerve, and not the intraocular portion; primary nerve tumors are rarely observed on the disc
6. Optic nerve avulsion	Blind eye	–	Sludged	Pale	±	–	±	Contralateral eye normal	Contre-coup or direct trauma

Blurred optic nerve heads (Continued)

	Vision	Visual Fields	Retinal Veins	Color of Nerve Head	Retinal Hemorrhages	Peripapillary Retinal Edema	Vitreous Cells	Symmetry of Nerve Heads	Comments
7. Hyaline bodies of nerve head parents	Normal	Normal or a variety of field cuts	Normal	Normal	− (Very rarely +)	−	−	Often symmetric hyaline bodies sometimes seen at disc margins in one eye only	Often familial (examine and siblings)
8. Hypotony of eye (after trauma)	Slightly impaired	Usually normal	Distended	Pink ±	±	Peripheral edema	−	Unilateral	Soft eye; commotio retinae

Paton, D., and Goldberg, M.F.: *Injuries of the Eye, the Lids, and the Orbit.* Philadelphia, W.B. Saunders, 1968.

(Neuritis) papillitis and retrobulbar neuritis

	Multiple Sclerosis	Temporal Arteritis	Sinusitis	Diabetes Mellitus	Hyperthyroidism	Chronic Glomerulonephritis	Paget's Disease	Fibrocystic Disease of Pancreas	Oral Contraceptives
History									
1. Familial				U					
2. Greater in children						S			
3. Greater in elderly									
4. Greater in females					S				
5. Greater in men							U		
6. Greater in young individuals	U		U						
7. Greater over age 40				U					
8. Headache, tender temporal arteries and jaw claudication		U							
9. Hereditary						S	U	U	
10. Oral contraceptive history									U
11. Orbital ache (deep)									
12. Possible early viral infection	S								
Physical Findings									
1. Angioid streaks							S		
2. Anisocoria	U				S				
3. Asteroid hyalosis				S					
4. Blue sclera				S				S	
5. Cataract								S	
6. Central retinal artery occlusion		U							
7. Convergent weakness	S				S				
8. Corneal ring opacities							U		
9. Cotton wool spots			U	U		U			
10. Decreased or absent pupillary reaction to light	U	S							
11. Dilation of retinal veins				U		U		U	
12. Diplopia	S								S
13. Discoloration of upper eyelids					S				
14. Extropion uvea				R					
15. Exophthalmos					U		S		
16. Gaze palsy	S								
17. Glaucoma				R	R				
18. Hard yellow exudates				U					
19. Hypotony of the globe			S	R					
20. Hippus of pupil	U								
21. Impaired fixation on extreme lateral gaze	R				S				
22. Iritis			S						
23. Irregular sheathing of retinal veins				S					
24. Ischemic optic neuropathy		U		S				U	
25. Ischemic retinopathy	R			U					
26. Keratitis					S				
27. Keratoconjunctivitis sicca									S
28. Lid lag					U				
29. Lid trembling on gentle closure					U				
30. Lipemia retinalis				U					
31. Macular degeneration							S	S	

(Neuritis) papillitis and retrobulbar neuritis (Continued)

	Multiple Sclerosis	Temporal Arteritis	Sinusitis	Diabetes Mellitus	Hyperthyroidism	Chronic Glomerulonephritis	Paget's Disease	Fibrocystic Disease of Pancreas	Oral Contraceptives
Physical Findings									
32. Macular edema				U					
33. Marcus Gunn pupil sign	U	U							
34. Microaneurysms of retina				U					
35. Myopia									S
36. Myokymia	S								
37. Neuroretinal edema				S	U	S			
38. Nystagmus	U								
39. Ophthalmoplegia		S							
40. Optic atrophy	S			S			S	S	
41. Pain and tenderness of the brows			U						
42. Paralysis of 3rd or 6th nerve	S			S			S		
43. Photophobia					S				
44. Prolapse of lacrimal gland					U				
45. Pseudo-Foster Kennedy syndrome	R	U							
46. Ptosis	S	S							
47. Reduced blinking					S				
48. Retinal hemorrhages		S		U		U	S	S	
49. Retinal periphlebitis	R								
50. Retinal neovascularization				S					
51. Retraction of upper lid					U				
52. Rubeosis iridis				S					
53. Scleritis		S							
54. Shallow orbits					S				
55. Swelling of eyelids					U				
56. Tearing, excessive					S				
57. Tonic pupil		U							
58. Uveitis	S								
59. Vitreal hemorrhages				S					R
60. Xerosis of conjunctiva								S	
Lab Data									
1. CT scan of optic foramina and parasellar areas abnormal									
2. Dense, expanded bones on X ray								U	
3. E.S.R. elevated		U							
4. Fluorescein angiography abnormal	R	U		U					
5. Glycosuria				U					
6. Hematuria						U			
7. Hyperglycemia				U					
8. Ketonuria				U					
9. Proteinuria				R		U			
10. T4, radio T3 resin uptake and radioiodine uptake elevated								U	
11. Temporal artery biopsy with cellular infiltration and giant cells		U							
12. Urinary hydroxyproline elevated								U	

R = rarely; S = sometimes; U = usually.

PSEUDOOPTIC NEURITIS (LESIONS THAT MIMIC OPTIC NEURITIS)

1. Congenital retinoschisis
2. Hematoma
3. Ischemic optic neuropathy
4. Papilledema (see p. 593)
5. Retinal lesions that also exhibit metamorphopsia, e.g., serous or angiospastic retinopathy
6. Tumors
   A. Disc
      (1) Gliomas
      (2) Meningiomas
      (3) Metastatic carcinoma
      (4) Neurofibromas
   B. Expanding lesions of anterior and middle cranial fossa producing central scotoma
      (1) Craniopharyngiomas
      (2) Ectopic pinealomas
      (3) Meningiomas
      (4) Metastatic carcinomas
      (5) Myeloproliferative diseases
         a. Hodgkin disease
         b. Lymphomas
         c. Plasmocytoma
      (6) Nasopharyngeal carcinomas
      (7) Pituitary adenomas

Huber A. *Eye symptoms in brain tumors*, 2nd ed. St. Louis: CV Mosby, 1971.

Roy FH. *Ocular syndromes and systemic diseases*, 3rd ed. Philadelphia: Lippincott Williams & Wilkins, 2002.

OPTICOCILIARY SHUNTS (TORTUOUS, ECTATIC CHANNELS FROM OPTIC NERVE TO CHOROID)

1. Arachnoid cyst of the optic nerve
2. Central retinal vein occlusion (see p. 468–472)
3. Chronic atrophic papilledema
4. Drusen of the optic nerve
5. Optic-nerve glioma
6. Primary nerve sheath meningioma
7. Sickle cell trait
8. Sphenoorbital meningioma

Dowhan TP, et al. Opticiliary shunts and sickle retinopathy in a woman with sickle cell trait. *Ann Ophthalmol* 1990;22:66–69.

Mendoza RM, et al. Optociliary veins in optic nerve sheath meningioma. *Ophthalmology* 1999;106:311–318.

PAPILLEDEMA (SWELLING OF OPTIC DISC)

1. Drugs, poisons, and vaccines
   A. Drugs (those in all capitalized letters are drugs that also cause pseudotumor cerebri):

acetophenazine
ADRENAL CORTEX INJECTION
ALDOSTERONE
allobarbital
amiodarone
amobarbital
AMPHOTERICIN B
antimony lithium thiomalate
antimony potassium tartrate
antimony sodium tartrate
antimony sodium thioglycollate
aprobarbital
aspirin
auranofin (?)
aurothioglucose (?)
aurothioglycanide (?)
Azathioprine
barbital
benzathine penicillin G
bromide (?)
bupivacaine (?)
butabarbital
butalbital
butallylonal
butaperazine
butethal
calcitriol
carbamazepine
carbon dioxide
carphenazine
cephaloridine (?)
chlorambucil
chloramphenicol (?)
chloroprocaine (?)
chlorpromazine
CHLORTETRACYCLINE
cholecalciferol
cisplatin
colchicine
CORTISONE
cyclobarbital
cyclopentobarbital
DANAZOL

DEMECLOCYCLINE
DESOXYCORTICOSTERONE
DEXAMETHASONE
DEXTROTHYROXINE
didanosine
diethazine
DOXYCYCLINE
ELTROXIN
ethambutol
ethopropazine
etidocaine (?)
etoposide
FLUDROCORTISONE
fluorometholone
fluphenazine
FLUPREDNISOLONE
GENTAMICIN
glutethimide
gold Au 198
gold sodium thiomalate (?)
gold sodium thiosulfate (?)
heptabarbital
HEXACHLOROPHENE
hexethal
hexobarbital
hydrabamine phenoxymethyl penicillin
HYDROCORTISONE
IBUPROFEN
INDOMETHACIN
INSULIN-LIKE GROWTH FACTOR I
interferon
interferon alpha, beta, or gamma
isocarboxazid (?)
isoniazid
ISOTRETINOIN
KETOPROFEN
LEVODOPA
LEVOTHYROXINE
lidocaine
LIOTHYRONINE
LITHIUM CARBONATE
LITHIUM CITRATE
MANGANESE

mephobarbital

mepivacaine (?)

MEPREDNISONE

mesoridazine

METHACYCLINE

methaqualone (?)

metharbital

methdilazine

methitural

methohexital

methotrimeprazine

methyl alcohol

methylene blue

METHYLPREDNISOLONE

methyprylon

mitotane

nadolol (?)

NALIDIXIC ACID

Naproxen (?)

NITROFURANTOIN

NITROGLYCERIN

NORPLANT

ofloxacin

ORAL CONTRACEPTIVES

OXYTETRACYCLINE

PARAMETHASONE

penicillamine

pentobarbital

perazine

PERHEXILINE

pericyazine

perphenazine

phenelzine (?)

phenobarbital

phenoxymethyl penicillin

PHENYLPROPANOLAMINE

PHENYTOIN

piperacetazine

POTASSIUM PENICILLIN G

POTASSIUM PENICILLIN V

POTASSIUM PHENETHICILLIN

PREDNISOLONE

PREDNISONE

prilocaine (?)

primidone

probarbital

procaine (?)

PROCAINE PENICILLIN G

procarbazine

prochlorperazine

promazine

promethazine

propiomazine

propoxycaine (?)

PYRIDOXINE

quinine

RETINOIDS

secobarbital

sodium antimonylgluconate

sodium salicylate

stibocaptate

stibogluconate

stibophen

sulfacetamide

sulfachlorpyridazine

sulfacytine

sulfadimethoxine

sulfamerazine

sulfameter

sulfamethazine

sulfamethizole

sulfamethoxazole

sulfamethoxypyridazine

sulfanilamide

sulfaphenazole

sulfapyridine

sulfasalazine

sulfathiazole

sulfisoxazole

sulthiame

talbutal

tamoxifen

TETRACYCLINE

thiamylal

thiethylperazine

thiopental

thiopropazate

thioproperazine

thioridazine

THYROGLOBULIN

THYROID

tranylcypromine (?)

trifluoperazine

triflupromazine

trimeprazine

vinbarbital

VITAMIN A (RETINOL)

vitamin D (calcitriol)

vitamin D_2 (ergocalciferol)

vitamin D_3 (cholecalciferol)

    B. Poisons (inhalation, skin absorption, or ingestion)

        (1) Carbon dioxide

        (2) Lead

        (3) Methyl alcohol

    C. Vaccines

        (1) Diphtheria–tetanus toxoids–pertussis vaccine (absorbed)

        (2) Influenza virus vaccine

        (3) Measles or mumps or rubella live vaccine

  2. Intracranial causes—usually bilateral

    A. Tumors

      *(1) Frontal lobe lesion—mental changes (apathy, euphoria, and social behavioral changes); normal visual field if confined to frontal lobe; most likely, tumors are medulloblastoma, meningioma, astrocytoma, glioblastoma, or metastasis from lung or breast

      *(2) Temporal lobe lesions—formed hallucinations, superior homonymous quadrantanopia, or homonymous hemianopia, ipsilateral mydriatic fixed pupil and oculomotor paresis, and contralateral facial palsy; most likely, tumors are medulloblastoma, meningioma, astrocytoma, glioblastoma, or metastasis from lung or breast

      *(3) Parietal lobe lesions—visual agnosia such as alexia or dyslexia, complete homonymous hemianopia, or inferior homonymous quadrantanopia, disturbances of trigeminal nerve, including decreased corneal sensation and positive (asymmetric response) optokinetic nystagmus; most likely caused by:

        a. Astrocytoma

        b. Glioblastoma

        c. Medulloblastoma

        d. Meningioma

        e. Metastasis from lung or breast

      (4) Occipital lobe lesions—unformed visual hallucinations and homonymous congruous visual field defect; most likely caused by the following:

        a. Astrocytoma

        b. Glioblastoma

        c. Hemangioma

        d. Meningioma

        e. Metastasis from lung or breast

      (5) Third-ventricle and sellar lesions—visual field of bitemporal hemianopia or unilateral blindness and contralateral temporal hemianopia; most likely, tumors are craniopharyngioma

      (6) Fourth-ventricle and cerebellum lesions—ataxia, asynergy, dysmetria, hypotonia, and acquired jerk nystagmus, usually horizontal and more pronounced in lateral gaze; most likely caused by:

        a. Astrocytoma

        b. Hemangioblastoma

        c. Medulloblastoma

        d. Metastasis from lung or breast

* = most important

(7) Cerebellar-pontine angle tumor such as Cushing syndrome II (acoustic neuroma syndrome)

(8) Base skull tumor, such as Garcin syndrome (half-base syndrome)

(9) Chiasmal tumor such as Fröhlich syndrome (dystrophia adiposogenitalis)

(10) Neuroblastoma

(11) Russell syndrome (diencephalic syndrome)

(12) Zollinger–Ellison syndrome (polyglandular adenomatosis syndrome)

B. Decreased intracranial capacity, such as in acrocephalosyndactyly (Apert disease), Arnold–Chiari syndrome (cerebellomedullary malformation syndrome), craniofacial dysostosis (Crouzon disease), craniostenosis, hypertelorism, and tower skull (oxycephaly)

C. Pseudotumor cerebri (Symonds syndrome)—bilateral papilledema and increased intracranial pressure but negative neurologic and general physical findings

(1) Addison disease (adrenal cortical insufficiency)

(2) Autosomal dominant endosteal hyperostosis

(3) Chronic respiratory insufficiency

(4) Familial Mediterranean fever

(5) Hypertension

(6) Multiple sclerosis

(7) Polyangiitis overlap syndrome

(8) Psittacosis

(9) Renal disease

(10) Reye syndrome

(11) Sarcoidosis

(12) SLE

(13) Thrombocytopenia purpura

(14) Vitamin A (excessive) after overeating carrots in a weight loss program

(15) Drugs including the following:

(absorbed) levodopa (?)	hexachlorophene	nitrofurantoin
adrenal cortex injection	hydrabamine penicillin V	nitroglycerin
aldosterone	hydrocortisone	ofloxacin
amiodarone	ibuprofen (?)	oral contraceptives
benzathine penicillin G	indomethacin	oxytetracycline
betamethasone	isotretinoin	paramethasone
chlorambucil	ketoprofen	penicillin G
chlortetracycline	leuprolide acetate	penicillin V
cortisone	levonorgestrel	perhexiline
danazol	levothyroxine	phenylpropanolamine
demeclocycline	liothyronine	phenytoin
desoxycorticosterone	liotrix	potassium
dexamethasone	lithium carbonate	potassium phenethicillin
diptheria and tetanus toxoids	manganese	prednisolone
and pertussis vaccine	medroxyprogesterone	prednisone
doxycycline	medrysone	procaine
etretinate	meprednisone	tetracycline
fludrocortisone	methacycline	thyroglobulin
fluprednisolone	methylprednisolone	thyroid
gentamicin	minocycline	triamcinolone
griseofulvin	nalidixic acid	vitamin A

       (16) Frankl–Hochwart syndrome (pineal–neurologic–ophthalmic syndrome)

       (17) Glomus jugulare tumor

       (18) Iron-deficiency anemia

       (19) Menarche

       (20) Pregnancy

       (21) Thrombosis of the sagittal or lateral sinus, such as that following otitis media in children

       (22) *Yersinia pseudotuberculosis*

3. Neurologic disorders
   A. Cerebral palsy
   B. Foster–Kennedy syndrome
   - (1) Aneurysm of internal carotid, anterior cerebral, or anterior communicating artery
   - (2) Arteriosclerotic plaques of internal carotid or anterior cerebral arteries
   - (3) Chiasmal arachnoiditis secondary to trauma, spinal anesthesia, or syphilis
   - (4) Craniopharyngioma with forward extension
   - (5) Frontal lobe tumors or abscess
   - (6) Glioma of the intracranial portion of optic nerve
   - (7) Internal hydrocephalus because of tumor of posterior fossa
   - (8) Old unilateral optic nerve atrophy (e.g., consecutive ischemic optic neuropathies)
   - (9) Olfactory groove, sphenoid ridge and suprasellar meningioma
   C. High cerebrospinal fluid protein content and defective absorption (e.g., Guillain–Barré syndrome (Acute Infectious Neuritis))
   D. Muscular dystrophy
   E. Parkinson syndrome (shaking palsy)
   F. Status dysraphicus syndrome (Passow syndrome, syringomyelia)
   G. Subdural or subarachnoid hemorrhage
4. Miscellaneous
   A. Abscess
   B. Angioedema
   C. Brown–Séquard syndrome
   D. Camurati–Engelmann syndrome (progressive diaphyseal dysplasia)
   E. Chediak–Higashi syndrome (anomalous leukocytic inclusions with constitutional stigma)
   F. Churg–Strauss syndrome (allergic granulomatosis and angiitis)
   G. Citrullinemia (late onset)
   H. Degos syndrome (malignant atrophic papulosis)
   I. Fabry disease (angiokeratoma corporis diffusum)
   J. Hydrocephalus
   K. Kenny syndrome
   L. McCune–Albright syndrome (fibrosus dysplasia)
   M. Nocturnal hypoventilation
   N. Pelizaeus–Merzbacher syndrome (aplasia axialis extracorticalis congenita)
   O. Polymyalgia rheumatica
   P. Primary hyperoxaluria type
   Q. Renal insufficiency

5. Ocular cause—usually unilateral
   A. Acute glaucoma
   B. ACME (Irvine–Gass syndrome)
   C. Central retinal vein or artery occlusion
   D. Hypotony, including that following intraocular surgery
   E. Inflammatory
      (1) Bird-shot retinochoroidenopathy
      (2) Gumma of nerve head
      (3) Juxtapapillary choroiditis
      (4) Neuroretinitis (see p. 563)
      (5) Retinal vasculitis
      (6) Rocky Mountain spotted fever
      (7) Sarcoidosis
      (8) Tuberculoma of nerve head
      (9) Uveitis
      (10) Vasculitis
   F. Trauma
   G. Tumors
      (1) Glioma
      (2) Hemangioma
      (3) Melanocytoma
      (4) Melanotic sarcoma
      (5) Neurofibromatosis (von Recklinghausen disease)
      (6) Periocular and ocular metastatic tumors
      (7) Secondary carcinoma
      (8) Tuberous sclerosis

6. Orbital cause—usually unilateral, may have exophthalmos
   A. Aneurysm of the ophthalmic artery
   B. Orbital abscess
   C. Rollet syndrome (orbital apex syndrome)
   D. Scaphocephaly syndrome (craniofacial dysostosis)
   E. Sinusitis
   F. Superior orbital fissure syndrome (Rochon–Duvigneaud syndrome)
   G. Trauma
   H. Tumors
      (1) Benign
         a. Cystic adenoma
         b. Dermoid cyst
         c. Osteopetrosis (Albers–Schonberg disease)
         d. Paget disease
      (2) Malignant
         a. Fibrosarcoma
         b. Glioma
         c. Hutchinson–Pepper syndrome
         d. Lacrimal gland
         e. Lymphosarcoma
         f. Myosarcoma

        g. Osteosarcoma

        h. Secondary metastasis and extension from nasopharynx or sinuses

    (3) Orbital invasion by intracranial tumor (e.g., chordoma)

7. Systemic diseases—usually bilateral

  A. Blood dyscrasias

    (1) Iron-deficiency anemias

    (2) Pernicious anemia

    (3) Thrombocytopenic purpura

  B. Carbohydrate metabolisms disorders

    (1) Diabetes mellitus

    (2) ML III

    (3) MPS II (Hunter syndrome)

    (4) MPS VI (Maroteaux–Lamy syndrome)

  C. Cardiopulmonary insufficiency

    (1) Chronic bronchitis

    (2) Congenital heart disease

    (3) Cystic fibrosis of lungs

    (4) Pickwickian syndrome

    (5) Pulmonary emphysema

  D. Collagen diseases

    (1) Polyarteritis nodosa

    (2) PSS (scleroderma)

    (3) Relapsing polychondritis

    (4) SLE

  E. Endocrine

    (1) Addison disease (adrenal cortical insufficiency)

    (2) Diabetes mellitus (Willis disease)

    (3) Hyperparathyroidism

    (4) Hyperthyroidism (Basedow syndrome)

    (5) Hypothyroidism

    (6) Hypocalcemia

    (7) Hypoparathyroidism

    (8) Hypophosphatasia

    (9) Idiopathic hypercalcemia (Drummond syndrome)

    (10) Menses

    (11) Pituitary deficiency

    (12) Pregnancy

    (13) Pseudohypoparathyroidism syndrome

    (14) Suppression of adrenal function from prolonged use of steroids

    (15) Suprarenal–sympathetic syndrome

  F. Giant cell (temporal arteritis)

  G. Hypertension/arteriosclerosis

  H. Infectious (rare usually optic neuritis)

    (1) AIDS

    (2) Anterior poliomyelitis

    (3) Bang disease (brucellosis)

    (4) Chickenpox

    (5) Coccidioidomycosis

    (6) Echinococcosis (hydatid cyst)

  (7) Encephalitis

  (8) Infectious mononucleosis

  (9) Lyme disease (borreliosis, relapsing fever)

  (10) Malaria

  (11) Meningitis

  (12) Mycoplasma pneumoniae

  (13) Parasitic infections (e.g., cysticercosis, cryptococcus)

  (14) Parinaud syndrome (divergence paralysis)

  (15) Pertussis (whooping cough)

  (16) Presumed ocular histoplasmosis

  (17) Psittacosis

  (18) Sandfly fever (Pappataci fever)

  (19) Trichinellosis

  (20) Whipple disease (intestinal lipodystrophy)

 I. Postinfectious

  (1) Guillain-Barré syndrome (acute infectious neuritis)

  (2) Reye syndrome (acute encephalopathy syndrome)

  (3) Subacute sclerosing panencephalitis (Dawson disease)

  (4) Vogt–Koyanagi–Harada syndrome (uveitis–vitiligo–alopecia–poliosis)

 J. Myeloproliferative diseases

  (1) Histiocytosis X (lipoid granuloma)

  (2) Hodgkin disease

  (3) Leukemia

  (4) Multiple myeloma

  (5) Mycosis fungoides (Sézary syndrome)

  (6) Polycythemia vera

 K. Paraproteinemias

  (1) Cryoglobulinemia

  (2) Macroglobulinemia

  (3) Mediterranean fever

  (4) POEMS syndrome (polyneuropathy, organomegaly, endocrinopathy, M protein, and skin changes)

 L. Nutritional diseases

  (1) Beriberi (thiamine deficiency)

  (2) Pellagra (niacin deficiency)

  (3) Plummer–Vinson syndrome (deficiency of vitamin B complex and iron)

  (4) Vitamin B_{12} deficiency

 M. Sarcoidosis (Heerford syndrome, Schaumann syndrome)

8. Trauma

 A. Battered/shaken baby syndrome

 B. Cerebral hemorrhage

 C. Purtscher syndrome

9. Vascular malformations

 A. Arteriovenous fistula

 B. Aneurysms

  (1) Bonnet–Dechaume–Blanc syndrome (neuroretinoangiomatosis)

  (2) Foramen lacerum syndrome (aneurysm of internal carotid artery syndrome)

  (3) Superior vena cava syndrome

 C. Cavernous sinus thrombosis (Foix syndrome)

Brodsky MC, Vaphiades M. Magnetic resonance imaging in pseudotumor cerebri. *Opthalmology* 1998;105: 1686–1693.

Donahue SP. Recurrence of idiopathic intracranial hypertension after weight loss. The carrot craver. *Am J Ophthalmol* 2000;130:850–851.

Fraunfelder FT, Fraunfelder FW. *Drug-induced ocular side effects and drug interactions.* Woburn, MA: Butterworth-Heinemann, 2001.

Miller N, Newman N. *Walsh & Hoyt's clinical neuro-ophthalmology.* Philadelphia: Lippincott Williams & Wilkins, 1999.

Roy FH. *Ocular syndromes and systemic diseases*, 3rd ed. Philadelphia: Lippincott Williams & Wilkins, 2002.

PSEUDOPAPILLEDEMA (MAY BE MISTAKEN FOR SWELLING OF OPTIC NERVE)

1. Arteriovenous aneurysms (racemose aneurysms) of the retina (Wyburn–Mason syndrome)
2. Bergmeister papilla
3. Cervicooculoacousticus syndrome
4. Down syndrome
5. Drusen of optic nerve (see p. 559)
6. Epipapillary membrane and Bergmeister papilla
7. Fuchs coloboma (partial)
8. Hematoma
9. High hyperopia or astigmatism
10. Juvenile diabetes mellitus (Mauriac syndrome)
11. Medullated nerve fibers (opaque nerve fibers)
12. Normal variant
13. Opacities or haziness of the media, especially nuclear sclerosis of the lens
14. Optic neuritis or papillitis (see p. 578)
15. Peripapillary retinal hemangioma
16. Sarcoidosis (Schaumann syndrome)
17. Tilted disc (partial)
18. Tortuosity and anomalous early branching of the retinal vessels
19. Tumors of disc
    A. Gliomas
    B. Meningiomas
    C. Metastatic
    D. Neurinoma
    E. Neurofibroma

Catalano RA, Simon JW. Optic disk elevation in Down's syndrome. *Am J Ophthalmol* 1990;110:28–32.

Perkins ES, Dobree JH. *The differential diagnosis of fundus conditions.* St. Louis: CV Mosby, 1972.

PERIPAPILLARY SUBRETINAL NEOVASCULARIZATION

1. Excessive laser treatment
2. Optic disc drusen
3. Optic nerve coloboma

Unilateral papilledema (swelling of optic disc)

	Hypotony	Acute Glaucoma*	Ocular Inflammation as Sarcoid	Retinoblastoma	Central Retinal Vein Occlusion*	Central Retinal Artery Occlusion*	Ocular Trauma	Orbital Benign Tumor as Paget Disease	Orbital Malignant Tumor as Lacrimal Gland	Orbital Infection as Abscess
History										
1. Common in blacks		U	U					S		
2. Common in females			U	S		R				
3. Common in males		S						U	U	S
4. Common over fourth decade		U			S	U		U		
5. Familial		S		S						
6. Hereditary				S				U		
7. Lacrimation							S	S	S	
8. Ocular pain	U						S		S	U
9. Painless				U						
10. Trauma/surgery	U						U			S
Physical Findings										
1. Anterior/posterior synechiae	S	U	S				S			
2. Associated with neurofibromatosis				R						
3. Blue sclera								R	S	
4. Cataract	S	U	S				U	S		
5. Chemosis of conjunctiva		U							S	U
6. Cherry-red spot of macula						U				
7. Choroidal detachment	U									
8. Choroidal folds	U		S	S					S	S
9. Choroidal rupture							S			
10. Closed anterior chamber angle		U								
11. Cotton-wool spots					S					
12. Cyclodialysis cleft	S									
13. Dacryoadenitis			S							
14. Dacryocystitis			S							
15. Decreased intraocular pressure	U				S		S			
16. Disc pallor				S						
17. Endothelial corneal damage							S			
18. Epithelial corneal edema		U					S			
19. Exophthalmos			S	S			S	S	S	
20. Extraocular muscle paralysis			S	S			S		S	U
21. Folds in Bowman Descemet membrane	U	U								
22. Globe displacement								R	S	
23. Hard exudates					S					
24. Hypermetropia				S						
25. Hyphema							S			
26. Hypopyon			R							
27. Increased intraocular pressure		U	S	S	S	R	S	S		S
28. Involvement of trigeminal nerve									S	S
29. Iridodialysis							S			
30. Keratopathy	U	S								S
31. Macular edema	S				S	S	R			S
32. Macular hemorrhage			R		S		S			
33. Marcus-Gunn pupil				S			S			

Unilateral papilledema (swelling of optic disc) (Continued)

	Hypotony	Acute Glaucoma*	Ocular Inflammation as Sarcoid	Retinoblastoma	Central Retinal Vein Occlusion*	Central Retinal Artery Occlusion*	Ocular Trauma	Orbital Benign Tumor as Paget Disease	Orbital Malignant Tumor as Lacrimal Gland	Orbital Infection as Abscess
Physical Findings										
34. Milky appearance of retina						U	S			
35. Nystagmus				S						
36. Optic neuritis			S							S
37. Orbital mass				U					U	
38. Orbital myositis								R	S	
39. Panophthalmitis									R	
40. Pigmentary iris degeneration	S	U								
41. Pigmentary retinopathy								S	S	
42. Pseudoretinitis pigmentosa								S		
43. Pupil dilated and fixed		U	S			S		S		
44. Recessed chamber angle								S		
45. Retinal detachment			S					S		
46. Retinal folds	U									
47. Retinal hemorrhages			S		U	R	U	S		
48. Retinal microaneurysms					S					
49. Retinal neovascularization					S					
50. Retinal tractional tear								S		
51. Rubeosis iridis					S	R				
52. Scleral rupture								S		
53. Shallow anterior chamber	U	U								
54. Shallow orbits								S		
55. Strabismus				S						
56. Subluxed lens	S							S		
57. Uveitis	S		S	R						S
58. Visual field defects		U			S	U	U	S		
59. Vitreous hemorrhage			S					S		
Laboratory Data										
1. Abnormal glucose tolerance test					S					
2. Biopsy of inferior forniceal follicles			U							
3. Computed tomography of orbit				U				U	S	U
4. Cerebrospinal fluid protein level elevated			U							S
5. Chest roentgenogram			U						S	S
6. Fluorescein angiography	S				U	U	U	S	R	S
7. Lipid profile elevated					S					
8. Orbit roentgenogram			S	U				S	R	S
9. Visual field test		U		S				S		
10. Ultrasonography	S		S	U			U	S	S	S

R = rarely; S = sometimes; and U = usually.

Bilateral papilledema (swelling of optic disc)

	Frontal Lobe Tumor as Meningioma	Temporal Lobe Tumor as Medulloblastoma	Parietal Lobe Tumor as Astrocytoma	Occipital Lobe Tumor as Glioblastoma	Third Ventricle and Sellar Tumor as Craniopharyngioma	Fourth Ventricle and Cerebellum Tumor as Hemangioblastoma	Infection as Meningitis	Pseudotumor Cerebri	Blood Dyscrasias	Hypertension	Cystic Fibrosis	Hyperthyroidism	Diabetes Mellitus	Collagen Disorders as Polyarteritis Nodosa
History														
1. Common in children		U	U		R	U	S		S		U			
2. Common in females	U							U				U		
3. Common in males				U		R	R		S					U
4. Congenital					U						U			
5. Familial										R	S	U	U	
6. Hereditary						R					U			
7. Occurs in blacks								U						
8. Occurs in whites								U			U			
9. Visual hallucinations		S		U										
10. Visual object agnosia				S										
Physical Findings														
1. Associated with neurofibromatosis	S													
2. Cataract													U	S
3. Cotton-wool spots									S	S			S	S
4. Edema of lids/conjunctiva	S											S		S
5. Exophthalmos	S	S	S			S								S
6. Extraocular muscle paralysis	U	S			S	S	S	S	S			S		S
7. Glaucoma						S				S			S	
8. Hypermetropia	S													
9. Infrequent blinking												U		
10. Intraorbital bleeding										U				
11. Keratitis	S					S	S					U		S
12. Lid lag												U		
13. Macular edema									S	S		U		
14. Marcus-Gunn pupil	S				S									
15. Nystagmus	S	S	U		S									S
16. Optic neuritis		S		S	S			U	S		S	R		
17. Opticocilary venous shunts	S													
18. Orbital mass	U					S			U					
19. Orbital myositis				S										
20. Peripheral retinal neovascularization									S				S	
21. Ptosis						S			R					S
22. Retinal angioma						U								
23. Retinal detachment						S			S	S			S	R
24. Retinal hemorrhages									S	S	S		U	
25. Retinal microaneurysms									S	S			U	
26. Venous sheathing									S	R			S	R
27. Retinal vein occlusion										S			S	S
28. Retraction of upper lid												U		
29. Rubeosis iridis													S	
30. Scleritis														S

Bilateral papilledema (swelling of optic disc) (Continued)

	Frontal Lobe Tumor as Meningioma	Temporal Lobe Tumor as Medulloblastoma	Parietal Lobe Tumor as Astrocytoma	Occipital Lobe Tumor as Glioblastoma	Third Ventricle and Sellar Tumor as Craniopharyngioma	Fourth Ventricle and Cerebellum Tumor as Hemangioblastoma	Infection as Meningitis	Pseudotumor Cerebri	Blood Dyscrasias	Hypertension	Cystic Fibrosis	Hyperthyroidism	Diabetes Mellitus	Collagen Disorders as Polyarteritis Nodosa
Physical Findings														
31. Superficial strawberry hemangioma						S								
32. Strabismus						S								
33. Tremor of closed eyelids												U		
34. Uveitis							R		R					S
35. Visual field defects	S	S	U	U	U			U						S
36. Vitreous hemorrhage									S	S			S	
Laboratory Data														
1. Angiography, cerebral	R	R	R	R	R	R		R						
2. Biopsy, muscle														U
3. Blood cell count							U		U					U
4. Blood sugar elevated													U	
5. Bone marrow puncture									U					
6. Computed tomography	U	U	U	U	U	U						U		
7. Cerebral spinal fluid							U	U	U					
8. Chest roentgenogram											U			
9. Fluorescein angiography						S				U			U	
10. Lipid profile										U			S	
11. Sed rate							U							S
12. Ultrasonography, orbit	S					S						U		
13. MRI	U	U	U	U	U	U	S	U	R					

R = rarely; S = sometimes; and U = usually.

4. Presumed histoplasmosis syndrome
5. Presumed sarcoidosis
6. Serpiginous peripapillary choroiditis

Gragoudas ES, Regan CDJ. Peripapillary subretinal neovascularization in presumed sarcoidosis. *Arch Ophthalmol* 1981;99:1194.

Yedavally S, Frank RN. Peripapillary subretinal neovascularization associated with coloboma of the optic nerve. *Arch Ophthalmol* 1993;111:552–553.

PIGMENTED TUMORS OF OPTIC DISC

1. Drusen
2. Bourneville syndrome (tuberous sclerosis)
3. Hemangioma of the disc with hemorrhages and secondary pigmentation
4. Malignant melanoma
5. Melanocytomas
6. Metastases

Apple DJ, et al. Congenital anomalies of the optic disc. *Surv Ophthalmol* 1982;27:3.

PSEUDOGLAUCOMATUS ATROPHY OF OPTIC DISC

This condition involves cupping of the nerve head with optic atrophy and field defects simulating true glaucoma but without ocular hypertension.

1. Arteriosclerosis
2. Congenital anomalies of the optic disc
    A. Branching of vessels behind the lamina so that the individual branches appear at the disc margins
    B. Coloboma within the nerve sheath
    C. Congenital coloboma of the optic disc
    D. Morning-glory anomaly
    E. Oblique insertion of the optic nerve
    F. Traction of the disc with bowing of the scleral crescent
3. Giant cell (temporal) arteritis
4. Optic pit
5. Patients using digitalis
6. Reduced blood supply to optic nerve (e.g., acute hypotension, blood loss [severe] carotid insufficiency, gastrointestinal bleeding, ischemic optic neuropathy, myocardial infarction, pernicious anemia)
7. Schnobel cavernous atrophy
8. Syphilitic optic-nerve atrophy
9. Tumors arising near the chiasm

Jonas JB, et al. Pseudoglaucomatous physiologic large cups. *Am J Ophthalmol* 1989;107:137–144.

Kolker AE, Hetherington J. *Becker-Schaffer's diagnosis and therapy of the glaucomas*, 6th ed. St. Louis: CV Mosby, 1989.

Moore M, et al. Progressive optic nerve cupping and neural rim decrease in a patient with bilateral autosomal dominant optic nerve colobomas. *Am J Opthalmol* 2000;129:517–520.

Vaughan D, et al. *General ophthalmology*, 12th ed. Norwalk, CT: Appleton & Lange, 1989.

TEMPORALLY DISPLACED DISC (DRAGGED DISC)

1. Abnormal tortuous retinal vessels temporally
2. Ectopic macula
3. ROP
4. Temporally displaced vessels

Gow J, Oliver GL. Familial exudative vitreoretinopathy. *Arch Ophthalmol* 1971;86:150–155.

18

Visual-Field Defects

CONTENTS

PSEUDO–VISUAL-FIELD DEFECTS

1. Facial contour
   A. Prominent nose
   B. Bushy, projecting eyebrows
   C. High cheekbones
   D. Ptosis or blepharochalasis
   E. Sunken globes
   F. Fracture of orbit
2. Corneal opacities
3. Lenticular opacities, especially if miotics are used, will depress fields and exaggerate existing scotomas
4. Aphakia without lens or with convex lens; little distortion with contact lens or intraocular lens
5. Dull patient; patient may be mentally defective, have toxemia, arteriosclerosis, cerebral tumor, brain abscess, or increased intracranial pressure
6. Pupillary size
   A. Decrease in miotic field, especially with opacities of ocular media
7. Uncorrected refractive errors—correct for distance testing
8. Head tilting when the head is tilted toward the left shoulder; the right blind spot is elevated; when the head is tilted toward the right shoulder, the right blind spot is lowered

9. Environmental artifacts
   A. Reduction in illumination of screen and test objects magnifies field defect
   B. Variation in size of test object changes field defect
   C. Standard distance of patient from screen
   D. Attention of patient
   E. Technique of examiner
10. Psychologic artifacts
    A. Patient's misunderstanding of test
    B. Tiring of patient by prolonged testing
    C. Malingering—isopters at different distances are inconsistent
    D. Hysteria—spiral field defects may be found
11. Frames of glasses and segments of multifocal lenses
12. Colored contact lenses

Insler MS, et al. Visual field constriction caused by colored contact lenses. *Arch Ophthalmol* 1988;106:1680–1682.

Meyer DR, et al. Evaluating the visual field effects of blepharoptosis using automated static perimetry. *Ophthalmology* 1993;100:651–659.

Pau H. *Differential diagnosis of eye diseases*, 2nd ed. New York: Thieme Medical, 1988.

BILATERAL CENTRAL SCOTOMAS

These are bilateral macular defects with decreased visual acuity; scotomas may be central or centrocecal.

1. Bilateral macular lesions, such as cysts or those due to hemorrhage, edema, degeneration, detachment, hole, or infection (see p. 439)
2. Bilateral optic-nerve lesions
   A. Papilledema with macular edema (see p. 593)
   B. Bipituitary adenoma compressing the prechiasmatic segment of the distal optic nerve
   C. Papillitis (see p. 578)
   D. Retrobulbar neuritis (see p. 578)
3. Diabetes mellitus
4. Familial optic atrophies (see p. 564)
5. Hyperbaric oxygen
6. Migraine—forerunner of visual aurae
*7. Nutritional deficiency, such as thiamine or vitamin B_{12} deficiency
8. Pernicious anemia
9. Occipital cortex lesions
10. Toxic agents
    A. Aromatic aminocompounds and nitrocompounds—aniline, nitrobenzene, trinitrotoluene
    B. Carbon disulfide
    C. Drugs, including:

acetophenazine	aluminum nicotinate (?)	aspirin
acetyldigitoxin	aminosalicylic acid (?)	barbital
adrenal cortex injection	amiodarone	beclomethasone
alcohol	amobarbital	betamethasone
aldosterone	amodiaquine	bromide
alkavervir	antazoline	bromisovalum
allobarbital	aprobarbital	brompheniramine

* = most important

butabarbital
butalbital
butallylonal
butaperazine
butethal
caramiphen (?)
carbinoxamine
carbon dioxide
carbromal
carisoprodol
carphenazine
chloramphenicol
chloroquine
chlorpheniramine
chlorpromazine
chlorpropamide (?)
chlortetracycline
ciprofloxacin
cisplatin
clemastine
clomiphene
cobalt (?)
contraceptives
cortisone
cyclobarbital
danazol
dapiprazole hydrochloride
deferoxamine
demeclocycline
deslanoside
desoxycorticosterone
dexamethasone
dexbrompheniramine
dexchlorpheniramine
diatrizoate meglumine and
　sodium
diazoxide
diethazine
diethylcarbamazine
digitalis
digitoxin
digoxin
dimethindene
diphenhydramine
diphenylpyraline
diphtheria and tetanus
　toxoids absorbed
disulfiram
doxylamine

emetine
epinephrine
ergonovine
ergot
ergotamine
ethambutol
ethchlorvynol
ethopropazine
fludrocortisone
fluorometholone
fluphenazine
fluprednisolone
gitalin
heptabarbital
hexamethonium
hexethal
hexobarbital
hydrocortisone
hydroxychloroquine
ibuprofen
indomethacin (?)
influenza virus vaccine
interleukin 2, 3, and 6
iodide and iodine solutions
　and compounds
iothalamic acid
isoniazid
lanatoside C
lidocaine
lithium carbonate
medrysone
mephobarbital
meprednisone
meprobamate
mesoridazine
methacycline
metharbital
methdilazine
methitural
methohexital
methotrimeprazine
methoxsalen
methyldopa
methylergonovine
methylprednisolone
methysergide
morphine (?)
naproxen
niacinamide (?)

nicotinic acid (?)
nicotinyl alcohol (?)
ofloxacin
opium
oral contraceptives
ouabain
oxygen
oxyphenbutazone
paramethadione
paramethasone
pentobarbital
perazine
pericyazine
perphenazine
phenobarbital
piperacetazine
prednisolone
prednisone
primidone
probarbital
prochlorperazine
promazine
promethazine
propiomazine
quinacrine
quinidine
quinine
radioactive iodides
secobarbital
sodium
sodium salicylate
streptomycin
sulfacetamide
sulfachlorpyridazine
sulfadiazine
sulfadimethoxine
sulfamerazine
sulfameter
sulfamethizole
sulfamethoxazole
sulfamethoxypyridazine
sulfanilamide
sulfaphenazole
sulfisoxazole
talbutal
thiamylal
thiethylperazine
thiopental
thiopropazate

thioproperazine	trichloroethylene	trimethadione
thioridazine	trifluoperazine	vinbarbital
thyroid (?)	triflupromazine	
triamcinolone	trimeprazine	

    D. Ethyl alcohol

    E. Halogenated hydrocarbons—methyl chloride, methyl bromide, iodoform, trichloroethylene

    F. Metals—lead, thallium (inorganic), arsenic

    G. Methyl alcohol

    H. Tobacco

Fraunfelder FT, Fraunfelder FW. *Drug-induced ocular side effects.* Woburn, MA: Butterworth-Heinemann, 2001.

Harrington DO, Drake MV. *The visual fields: text and atlas of clinical perimetry,* 6th ed. St. Louis: CV Mosby, 1990.

Karanjia N, Dacobson DM. Compression of the prechiasmatic optic nerve produces a junctional scotoma. *Am J Ophthalmol* 1999;128,2:256–258.

ENLARGEMENT OF BLIND SPOT

    1. Blind spot syndrome (multiple evanescent white-dot syndrome [MEWS])

    2. Coloboma of the optic nerve

    3. Drugs, including the following:

adrenal cortex injection	ergot	oxytetracycline
aldosterone	fludrocortisone	paramethasone
betamethasone	fluorometholone	prednisolone
carbon dioxide	fluprednisolone	prednisone
chlortetracycline	hydrocortisone	quinacrine
cortisone	indomethacin (?)	tetracycline
demeclocycline	medrysone	triamcinolone
desoxycorticosterone	methacycline	trichloroethylene
dexamethasone	methylprednisolone	vigabatrin
doxycycline	minocycline	vitamin A

    3. Drusen of the optic nerve (see p. 559)

    4. Glaucoma

    5. Inferior conus

    6. Inverted disc or nasally directed scleral canal

    7. Juxtapapillary choroiditis

    8. Medullated nerve fibers

    9. Multifocal choroiditis

    10. Multifocal evanescent white-dot syndrome

*11. Papilledema (pseudotumor cerebri) (see p. 593)

    12. Papillitis (see p. 578)

    13. Progressive myopia with a temporal crescent

    14. Senility—senile halo

    15. High-resistance instrument players

Fraunfelder FT, Fraunfelder FW. *Drug-induced ocular side effects.* Woburn, MA: Butterworth-Heinemann, 2001.

Poinoosawmy D, et al. Frequency of asymmetric visual field defects in normal tension and high tension glaucoma. *Ophthalmology* 1998;105:988–991.

* = most important

Rebolleda G, et al. Screening of patients taking Vigabatrin. *Ophthalmology* 2000;107:1219–1220.

Singh K, et al. Acute idiopathic blind spot enlargement. *Ophthalmology* 1991;98:497–502.

ARCUATE (CUNEATE) SCOTOMA

In this condition, scotoma follows the lines of the nerve fibers in the retina with the narrow end at the blind spot and broad end at horizontal raphe.

1. Acute bleeding episode
2. Branch artery occlusion
3. Branch vein occlusion
4. Chorioretinitis juxtapapillaris
5. Coloboma of the disc
6. Drusen of optic nerve
*7. Glaucoma
8. High myopia
9. Inferior conus
10. Ischemic optic neuropathy
11. Myelinated nerve fibers

Greve EL, Verriest G. *Fourth International Visual Field Symposium*. The Hague, Netherlands, 1981.

Harrington DO, Drake MV. *The visual fields: text and atlas of clinical perimetry*, 6th ed. St. Louis: CV Mosby, 1990.

UNILATERAL SECTOR-SHAPED DEFECTS

In this condition, the narrow end of scotoma characteristically touches the physiologic blind spot.

1. Optic disc involvement
   A. Glaucoma (early stages primarily on nasal side)
   B. Papillitis
   C. Secondary optic atrophy after choked disc (more on nasal side)
2. Retina
   A. Branch artery occlusion (see p. 468–472)
   B. Juxtapapillary chorioretinitis
3. Optic nerve—between disc and chiasm
   A. Aneurysm
   B. Drusen
   C. Tumor

Hart WM, Becker B. The onset and evolution of glaucomatous visual field defects. *Ophthalmology* 1982;89:268.

Spekreijse H, Apkarian PA. *Visual pathways*. The Hague, Netherlands: Dr. Junk, 1981.

PERIPHERAL-FIELD CONTRACTION

Central vision is present; the patient may complain of poor night vision.

1. Choroiditis—periphery of fundus
*2. Chronic atrophic papilledema (pseudotumor cerebri)
3. Bilateral homonymous hemianopia (if the macular sparing in one homonymous hemia-

nopia is larger than that in the other homonymous hemianopia, the spared central portion of the field has small vertical steps, above and below fixation, where the two areas of macular sparing do not quite coincide.)

  A. Cortical blindness with damage to occipital lobe and macular recovery
    (1) Anoxia
    (2) Carbon monoxide poisoning
    (3) Cardiac arrest
    (4) Cerebral angiography
    (5) Exsanguination
    (6) Trauma
  B. Stroke of infarction of occipital lobe
  4. Drugs, including the following:

acetophenazine
acridine
alcohol
allobarbital
amobarbital
amodiaquine
aprobarbital
arsenic
aspirin
barbital
bromisovalum
butalbital
butallylonal
butaperazine
butethal
carbon dioxide
carbon monoxide
carbromal
carisoprodol
carphenazine
chloramphenicol
chloroquine
chlorpromazine
chlorpropamide (?)
clomiphene
cobalt
cortisone

cyclobarbital
deslanoside
desoxycorticosterone
dexamethasone
diethazine
digitalis
digoxin
disulfiram
emetine
epinephrine
ergot
ethambutol
ethchlorvynol
ethopropazine
ethylhydrocupreine
filax mas
fludrocortisone
fluorometholone
fluphenazine
fluprednisolone
gitalin
heptabarbital
hexamethonium
hexethal
hexobarbital
hydrocortisone
hydroxychloroquine

ibuprofen
indomethacin
iodide and iodine solutions
  and compounds
isoniazid
lanatoside C
lithium carbonate
medrysone
mephobarbital
mesoridazine
metharbital
methdilazine
methitural
methohexital
methotrimeprazine
methylprednisolone
methysergide
morphine (?)
niacinamide (?)
nicotinic acid (?)
nicotinyl alcohol (?)
opium
oral contraceptives
ouabain
oxygen
paramethadione
pomas

  5. Drusen of optic disc
  6. Frontal-lobe tumors
  7. General apathy in a lackadaisical subject
 *8. Glaucoma
  9. Hysteria and malingering
 10. Many conditions in which night blindness occurs (see p. 656)
 11. Optic atrophy (see p. 564)
 12. Papillitis (see p. 578)
 13. Post vitrectomy with fluid–air exchange

* = most important

14. Retinitis—periphery of fundus
15. Retinitis pigmentosa
16. Unilateral concentric constriction, excluding diseased retina or glaucoma, suggests lesion of optic nerve and chiasm
    A. Meningioma of tuberculum sellae, sphenoid ridge, or the olfactory groove
    B. Tumor of optic nerve

Fraunfelder FT, Fraunfelder FW. *Drug-induced ocular side effects and drug interactions.* Woburn, MA: Butterworth-Heinemann, 2001.

Grover S, et al. Patterns of visual field progression in patients with retinitis pigmentosa. *Ophthalmology* 1998;105: 1060–1075.

Harrington DO, Drake MV. *The visual fields: text and atlas of clinical perimetry*, 6th ed. St. Louis: CV Mosby, 1990.

Kokame GT. Visual field defects after vitrectomy with fluid-air exchange. *Am J Ophthalmol* 2000;129:653–654.

ALTITUDINAL HEMIANOPIA

This condition comprises defective vision or blindness in the upper or lower horizontal half of the visual field. It may be unilateral or bilateral; unilateral field defect is prechiasmal.

1. Anemia—produces bilateral inferior altitudinal hemianopia
*2. Anterior ischemic optic neuropathy
3. Bilateral branch retinal artery occlusion
4. Fusiform aneurysms (arteriosclerotic or congenital)—may produce inferior altitudinal hemianopia by pressure against the lateral halves of the optic chiasm or nerve
5. Herpes zoster
6. Lesion that presses the chiasm upward against the superior margin of the optic foramen
7. Occipital lobe lesions
    A. Hypoxia
    B. Stroke
8. Olfactory groove meningioma extending posteroinferior to compress the intracranial portion of the optic nerve
9. Optic-nerve lesion
    A. Anterior ischemia optic neuropathy
    B. Coloboma
    C. Glaucoma
    D. Optic neuritis
    E. Papilledema
    *F. Trauma
    G. Tumor
10. Sclerotic plaques of internal carotid artery or anterior cerebral arteries—pressure of plaques on optic nerve results in inferior altitudinal hemianopia
11. Following pars plana vitrectomy

Harrington DO, Drake MV. *The visual fields: a text and atlas of clinical perimetry*, 6th ed. St. Louis: CV Mosby, 1990.

Miyashita K, et al. Superior altitudinal hemianopia and herpes zoster. *Ann Ophthalmol* 1993;25:20–23.

BINASAL HEMIANOPIA

This condition comprises defects in the nasal half of visual fields, usually incomplete. This condition is due to lateral involvement of chiasm; it presupposes bilateral lesions.

1. Bilateral occipital lesion (thrombosis)
2. Chiasmic arachnoiditis, postneuritic optic atrophy, and bilateral retrobulbar neuritis of multiple sclerosis
3. Damage to chiasm
4. Drusen of optic nerve (see p. 559)
5. Fusiform aneurysms—arteriosclerotic or congenital—of internal carotid artery
6. Glaucoma
7. Meningiomas, especially from the lesser wing of the sphenoid bone
8. Nasal quadrant peripheral depression of glaucoma—bilateral and reasonably symmetrical
9. Pituitary tumor with third ventricle dilatation pushing laterally
10. Retinal damage
11. Severe exsanguination
12. Sclerotic plaques of internal carotid artery or anterior cerebral arteries
13. Symmetric lesions in the temporal halves of both retinas, such as severe retinal edema associated with diabetic retinopathy
14. Trauma

Cox TA, et al. Unilateral nasal hemianopia as a sign of intracranial optic nerve compression. *Am J Ophthalmol* 1981;92:230–232.

Harrington DO, Drake MV. *The visual fields: text and atlas of clinical perimetry*, 6th ed. St. Louis: CV Mosby, 1990.

Pau H. *Differential diagnosis of eye diseases*, 2nd ed. New York: Thieme Medical, 1988.

BITEMPORAL HEMIANOPIA

This condition involves defects in the temporal half of the visual field, usually incomplete; it is due to pressure on the optic chiasm.

1. Chiasmal lesions
    A. Congenital defect such as de Morsier syndrome (septooptic dysplasia); autosomal dominant
    B. Inflammatory lesions
        *(1) Basal meningitis, including: chronic chiasmal syphilitic, tuberculous, actinomycotic, and cysticercal arachnoiditis
        (2) Chiasmal neuritis
    C. Tumors of the chiasm
        *(1) Primary tumors, including gliomas in childhood
        *(2) Secondary tumors (rare), including meningiomas, retinoblastoma, pinealoma, and ependymoma
    D. Vascular lesions
        (1) Arterial compression
        (2) Arteriosclerosis
        (3) Ectasia of the intracranial carotid arteries
        *(4) Intracranial aneurysms, such as congenital, endocardial emboli, traumatic, atheromatous, or syphilitic, especially intrasellar aneurysms
        (5) Thrombosis of the carotid artery
2. Perisellar lesions
    A. Parasellar tumors
        (1) Injuries to the chiasmal pathway, such as from trauma
        *(2) Meningioma of the sphenoid ridge

* = most important

    (3) Migraine
    (4) Sudden onset without apparent cause
        a. Arteriosclerotic or giant cell arteritic occlusion of nutrient vessels of the chiasm in older patients
        b. Disseminated sclerosis
    (5) Tumors of the basal meninges
    (6) Tumors of the sphenoid bone including osteochondroma, sarcoma, anaplastic carcinoma

  B. Presellar tumors
    *(1) Meningioma of the olfactory groove
    (2) Neuroblastoma of the olfactory groove

  C. Suprasellar tumors
    (1) Chordoma
    *(2) Craniopharyngioma—manifestations may include diabetes insipidus, infantilism, and calcification of hypophyseal-pituitary region
    (3) Epidermoids
    (4) Lymphoblastoma
    (5) Pinealoma
    *(6) Suprasellar meningioma
    (7) Teratoma
    (8) Tumors of the frontal lobe, including porencephaly (cystic cavity in brain substance) and glioma
    (9) Tumors of the third ventricle and internal hydrocephalus, such as glioma and epidymoma

3. Pituitary lesions
  A. Pituitary hyperplasia
  B. Pituitary tumors
    (1) Adenoma
        a. Acidophilic adenoma—varies from gigantism to acromegaly
        b. Basophilic adenoma—hyperadrenalism (Cushing disease), Nelson syndrome
        c. Chromophobe adenoma—varies from no endocrine symptoms to panhypopituitarism; most common type of pituitary tumor, Fröhlich syndrome
    (2) Adenocarcinoma (rare)
    (3) Metastatic tumors as from breast (rare)

Kerrison JB, Lee AG. Acute loss of vision during pregnancy due to a suprasellar mass. *Surv Ophthalmol* 1997;41: 400–401.

Pomerantz HD, Lessell S. A hereditary chiasmal optic neuropathy. *Arch Ophthalmol* 1999;117:128–131.

Roy FH. *Ocular syndromes and systemic diseases*, 3rd ed. Philadelphia: Lippincott Williams & Wilkins, 2002.

HOMONYMOUS QUADRANTANOPIA

In this condition, one quadrant is involved in upper or lower and right or left visual fields; etiology may include tumor, vascular lesion, or infection.

1. Superior homonymous quadrantanopia
  A. Inferior lip of the calcarine fissure—congruous
  B. Temporal lobe—incongruous
2. Inferior homonymous quadrantanopia
  A. Anton syndrome (denial—visual hallucination)

B. Superior radiation in parietal lobe—incongruous

C. Upper lip of the calcarine fissure in the occipital lobe—congruous

Bosley TM, et al. Neuro-imaging and positron emission tomography of congenital homonymous hemianopsia. *Am J Ophthalmol* 1991;111:413–418.

Harrington DO, Drake MV. *The visual fields: textbook and atlas of clinical perimetry*, 6th ed. St. Louis: CV Mosby, 1990.

CROSSED QUADRANTANOPIA

In this condition, the upper quadrant of one visual field is along with the lower quadrant of opposite visual field.

*1. Asymmetric homonymous hemianopia, such as vascular lesion of the upper lip of the calcarine area on one side and the lower lip of the opposite calcarine cortex

2. Chiasm compression from lesion below compressing it against contiguous arterial structure

3. Glaucoma

4. Inflammatory lesion, such as choroiditis juxtapapillaris

Harrington DO, Drake MV. *The visual fields: text and atlas of clinical perimetry*, 6th ed. St. Louis: CV Mosby, 1990.

HOMONYMOUS HEMIANOPIA

This type of hemianopia affects the right or left halves of the visual fields; the lesion is posterior to the optic chiasm,

1. Optic tract lesions—visual conduction system posterior to optic chiasm and anterior to lateral geniculate body; lesion demonstrates incongruous field defect on side opposite to defect, often with decreased vision, optic atrophy and afferent pupil.
   A. Demyelinative disease—retrobulbar, multiple sclerosis, and Schilder disease
   B. Migraine
   C. Pituitary adenomas and craniopharyngiomas (most common); nasopharyngeal carcinomas, chordomas, infundibulomas, and gliomas (less common)
   D. Saccular aneurysms of internal carotid or posterior communicating artery
   E. Trauma
2. Temporoparietal lesions—temporal lobe lesions are manifest initially in the upper visual fields, whereas lesions of the parietal lobe are first manifest in the lower visual fields
   A. Diffuse demyelinative diseases
      (1) Krabbe type (Sturge–Weber–Krabbe syndrome)
      (2) Metachromatic leukoencephalopathy
      (3) Pelizaeus–Merzbacher type (aplasia axialis extracorticalis congenita)
      (4) Progressive multifocal leukoencephalopathy
      (5) Schilder type (encephalitis periaxialis diffusa)
      (6) Spongy degeneration of the brain (Canavan disease)
   B. Migraine
   C. Tumor—gradual onset of symptoms—lesions include intrinsic astrocytoma and glioblastoma, extrinsic meningioma, and lung metastasis
   D. Vascular lesions—sudden onset
      (1) Embolism—may be associated with rheumatic or arteriosclerotic heart disease, bacterial endocarditis, myocardial infarction, or septic focus in lungs

* = most important

    (2) Occlusion—middle cerebral occlusion affects primarily the arm and face; anterior cerebral occlusion affects primarily the leg

    (3) Subdural hematoma—spontaneous or following trauma

    (4) Thrombosis—premonitory symptoms include unilateral blackouts in one eye

  E. Trauma (surgical)

3. Occipital lesions—congruous field defect and macular sparing most likely

  A. Demyelinative disease

    (1) Creutzfeldt–Jakob disease

    (2) Krabbe type (Sturge–Weber–Krabbe syndrome)

    (3) Metachromatic leukoencephalopathy

    (4) Pelizaeus–Merzbacher type (aplasia axialis extracorticalis congenita)

    (5) Progressive multifocal leukoencephalopathy

    (6) Schilder type (encephalitis periaxialis diffusa)

    (7) Spongy degeneration of the brain (Canavan disease)

  B. Migraine

  C. Poisons, such as carbon monoxide, digitalis, mescal, opium, lysergic acid diethylamide

  D. Trauma

    (1) Direct—penetrating missiles and depressed bone fragments

    (2) Indirect—general concussion syndrome

    (3) Temporal lobectomy

  E. Tumors—gradual onset of symptoms—lesions include intrinsic astrocytoma and glioblastoma, extrinsic meningioma, and lung metastasis

  F. Vascular lesion—sudden onset

    (1) Arteriovenous anomalies

    (2) Aneurysms (rare)

    (3) Occlusion of posterior cerebral artery—thrombotic or embolic

    (4) Subclavian steal syndrome, with reversal of blood flow through the vertebral artery

Harrington DO, Drake MV. *The visual fields: text and atlas of clinical perimetry*, 6th ed. St. Louis: CV Mosby, 1990.

Roy FH. *Ocular syndromes and systemic diseases*, 3rd ed. Philadelphia: Lippincott Williams & Wilkins, 2002.

Vargas ME, et al. Homonymous field defect as the first manifestation of Creutzfeldt-Jakob disease. *Am J Ophthalmol* 1995;119:497–504.

SPIRAL-FIELD DEFECTS

*1. Hysteria

2. Radiation therapy in or about the retina, optic nerve, and anterior visual pathways

Fitzgerald CR, et al. Radiation therapy in and about the retina, optic nerve, and anterior visual pathway. *Arch Ophthalmol* 1981;99:611–623.

DOUBLE HOMONYMOUS HEMIANOPIA

This condition involves peripheral constriction with small vertical steps above and below fixation as a result of lesions of the occipital area and probable involvement of striate cortex of both occipital lobes.

1. Bilateral central retinal artery occlusion

2. Bilateral central retinal vein occlusion

* = most important

3. Bilateral vascular lesions involving a calcarine fissure
4. Increased intracranial pressure with shift of uncal portion of temporal lobe down over edge of tentorium with compression of posterior cerebral arteries and infarction in calcarine cortex.
5. Partial recovery from cortical blindness (see p. 632) from trauma, anoxia, carbon monoxide poisoning, cerebral angiography, cardiac arrest, exsanguination, and other similar conditions
6. Severe end-stage glaucoma
7. Severe trauma with massive brain damage as in depressed fracture of occiput

Harrington DO, Drake MV. *The visual fields: text and atlas of clinical perimetry*, 6th ed. St. Louis: CV Mosby, 1990.

PART II

General Signs and Symptoms

19

Visual Disturbance

CONTENTS

ACQUIRED MYOPIA*

This condition comprises an error of refraction in which parallel rays of light focus in front of the retina, usually producing blurred distant vision and clear near vision.

*1. Conditions such as diabetes mellitus or nuclear sclerotic cataract in which there is increased index of refraction of lens
*2. Refractive myopia—increased curvature of the refracting surfaces because of the following:
   A. Ciliary muscle spasm
      (1) Functional—adolescence, hysteria
      (2) Miotics such as carbachol, demecarium, echothiophate, isoflurophate, neostigmine, and physostigmine
      (3) Trauma—ocular contusion or anterior dislocation of the lens
      (4) Mushroom (*Amanita muscaria*) poisoning

619   * = most important

B. Lens hydration changes—diabetes mellitus, dysentery, or toxemia of pregnancy

C. Drug reaction—probably because of ciliary body edema, including the following:

acetazolamide
acetophenazine
adrenal cortex injection
alcohol
aldosterone
aspirin
beclomethasone
bendroflumethiazide
benzthiazide
betamethasone
betaxolol
butaperazine
carbachol
carphenazine
chlorothiazide
chlorpromazine
chlortetracycline
chlorthalidone
cimetidine (?)
clofibrate
codeine
cortisone
cyclothiazide
demecarium
demeclocycline
desoxycorticosterone
dexamethasone
dichlorphenamide
diethazine
digitalis (?)
doxycycline
droperidol (?)
echothiophate
ethopropazine
ethosuximide
ethoxzolamide
etretinate
fludrocortisone
fluorometholone
fluphenazine
fluprednisolone
glibenclamide

haloperidol (?)
hyaluronidase
hyaluronic acid
hydrochlorothiazide
hydrocortisone
hydroflumethiazide
hydroxypropyl
ibuprofen
indapamide
isoflurophate
isosorbide dinitrate
isotretinoin
levobunolol
medrysone
meprednisone
mesoridazine
methacholine
methacycline
methazolamide
methdilazine
methotrimeprazine
methsuximide
methyclothiazide
methylcellulose
methylprednisolone
metolazone
minocycline
morphine
neostigmine
opium
oral contraceptives
oxygen
oxytetracycline
paramethasone
penicillamine
perazine
pericyazine
perphenazine
phenformin
phensuximide
physostigmine
pilocarpine

piperacetazine
polythiazide
prednisolone
prednisone
prochlorperazine
promazine
promethazine
propiomazine
quinethazone
quinine
sodium salicylate
spironolactone
sulfacetamide
sulfachlorpyridazine
sulfacytine
sulfadiazine
sulfadimethoxine
sulfamerazine
sulfameter
sulfamethazine
sulfamethizole
sulfamethoxazole
sulfamethoxypyridazine
sulfanilamide
sulfaphenazole
sulfapyridine
sulfasalazine
sulfathiazole
sulfisoxazole
tetracycline
thiethylperazine
thiopropazate
thioproperazine
thioridazine
timolol
triamcinolone
trichlormethiazide
trifluoperazine
trifluperidol (?)
triflupromazine
trimeprazine

    D. Elongated globe

    E. Paralysis of accommodation for distance (sympathetic paralysis)—young patient with unilateral Homer syndrome or migraine

    F. Retinopathy of prematurity (retrolental fibroplasia)

    G. Congenital glaucoma

    H. Albinism

    I. Gyrate atrophy (ornithine ketoacid aminotransferase deficiency)

    J. Hypoparathyroidism

    K. Malaria

    L. Inherited

        (1) Cochlear deafness with myopia and intellectual impairment—autosomal recessive

        (2) Epiphyseal dysplasia of femoral heads, myopia, deafness—autosomal recessive

        (3) Epiphyseal dysplasia, multiple, with myopia and conductive deafness—autosomal dominant

        (4) Microcornea and cataract—autosomal dominant

        (5) Microphthalmos with myopia and corectopia—autosomal dominant

        (6) Myopia—autosomal recessive or dominant or less often X-linked

        (7) Night blindness, congenital stationary with myopia (nyctalopia–myopia)—X-linked

        (8) Night blindness with high-grade myopia—autosomal recessive

        (9) Pinguecula blindness (total color blindness with myopia, achromatopsia with myopia)—autosomal recessive

    M. With scleral buckling surgery

3. Syndromes associated with myopia

    A. Aberfeld syndrome (congenital blepharophimosis)

    B. Achard syndrome (Marfan syndrome with mandibulofacial dysostosis)

    C. Alport syndrome (hereditary familial congenital hemorrhagic nephritis)

    D. Bloch–Sulzberger syndrome

    E. Chromosome partial deletion (long-arm) syndrome

    F. Cohen syndrome

    G. Cri-du-chat syndrome

    H. de Lange syndrome (congenital muscular hypertrophy cerebral syndrome)

    I. Down syndrome (trisomy syndrome)

    J. Ehlers–Danlos syndrome (fibrodysplasia elastica generalisata)

    K. Fetal alcohol syndrome

    L. Forsius–Eriksson syndrome (Aland disease)

    M. Gansslen syndrome (familial hemolytic icterus)

    N. Haney–Falls syndrome (congenital keratoconus posticus circumscriptus)

    O. Homocystinuria

    P. Hypomelanosis of Ito syndrome

    Q. Kartagener syndrome (sinusitis, bronchiectasis, situs inversus syndrome)

    R. Kniest syndrome

    S. Laurence–Moon–Bardet–Biedl syndrome (retinitis pigmentosa–polydactyly–adiposogenital syndrome)

    T. Marchesani syndrome (brachymorphy with spherophakia)

    U. Marfan syndrome (arachnodactyly dystrophia mesodermalis congenita)

V. Marshall syndrome (atypical ectodermal dysplasia)

W. Matsoukas syndrome (oculocerebroarticuloskeletal syndrome)

X. Myasthenia gravis (Erb–Goldflam syndrome)

Y. Noonan syndrome (male Turner syndrome)

Z. Obesity-cerebral-ocular-skeletal anomalies syndrome

AA. Oculodental syndrome (Peter syndrome)

BB. Pierre Robin syndrome (micrognathia–glossoptosis syndrome)

CC. Pigmentary ocular dispersion syndrome

DD. Rubinstein–Taybi syndrome (broad-thumbs syndrome)

EE. SED congenita (spondyloepiphyseal dysplasia, congenital type)—autosomal dominant

FF. Scheie syndrome

GG. Schwartz syndrome (glaucoma associated with retinal detachment)

HH. Siemens syndrome (hereditary ectodermal dysplasia syndrome)—autosomal recessive

II. Smith–Magenis syndrome

JJ. Stickler syndrome (hereditary progressive arthroophthalmopathy)—autosomal dominant

KK. Trisomy 20p syndrome

LL. Trisomy syndrome

MM. Tuomaala–Haapanen syndrome (unknown etiology, similar to pseudohypoparathyroidism)

NN. Van Bogaert–Hozoy syndrome (similar to Rubinstein–Taybi syndrome)

OO. Wagner syndrome (hyaloideoretinal degeneration)

PP. Weill–Marchesani syndrome (brachymorphy with spherophakia)

QQ. Wrinkly-skin syndrome

RR. XXXXY syndrome (hypogenitalism, limited elbow pronation, low dermal finger tip ridge count)

4. Transient myopia

A. Chemical agents and disease

*B. Diabetes

*C. After surgery

D. Trauma

Chow DR, et al. Refractive changes associated with scleral buckling and division in retinopathy of prematurity. *Arch Ophthalmol* 1998;116:1446–1450.

Finucane BM, Jaeger ER. Smith-Magenis syndrome. *Ophthalmology* 1997;104:732–733.

Fraunfelder FT, Fraunfelder FW. *Drug-induced ocular side effects.* Woburn, MA: Butterworth-Heinemann, 2001.

McKusick VA. *Mendelian inheritance in man*, 12th ed. Baltimore: Johns Hopkins University Press, 1998.

Roy FH. *Ocular syndromes and systemic diseases*, 3rd ed. Philadelphia: Lippincott Williams & Wilkins, 2002.

Sorenson AL, et al. Ultrasonographic measurement of induced myopia associated with capsular bag distention syndrome. *Ophthalmology* 2000;107:902–908.

ACQUIRED HYPEROPIA

This condition comprises far-sightedness and error of refraction in which parallel rays of light focus behind the retina, usually producing clear distant vision and blurred near vision.

1. Aarskog syndrome (facial–digital–genital syndrome)

2. Adie syndrome (tonic pupil)

*3. Aphakia
4. Best syndrome (vitelliform dystrophy)
*5. Diabetes mellitus (poorly controlled to controlled)
6. Down syndrome (mongolism)
7. Drugs, including the following:

antihistamines	sulfachlorpyridazine (?)	sulfanilamide (?)
cannabis	sulfadiazine (?)	sulfaphenazole (?)
chloroquine	sulfadimethoxine (?)	sulfapyridine (?)
ergot	sulfamerazine	sulfasalazine (?)
imipramine	sulfameter (?)	sulfathiazole (?)
meprobamate	sulfamethazine	sulfisoxazole (?)
parasympatholytic drugs	sulfamethizole	tolbutamide (?)
penicillamine	sulfamethoxazole	
phenothiazine	sulfamethoxypyridazine (?)	

8. Flat cornea
9. Gorlin–Chaudhry–Moss syndrome (multiple basal cell nevi syndrome)
*10. Hyperopia—refractive or axial
11. Hypoglycemia
12. Kenny syndrome (nanophthalmos with hyperopia)
13. Leber congenital amaurosis
14. Lesions causing internal ophthalmoplegia with paralysis of accommodation
15. Macular edema
16. Orbital tumor with extraocular globe pressure and retinal striae
17. Postsurgical correction of myopia (retinal keratotomy, automated lamella keratoplasty, photoreactive keratectomy)
*18. Presbyopia
19. Rubinstein–Taybi syndrome
20. Sorsby syndrome (hereditary macular coloboma syndrome)
20. Toxin of *Clostridium botulinum*
21. Trauma to the eye with posterior dislocation of the lens, macular edema, or ciliary body contusion

Fraunfelder FT, Fraunfelder FW. *Drug-induced ocular side effects.* Woburn, MA: Butterworth-Heinemann, 2001.

John ME. High hyperopia after radial keratotomy. *J Cataract Refract Surg* 1993;19:446–448.

Newell FW. *Ophthalmology: principles and concepts,* 8th ed. St. Louis: CV Mosby, 1992.

Roy FH. *Ocular syndromes and systemic diseases,* 3rd ed. Philadelphia: Lippincott Williams & Wilkins, 2002.

DYSMEGALOPSIA—OPTICAL ILLUSIONS OF SIZE

1. Macropsia (objects appear larger)
   *A. Miotics
   *B. Spasm of accommodation (see p. 416–417)
   C. Use of excessive plus lenses
2. Metamorphopsia (objects appear distorted)
   A. Cerebral
      (1) Drug intoxications
      (2) Epilepsy
      (3) Focal lesions such as thrombosis of right middle cerebral artery

* = most important

*(4) Migraine
(5) Parietal lobe lesion, including tumor and vascular lesion
(6) Schizophrenia
B. Hysteria
C. Ocular
(1) Astigmatism
*(2) Macular lesions, including orbital tumor with macular striae and macular edema, inflammation, heterotopia or hole
(3) Posterior vitreous separation and residual vitreoretinal macular traction
(4) Retinal detachment
D. Paget disease (osteitis deformans)
3. Micropsia (objects appear smaller)
A. Accommodative paralysis and subnormal accommodation
B. Atropinization
C. Botulism
D. Diphtheria
*E. Presbyopia
F. Use of excessive minus lenses
G. Use of scopolamine
4. Teleopsia (objects appear farther away than they actually are)
A. Bilateral parietal lesion
B. Parietal lesion in nondominant hemisphere

Pau H. *Differential diagnosis of eye diseases*, 2nd ed. New York: Thieme Medical, 1988.

Saito Y, et al. The visual performance and metamorphopsia of patients with macular holes. *Arch Ophthalmol* 2000; 118:41–44.

Walsh FB, Hoyt WF. *Clinical neuro-ophthalmology*, vol 1, 4th ed. Baltimore: Williams & Wilkins, 1985.

BILATERAL TRANSIENT LOSS OF VISION (TRANSIENT DARKENING OF VISION)

*1. Circulatory disturbances when bending over or straining (postural hypotension)
2. Essential hypotension
A. Arteriosclerosis
B. Chronic hypotension
*C. Fatigue
D. Hormonal disorders
E. Hunger
F. Vitamin deficiency
3. Fainting with vasomotor collapse
4. Heart failure
5. Transurethral resection of the prostate

Creel DJ, et al. Transient blindness associated with transurethral resection of the prostate. *Arch Ophthalmol* 1987; 105:1537–1539.

Levin LA, Moohta V. Postprandial transient visual loss. *Ophthalmology* 1997;104:397–401.

Pau H. *Differential diagnosis of eye diseases*, 2nd ed. New York: Thieme Medical, 1988.

AMAUROSIS FUGAX (TRANSIENT MONOCULAR BLACKOUT OF VISION)

1. Amaurosis fugax syndrome

2. Arteriosclerosis, hypertension, and hypertensive crisis
3. Canalis opticus syndrome: functional—hysteria, neurasthenia
*4. Cerebrovascular insufficiency
    A. Arterial aneurysms
    B. Congenital or acquired arteriovenous malformations
    C. Fibromuscular hyperplasia
    D. Post-traumatic acute and chronic arterial occlusion
    E. Takayasu syndrome (pulseless disease)
    *F. Unilateral occlusive carotid disease
5. Compressive optic neuropathy
6. Corneal surface problems
7. Functional—hysteria, neurasthenia
8. Hematologic causes
    A. Emboli
        (1) Infective, such as subacute bacterial endocarditis
        (2) Gas in dysbarism
    B. Idiopathic thrombocytosis
    C. Multiple myeloma (Kahler disease)
    D. Polycythemia (Vaquez disease)
    E. Severe anemia
    F. Sickle cell disease (Herrick syndrome)
9. Hypotension of fundus
    A. Cardiac arrhythmia
    B. Glaucoma, narrow angle, pigment dispersion
    C. Gaze-evoked amaurosis (transient monocular loss of vision occurring in a particular direction of eccentric gaze)
        *(1) Bone fragment adjacent to optic nerve following orbital fracture
        *(2) Central retinal artery occlusion
        (3) Optic nerve sheath meningiomas
        (4) Orbital cavernous hemangiomas
        (5) Orbital osteoma
    B. Impending vascular occlusion, retinal vasospasm associated with systemic vasospastic disease (migraine)
    C. Increased intracranial pressure, such as from intracranial tumors that interfere with vascular supply to the optic nerve
    D. Increased venous pressure
        (1) Impending central retinal vein occlusion (see p. 468–472)
        (2) Intermittent elevation of intraocular pressure (glaucoma)
    E. Negative G-force in pilots—circular maneuver with head toward the center of the circle
    F. Ocular ischemic syndrome
    G. Orbital vascular insufficiency with giant cell arteritis
    H. Papilledema—lasts for to seconds (see p. 593)
    I. Positive G-force in pilots—circular maneuver with feet toward center of circle
    J. Vasospasm including temporal arteritis, polyarteritis nodosa, eosinophilic vasculitis, migraine and cluster headache
10. Large vitreous floater
11. Optic disc anomalies (congenital)
12. Ornithine transcarbamoylase deficiency

* = most important

13. Pituitary tumor
14. Polymyalgia rheumatica
15. Quinine poisoning
16. Raynaud disease (paroxysmal digital cyanosis)
17. Retrobulbar anesthesia
18. Schleral buckling procedure
19. Spontaneous bleeding from a normal-appearing iris or intraocular lens iris touch
20. Taveras syndrome (progressive intracranial arterial occlusion syndrome)
21. Uhthoff symptom—vision decreased with exercise or ocular hyperthermia can occur with:
    A. Friedreich ataxia
    B. Insufficiency of posterior cerebral arteries
    C. Intrasellar and parasellar tumor
    D. Multiple sclerosis (disseminated sclerosis)
22. Uremic amaurosis—with eclampsia
23. Vasospasm
24. Wasp sting

Bernard GA, et al. Vasospastic amaurosis fugax. *Arch Ophthalmol* 1999;117:1568.

Fineman MS, et al. Transient visual loss and decreased ocular blood flow velocities following a schleral buckling procedure. *Arch Ophthalmol* 1999;117:1647–1648.

Knapp ME, et al. Gaze-induced amaurosis from central artery compression. *Ophthalmology* 1992;99:238–240.

Roy FH. *Ocular syndromes and systemic diseases*, 3rd ed. Philadelphia: Lippincott Williams & Wilkins, 2002.

Slavin M. Clinical challenges. *Surv Opthalmol* 1997;41:6,481–487.

SUDDEN PAINLESS LOSS OF VISUAL ACUITY—ONE EYE

1. Acute keratoconus
2. Complication of retrobulbar block
3. Injury to the optic nerve
4. Meningeal carcinomatosis
5. Occlusion of central retinal artery
*6. Retinal detachment
7. Vitreous or retinal hemorrhage

Appen RE, et al. Meningeal carcinomatosis with blindness. *Am J Ophthalmol* 1978;86:661–665.

Brookshire GL, et al. Life-threatening complication of retrobulbar block. *Ophthalmology* 1986;93:1476–1478.

Kearne JR. Sudden blindness after ventriculography: bilateral retinal vascular occlusion superimposed on papilledema. *Am J Ophthalmol* 1974;78:275–278.

POSTTRAUMATIC LOSS OF VISION

*1. Acute (angle-closure) glaucoma precipitated by emotional trauma of recent accident or from intumescent lens capsular trauma or other blunt trauma
2. Avulsion of optic nerve by lateral orbital wall trauma or contrecoup blow to head
3. Central retinal artery or vein occlusion (from markedly increased orbital pressure or embolus)
4. Cortical blindness from hematoma, ischemia, or anoxia (patient may be unaware of blindness)
5. Hyphema, vitreous hemorrhage
6. Hysteria

7. Indirect trauma to optic nerves or chiasm
8. Intracranial interruption of visual pathways (hemorrhage, foreign body)
*9. Lid swelling, blood or foreign material covering cornea, corneal damage
10. Malingering
*11. Retinal detachment
12. Traumatic cataract, luxation of the lens (see p. 401)
13. Traumatic retinal edema and hemorrhages of retina from direct or contrecoup blows

Deutsch TA, Feller DB. *Paton and Goldberg's management of ocular injuries.* Philadelphia: WB Saunders, 1985.

DECREASED VISUAL ACUITY

1. Achromatopsia
2. Amblyopia ex anopsia—disuse
   A. Anisometropia—difference in refractive error between the eyes
   B. Monocular occlusion
   C. Strabismus—esotropia, exotropia, or hypertropia
   D. Unilateral atropinization
3. Anomalous elevation of optic disc with hyperplastic glial tissue and anomalous retinal vessels
4. Apparently normal eye with central fixation with poorer visual acuity in one than other eye—anisometropia
5. Apparently normal eye with normal fixation with disparity between near and distance vision—amblyopia, hysteria, malingering, retrobulbar neuritis, presbyopia, and micronystagmus
6. Apparently normal eye with normal fixation with poor distance and near vision astigmatism, amblyopia, hyperopia in older persons
7. Drugs, including the following:

acebutolol
aceclidine
acetaminophen
acetanilid
acetazolamide
acetohexamide
acetophenazine
acetyldigitoxin
acid bismuth sodium tartrate (?)
acyclovir
adiphenine
adrenal cortex injection
albuterol
alcohol
aldosterone
alkavervir
allobarbital
allopurinol
alprazolam
alseroxylon
aluminum nicotinate

amantadine
ambenonium
ambutonium
aminosalicylate (?)
aminosalicylic acid (?)
amiodarone
amithiozone
amitriptyline
amobarbital
amodiaquine
amoxapine
amphetamine
amphotericin B
amyl nitrite
anisindione
anisotropine
antazoline
antimony lithium thiomalate
antimony potassium tartrate
antimony sodium tartrate
antimony sodium thioglycollate

antipyrine
aprobarbital
aspirin
atenolol
atropine
azatadine
bacitracin
baclofen
barbital
bacille Calmette–Guérin (bCG) vaccine
belladonna
bendroflumethiazide
benoxinate
benzathine penicillin G
benzphetamine
benzthiazide
benztropine
betamethasone
betaxolol
biperiden
bismuth oxychloride

* = most important

bismuth sodium tartrate (?)
bismuth sodium
   thioglycollate (?)
bismuth sodium
   triglycollamate (?)
bismuth subcarbonate (?)
bismuth subsalicylate (?)
bromide
bromisovalum
brompheniramine
broxyquinoline
bupivacaine
busulfan
butabarbital
butacaine
butalbital
butallylonal
butaperazine
capreomycin
captopril
carbachol
carbamazepine
carbinoxamine
carbon dioxide
carbromal
carisoprodol
carmustine
carphenazine
cefaclor (?)
cefadroxil (?)
cefamandole (?)
cefazolin (?)
cefonicid (?)
cefoperazone (?)
ceforanide (?)
cefotaxime (?)
cefotetan (?)
cefoxitin (?)
cefsulodin (?)
ceftazidime (?)
ceftizoxime (?)
ceftriaxone(?)
cefuroxime(?)
cephalexin(?)
cephaloglycin (?)
cephaloridine (?)
cephalothin (?)
cephapirin (?)
cephradine (?)

chloral hydrate
chlorambucil
chloramphenicol
chlorcyclizine
chlordiazepoxide
chloroform
chloroprocaine
chloroquine
chlorothiazide
chlorpheniramine
chlorphenoxamine
chlorphentermine
chloroprocaine
chlorpromazine
chlorpropamide
chlorprothixene
chlortetracycline
chlorthalidone
cimetidine
cisplatin
clemastine
clidinium
clofazimine
clofibrate
clomiphene
clomipramine
clonazepam
clonidine
clorazepate
cobalt
cocaine
codeine
colchicine
colloidal silver
cortisone
cryptenamine
cyclizine
cyclobarbital
cyclopentobarbital
cyclopentolate
cyclophosphamide
cycloserine
cyclosporine
cyclothiazide
cycrimine
cyproheptadine
cytarabine
dacarbazine
danazol

dantrolene
dapsone
deferoxamine
demecarium
demeclocycline
deserpidine
desipramine
deslanoside
desoxycorticosterone
dexamethasone
dexbrompheniramine
dexchlorpheniramine
dextroamphetamine
dextrothyroxine
diatrizoate meglumine and
   sodium
diazepam
diazoxide
dibucaine
dichlorphenamide
dicumarol
dicyclomine
diethazine
diethylpropion
digitalis
digitoxin
digoxin
diltiazem
dimethindene
diphemanil
diphenadione
diphenhydramine
diphenylpyraline
diphtheria and tetanus
   toxoids adsorbed
diphtheria and tetanus
   toxoids and pertussis
   (adsorbed)
diphtheria toxoid (adsorbed)
dipivefrin
disopyramide
disulfiram
doxepin
doxycycline
doxylamine
dronabinol
droperidol
dyclonine
echothiophate

edrophonium
emetine
enalapril
ephedrine
epinephrine
ergonovine
ergot
ergotamine
erythrityl tetranitrate
ethacrynic acid
ethambutol
ethchlorvynol
ether
ethionamide
ethopropazine
ethosuximide
ethoxzolamide
etidocaine
etretinate
fenfluramine
fenoprofen
flecainide
floxuridine
fludrocortisone
fluorometholone
fluorouracil
fluphenazine
fluprednisolone
flurazepam
flurbiprofen
furosemide
gentamicin
gitalin
glutethimide
glyburide
glycerin
glycopyrrolate
griseofulvin
guanethidine
halazepam
haloperidol
hashish
heparin
heptabarbital
hexachlorophene
hexamethonium
hexethal
hexobarbital
hexocyclium

homatropine
hydrabamine penicillin V
hydralazine
hydrochlorothiazide
hydrocortisone
hydroflumethiazide
hydromorphone
hydroxyamphetamine
hydroxychloroquine
ibuprofen
imipramine
indapamide
indomethacin
influenza virus vaccine
insulin
interferon
iodide and iodine solutions
    and compounds
iodochlorhydroxyquin
iodoquinol
iophendylate
iothalamate meglumine and
    sodium ophthalmic
    acid
iron dextran
isocarboxazid
isoflurophate
isoniazid
isopropamide
isosorbide
isosorbide dinitrate
isotretinoin
kanamycin
ketamine
ketoprofen
labetalol
lanatoside C
levallorphan
levobunolol
levodopa
levothyroxine
lidocaine
liothyronine
liotrix
lithium carbonate
lomustine
lorazepam
lysergide
mannitol

mannitol hexanitrate
maprotiline
marihuana
measles and rubella virus
    vaccine (live)
measles, mumps and rubella
    virus vaccine (live)
measles virus vaccine (live)
mecamylamine
mechlorethamine
meclizine
medrysone
mefenamic acid
melphalan
mepenzolate
meperidine
mephenesin
mephobarbital
mepivacaine
meprednisone
meprobamate
mescaline
mesoridazine
methacycline
methadone
methamphetamine
methantheline
methaqualone
metharbital
methazolamide
methdilazine
methitural
methixene
methocarbamol
methohexital
methotrexate
methotrimeprazine
methscopolamine
methsuximide
methyclothiazide
methyl alcohol
methylatropine nitrate
methyldopa
methylene blue
methylergonovine
methylphenidate
methylprednisolone
methyprylon
methysergide

metoclopramide
metolazone
metoprolol
metrizamide
metronidazole
mexiletine
mianserin
midazolam
minocycline
minoxidil
mitomycin
mitotane
morphine
moxalactam (?)
mumps virus vaccine (live)
nadolol
nalidixic acid
nalorphine
naloxone
naltrexone
naphazoline
naproxen
neostigmine
niacin
niacinamide
nialamide
nicotinyl alcohol
nifedipine
nitrazepam
nitrofurantoin
nitroglycerin
nitrous oxide
nortriptyline
nystatin
opium
oral contraceptives
orphenadrine
ouabain
oxazepam
oxprenolol
oxygen
oxymorphone
oxyphenbutazone
oxyphencyclimine
oxyphenonium
oxytetracycline
paraldehyde
paramethasone
pemoline

pentaerythritol tetranitrate
pentazocine
pentobarbital pentolinium
perazine
perhexiline
pericyazine
perphenazine
phenacaine
phenacetin
phencyclidine
phendimetrazine
phenelzine
phenindione
pheniramine
phenmetrazine
phenobarbital
phensuximide
phentermine
phenylbutazone
phenylephrine
phenylpropanolamine
phenytoin
physostigmine
pilocarpine
pimozide
pindolol
pipenzolate
piperacetazine
piperazine
piperidolate
piperocaine
piroxicam
poldine
poliovirus vaccine
polymyxin B
polythiazide
potassium penicillin G
potassium penicillin V
potassium phenethicillin
practolol
pralidoxime
prazepam
prazosin
prednisolone
prednisone
prilocaine
primidone
probarbital
procaine

procaine penicillin G
prochlorperazine
procyclidine
promazine
promethazine
propantheline
proparacaine
propiomazine
propoxycaine
propoxyphene
propanolol
protoveratrines A and B
protriptyline
psilocybin
pyridostigmine
pyrilamine
quinacrine
quinethazone
quinidine
quinine
rabies immune globulin
rabies vaccine
radioactive iodides
ranitidine
rauwolfia serpentina
rescinnamine
reserpine
rifampin
rubella and mumps virus
 vaccine (live)
rubella virus vaccine (live)
scopolamine
secobarbital
semustine
silver nitrate
silver protein
smallpox vaccine
sodium antimonylgluconate
sodium salicylate
spironolactone
stibocaptate
stibogluconate
stibophen
streptomycin
streptozocin
sulfacetamide
sulfachlorpyridazine
sulfacytine
sulfadiazine

sulfadimethoxine
sulfamerazine
sulfameter
sulfamethazine
sulfamethizole
sulfamethoxazole
sulfamethoxypyridazine
sulfanilamide
sulfaphenazole
sulfapyridine
sulfasalazine
sulfathiazole
sulfisoxazole
sulindac
sulthiame
syrosingopine
talbutal
tamoxifen
temazepam
tetracaine
tetracycline
tetraethylammonium
tetrahydrocannabinol

tetrahydrozoline
thiabendazole
thiamylal
thiethylperazine
thiopental
thiopropazate
thioproperazine
thioridazine
thiothixene
thyroglobulin
thyroid
timolol
tobramycin
tocainide
tolazamide
tolbutamide
tranylcypromine
trazodone
triamcinolone
triazolam
trichlormethiazide
trichloroethylene
tridihexethyl

triethylenemelamine
trifluoperazine
trifluperidol
triflupromazine
trihexyphenidyl
trimeprazine
trimethaphan
trimethidinium
trimipramine
tripelennamine
triprolidine
trolnitrate
tropicamide
tryparsamide
uracil mustard
urea
urethan
verapamil
veratrum viride alkaloids
vinbarbital
vinblastine
warfarin

8. Hysteria
9. Irregular astigmatism—distortions in the anterior corneal surface (scarring, ectasia, edema, ulcer, postinflammatory processes)
10. Macular pathology (including edema, hemorrhage, or scar tissue)
11. Malingering
*12. Myopia
13. Myotonic dystrophy—exertional vision loss
14. Nystagmus
15. Opacities of cornea, lens, or vitreous precluding good vision
16. Optic neuritis—retrobulbar and papillitis, including toxic causes such as those due to tobacco, alcohol, and quinine (see p. 564)
17. Sphenoid sinus mucocele
18. Transient refractive errors
 *A. Hyperopia
 B. Myopia—diabetes

Cohen DB, Glasgow BJ. Bilateral optic nerve cryptococcosis in sudden blindness in patients with acquired immune deficiency syndrome. *Ophthalmology* 1993;100:1689–1694.

Fraunfelder FT, Fraunfelder FW. *Drug-induced ocular side effects.* Woburn, MA: Butterworth-Heinemann, 2001.

Pau H. *Differential diagnosis of eye diseases*, 2nd ed. New York: Thieme Medical, 1988.

BILATERAL BLURRING OF VISION

1. Drug-induced (see paresis of accommodation, p. 631–632)
2. Intracranial hypertension and advanced papilledema (see p. 593)
*3. Migraine—attacks last 15 to 20 minutes

* = most important

4. Narcolepsy
5. Refractive error (myopia, hyperopia, presbyopia)
6. Retinal "blackout" experienced by pilots
7. Severe systemic hypertension
8. Systemic hypotension
9. Vertebrobasilar insufficiency

Norman ME, Dyer JA. Ophthalmic manifestations of narcolepsy. *Am J Ophthalmol* 1987;103:81–86.

Wylie EJ, Ehrenfeld WK. *Extracranial occlusive cerebrovascular disease: diagnosis and management.* Philadelphia: WB Saunders, 1970.

CORTICAL BLINDNESS (CEREBRAL BLINDNESS)

This condition involves a complete loss of all visual sensation, including all appreciation of light and dark and a loss of reflex lid closure to bright illumination and to threatening gestures; retention of pupil constriction to light and accommodation; normal ophthalmoscopic examination; and normal motility. It may be associated with hemiplegia, sensory disorders, aphasia, and disorientation.

1. Degenerative conditions
   A. Alper progressive gray matter
   B. Cerebral dysgenesis associated with dementia
   C. Creutzfeldt-Jakob disease (corticostriatospinal degeneration)
   D. Cytomegalic inclusion disease (rare)
   E. Galactosemia
   F. Hodgkin disease
   G. Infantile neuroaxonal dystrophy
   H. Krabbe syndrome
   I. Phenylpyruvic oligophrenia
   J. Pompe disease (generalized glycogenesis)
   K. Porencephaly
   L. Renal failure
   M. Schilder disease (encephalitis periaxialis diffusa)
   N. Scholz subacute cerebral sclerosis
   O. Spongy degeneration of the brain
   P. Subacute sclerosing panencephalitis
   Q. Tay–Sachs disease (familial amaurotic idiocy)
   R. Toxoplasmosis (rare)
2. Drugs, including the following:

alcohol	cyclothiazide (?)	indapamide (?)
bendroflumethiazide (?)	diatrizoate meglumine or	iopamidol
benzthiazide (?)	sodium estradiol	iothalamate meglumine or
carbon dioxide	ether (?)	sodium iothalanuc
carbon monoxide	etoposide	ketamine (?)
chloroform (?)	etretinate	lead poisoning
chlorothiazide	FK506	meglumine
chlorthalidone	glycine	methadone
cisplatin	hexamethonium chloride	methyclothiazide (?)
corticotropin	hydrochlorothiazide (?)	methylergonovine (?)
cyclosporin	hydroflumethiazide (?)	metolazone (?)

metrizamide

nifedipine

nitroglycerin

nitrous oxide (?)

polythiazide (?)

quinethazone

sulfacetamide

sulfachlorpyridazine

sulfacytine

sulfadiazine

sulfadimethoxine

sulfamerazine

sulfameter

sulfamethazine

sulfamethizole

sulfamethoxazole

sulfamethoxypyridazine

sulfanilamide

sulfaphenazole

sulfapyridine

sulfasalazine

sulfathiazole

sulfisoxazole

tansy poisoning

thiopental (?)

trichlormethiazide (?)

vinblastine

vincristine

*3. Inflammatory lesions
   A. Bacterial endocarditis
   B. Encephalitis (including that due to measles and pertussis) and subacute sclerosing panencephalitis
   C. Influenza
   D. Meningococcal meningitis
   E. Mumps
   F. Pneumococcal meningitis
   G. Syphilitic meningitis
 4. Space-taking lesions, such as tumors, gummas, abscesses, and cysts
*5. Trauma
   A. Birth trauma, including heart dysfunction, postictal, and vertebral artery injury
   B. Chiropractic manipulation of the neck and odontotic subluxation
   C. Posthypoxic syndrome
   D. Subdural hematoma with cerebral edema
   E. Occipital region
   F. Ventriculography and ventriculoatrial shunt operation
*6. Vascular lesions
   A. Air embolism
   B. Angioma of occipital region
   C. Angiospastic lesions, including hypertension, nephritis, eclampsia, uremia, and chronic lead poisoning (saturnism)
   D. Anoxia from chronic respiratory insufficiency
   E. Anoxia from high altitude
   F. Basilar artery thrombosis
   G. Bilateral posterior cerebral artery occlusion
   H. Blood loss syndrome (acute cerebral hypotension)
    I. Blood transfusion reaction
   J. Cardiac arrest
   K. Cerebral hemorrhage
   L. Electroshock
   M. Following burns and sunstroke
   N. Following cardiac, cerebral or vertebral angiography
   O. Hemorrhage in spastic paralysis
   P. Herniation of hippocampal gyrus associated with subdural hematoma
   Q. Hydrocephalus and microcephaly
   R. Malaria
   S. Obstruction of the local venous sinus, such as from septic thrombosis of superior longitudinal sinus

* = most important

T. Periarteritis nodosa

U. Subarachnoid hemorrhage

V. "Subclavian steal syndrome" with reversal of blood flow through the vertebral artery

W. Thrombotic thrombocytopenic purpura

Fraunfelder FT, Fraunfelder FW. *Drug-induced ocular side effects*. Woburn, MA: Butterworth-Heinemann, 2001.

Rama BN, et al. Cortical blindness after cardiac catheterization: effect of rechallenge with dye. *Cathet Cardiovasc Diagn* 1993;28:149–151.

Roy FH. *Ocular syndromes and systemic diseases*, 3rd ed. Philadelphia: Lippincott Williams & Wilkins, 2002.

Wong VC. Cortical blindness in children: a study of etiology and prognosis. *Pediatr Neurol* 1991;7:178–185.

Cortical blindness

	Trauma (Subdural Hematoma)	Space-occupying Lesions (Occipital Tumors)	Inflammatory Lesions as Meningitis	Vascular Lesion (Subarachnoid Hemorrhage)	Drugs (Alcohol [Methanol])	Degenerative Condition (Renal Failure)
History						
1. Accidental ingestion					U	
2. Diplopia	S	S	S		U	
3. Formed hallucinations		S		R		
4. Head injury	U			S		
5. Photophobia			U	U		
6. Photopsia			U			
7. Systemic bacterial infection			U			
8. Systemic hypertension				S		U
9. Unformed hallucination		U				
10. Usually in elderly persons		U				
Physical Findings						
1. Blepharoptosis				S		
2. Cataract						S
3. Choroidal ischemic infarcts						S
4. Conjunctivitis			U			
5. Cotton-wool spots						U
6. Exophthalmos				S		
7. Failing visual acuity		U			U	
8. Fixed dilated pupil	U			S		
9. Glaucoma						S
10. Keratitis			U			
11. Lid edema						U
12. Macular edema			S			
13. Miosis			S			
14. Nonrhegmatogenous retinal detachment						S
15. Nystagmus			S		U	
16. Oculomotor paralysis				S		
17. Optic nerve atrophy			U		U	
18. Optic neuritis			S			
19. Panophthalmitis			S			
20. Papilledema	U	U	S	U	U	U
21. Paralysis of sixth cranial nerve	S		S			
22. Paresis of seventh cranial nerve			S			
23. Retinal edema						U
24. Retinal hemorrhage	S			U		U
25. Subhyaloid hemorrhage						
26. Unilateral central retinal vein occlusion				U		S
27. Uveitis			U			

Cortical blindness (Continued)

Laboratory Data	Trauma (Subdural Hematoma)	Space-occupying Lesions (Occipital Tumors)	Inflammatory Lesions as Meningitis	Vascular Lesion (Subarachnoid Hemorrhage)	Drugs (Alcohol [Methanol])	Degenerative Condition (Renal Failure)
1. Cerebral angiography	U	U	S	U		
2. Cerebrospinal fluid abnormal			U	U		
3. Computed tomographic scan of head	U	U		U		
4. Electroencephalogram	R					
5. Pneumoencephalogram	S					
6. Proteinuria/hematuria						U
7. Red blood cell count, white blood cell count, hemoglobin, hematocrit			U		U	
8. Serum blood-urea nitrogen, creatinine potassium, phosphate, sulfate increased						U
9. Serum sodium, calcium CO_2, decreased						U
10. Skull roentgenogram	S	S	S			
11. Subdural tap—children	U					

R = rarely; S = sometimes; and U = usually.

BLINDNESS IN CHILDHOOD

1. Cornea
    A. Hereditary dystrophies
    B. Inflammations such as varicella, rubeola, vaccinia, and gonorrhea, ophthalmia neonatorum, and pemphigus
    C. Trauma (abrasion or laceration)
2. Cortical blindness (see p. 632)
3. Globe
    A. Anophthalmos (see p. 228)
    B. Buphthalmos (see p. 222)
    C. Congenital, primary infantile, or secondary glaucoma (see p. 305)
    D. Hydrophthalmos
    E. Microphthalmos (see p. 220)
4. Lens
    A. Aphakia
    B. Congenital cataracts (see syndromes associated with cataracts, p. 410–416)
5. Optic nerve
    A. Aplasia
    B. Asphyxia at birth
    C. Associated with widespread disease such as mental deficiency, cerebral palsy, or epilepsy
    D. Atrophy (hereditary or secondary) (see p. 564)
    E. Cavernous sinus thrombosis (Foix syndrome)
    F. Cerebral hemorrhage (associated with major brain damage from accidental trauma, abuse or birth trauma)
    G. Crouzon syndrome (craniofacial dysostosis)
    H. Hydrocephalus
    I. Inflammatory damage—encephalomyelitis, encephalitis, tuberculous
    J. Osteopetrosis (Albers–Schönberg syndrome)
    K. Subdural hematoma
    L. Trauma—fracture at the orbital canal
    M. Tumors
6. Psychic blindness
    A. Agnosia
    B. Alexia
7. Retina
    A. Achromatopsia
    B. Albinism
    C. Coats disease (retinal telangiectasia)
    D. Early chorioretinal heredodegenerations, including Stargardt disease and pigmentary retinopathy (see pseudoretinitis pigmentosa, p. 497–499)
    E. Embryopathies, including rubella, toxoplasmosis, and syphilis
    F. High myopia
    G. Infantile macular degeneration
    H. Pseudoretinitis pigmentosa (see p. 497–499)
    I. Reese retinal dysplasia
    J. Retinal detachment
    K. Retinoblastoma

    L. Retinoschisis

    M. Retinopathy of prematurity

    N. Tapetoretinal degeneration

 8. Syndromes associated with amaurosis or blindness

    A. Adie syndrome

    B. Davidoff single ventricle

    C. Laurence–Moon–Bardet–Biedl syndrome (retinitis-pigmentosa-polydactyly-adi-posogenital syndrome)

    D. Malformative syndrome with cryptophthalmos

    E. Marfan syndrome (arachnodactyly dystrophia mesodermalis congenita)

    F. Metachromatic leukodystrophy (arylsulfatase A deficiency syndrome)

    G. Niemann–Pick syndrome (essential lipoid histiocytosis)

    H. Sandhoff disease

    I. Schilder disease (encephalitis periaxialis diffusa)

 9. Uveal tract

    A. Chorioretinitis

    B. Congenital coloboma

    C. Iridocyclitis

10. Vitreous

    A. Persistence of primary vitreous

    B. Pseudoglioma

Brownstein S, et al. Sandhoff's disease (Gmgangliosidosis type 2). *Arch Ophthalmol* 1980;98:1089.

Firth AY. Adie syndrome: evidence for refractive error and accommodative asymmetry as the cause of amblyopia. *Am J Ophthalmol* 1999;128:118–119.

Pau H. *Differential diagnosis of eye diseases*, 2nd ed. New York: Thieme Medical, 1988.

BINOCULAR DIPLOPIA (DOUBLE VISION USING BOTH EYES)

 1. Intractable postoperative diplopia

    A. Anomalous retinal correspondence with or without amblyopia (common), which is called *paradoxical diplopia*

    B. Cyclotropia due to oblique muscle operation

    C. Following surgical treatment of retinal detachment because of symblepharon or limitation of extraocular movement

    D. "Horror fusionis" (rare)—congenital or developmental deficiency of fusion (i.e., absence of sensory correspondence between two eyes (not the same as abnormal retinal correspondence, because visual directions are normal in these cases)

    E. Large surgical overcorrection

 2. Other

    A. Aniseikonia, including association with macular disease

    B. Divergence paresis

    C. Heterophoria—due to lesions such as orbital tumor and cellulitis

    D. Narcolepsy

    E. Physiologic diplopia

    F. Psychogenic causes

 3. Paralysis of one or more extraocular muscles

    A. Fourth-nerve palsy (rare) (see p. 158)

 *B. Sixth-nerve palsy—has no localizing value (see p. 161)

    C. Third-nerve palsy—with isolated muscle paralysis one must suspect a nuclear lesion (hemorrhage, syphilis, multiple sclerosis) or myasthenia gravis (see p. 153)

Benegas NM, et al. Diplopia secondary to aniseikonia associated with macular disease. *Arch Ophthalmol* 1999;117: 896–899.

Norman ME, Dyer JA. Ophthalmic manifestations of narcolepsy. *Am J Ophthalmol* 1987;103:81–86.

Schanzer B, Bordaberry M. The child with divergence paresis. *Surv Ophthalmol* 1998;42:571–574.

BINOCULAR TRIPLOPIA (UNIOCULAR DIPLOPIA)

1. Abnormal retinal correspondence with single image given two associations of direction so that the abnormal retinal point is brought into consciousness at the same time as the macula image
2. Central uniocular diplopia (rare)—systemic or neurologic causes include cerebral aneurysm, abscess or gross degenerative lesions, encephalitis lethargica, postencephalitis, multiple sclerosis, basal meningitis, cerebellar tumor, and vertebrobasilar insufficiency
*3. Malingering, hysteria, or psychogenic causes
4. Optical causes external to the eye
   A. Double or single prism placed in center of pupil before one eye
   *B. Improper correction of a high astigmatism
   *C. Looking through the edge of a bifocal or margin of lens
5. Optical causes in the eye
   A. Air bubbles or transparent foreign bodies in aqueous or vitreous
   B. Complete or partial contraction of the eyelids in which the eyelids impinge on the cornea (de Schweintz)
   C. Dislocation of the lens or misalignment of corneal and lenticular optical axis
   D. Double pupil
   E. High myopia, probably because of irregular astigmatism
   F. Irregular astigmatism, such as pressure on the globe
   G. Irregular spasm of the ciliary muscle
   H. Keratoconus (see p. 288)
   I. Lens abnormalities, such as fluid clefts or incipient cataract
   J. Looking through edge of intraocular lens
   *K. Map-dot fingerprint dystrophy
   L. Megalocornea (see p. 255)
   M. Migration of filtering bleb into the cornea
   N. Multifocal intraocular lens
   O. Post iridectomy
   *P. Refractive surgery
   Q. Retinal detachment
   R. Spherophakia (see p. 400–401)

Coffeen P, Guyton DL. Monocular diplopia accompanying ordinary refractive errors. *Am J Ophthalmol* 1988;105: 451–459.

Ellingson FT. Explanation of 3M diffractive intraocular lenses. *J Cataract Refract Surg* 1990;16:697–702.

Girard LJ. Monocular diplopia accompanying ordinary refractive errors. *Am J Ophthalmol* 1988;106:369.

Wyzinski P, O'Dell L. Subjective and objective findings after radial keratotomy. *Ophthalmology* 1989;96: 1608–1611.

DIPLOPIA FOLLOWING HEAD TRAUMA

1. Avulsion, contusion, or transection of extraocular muscles
2. Avulsion of the pulley of the superior oblique

* = most important

3. Decompensation of a preexisting ocular phoria, becoming a tropia
4. Edema or detachment of the macula (monocular diplopia)
*5. Hematoma in the orbit or the ocular muscles
*6. Orbital fracture (particularly blowout fracture of the floor, causing restricted function of inferior rectus and inferior oblique muscles)
7. Subluxation of the lens (monocular diplopia)
8. Third, fourth, or sixth cranial nerve palsies (orbital or intracranial) (see pp. 158, 161, 153)
9. "Whiplash" injury and the diplopias of obscure origin

Deutsch TA, Feller DB. *Paton's and Goldberg's management of ocular injuries.* Philadelphia: WB Saunders, 1985.

ECCENTRIC VISION

In this condition, vision is best when the individual is not looking directly at object of regard.

1. Central scotoma
2. Craniopharyngioma
3. Eccentric fixation with amblyopia
4. Ectopic macula, such as macula displaced by retinal scarring or fibrous strands, often a result of retinopathy of prematurity
5. Glaucoma—late with only eccentric field remaining
6. Homonymous hemianopia with macular involvement (see p. 613)
*7. Macular scar, such as with age-related macular degeneration.

Beyer-Machule C, von Noorden GK: *Atlas of ophthalmic surgery*, vol 1: *Lids, orbits, extraocular muscles.* New York: Thieme Medical, 1984.

Huber A. *Eye signs and symptoms in brain tumors*, 3rd ed. St. Louis: CV Mosby, 1976.

DECREASED DARK ADAPTATION (NYCTALOPIA; NIGHT BLINDNESS)

1. Choroideremia
2. Congenital night blindness
*3. May be due to drugs, including the following:

alcohol	hashish	methysergide
amodiaquine	hydroxychloroquine	oxygen
cantanidin	indomethacin (?)	pilocarpine
carbon dioxide	isotretinoin	psilocybin
chloroquine	lithium carbonate	silver nitrate
colloidal silver	lysergic acid diethylamide	silver protein
deferoxamine	(LSD)	tetrahydrocannabinol
dronabinol	lysergide	TI-iC
ergonovine	marihuana	vinblastine
ergotamine	mescaline	vincristine
etretinate	methylergonovine	

4. Progressive cone-rod dystrophy
5. Refsum syndrome (heredopathia atactica polyneuritiformis syndrome)
6. Retinitis pigmentosa (see p. 497)

Fraunfelder FT, Fraunfelder FW. *Drug-induced ocular side effects.* Woburn, MA: Butterworth-Heinemann, 2001.

Tasman W, Jaeger E, eds. *Duane's clinical ophthalmology.* Philadelphia: JB Lippincott, 1990.

ASTIGMATISM

In this condition, the refractive power of the eye varies along different meridians; its steepest meridian is vertical in "with the rule" (corrected with plus cylinder at 90 degrees) and horizontal in "against the rule."

  1. Adnexal masses
  2. Anterior segment surgery for cornea, lens, or glaucoma
*3. Chalazion
*4. Contact lens wear
*5. Corneal scars
*6. Following refractive surgery
  7. Keratoconus (see p. 288)
  8. May be dominant inheritance with incomplete penetrance
  9. Nuclear cataract with coloboma of lens, iris, and choroid
10. Oversized, rigid, anterior chamber, intraocular lens implant
11. Physiologic—about 0.5 diopters of "with the rule"
12. Retinal detachment procedures
13. Scleral infolding
14. Tilted intraocular lens

Abdel-Hakim AS. Corneal astigmatism induced by oversized rigid anterior chamber implants. *Am Intra Implant Soc J* 1985;11:474–482.

Bouzas AG. Anterior polar congenital cataract and corneal astigmatism. *J Pediatr Ophthalmol Strabismus* 1993; 29:210–212.

Fraunfelder FT, Roy FH. *Current ocular therapy*, 5th ed. Philadelphia: WB Saunders, 2000.

Hayashi H, et al. Corneal shape changes after scleral buckling surgery. *Opthalmology* 1997;104:831–837.

Inoue T, et al. Factors that influence the surgical effects of astigmatic keratotomy after cataract surgery. *Ophthalmology* 2001;108:1269–1274.

Kim T, et al. Induced corneal astigmatism after macular translocation surgery with scleral infolding. *Ophthalmology* 2001;108:1203–1208.

Plager DA, Snyder SK. Resolution of astigmatism after surgical resection of capillary hemangiomas in infants. *Ophthalmology* 1997;104:1102–1106.

VISUAL ALLESTHESIA

This condition involves displacement of image to opposite half of the visual field.

  1. Parietooccipital lobe disease
    A. Neoplasm
    B. Vascular insufficiency
    C. Trauma
    D. Seizure activity
  2. Occipital-lobe disease
    A. Neoplasm
    B. Vascular insufficiency
    C. Trauma
    D. Seizure activity

Bowen SF. Visual disorientation in allesthesia and palinopsia. *JAMA* 1978;239:56.

Jacobs L. Visual allesthesia. *Neurology* 1980;30:1059.

* = most important

VISUAL ACUITY LOSS AFTER GLAUCOMA SURGERY

1. Cystoid macular edema
*2. Hypotony maculopathy
3. Intraocular pressure spike
*4. Lens opacification
5. Postoperative capsule opacity
6. Retinal detachment
7. Suprachoroidal hemorrhage
8. Unknown
9. Vitreous hemorrhage
10. Wipeout (loss of central fixation)

Costa VP, et al. Loss of visual acuity after trabeculectomy. *Ophthalmology* 1993;100:599–612.

Cristiansson J. Ocular hypotony after fistulizing glaucoma surgery. *Acta Ophthalmol* 1967;45:837–845.

Watson RG, et al. The complications of trabeculectomy (a year follow-up). *Eye* 1990;4:425–438.

SUDDEN PAINFUL LOSS OF VISION

1. Acute-angle closure glaucoma
2. Fracture of the lesser wing of the sphenoid bone
3. Keratoconus
4. Optic neuritis
5. Temporal arteritis
6. Uveitis

Friedberg MA, Rapuano CJ. *Office and emergency room diagnosis and treatment of eye disease*. Philadelphia: JB Lippincott, 1990.

SUDDEN PAINLESS LOSS OF VISION—BOTH EYES

1. Brain injury
2. Brainstem arteriovenous malformations
3. Meningeal carcinomatosis
4. Quinine poisoning
5. Wood alcohol poisoning (methyl)

Friedberg MA, Rapuano CJ. *Office and emergency room diagnosis and treatment of eye disease*. Philadelphia: JB Lippincott, 1990.

Kerrison JB, Lee AG. Acute loss of vision during pregnancy due to a suprasellar mass. *Surv Ophthalmol* 1997;41:400–401.

GRADUAL PAINLESS LOSS OF VISION

1. Age-related macular degeneration
2. *Bartonella henselae*
3. Behcet disease
4. Cardiolipin antibody syndrome
5. Cataract
6. Chronic corneal disease
7. Diabetic retinopathy
8. Eales disease

* = most important

9. Glaucoma, open-angle
10. Herpetic viral infection
11. Idiopathic causes
12. Optic neuropathy/atrophy
13. Refractive error
14. Retinal disease, chronic
15. Systemic lupus erythematosus
16. Wegener granulomatosis

Friedberg MA, Rapuano CJ. *Office and emergency room diagnosis and treatment of eye disease.* Philadelphia: JB Lippincott, 1990.

Goldstein SM, et al. Cancer-associated retinopathy. *Arch Ophthalmol* 1999;117:1641–1645.

20

Visual Complaint

CONTENTS

PHOTOPSIA (SCINTILLATIONS, SPARKS, OR FLASHES OF LIGHT BEFORE THE EYES)

1. Associated with arteriovenous aneurysm
2. Auditory–visual synesthetic phenomena—optic nerve lesion; usually demyelinative
3. Brain concussion
4. Clomiphene citrate (Clomid)
5. Focal lesions of occipital region
6. Glaucoma
7. Idiopathic thrombocytosis
8. Impending retinal detachment
9. Lyme borreliosis
*10. Migraine and epilepsy
11. Moore lightning streak—traction of a partially liquefied vitreous on the retina
12. Oculodigital phenomenon (entopic phenomenon)
13. Paraneoplastic retinopathy
14. Phosphene of quick eye motion (Flick phosphene)

* = most important

15. Retinal microembolization
16. Retinitis
17. Vertebral basilar insufficiency

Mikkila HA, et al. The expanding clinical spectrum of ocular Lyme borreliosis. *Ophthalmology* 2000;107:581–587.

Pau H. *Differential diagnosis of eye diseases*, 2nd ed. New York: Thieme Medical, 1988.

Walsh FB, Hoyt WF. *Clinical neuro-ophthalmology*, 4th ed. Baltimore: Williams & Wilkins, 1985.

HALLUCINATIONS (FORMED IMAGES)

1. Blind persons (central or peripheral visual field loss)
2. Bilateral eye covering—such as may be required after an eye operation, especially in older patients
3. Ocular lesions, such as retinal hemorrhage, glaucoma, optic atrophy of tertiary syphilis, and choroidal neovascularization.
4. Psychoses
5. Central nervous system lesions
   A. Alzheimer disease
   B. Diffuse irritative lesion of parietotemporal area, including uncinate seizures of the temporal lobe, stimulation of superior colliculus, and optic radiation
   C. Encephalitis
   D. Hippocampus lesions
   E. Hypophyseal duct tumors
   F. Measles
   G. Medulloblastoma
   H. Myxedema
   I. Narcolepsy
   J. Occipital lobe seizures—moving lights and colors, visual and complex hallucinations with formed images
   K. Papilledema (see p. 593)
   L. Peduncular hallucinations with midbrain lesions from vascular, encephalitic, and mass lesions
   M. Pellagra
   N. Pituitary and optic chiasmal lesion
   O. Vertebrobasilar insufficiency/basilar artery migraine
6. Chronic mountain sickness (Monge syndrome)
7. Malignant melanoma
8. Poisonings, such as mushroom, psilocin, cannabis, hashish, hemp, camphor, mescaline from peyote, myristica (nutmeg), gasoline, mullet (Hawaiian fish), and ololiuqui (morning-glory seeds)
9. Drugs, including the following:

acebutolol	aldosterone	amyl nitrite
acetaminophen	allobarbital	antazoline
acetanilid	alprazolam	aprobarbital
acetophenazine	amantadine	aspirin
acid bismuth sodium tartrate	amitriptyline	atenolol
acyclovir	amobarbital	atropine
adrenal cortex injection	amodiaquine	azatadine
albuterol	amoxapine	baclofen
alcohol	amphetamine	barbital

belladonna
bendroflumethiazide
benzathine penicillin G
benzphetamine
benztropine
betamethasone
betaxolol
biperiden
bismuth oxychloride
bismuth sodium tartrate
bismuth sodium
    thioglycollate
bismuth sodium
    triglycollamate
bismuth subcarbonate
bismuth subsalicylate
bromide
brompheniramine
butabarbital
butalbital
butallylonal
butaperazine
butethal
calcitriol
capreomycin
captopril
carbamazepine
carbinoxamine
carbon dioxide
carphenazine
cefaclor
cefadroxil
cefamandole
cefazolin
cefonicid
cefoperazone
ceforanide
cefotaxime
cefotetan
cefoxitin
cefsulodin
ceftazidime
ceftizoxime
ceftriaxone
cefuroxime
cephalexin
cephaloglycin
cephaloridine
cephalothin

cephapirin
cephradine
chloral hydrate
chlorambucil
chlordiazepoxide
chloroquine
chlorpheniramine
chlorphenoxamine
chlorpromazine
chlortetracycline
chlorthalidone
cholecalciferol
cimetidine
clemastine
clomipramine
clonazepam
clonidine
clorazepate
cocaine
codeine
cortisone
cyclizine
cyclobarbital
cyclopentobarbital
cyclopentolate
cycloserine
cyclosporine
cyclothiazide
cycrimine
cyproheptadine
dantrolene
dapsone
demeclocycline
desipramine
desoxycorticosterone
dexamethasone
dexbrompheniramine
dexchlorpheniramine
dextroamphetamine
dextrothyroxine
diazepam
diethazine
diethylpropion
digitalis
digoxin
diltiazem
dimethindene
diphenhydramine
diphenylhydantoin

diphenylpyraline
disopyramide
disulfiram
ditaven
divalproex sodium
doxepin
doxycycline
dronabinol
droperidol
enalapril
ephedrine
ergocalciferol
ethchlorvynol
ethionamide
ethopropazine
ethosuximide
fenfluramine
flecainide
fludrocortisone
fluphenazine
fluprednisolone
flurazepam
furosemide
gentamicin
glutethimide
glycerin
griseofulvin
halazepam
haloperidol
hashish
heptabarbital
hexethal
hexobarbital
homatropine
hydrabamine penicillin V
hydrochlorothiazide
hydrocortisone
hydroflumethiazide
hydroxychloroquine
hydroxyurea
ibuprofen
imipramine
indapamide
indomethacin
interferon
iodide and iodine solutions
    and compounds
isoniazid
isosorbide

ketamine
ketoprofen
labetalol
levallorphan
levobunolol
levodopa
levothyroxine
lidocaine
liothyronine
liotrix
lithium carbonate
lorazepam
lysergide
mannitol
maprotiline
marihuana
meclizine
meperidine
mephentermine
mephobarbital
meprednisone
mescaline
mesoridazine
methacycline
methamphetamine
methaqualone
metharbital
methdilazine
methitural
methohexital
methotrimeprazine
methscopolamine
methsuximide
methyclothiazide
methyldopa
methylpentynol
methylphenidate
methylprednisolone
methyprylon
methysergide
metolazone
metoprolol
metrizamide
metronidazole
mexiletine
mianserin
midazolam
minocycline
morphine (?)

moxalactam
nadolol
nalidixic acid
nalorphine
naloxone
naltrexone
neostigmine
nialamide
nifedipine
nitrazepam
nitrofurantoin (?)
nitroglycerin (?)
nortriptyline
opium (?)
orphenadrine
oxazepam
oxprenolol
oxyphenbutazone
oxytetracycline
paraldehyde
paramethasone
pargyline
pemoline
penicillin
pentazocine
pentobarbital
pentylenetetrazol
perazine
perhexiline (?)
pericyazine
perphenazine
phenacetin
phencyclidine
phendimetrazine
phenelzine
pheniramine
phenobarbital
phensuximide
phentermine
phenoxymethyl
phenylbutazone
phenylephrine
phenylpropanolamine
phenytoin
pimozide
pindolol
piperacetazine
piperazine
piroxicam

polythiazide
potassium penicillin G
potassium penicillin V
phenoxymethyl penicillin
practolol
prazepam
prazosin
prednisolone
prednisone
primidone
probarbital
procaine penicillin G
prochlorperazine
procyclidine
promazine
promethazine
propiomazine
propoxyphene
propranolol
protriptyline
psilocybin
pyrilamine
quinacrine
quinethazone
quinidine
quinine
radioactive iodides
ranitidine
scopolamine
secobarbital
sodium salicylate
sulfacetamide
sulfachlorpyridazine
sulfacytine
sulfadiazine
sulfadimethoxine
sulfamerazine
sulfameter
sulfamethazine
sulfamethizole
sulfamethoxazole
sulfamethoxypyridazine
sulfanilamide
sulfaphenazole
sulfapyridine
sulfasalazine
sulfisoxazole
sulfathiazole
sulindac (?)

talbutal	thyroid	trimipramine
temazepam	timolol	tripelennamine
tetanus immune globulin	tobramycin	triprolidine
tetanus toxoid	tocainide	tropicamide
tetracycline	trazodone	urea
tetrahydrocannabinol	triamcinolone	valproate sodium
thiabendazole	triazolam	valproic acid
thiamylal	trichlormethiazide	verapamil
thiethylperazine	trichloroethylene	vidarabine
thiopental	trifluoperazine	vinbarbital
thiopropazate	trifluperidol	vinblastine
thioproperazine	triflupromazine	vincristine
thioridazine	trihexyphenidyl	vitamin D
thyroglobulin	trimeprazine	

10. Exercise induced with occipital lobe tumor
11. Patients in seclusion

Fisher CM. Visual hallucinations, atropine toxicity. *Am J Ophthalmol* 1991;112:368.

Fraunfelder FT, Fraunfelder FW. *Drug-induced ocular side effects*. Woburn, MA: Butterworth-Heinemann, 2001.

Lerner AJ, et al. Concomitants of visual hallucinations in Alzheimer's disease. *Neurology* 1994;44:523–527.

Loewenstein JI. Visual hallucinations in patients with choroidal neovascularization. *JAMA* 1994;272:243.

Scott IU, et al. Visual hallucinations in patients with retinal disease. *Am J Ophthalmol* 2001;131:590–598.

"SPOTS" BEFORE EYES (DOTS OR FILAMENTS THAT MOVE WITH MOVEMENT OF EYE)

*1. Vitreous opacities—muscae volitantes; associated with preretinal hemorrhage, myopia, posterior vitreous detachment, or intraocular inflammations
 2. Scotomatous defects
    A. Retinal lesions
    B. Myopia
 3. Corneal foreign-body reflection/corneal opacity
 4. Carbon tetrachloride poisoning
 5. Migraine

Grant WM. *Toxicology of the eye*, 2nd ed. Springfield, IL: Charles C Thomas, 1974.

Vaughan D, et al. *General ophthalmology*, 14th ed. Norwalk, CT: Appleton & Lange, 1995.

COLORED HALOS AROUND LIGHTS (BLUE AND VIOLET ARE NEXT TO THE STIMULATING LIGHT AND RED OUTERMOST)

1. Glaucoma
    A. Acute-angle closure with stretching of corneal lamellae
    B. Open-angle glaucoma—halo noted on awakening (intraocular pressure is highest in the morning)
2. Mucus on the cornea
3. Corneal scar/corneal edema
4. Krukenberg spindle
5. Lens opacities

6. Vitreous opacities (see p. 429–430)
7. Any haze of ocular media
8. Drugs probably affecting corneal epithelium, including the following:

acetophenazine
acetyldigitoxin
amiodarone
amodiaquine
amyl nitrite
butaperazine
carphenazine
chloroquine
chlorine dioxide
chlorpromazine
cortisone
deslanoside
dexamethasone
diethazine
digitalis
digitoxin
digoxin
ethopropazine
ethylene diamine

fluorometholone
fluphenazine
gitalin
hydrocortisone
hydroxychloroquine
lanatoside C
medrysone
mesoridazine
methdilazine
methotrimeprazine
methylprednisolone
nitroglycerin
nitronaphthalene
oral contraceptives
ouabain
paramethadione
perazine
pericyazine
perphenazine

piperacetazine
prednisolone
prochlorperazine
promazine
promethazine
propiomazine
quinacrine
sildenafil
thiethylperazine
thiopropazate
thioproperazine
thioridazine
trifluoperazine
triflupromazine
trimeprazine
trimethadione
water (sterile)

9. Physiologic halos—most common when lens acts as diffracting gradient
10. Too intense exposure to light, as in snow blindness
11. Asymmetric placement of the intraocular lens in relation to the pupillary aperture

Fraunfelder FT, Fraunfelder FW. *Drug-induced ocular side effects*. Woburn, MA: Butterworth-Heinemann, 2001.

Gabrieli CB, et al. Subjective visual halos after sildenafil (Viagra) administration. *Ophthalmology* 2001;108:877–881.

Mantyjarvi M, et al. Ocular side effects of amiodarone. *Surv Ophthalmol* 1998;42:360–366.

LIGHT STREAKS

1. Cataracts
2. Contact lenses
3. Excessive tear meniscus
4. Intraocular lens scratches
5. Lashes
*6. Migraine
7. Posterior capsules—lens fibers and debris-filled corrugations
8. Rapid eye movements (especially in a dark environment)
9. Reflection off edge of intraocular lens
10. Reflection off manipulation holes of intraocular lens
*11. Retinal break/tear or detachment
12. Spectacles
13. Windshields, windows

Holladay JT, et al. Diagnosis and treatment of mysterious light streaks seen by patients following extracapsular cataract extraction. *American Intraimplant Society Journal* 1985;11:21–23.

Holladay JT, et al. The optimal size of a posterior capsulotomy. *American Intraimplant Society Journal* 1985;11:18–20.

* = most important

PHOTOPHOBIA (PAINFUL INTOLERANCE OF THE EYES TO LIGHT)

1. Aniridia
*2. Ocular, including conjunctivitis, keratitis, iritis, iridocyclitis, uveitis, and corneal, lenticular, and vitreous opacities, Angelucci syndrome (critical allergic conjunctivitis), acute hemorrhagic conjunctiva, and cone-dysfunction syndrome
3. Albinism
4. Total color blindness (achromatopsia)
5. Patients with corneal lesions having diseases characterized by photosensitization (xeroderma pigmentosa, hydroa vacciniforme, and smallpox)
6. Systemic diseases, including botulism, cystinosis, erythropoietic porphyria, hypoparathyroidism, rabies, psittacosis, and schistosomiasis
7. Toxic causes, including mercury poisoning
8. Drugs, including the following:

acetohexamide
acetophenazine
adiphenine
adrenal cortex injection
alprazolam
allobarbital
ambutonium
amiodarone
amitriptyline
amobarbital
amodiaquine
anisotropine
antazoline
atropine
auranofin
aurothioglucose
aurothioglycanide
beclomethasone
belladonna
bendroflumethiazide
benzthiazide
betamethasone
botulinum A toxin
brimonidine tartrate
brinzolamide
bromide
brompheniramine
butaperazine
capecitabine
captopril (?)
carbon dioxide
carphenazine
chlordiazepoxide
chloroquine

chlorpromazine
chlorpropamide
chlortetracycline
cimetidine·
clidinium
clonazepam
clomiphene
clorazepate
dapiprazole hydrochloride
deferoxamine
demeclocycline
desipramine
dextran
dextrothyroxine
diacetylmorphine
diazepam (?)
dicyclomine
diethylcarbamazine
diethazine
digitalis
digitoxin
dimethyl sulfoxide
diphemanil
dipivalyl epinephrine (DPE)
dipivefrin
disopyramide
doxepin
doxycycline
dronabinol
edrophonium
enalapril
ethambutol
ethionamide
ethopropazine

ethosuximide
ethotoin
ferrocholinate
ferrous fumarate
ferrous gluconate
ferrous succinate
ferrous sulfate
flecainide
floxuridine
fludrocortisone
fluorometholone
fluorouracil
fluoxetine hydrochloride
fluphenazine
fluprednisolone
flurazepam
fluvoxamine maleate
furosemide (?)
glyburide
glycopyrrolate
gold Au 198
gold sodium thiomalate
gold sodium thiosulfate
guanethidine
halazepam
hashish
hexethal
hexobarbital
hexocyclium
homatropine
hydralazine
hydroxyamphetamine
   indomethacin
hydroxychloroquine

* = most important

ibuprofen
imipramine
indomethacin
iron dextran
iron sorbitex
isocarboxazid
isoniazid
isopropamide
labetalol
latanoprost
levarterenol
levothyroxine
liothyronine
liotrix
lithium carbonate
lorazepam
marihuana
midazolam
mepenzolate
mephenytoin
mesoridazine
methacycline
methantheline
methdilazine
methixene
methotrimeprazine
methoxsalen
methsuximide
methyl alcohol
methylatropine nitrate
methyldopa
metoclopramide
metrizamide

metronidazole
minocycline
nalidixic acid
naltrexone
nialamide
norfloxacin
norepinephrine
nortriptyline
oral contraceptives
oxazepam
oxprenolol
oxyphenbutazone
oxyphencyclimine
oxyphenonium
oxytetracycline
paramethadione
perazine
pericyazine
perphenazine
phenelzine
phensuximide
phenylbutazone
pipenzolate
piperacetazine
piperidolate
poldine
practolol
procarbazine
prochlorperazine
promazine
promethazine
propantheline
propiomazine
protriptyline

quinacrine
quinidine
quinine
rabies immune globulin
rabies vaccine
scopolamine
sildenafil citrate
streptomycin
temazepam
tetanus immune globulin
tetanus toxoid
tetracycline
thiethylperazine
thiopropazate
thioproperazine
thioridazine
thyroglobulin thyroid
tolazamide
tolbutamide
tranylcypromine
trichloroethylene
tridihexethyl
trifluoperazine
triflupromazine
trimeprazine
trimethadione
trioxsalen
tripelennamine
vancomycin
vinbarbital
vinblastine
vincristine

9. Normal ocular findings with photophobia
   A. Trigeminal neuralgia (Charlin syndrome)
   B. Migraine
   C. Neurasthenia
   D. Meningitis
   E. Subarachnoid hemorrhage
   F. Acromegaly
   G. Associated with hypophyseal tumor and craniopharyngioma
   H. During and following retrobulbar neuritis
   I. Acrodynia (Feer syndrome)
   J. Following severe head injury
   K. Hypoparathyroidism
   L. Lesions of gasserian ganglion

    M. Tumors of ophthalmic branch of the trigeminal nerve, such as neuroma, middle fossa tumor, and posterior fossa tumor, such as meningioma or acoustic neuroma

    N. Increased intracranial pressure, including subdural hematomas

10. Acrodermatitis chronica atrophicans
11. Avitaminosis B (pellagra)
12. Chédiak–Higashi syndrome (anomalous leukocytic inclusions with constitutional stigmata)
13. Danbolt–Closs syndrome (acrodermatitis enteropathica)
14. Elschnig syndrome (meibomian conjunctivitis)
15. Feer syndrome (acrodynia)
16. Folling syndrome (phenylketonuria)
17. Following refractive surgery
18. Gradenigo syndrome (temporal syndrome)
19. Hanhart syndrome (pseudoherpetic keratitis)
20. Hartnup syndrome (niacin deficiency)
21. Hysteria
22. Infantile globoid cell leukodystrophy (Krabbe disease)
23. Keratodermia palmaris et plantaris
24. Photosensitivity and sunburn
25. Reiter syndrome (polyarthritis enterica)

Fraunfelder FT, Fraunfelder FW. *Drug-induced ocular side effects*. Woburn, MA: Butterworth-Heinemann, 2001.

Pau H. *Differential diagnosis of eye diseases*, 2nd ed. New York: Thieme Medical, 1988.

Roy FH. *Ocular syndromes and systemic diseases*, 3rd ed. Philadelphia: Lippincott Williams & Wilkins, 2002.

ASTHENOPIA (UNCOMFORTABLE OCULAR SENSATION OR EYE ACHE)

1. Dazzling from bright light
2. Episcleritis or scleritis
3. Glaucoma
4. Iritis or iridocyclitis
5. Neurasthenia or hysteria
6. Passive congestion
7. Phoria or tropia
8. Retrobulbar neuritis
9. Sinus disease
10. Spasm from muscles held too long in a restricted position
11. Subclinical open-angle glaucoma
12. Uncorrected refractive errors, especially hyperopia or astigmatism
13. Unknown
14. Use of miotics
15. Weak accommodation

Otto J. Asthenopia and wide-angle glaucoma. *Glaucoma* 1986;8:75–77.

Pau H. *Differential diagnosis of eye diseases*, 2nd ed. New York: Thieme Medical, 1988.

DAZZLING OR GLARE DISCOMFORT

1. Altered pupillary response

2. Asymmetric placement of the intraocular lens in relation to the pupillary aperture
3. Corneal scars or foreign bodies
4. Drugs, such as chloroquine, acetazolamide, or trimethadione (Tridione)
5. Emotional disorders
6. Following refractive surgery
7. Idiopathic
8. Lenticular changes

Brems RN, et al. Posterior chamber intraocular lenses in a series of autopsy eyes. *J Cataract Refract Surg* 1986; 12:367–375.

Vaughan D, et al. *General ophthalmology*, 12th ed. Norwalk, CT: Appleton & Lange, 1989.

CHROMATOPSIA (COLORED VISION, OBJECTS ARE ABNORMALLY COLORED)

1. Blue color (cyanopsia)
   A. Drugs, including the following:

acetyldigitoxin	deslanoside	methylene blue
alcohol	digitalis	nalidixic acid
amodiaquine	digitoxin	oral contraceptives
amphetamine	digoxin	ouabain
chloroquine	gitalin	quinacrine
combination products of estrogens and progestogens	hydroxyamphetamine hydroxychloroquine lanatoside C	sildenafil citrate

   B. Pseudophakia
   C. Optic atrophy of tertiary syphilis
2. Red color (erythropsia)
   A. Drugs, including the following:

acetyldigitoxin	methylergonovine	sulfamethazine
atropine	methysergide	sulfamethizole
belladonna	naproxen	sulfamethoxazole
deslanoside	ouabain	sulfamethoxypyridazine
digitalis	quinine	sulfanilamide
digitoxin	sulfacetamide	sulfaphenazole
digoxin	sulfachlorpyridazine	sulfapyridine
ergonovine	sulfacytine	sulfasalazine
ergotamine	sulfadiazine	sulfathiazole
gitalin	sulfadimethoxine	sulfisoxazole
homatropine	sulfamerazine	sulthiame
lanatoside C	sulfameter	

   B. Hysteria
   C. Optic atrophy of tertiary syphilis
   D. Vitreous or retinal hemorrhage (see p. 473–478)
   E. Pseudophakia and aphakia
   F. Snow blindness or blindness following electric shock
   G. After working with green monochrome video display terminals
   H. Welding arc maculopathy

3. Yellow color (xanthopsia)
   A. Drugs, including the following:

acetaminophen
acetanilid
acetophenazine
acetyldigitoxin
allobarbital
alseroxylon
amobarbital
amodiaquine
amyl nitrite
aprobarbital
aspirin
barbital
bendroflumethiazide
benzthiazide
butabarbital
butalbital
butallylonal
butaperazine
butethal
carbachol (?)
carbon dioxide
carphenazine
chloramphenicol
chloroquine
chlorothiazide
chlorpromazine
chlortetracycline
chlorthalidone
cimetidine (?)
colloidal silver
cyclobarbital
cyclopentobarbital
cyclothiazide
deserpidine
deslanoside
diethazine
digitalis
digitoxin
digoxin
dronabinol
ethopropazine
fluorescein
fluphenazine

furosemide
gitalin
hashish
heptabarbital
hexethal
hexobarbital
hydrochlorothiazide
hydroflumethiazide
hydroxychloroquine
indapamide
lanatoside C
marijuana
mephobarbital
mesoridazine
methaqualone
metharbital methazolamide
methdilazine
methitural
methohexital
methotrimeprazine
methyclothiazide
metolazone
mild silver protein
nalidixic acid
nitrofurantoin (?)
ouabain
pentobarbital
pentylenetetrazol
perazine
pericyazine
perphenazine
phenacetin
phenobarbital
piperacetazine
polythiazide
primidone
probarbital
prochlorperazine
promazine
promethazine
propiomazine
quinacrine
quinethazone
rauwolfia serpentina

rescinnamine
reserpine
secobarbital
silver nitrate
silver protein
sodium salicylate
streptomycin
sulfacetamide
sulfachlorpyridazine
sulfacytine
sulfadiazine
sulfadimethoxine
sulfamerazine
sulfameter
sulfamethazine
sulfamethizole
sulfamethoxazole
sulfamethoxypyridazine
sulfanilamide
sulfaphenazole
sulfapyridine
sulfasalazine
sulfathiazole
sulfisoxazole
syrosingopine
talbutal
tetrahydrocannabinol
tetrahydrocannabinol (THC)
thiabendazole
thiamylal
thiethylperazine
thiopental
thiopropazate
thioproperazine
thioridazine
trichlormethiazide
trifluoperazine
triflupromazine
trimeprazine
vinbarbital
vitamin A

   B. Lenticular change
   C. Aphakia
   D. Poisons, including aconite, dichlorodiphenyl trichloroethane, carbon disulfide,
      chromic acid, methyl salicylate, aspidium (Felix mas), santonin, picric acid
   E. Jaundice
   F. Hysteria

4. Green color (chloropsia)
    A. Drugs, including the following:

acetyldigitoxin
allobarbital
amobarbital
amodiaquine
aprobarbital
barbital
butabarbital
butalbital
butallylonal
butethal
chloroquine
cyclobarbital
cyclopentobarbital
deslanoside
digitalis
digitoxin

digoxin
epinephrine
gitalin
griseofulvin
heptabarbital
hexethal
hexobarbital
hydroxychloroquine
iodide and iodine solutions
    and compounds
lanatoside C
mephobarbital
metharbital
methitural
methohexital
nalidixic acid

naproxen
ouabain
pentobarbital
phenobarbital
primidone
probarbital
quinacrine
quinine
radioactive iodides
secobarbital
talbutal
thiamylal
thiopental
vinbarbital

    B. Poisons such as santonin

5. Violet color (ianthinopsia)
    A. Drugs, including the following:

dronabinol
hashish

marihuana
nalidixic acid

quinacrine
tetrahydrocannabinol

    B. Pseudophakia and aphakia
    C. Intracameral air

6. Brown color
    A. Drugs, including the following:

acetophenazine
butaperazine
carphenazine
chlorpromazine
diethazine
ethopropazine
fluphenazine
mesoridazine
methdilazine

methotrimeprazine
perazine
pericyazine
perphenazine
piperacetazine
prochlorperazine
promazine
promethazine
propiomazine

THC
thiethylperazine
thiopropazate
thioproperazine
thioridazine
trifluoperazine
triflupromazine
trimeprazine

    B. Lenticular change

7. White color
    A. Drugs, including the following:

capreomycin
diphenylhydantoin

paramethadione trimethadione
phenytoin

    B. Pseudophakia and aphakia

Fraunfelder FT, Fraunfelder FW. *Drug-induced ocular side effects.* Woburn, MA: Butterworth-Heinemann, 2001.

Uniat L, et al. Welding arc maculopathy. *Am J Ophthalmol* 1986;102:394–395.

Walsh FB, Hoyt WF. *Clinical neuro-ophthalmology*, vol 1, 4th ed. Baltimore: Williams & Wilkins, 1985.

HEIGHTENED COLOR PERCEPTION

1. Heightened color perception is due to drugs, including the following:

dronabinol	lysergide	psilocybin
ethionamide	marihuana	tetrahydrocannabinol
hashish	mescaline	THC
LSD	oxygen	

Fraunfelder FT, Fraunfelder FW. *Drug-induced ocular side effects.* Woburn, MA: Butterworth-Heinemann, 2001.

NYCTALOPIA (NIGHT BLINDNESS)

1. Anemia
2. Carbon monoxide poisoning
3. Congenital high myopia
4. Diffuse opacities of media including corneal edema, keratitis and nuclear cataract
5. Following refractive surgery
6. Glaucoma—especially open-angle and angle-closure glaucoma
7. Paraneoplastic retinopathy including melanoma-associated retinopathy and cancer-associated retinopathy
8. Psychologic causes—malingering or psychoses
9. Optic atrophy
10. Refsum syndrome (phytanic acid oxidase deficiency)
11. Tapetoretinal degenerations
    A. Choroideremia
    B. Congenital night blindness
       (1) Dominant form
       (2) Recessive form
       (3) Recessive, sex-linked
    C. Detachment of retina, including malignant melanoma
    D. Drugs, including the following:

acetophenazine	mesoridazine	propiomazine
amodiaquine	methdilazine	quinidine
butaperazine	methotrimeprazine	quinine
carphenazine	paramethadione	thiethylperazine
chloroquine	perazine	thiopropazate
chlorpromazine	pericyazine	thioproperazine
diethazine	perphenazine	thioridazine
ethopropazine	piperacetazine	trifluoperazine
fluphenazine	prochlorperazine	triflupromazine
hydroxychloroquine	promazine	trimeprazine
indomethacin	promethazine	trimethadione

    E. Drusen (familial)—minimal
    F. Fleck retina—nonprogressive, congenital, rare
    G. Fundus flavimaculatus—minimal
    H. General choroidal sclerosis
    I. Gyrate atrophy
    J. Retinitis pigmentosa
    K. Retinitis punctata albescens

  L. Miner nystagmus

  M. Oguchi disease—may be abnormal

12. Visual field defects

13. Vitamin A deficiency

  A. Dietary deficiencies, including malnutrition, alcoholism and cystic fibrosis

  B. Digestive tract disturbance

    (1) Colitis and enteritis

    (2) Crohn disease

    (3) Jejunoileal bypass surgery

    (4) In pancreas—such as chronic pancreatitis

    (5) In stomach—achlorhydria, chronic gastritis or diarrhea, peptic ulcer

    (6) Abetalipoproteinemia

  C. Liver disease, such as chronic cirrhosis

  D. Malaria

  E. Pregnancy

  F. Pulmonary tuberculosis

  G. Skin disorders, such as pityriasis rubra pilaris

  H. Thyroid gland disorders, such as hyperthyroidism

14. Vitreous opacities, including hemorrhage

15. Vitreotapetoretinal degeneration—sex-linked recessive and autosomal recessive

Berson EL, Lessell S. Paraneoplastic night blindness with malignant melanoma. *Am J Ophthalmol* 1988;106: 307–311.

Dryja TP. Molecular genetics of Oguchi disease, fundus albipunctatus, and other forms of stationary night blindness: LVII Edward Jasckson Memorial Lecture. *Am J Ophthalmol* 2000;130:547–563.

Fraunfelder FT, Fraunfelder FW. *Drug-induced ocular side effects*. Woburn, MA: Butterworth-Heinemann, 2001.

Gans M, Taylor C. Reversal of progressive nyctalopia in a patient with Crohn' disease. *Can J Ophthalmol* 1990; 25:156–158.

HEMERALOPIA

This condition involves day blindness, that is, an inability to see as distinctly in a bright light as in a dim one.

 1. Adie pupil

 2. Albinism

 3. Aniridia

 4. Central opacities of the lens—nuclear or perinuclear cataracts

 5. Central scotoma

 6. Congenital—autosomal recessive trait usually associated with amblyopia and color deficiency

 7. Hereditary retinoschisis

 8. Intraocular iron

 9. Partial occlusion of the central retinal artery (see p. 457–461)

10. Refsum syndrome (phytanic acid oxidase deficiency)

11. Total color blindness

Gehrs K, Tiedeman J. Hemeralopia in an older adult. *Surv Ophthalmol* 1992;37:185–189.

Pau H. *Differential diagnosis of eye diseases*, 2nd ed. New York: Thieme Medical, 1988.

OSCILLOPSIA

This condition involves illusionary movement of the environment; it may be unilateral or bilateral and usually occurs because of acquired nystagmus.

1. Drugs, including the following:

alcohol	cyclopentobarbital	phenobarbital
allobarbital	diphenylhydantoin	primidone
amobarbital	gentamicin	probarbital
aprobarbital	heptabarbital	secobarbital
barbital	hexethal	talbutal
butabarbital	hexobarbital	thiamylal
butalbital	mephobarbital	thiopental
butallylonal	metharbital	valproate sodium
butethal	methitural	valproic acid
carbamazepine	methohexital	vinbarbital
cyclobarbital	pentobarbital	

2. Fixation and voluntary nystagmus
3. Defective vestibuloocular reflex/vestibular pathway lesion occurs during movement of the head or body
   A. Sectioning of vestibular (VIII) nerve for vertigo
   B. Streptomycin toxicity
   C. Spontaneous loss
4. Head trauma/seizures
5. Intermittent exotropia
6. Involvement of medial longitudinal fasciculus affecting ipsilateral medial rectus in internuclear ophthalmoplegia—monocular oscillopsia
7. Myokymia of the eyelid
8. Opsoclonus and ocular flutter
9. Vertebral artery dissection

Chrousos GA, et al. Two cases of downbeat nystagmus and oscillopsia associated with carbamazepine. *Am J Ophthalmol* 1987;103:221–224.

Fraunfelder FT, Fraunfelder FW. *Drug-induced ocular side effects.* Woburn, MA: Butterworth-Heinemann, 2001.

Glaser JS. *Neuro-ophthalmology*, 2nd ed. Philadelphia: JB Lippincott, 1989.

Hertle RW, et al. Onset of oscillopsia after visual maturation in patients with congenital nystagmus. *Ophthalmology* 2001;108:2301–2308.

Hicks PA, et al. Ophthalmic manifestation of vertebral artery dissection: patients seen at Mayo Clinic from 1976–1992. *Ophthalmology* 1994;101:1786–1792.

COLOR BLINDNESS

1. Inherited—stable defect, affecting both eyes
   A. Bassen–Kornzweig syndrome (abetalipoproteinemia)
   B. Congenital dyslexia syndrome (developmental dyslexia syndrome)
   C. Down syndrome (mongolism)
   D. Duane retraction syndrome (Stilling syndrome)
   E. Duchenne muscular dystrophy
   F. Glucose-6-phosphate dehydrogenase deficiency (glycogen storage disease type I)
   G. Guillain–Barré syndrome (acute infectious neuritis)
   H. Hemophilia

I. "Intrinsic" defect
    (1) Dichromat—two colors mixed to see white
        a. Deuteranope—green deficiency
        b. Protanope—red deficiency
        c. Tritanope—blue deficiency
    (2) Monochromat—one color mixed to see white
        a. Cone deficient
        b. Rod deficient
    (3) Trichromat—three colors mixed to see white
        a. Deuteranomaly—green anomaly
        b. Protanomaly—red anomaly
        c. Tritanomaly—blue anomaly
  J. Kallman syndrome (hypogonadotrophic hypogonadism–anosmia syndrome)
  K. Klinefelter syndrome (XXY) (gynecomastia–aspermatogenesis syndrome)
  L. Turner syndrome (XO) (gonadal dysgenesis)
2. Acquired—defect can increase or decrease; may affect only one eye; impairment of other visual function; often characterized by chromatopsia; hue discrimination primarily affected; yellow-blue defects more common in retinal disease; red–green defects in optic nerve disease
  A. Advanced hypertensive retinopathy
  B. Albinism
  C. Amblyopia
  D. Blue-yellow defect with retinal disorders from drugs, including the following:

acetophenazine	deferoxamine	piperacetazine
amiodarone (?)	diethazine	prazosin (?)
amodiaquine	diethylcarbamazine	prochlorperazine
azathioprine	ethambutol	procyclidine (?)
benztropine (?)	ethopropazine	promazine
biperiden (?)	fluphenazine	promethazine
butaperazine	hydroxychloroquine	propiomazine
carbamazepine	indomethacin (?)	quinacrine (?)
carphenazine	ketoprofen (?)	quinine
cephaloridine (?)	mesoridazine	sulindac (?)
chloramphenicol	methdilazine	tamoxifen
chloroquine	methotrexate	thiethylperazine
chlorphenoxamine (?)	methotrimeprazine	thiopropazate
chlorpromazine	minoxidil (?)	thioproperazine
chlorprothixene	mitotane	thioridazine
cisplatin	naproxen (?)	thiothixene
clofazimine	penicillamine	trifluoperazine
clonidine (?)	perazine	triflupromazine
cobalt (?)	pericyazine	trihexyphenidyl(?)
cycrimine (?)	perphenazine	trimeprazine

  E. Chorioretinitis
  F. Color anomia—inability to name colors; may be associated with homonymous hemianopia resulting from infarct of posterior parietal and corpus callosum
  G. Diabetic retinitis
  H. Dominantly inherited juvenile optic atrophy

I. Drugs and chemical substances causing optic neuropathy with red–green defect, including the following:

acetophenazine
alcohol
allobarbital
alseroxylon (?)
aminosalicylate (?)
aminosalicylic acid (?)
amobarbital
amodiaquine
antimony lithium thiomalate
antimony potassium tartrate
antimony sodium tartrate
antimony sodium
   thioglycollate
antipyrine
aprobarbital
aspirin
barbital
betamethasone
bromide (?)
bromisovalum
broxyquinoline
bupivacaine (?)
butabarbital
butalbital
butallylonal
butaperazine
butethal
calcitriol
carbromal
carphenazine
chloramphenicol
chloroprocaine (?)
chloroquine
chlorpromazine
cholecalciferol
clindamycin
cobalt (?)
cortisone
cyclobarbital
cyclopentobarbital
cycloserine (?)
dapsone
deferoxamine
deserpidine (?)
dexamethasone
dextrothyroxine (?)

diethazine
ergocalciferol
ergonovine (?)
ergot (?)
ergotamine (?)
ethambutol
ethopropazine
etidocaine (?)
ferrocholinate (?)
ferrous fumarate (?)
ferrous gluconate (?)
ferrous succinate (?)
ferrous sulfate (?)
fluorometholone
fluphenazine
gentamicin
heptabarbital
hexachlorophene
hexamethonium
hexethal
hexobarbital
hydrocortisone
hydroxychloroquine
iodide and iodine solutions
   and compounds
iodochlorhydroxyquin
iodoquinol
iron dextran (?)
iron sorbitex (?)
isoniazid
levothyroxine (?)
lidocaine (?)
liothyronine(?)
liotrix (?)
medrysone
mephobarbital
mepivacaine (?)
mesoridazine
metharbital
methdilazine
methitural
methohexital
methotrexate (?)
methotrimeprazine
methyl alcohol
methylene blue

methylergonovine
methysergide (?)
nitroglycerin (?)
oxyphenbutazone
pentobarbital
perazine
pericyazine
perphenazine
phenobarbital
phenylbutazone
piperacetazine
polysaccharide–iron complex
   (?)
prednisolone
prilocaine (?)
primidone
probarbital
procaine (?)
prochlorperazine
promazine
promethazine
propiomazine
propoxycaine (?)
propoxyphene
quinine
radioactive iodides
rauwolfia serpentina (?)
rescinnamine (?)
reserpine (?)
secobarbital
sodium antimonylgluconate
sodium salicylate
stibocaptate
stibogluconate
stibophen
streptomycin
sulfacetamide (?)
sulfachlorpyridazine (?)
sulfacytine (?)
sulfadiazine (?)
sulfadimethoxine (?)
sulfamerazine (?)
sulfameter (?)
sulfamethazine
sulfamethizole (?)
sulfamethoxazole (?)

sulfamethoxypyridazine (?)	thiamylal	trifluoperazine
sulfanilamide (?)	thiethylperazine	triflupromazine
sulfaphenazole (?)	thiopental	trimeprazine
sulfapyridine (?)	thiopropazate	tryparsamide
sulfasalazine (?)	thioproperazine	vinbarbital
sulfathiazole (?)	thioridazine	vinblastine
sulfisoxazole (?)	thyroglobulin (?)	vincristine
suramin	thyroid (?)	vitamin A
syrosingopine (?)	tobramycin	vitamin D
talbutal	trichloroethylene	

J. Friedreich ataxia

K. Glaucoma, including narrow and open angle

L. Hepatic cirrhosis

M. Hysteria

N. Macular lesions, including juvenile degeneration, senile degeneration dystrophy, and edema

O. Night blindness

P. Occlusion of retinal vessels

Q. Oguchi disease

R. Open-angle glaucoma

S. Ophthalmologist who use argon blue–green lasers or operating microscopes

T. Optic atrophy

U. Optic pathways, including brain tumor

V. Papillitis

W. Peripheral chorioretinal degeneration

X. Retinal detachment

Y. Retinitis pigmentosa

Z. Retrobulbar optic neuritis

AA. Snow blindness

Fraunfelder FT, Fraunfelder FW. *Drug-induced ocular side effects*. Woburn, MA: Butterworth-Heinemann, 2001.

Nousiainen I, et al. Color vision in epilepsy patients treated with vigabatrin or carbamazepine monotherapy. *Ophthalmology* 2000;107:884–888.

Pau H. *Differential diagnosis of eye diseases*, 2nd ed. New York: Thieme Medical, 1988.

Roy FH. *Ocular syndromes and systemic diseases*, 3rd ed. Philadelphia: Lippincott Williams & Wilkins, 2002.

Sample PA, et al. Isolating the color vision loss in primary open angle glaucoma. *Am Ophthalmol* 1988;106:686–691.

PALINOPSIA

This condition involves persistence or recurrence of visual images after exciting stimulus object has been removed; the patient has a hemianopic field defect. Polyopia (visual trailing effect with movement) may be present.

1. Acute migraine

2. Demyelinative optic neuritis

3. Encephalitis

4. Epilepsy

5. Intoxications, such as mescal delirium, LSD, trazodone-induced and clomiphene citrate.

6. Kartagener syndrome

7. Laser treatment of diabetic macular edema

8. Leber hereditary optic neuropathy
9. Temporal–parietal–occipital lesion
    A. Degenerative
    B. Neoplastic
    C. Traumatic
    D. Vascular
10. Schizophrenia
11. Drug, such as nefazodone (akinetopsia—persistence of moving objects)

Horton JC, Trobe JD. Akinetopsia from nefazodone toxicity. *Am J Ophthalmol* 1999;128,4:530–531.

Kawasaki A, Purvin V. Persistent palinopsia following ingestion of LSD. *Arch Ophthalmol* 1996;114:47–50.

Marneros A, Korner J. Chronic palinopsia in schizophrenia. *Psychopathology* 1993;26:236–239.

Pomeranz HD, Lessell S. Palinopsia and polyopia in the absence of drugs or cerebral disease. *Neurology* 2000;54: 855–859.

Purvin VA. Visual disturbance secondary to clomiphene citrate. *Arch Ophthalmol* 1995;113:482–484.

VERTICAL READING (PATIENT READS FROM ABOVE DOWNWARD)

1. Astigmatism—high error of refraction
2. Homonymous hemianopia (see p. 613)
3. Voluntary as oriental script written vertically

O'Brien CS. *Ophthalmology: notes for students.* Iowa City: Athens Press, 1930.

VISUAL AGNOSIA

This condition involves a failure to recognize objects by sight for animate and inanimate objects, but ot does not interfere with recognition of language symbols.

1. Drugs
2. Kluver–Bucy syndrome (temporal lobectomy behavior syndrome)
3. Lesion of Brodmann area 18

Fraunfelder FT, Fraunfelder FW. *Drug-induced ocular side effects.* Woburn, MA: Butterworth-Heinemann, 2001.

Scheie HG. *Textbook of ophthalmology*, 10th ed. Philadelphia: WB Saunders, 1986.

OCULAR LATEROPULSION

The eyes feel as though they are being drawn toward one side, but this problem can be overcome with conscious effect; full range of extraocular muscle movements is maintained.

1. Lateral medullary disease, including infarction of lateral medullary plate, acoustic neurinoma, posterior fossa meningioma, or multiple sclerosis
2. Peripheral vestibular disease

Meyer KT, et al. Ocular lateropulsion. *Arch Ophthalmol* 1980;98:1614–1616.

PAIN IN AND ABOUT EYE

1. Ocular
    A. Angle-closure glaucoma
    B. Chronic ocular hypoxia, carotid occlusive disease
    C. Dry-eye and tear-deficiency syndrome

      D. Local lid, conjunctival, and anterior segment disease

      E. Ocular inflammation including lyme borreliosis

2. Ophthalmic division

      A. Herpes zoster

      B. Migraine, cluster headache

      C. Painful ophthalmoplegia syndrome

      D. Raeder paratrigeminal neuralgia

      E. Referred (dural) pain, including occipital infarction

      F. Sinusitis

      G. Tic douloureux (infrequent in V1)

3. Mandibular division

      A. Dental disease

      B. Tic douloureux

4. Maxillary division

      A. Dental disease

      B. Nasopharyngeal carcinoma

      C. Sinusitis

      D. Temporomandibular syndrome

      E. Tic douloureux

5. Miscellaneous

      A. Atypical facial neuralgias

      B. Cranial arteritis

      C. Pain with medullary lesions

      D. Trigeminal tumors

Glaser JS. *Neuro-ophthalmology*, 2nd ed. Philadelphia: JB Lippincott, 1989.

Hill LM, Hasting G. Carotidynia: a pain syndrome. *J Family Practice* 1994;39:71–75.

HEADACHE

1. Vascular headache of migraine type

      A. Cephalalgia migraine (migraine equivalent)—migraine aura without headache

      B. Classic migraine—migraine with aura

      C. Common migraine—migraine without aura

      D. Complicated migraine—hemiplegic migraine and ophthalmoplegia migraine

      E. Cluster headache

      F. Lower-half headache

2. Muscle-contraction headache

3. Combined (skeletal vascular)

4. Headache of nasal vasomotor reaction

5. Headache of delusional, conversion, or hypochondriacal states

6. Nonmigraine vascular headaches

      A. Primary or metastatic tumors of meninges, vessels, or brain

      B. Hematomas (epidural, subdural, or parenchymal)

      C. Abscesses (epidural, subdural, or parenchymal)

      D. Post lumbar puncture headache (leakage, headache)

      E. Pseudomotor cerebri and various causes of brain swelling

7. Headache due to overt cranial inflammation

      A. Intracranial disorders

         (1) Mass

(2) Meningitis

(3) Subarachnoid hemorrhage

 B. Extracranial disorders (temporal arteritis)

 8. Headache because of diseases of ocular structures

 9. Headache because of diseases of aural structures

10. Headache because of diseases of the nasal and sinus structures

11. Headache because of diseases of dental structures

12. Headache because of diseases of other cranial and neck structures

13. Cranial neuritides

14. Cranial neuralgia

 A. Glossopharyngeal neuralgia

 B. Trigeminal neuralgia

15. Analgesic/ergotamine rebound headache

Friedman AP, et al. Classification of headache. *Neurology* 1962;12:173.

Glaser JS. *Neuro-ophthalmology*, 2nd ed. Philadelphia: JB Lippincott, 1989.

Mikkila HA, et al. The expanding clinical spectrum of ocular lyme borreliosis. *Ophthalmology* 2000;107:581–587.

PULFRICH PHENOMENON

This condition involves a three-dimensional illusion in which a moving object that is viewed binocularly with a light attenuating filter in front of one eye appears to transcribe an anomalous pathway.

 1. Age-related macular degeneration

 2. Anisocoria

 A. Induced

 B. Traumatic

 3. Anisometropic amblyopia

 4. Cataract

 5. Central serous retinopathy

 6. Corneal Opacity

 7. Hemianopia

 8. Multiple Sclerosis

 9. Optic Neuritis

10. Postretinal detachment repair

Larkin EB, Dutton GN, Heron G. Impaired perception of moving objects after minor injuries to the eye midface: the pulfrich phenomenon. *Br J Oral Maxillofac Surg* 1994;32:360–362.

Rubin ML. Perspectives in refraction. *Surv Opthalmology* 1997;41:6,493–499.

Scotcher SM, Canning CR, Weal MJ, et al. Pulfrich's phenomenon in patients with unilateral cataract: a previously unrecognized cause of visual disability. *Invest Opthalmol Vis Sci* 1995;36[Suppl]:s794(abst).

21

Head Position

CONTENTS

HEAD TURN (FACE TURN)

1. Head turned toward right (gaze left)
   A. Left Brown syndrome
   B. Left inferior oblique muscle palsy
   C. Left medial rectus muscle palsy
   D. Left superior oblique muscle palsy
   E. Right Duane syndrome
   F. Right jerk nystagmus
   G. Right inferior rectus muscle palsy
   H. Right lateral rectus muscle palsy
   I. Right superior rectus muscle palsy
   J. Right supranuclear gaze paresis
2. Head turned toward left (gaze right)
   A. Left Duane syndrome
   B. Left jerk nystagmus
   C. Left inferior rectus muscle palsy
   D. Left lateral rectus muscle palsy
   E. Left superior rectus muscle palsy
   F. Left supranuclear gaze paresis
   G. Right Brown syndrome
   H. Right inferior rectus muscle palsy
   I. Right medial rectus muscle palsy
   J. Right superior oblique muscle palsy
3. Head turned toward either left or right
   A. Congenital jerk nystagmus—head turned away from field with least amplitude of nystagmus (i.e., left jerk nystagmus improves in right gaze; left head turn)
   B. Esotropia—head turned in the direction of convergent eye (cross fixation)
   C. Hearing defect
   D. One blind eye—head turn away affected side (good eye fixates in adduction)

   E. Photophobia (see p. 650)
   F. Progressive intracranial arterial occlusion syndrome (Taveras syndrome)
   G. Strabismus fixus (general fibrosis syndrome)
   H. Under corrected myope

Hiatt RL, Cope-Troupe C. Abnormal head positions due to ocular problems. *Ann Ophthalmol* 1978;10:881–892.

Kushner BJ. Ocular causes of abnormal head postures. *Ophthalmology* 1979;86:2115–2125.

Walsh FB, Hoyt WF. *Clinical neuro-ophthalmology*, 4th ed. Baltimore: Williams & Wilkins, 1985.

HEAD TILT (HEAD TILTED TOWARD EITHER SHOULDER OR AROUND AN ANTEROPOSTERIOR AXIS)

1. Head tilted toward right
   A. Left superior oblique muscle palsy
   B. Left superior rectus muscle palsy
   C. Right inferior oblique muscle palsy
   D. Right inferior rectus muscle palsy
2. Head tilted toward left
   A. Left inferior oblique muscle palsy
   B. Left inferior rectus muscle palsy
   C. Right superior oblique muscle palsy
   D. Right superior rectus muscle palsy
3. Head tilted toward either right or left
   A. Astigmatism
   B. Beckwith–Wiedemann syndrome
   C. Blowout fracture
   D. Incorrectly aligned cylinder axis
   E. Monocular torticollis—patching of eyes does not eliminate problem; roentgenogram may help
      (1) Congenital malformation of fracture of cervical spine or vertebral processes
      (2) Fracture of clavicle
      (3) Functional habit and hysteria
      (4) Pain from infection
         a. Adenitis
         b. Arthritis
         c. Mastoiditis
         d. Synovitis
      (5) Paralysis of absent muscles on opposite side of head tilt
      (6) Sandifer syndrome (hiatus hernia–torticollis syndrome)
      (7) Spasm of sternocleidomastoid or contracture of sternocleidomastoid muscle on side of head tilt
      (8) Vestibular defect
         a. Acoustic neuroma
         b. Labyrinthitis
         c. Otitis media
   F. Nystagmus—turned away from field with least amplitude of nystagmus
   G. Superior oblique tendon sheath syndrome (Brown syndrome)

Greenberg MF, Pollard ZF. Ocular plagiocephaly: ocular torticellis with skull and facial asymmetry. *Ophthalmology* 2000;107:173–179.

Kattah JC, Dagi TF. Compensatory head tilt in upbeating nystagmus. *J Clin Neuro-Ophthalmol* 1990;10:27–31.

Levine RM. Ocular plagiocephaly. *Ophthalmology* 2000;107:2123–2124.

Rubin SE, et al. Ocular torticolis. *Surv Ophthalmol* 1986;30:366.

CHIN ELEVATION

1. Adaptive symptom of contact lens wearer
2. A-esotropia with fusion in downward gaze
3. Blowout fracture of orbit
4. Brown syndrome (superior oblique tendon sheath syndrome)
5. Double elevator palsy
6. General fibrosis syndrome (strabismus fixus)
7. Incomplete bilateral ptosis
8. Inferior oblique muscle palsy
9. Parinaud syndrome (dorsal midbrain syndrome)
10. Superior rectus muscle palsy
11. Supranuclear lesion (upgaze palsy)
12. Thyroidectomy
13. ''V'' pattern exotropia with fusion in downward gaze

Beyer-Machule C, von Noorden GK: *Atlas of ophthalmic surgery*, vol 1: *Lids, orbits, extraocular muscles*. New York: Thieme Medical, 1984.

Hiatt RL, Cope-Troupe C. Abnormal head positions due to ocular problems. *Ann Ophthalmol* 1978;10:881–892.

CHIN DEPRESSION

1. ''A'' pattern exotropia with fusion in upward gaze (A pattern)
2. Inferior rectus muscle palsy
3. Photophobia
4. Progressive supranuclear palsy
5. Superior oblique muscle palsy (bilateral)
6. Supranuclear lesion (down gaze palsy)
7. Uncorrected myope of low degree
8. ''V'' pattern esotropia with fusion in upward gaze

Beyer-Machule C, von Noorden GK. *Atlas of ophthalmic surgery*, vol 1: *Lids, orbits, extraocular muscles*. New York: Thieme Medical, 1984.

Kushner BJ. Ocular causes of abnormal head postures. *Ophthalmology* 1979;86:2115–2125.

HEAD NODDING

1. Benign or familial tremor
2. Bobble head doll syndrome—to-and-fro bobbing of the head and trunk, at 2- to 3-second intervals because of cyst of third ventricle
3. Congenital nystagmus
4. Extrapyramidal dysfunction, such as paralysis agitans (Parkinson syndrome)
5. Habit spasm
6. Spasms nutans

Gottlob I, et al. Head nodding is compensatory in spasmus nutans. *Ophthalmology* 1992;99:1024–1031.

Rubin SE, Slavin ML. Head nodding associated with intermittent esotropia. *J Pediatr Ophthalmol Strabismus* 1990; 27:250–251.

HEAD TREMOR

1. Cerebellar system afflictions (benign essential senile tremor)—most common
2. Extrapyramidal disorder
3. Hereditary postural tremor (familial tremor)
4. Postural tremor

Hughes AJ, et al. Paroxysmal dystonic head tumor. *Mov Disord* 1991;6:85–86.

Klawans HL. Rhythmic head tremor. *JAMA* 1982;248:1510.

HEAD THRUST

1. Oculomotor apraxia—defect or horizontal voluntary movements
2. Ataxia-telangiectasia syndrome
3. Isolated
4. Male predominance
5. Oral–facial–digital syndrome type II

Isenberg SJ. *The eye in infancy*. Chicago: Year Book Medical, 1989.

Subject Index

Page numbers followed by *t* indicate tabular material.